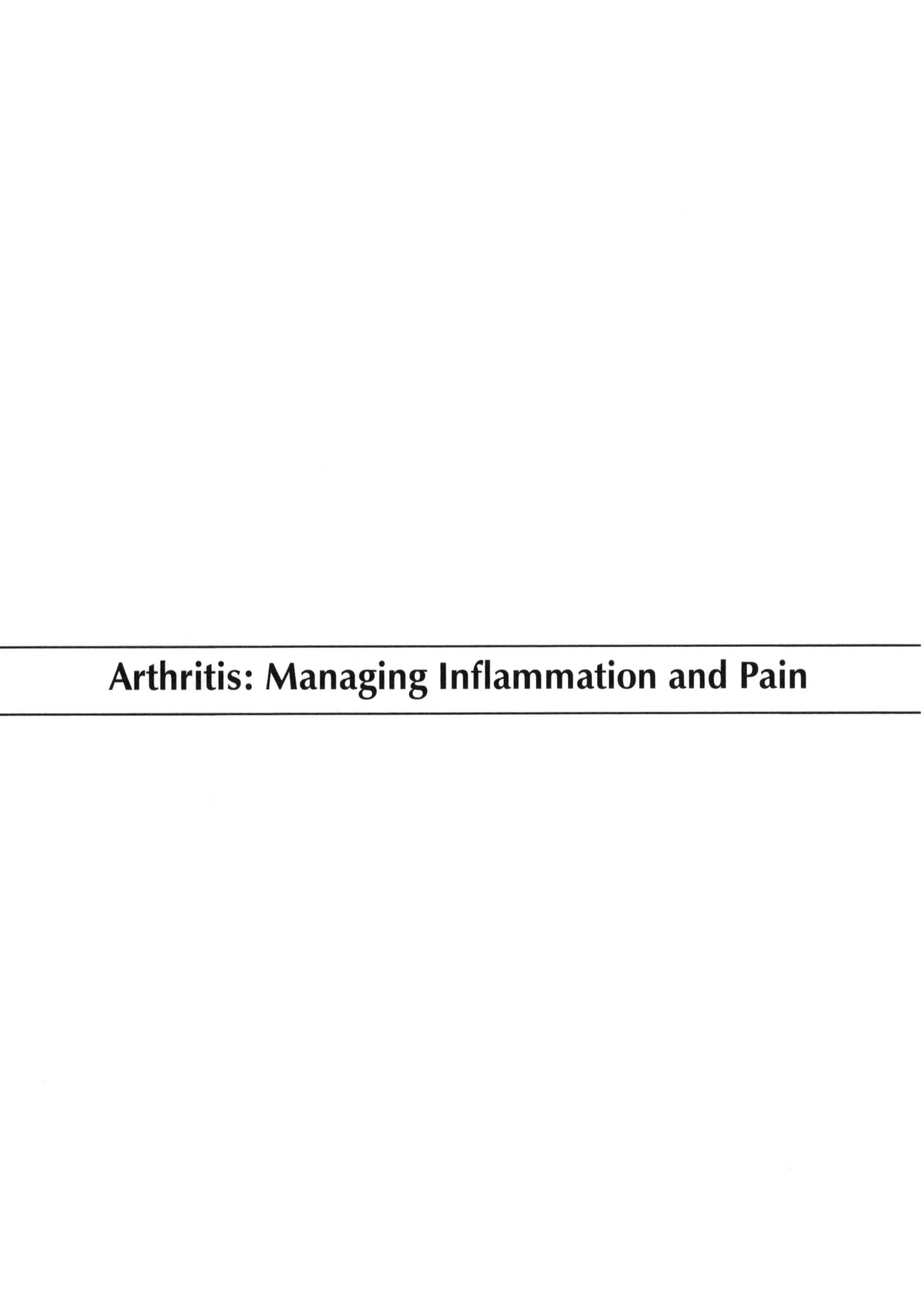

Arthritis: Managing Inflammation and Pain

Arthritis: Managing Inflammation and Pain

Editor: Ritchie Donovan

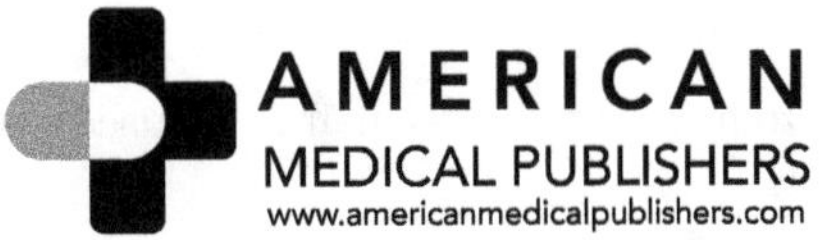

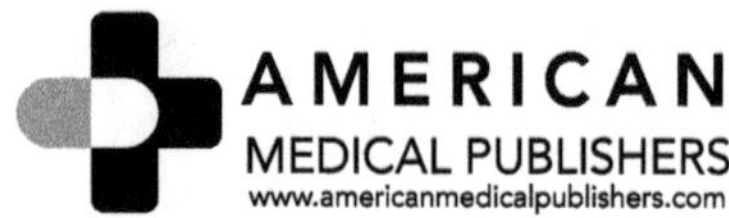

Cataloging-in-Publication Data

Arthritis : managing inflammation and pain / edited by Ritchie Donovan.
p. cm.
Includes bibliographical references and index.
ISBN 978-1-63927-896-1
1. Arthritis. 2. Inflammation. 3. Pain--Treatment. 4. Joints--Diseases. I. Donovan, Ritchie.
RC933 .A78 2023
616.722--dc23

American Medical Publishers,
41 Flatbush Avenue,
1st Floor, New York,
NY 11217, USA

ISBN 978-1-63927-896-1 (Hardback)

Contents

Preface IX

Chapter 1 **Factors associated with ASDAS remission in a long-term study of ankylosing spondylitis patients under tumor necrosis factor inhibitors** 1
Andrea Y. Shimabuco, Celio R. Gonçalves, Julio C. B. Moraes, Mariana G. Waisberg, Ana Cristina de M. Ribeiro, Percival D. Sampaio-Barros, Claudia Goldenstein-Schainberg, Eloisa Bonfa and Carla G. S. Saad

Chapter 2 **Psychoanalytic psychotherapy improves quality of life, depression, anxiety and coping in patients with systemic lupus erythematosus** 9
Céu Tristão Martins Conceição, Ivone Minhoto Meinão, José Atilio Bombana and Emília Inoue Sato

Chapter 3 **Association of anti-nucleosome and anti C1q antibodies with lupus nephritis in an Egyptian cohort of patients with systemic lupus erythematosus** 19
Imman Mokhtar Metwally, Nahla Naeem Eesa, Mariam Halim Yacoub and Rabab Mahmoud Elsman

Chapter 4 **$CD4^{+}CD69^{+}$ T cells and $CD4^{+}CD25^{+}FoxP3^{+}$ Tregcells imbalance in peripheral blood, spleen and peritoneal lavage from pristane-induced systemic lupus erythematosus (SLE) mice** 27
Tatiana Vasconcelos Peixoto, Solange Carrasco, Domingos Alexandre Ciccone Botte, Sergio Catanozi, Edwin Roger Parra, Thaís Martins Lima, Natasha Ugriumov, Francisco Garcia Soriano, Suzana Beatriz Verissímo de Mello, Caio Manzano Rodrigues and Cláudia Goldenstein-Schainberg

Chapter 5 **Comparison among ACR1997, SLICC and the new EULAR/ACR classification criteria in childhood-onset systemic lupus erythematosus** 40
Adriana Rodrigues Fonseca, Marta Cristine Felix Rodrigues, Flavio Roberto Sztajnbok, Marcelo Gerardin Poirot Land and Sheila Knupp Feitosa de Oliveira

Chapter 6 **Risk factors for cytomegalovirus disease in systemic lupus erythematosus (SLE)** 49
Hui Min Charlotte Choo, Wen Qi Cher, Yu Heng Kwan and Warren Weng Seng Fong

Chapter 7 **The diagnostic benefit of antibodies against ribosomal proteins in systemic lupus erythematosus** 56
Zhen-rui Shi, Yan-fang Han, Jing Yin, Yu-ping Zhang, Ze-xin Jiang, Lin Zheng, Guo-zhen Tan and Liangchun Wang

Chapter 8 **Machine learning techniques for computer-aided classification of active inflammatory sacroiliitis in magnetic resonance imaging** 63
Matheus Calil Faleiros, Marcello Henrique Nogueira-Barbosa, Vitor Faeda Dalto, José Raniery Ferreira Júnior, Ariane Priscilla Magalhães Tenório, Rodrigo Luppino-Assad, Paulo Louzada-Junior, Rangaraj Mandayam Rangayyan and Paulo Mazzoncini de Azevedo-Marques

Chapter 9 **Comparison of lupus patients with early and late onset nephritis: A study in 71 patients from a single referral center** 72
Juliana Delfino, Thiago Alberto F. G. dos Santos and Thelma L. Skare

Chapter 10 **Impact of *C4*, *C4A* and *C4B* gene copy number variation in the susceptibility, phenotype and progression of systemic lupus erythematosus** 77
Kaline Medeiros Costa Pereira, Sandro Perazzio, Atila Granado A. Faria, Eloisa Sa Moreira, Viviane C. Santos, Marcelle Grecco, Neusa Pereira da Silva and Luis Eduardo Coelho Andrade

Chapter 11 **Correlation of enthesitis indices with disease activity and function in axial and peripheral spondyloarthritis: A cross-sectional study comparing MASES, SPARCC and LEI** 85
Penélope Esther Palominos, Ana Paula Beckhauser de Campos, Sandra Lúcia Euzébio Ribeiro, Ricardo Machado Xavier, Jady Wroblewski Xavier, Felipe Borges de Oliveira, Bruno Guerra, Carla Saldanha, Aline Castello Branco Mancuso, Charles Lubianca Kohem, Andrese Aline Gasparin and Percival Degrava Sampaio-Barros

Chapter 12 **Human immunodeficiency virus in a cohort of systemic lupus erythematosus patients** 93
Vanessa Hax, Ana Laura Didonet Moro, Rafaella Romeiro Piovesan, Luciano Zubaran Goldani, Ricardo Machado Xavier and Odirlei Andre Monticielo

Chapter 13 **Autoimmune hepatitis in 847 childhood-onset systemic lupus erythematosus population** 99
Verena A. Balbi, Bárbara Montenegro, Ana C. Pitta, Ana R. Schmidt, Sylvia C. Farhat, Laila P. Coelho, Juliana C. O. Ferreira, Rosa M. R. Pereira, Maria T. Terreri, Claudia Saad-Magalhães, Nadia E. Aikawa, Ana P. Sakamoto, Kátia Kozu, Lucia M. Campos, Adriana M. Sallum, Virginia P. Ferriani, Daniela P. Piotto, Eloisa Bonfá and Clovis A. Silva

Chapter 14 **Diffuse alveolar hemorrhage in childhood-onset systemic lupus erythematosus: A severe disease flare with serious outcome** 105
Gabriela Blay, Joaquim C. Rodrigues, Juliana C. O. Ferreira, Gabriela N. Leal, Natali W. Gormezano, Glaucia V. Novak, Rosa M. R. Pereira, Maria T. Terreri, Claudia S. Magalhães, Beatriz C. Molinari, Ana P. Sakamoto, Nadia E. Aikawa, Lucia M. A. Campos, Taciana A. P. Fernandes, Gleice Clemente, Octavio A. B. Peracchi, Vanessa Bugni, Roberto Marini, Silvana B. Sacchetti, Luciana M. Carvalho, Melissa M. Fraga, Tânia C. M. Castro, Valéria C. Ramos, Eloisa Bonfá and Clovis A. Silva

Chapter 15 **Panniculitis in childhood-onset systemic lupus erythematosus** 111
Mônica Verdier, Pedro Anuardo, Natali Weniger Spelling Gormezano, Ricardo Romiti, Lucia Maria Arruda Campos, Nadia Emi Aikawa, Rosa Maria Rodrigues Pereira, Maria Teresa Terreri, Claudia Saad Magalhães, Juliana C. O. A. Ferreira, Marco Felipe Castro Silva, Mariana Ferriani, Ana Paula Sakamoto, Virginia Paes Leme Ferriani, Maraísa Centeville, Juliana Sato, Maria Carolina Santos, Eloisa Bonfá and Clovis Artur Silva

Chapter 16 **Nailfold capillaroscopy as a risk factor for pulmonary arterial hypertension in systemic lupus erythematosus patients** 116
Juliana Fernandes Sarmento Donnarumma, Eloara Vieira Machado Ferreira, Jaquelina Ota-Arakaki and Cristiane Kayser

Chapter 17 **Effect of food intake and ambient air pollution exposure on ankylosing spondylitis disease activity** ... **126**
Narjes Soleimanifar, Mohammad Hossein Nicknam, Katayoon Bidad, Ahmad Reza Jamshidi, Mahdi Mahmoudi, Shayan Mostafaei, Zahra Hosseini-khah and Behrouz Nikbin

Chapter 18 **Clinical and epidemiologic characterization of patients with systemic lupus erythematosus admitted to an intensive care unit in Colombia** ... **132**
Maria Fernanda Alvarez Barreneche, William Dario Mcewen Tamayo, Daniel Montoya Roldan, Libia Maria Rodriguez Padilla, Carlos Jaime Velasquez Franco and Miguel Antonio Mesa Navas

Chapter 19 **Axial Spondyloarthritis after bariatric surgery: A 7-year retrospective analysis** ... **139**
Thauana Luiza de Oliveira, Hilton Telles Libanori and Marcelo M. Pinheiro

Chapter 20 **The effect of therapies on the quality of life of patients with systemic lupus erythematosus** ... **144**
Tassia Catiuscia da Hora, Kelly Lima and Roberto Rodrigues Bandeira Tosta Maciel

Chapter 21 **The use of ultrasonography in the diagnosis of nail disease among patients with psoriasis and psoriatic arthritis** ... **151**
José Alexandre Mendonça, Sibel Zehra Aydin and Maria-Antonietta D'Agostino

Chapter 22 **Active human herpesvirus infections in adults with systemic lupus erythematosus and correlation with the SLEDAI score** ... **163**
Alex Domingos Reis, Cristiane Mudinutti, Murilo de Freitas Peigo, Lucas Lopes Leon, Lilian Tereza Lavras Costallat, Claudio Lucio Rossi, Sandra Cecília Botelho Costa and Sandra Helena Alves Bonon

Chapter 23 **Altered Tregs and oxidative stress in pregnancy associated lupus** ... **170**
Naveet Pannu, Rashmi Singh, Sukriti Sharma, Seema Chopra and Archana Bhatnagar

Chapter 24 **Comparison of urinary parameters, biomarkers and outcome of childhood systemic lupus erythematosus early onset-lupus nephritis** ... **178**
Daniele Faria Miguel, Maria Teresa Terreri, Rosa Maria Rodrigues Pereira, Eloisa Bonfá, Clovis Artur Almeida Silva, José Eduardo Corrente and Claudia Saad Magalhaes

Chapter 25 **Neutrophil/lymphocyte and platelet/lymphocyte ratios as potential markers of disease activity in patients with Ankylosing spondylitis** ... **183**
Mohammed Hadi Al-Osami, Nabaa Ihsan Awadh, Khalid Burhan Khalid and Ammar Ihsan Awadh

Chapter 26 **The Brazilian Society of Rheumatology guidelines for axial spondyloarthritis – 2019** 192
Gustavo Gomes Resende, Eduardo de Souza Meirelles, Cláudia Diniz Lopes Marques, Adriano Chiereghin, Andre Marun Lyrio, Antônio Carlos Ximenes, Carla Gonçalves Saad, Célio Roberto Gonçalves, Charles Lubianca Kohem, Cláudia Goldenstein Schainberg, Cristiano Barbosa Campanholo, Júlio Silvio de Sousa Bueno Filho, Lenise Brandao Pieruccetti, Mauro Waldemar Keiserman, Michel Alexandre Yazbek, Penelope Esther Palominos, Rafaela Silva Guimarães Goncalves, Ricardo da Cruz Lage, Rodrigo Luppino Assad, Rubens Bonfiglioli, Sônia Maria Alvarenga Anti, Sueli Carneiro, Thauana Luíza Oliveira, Valderílio Feijó Azevedo, Washington Alves Bianchi, Wanderley Marques Bernardo, Marcelo de Medeiros Pinheiro and Percival Degrava Sampaio-Barros

Permissions

List of Contributors

Index

Preface

In my initial years as a student, I used to run to the library at every possible instance to grab a book and learn something new. Books were my primary source of knowledge and I would not have come such a long way without all that I learnt from them. Thus, when I was approached to edit this book; I became understandably nostalgic. It was an absolute honor to be considered worthy of guiding the current generation as well as those to come. I put all my knowledge and hard work into making this book most beneficial for its readers.

Arthritis refers to joint inflammation which can impact a single joint or a number of joints. Rheumatoid arthritis (RA), metabolic arthritis, osteoarthritis and infectious arthritis are some of the different types of arthritis. It has various signs and symptoms such as stiffness, pain, swelling, redness, etc. The factors that contribute to the development of arthritis are aberrant metabolism, infections, injuries, immune system malfunction and genetic makeup. Some of the imaging techniques that are used to diagnose arthritis include computerized tomography (CT), ultrasound, X-rays and magnetic resonance imaging (MRI). Its treatment involves non-pharmacologic therapies, weight loss, surgery, drugs, occupational or physical therapy, etc. Physical activity improves mental health and movement, and reduces pain in people with arthritis. Nonsteroidal anti-inflammatory drugs (NSAIDs) are beneficial in reducing inflammation and relieving pain. Furthermore, putting ice packs on aching muscles can reduce inflammation and pain following intense activity among patients. The book aims to shed light on some of the unexplored aspects of arthritis and the recent researches on this medical condition. It includes some of the vital pieces of work being conducted across the world, on various topics related to the management of inflammation and pain. Researchers and students engaged in the study and management of this medical condition will be assisted by this book.

I wish to thank my publisher for supporting me at every step. I would also like to thank all the authors who have contributed their researches in this book. I hope this book will be a valuable contribution to the progress of the field.

Editor

Factors associated with ASDAS remission in a long-term study of ankylosing spondylitis patients under tumor necrosis factor inhibitors

Andrea Y. Shimabuco, Celio R. Gonçalves, Julio C. B. Moraes, Mariana G. Waisberg, Ana Cristina de M. Ribeiro, Percival D. Sampaio-Barros, Claudia Goldenstein-Schainberg, Eloisa Bonfa and Carla G. S. Saad*

Abstract

Objective: To determine the clinical and demographic factors associated with disease remission and drug survival in patients with ankylosing spondylitis (AS) on TNF inhibitors.

Methods: Data from a longitudinal electronic database of AS patients under anti-TNF therapy between June/2004 and August/2013. Demographic, clinical parameters, disease activity by ASDAS remission (< 1.3) and inactive/low (< 2.1) were analyzed to characterize reasons for drug survival and switching of anti-TNF.

Results: Among 117 AS patients, 69 (59%) were prescribed only one anti-TNF, 48 (41%) switched to a second anti-TNF and 13 (11%) to a third anti-TNF. Considering ASDAS-CRP < 1.3, 31 (39%) patients were inactive at the end of the study. Non-switchers ($P = 0.04$), younger age ($P = 0.004$), non-smoking ($P = 0.016$), shorter disease duration ($P = 0.047$), more frequent use of SSZ ($P = 0.037$) and lower BASDAI ($P = 0.027$), BASMI ($P = 0.034$) and BASFI ($P = 0.003$) at baseline were associated with remission. In the multivariate analysis younger age ($P = 0.016$) and lower BASDAI ($P = 0.032$) remained as remission predictors.

Conclusion: This study supports that ASDAS-CRP remission is an achievable goal not only for non-switchers but also for second anti-TNF, particularly in patients with younger age and lower BASDAI at baseline. Co-medication and non-smoker status seems to have a beneficial effect in anti-TNF response in this population.

Keywords: Ankylosing spondylitis, Anti-TNF, Co-medication, Remission, Switch

Introduction

Ankylosing spondylitis (AS), the most frequent disease in the spondyloarthritis (SpA) group, is a chronic rheumatic disorder characterized by inflammatory back pain, peripheral arthritis, enthesitis and extra-articular manifestations such as uveitis and inflammatory bowel disease [1]. Non-steroidal anti-inflammatory drugs (NSAIDs) are the first line drugs in the treatment of AS. Sulfasalazine (SSZ) and in some cases methotrexate (MTX) may be considered in patients with concomitant peripheral arthritis, but there is no evidence of the benefits of disease modifying anti-rheumatic drugs (DMARDs) for the treatment of axial involvement. According to the ASAS recommendations, treatment with anti-TNF drugs is indicated in patients who maintain persistent high disease activity [2].

Drug survival of anti-TNF agents in the long-term follow up is increased in patients with SpA, particularly AS, when compared to rheumatoid arthritis (RA) [3, 4]. In this setting, the identification of predictors of good response is important to optimize therapeutic decisions in AS. Previous studies have already demonstrated that younger age, lower Bath Ankylosing Spondylitis Functional Index (BASFI), increased disease activity with high C reactive protein (CRP) level, and even the presence of HLA-B27, are markers of good response to treatment [5–7]. In case of primary or secondary failure, switching to another anti-TNF is

* Correspondence: goncalves-carla@uol.com.br
Faculdade de Medicina da Universidade de São Paulo, Av. Dr. Arnaldo, 455 3° andar - sala 3131 - Cerqueira César, São Paulo, SP Cep: 01246-903, Brazil

currently the best therapeutic option. Although drug survival with the second anti-TNF is frequently lower than the first one, the clinical improvement with the first switch in AS can vary from 30 to 70% of patients, indicating that the lack or loss of response to a TNF blocker is not a predictor of failure to another one [8–10]. The Danish nationwide biologic registry (DANBIO) documented therapy with anti-TNF drugs in patients with AS and described that almost 30% of the 1436 patients switched to a second and 10% to a third anti-TNF medication during 10 years of follow up; switchers were more frequently women, with shorter disease duration and higher levels of Bath Ankylosing Spondylitis Disease Activity Index (BASDAI), BASFI and visual-analogue-scale (VAS) global at the beginning of the treatment. At the 2-year visit, 52% of switchers (number needed to treat – NNT = 1.9) and 63% of non-switchers (NNT = 1.6) achieved BASDAI 50 response, compared with the baseline visit of the first treatment [11]. There was no strong evidence of difference between switchers for failure or adverse events in relation to baseline characteristics and therapeutic response; however, studies with small group of patients have shown a slightly better response in those that switched due to adverse events than due to failure [12, 13].

Despite the well-known indication of DMARD associated with anti-TNF drugs in the treatment of RA, there is no such consensus in relation to SpA. ASAS recommendations do not support the mandatory use of conventional DMARDs associated with biological therapy, especially in cases of axial involvement [2]. As the formation of anti-drug antibodies is one of the possible mechanisms of lack or loss of blocking TNF response, co-medication with DMARDs has been suggested in many inflammatory diseases, including SpA [14, 15]. In the last decade, many studies have addressed the use of concomitant conventional DMARDs in patients with SpA, with contrasting results. Although two studies each have shown that MTX could be associated with longer anti-TNF drug survival in psoriatic arthritis [16, 17] and AS [18, 19], three other studies showed no benefits of this association [20–22]. Therefore, there is no definitive conclusion on the benefit of combined therapy with anti-TNF and DMARDs considering drug retention and effectiveness.

The primary aim of this study was to determine the clinical and demographic factors associated with disease remission and prolonged drug survival in patients with ankylosing spondylitis (AS) on anti-TNF inhibitors. We also evaluated the influence of co-medication in AS patients on anti-TNF switching, clinical response and remission.

Patients and methods

Patients

One hundred seventeen AS patients followed in the Spondyloarthritis Outpatient Clinic and referred to the Immunobiological Drugs Infusion Center (CEDMAC – *Centro de Dispensação de Medicação de Alto Custo*) with indication of biological therapy for disease activity refractory to conventional treatment were evaluated. Data of patients from an ongoing electronic database protocol that received anti-TNF therapy between June 2004 and August 2013 were retrospectively assessed. All patients fulfilled the modified New York classification criteria for definite AS [23]. Demographic characteristics as gender, age, HLA-B27 positivity, smoking (current or previous), and disease duration were recorded. Assessments also included parameters of previous and current treatment with DMARDs, NSAIDs and prednisone, as well as the presence of peripheral arthritis.

Study design

Patients were evaluated using an electronic chart database protocol established in 2000 with periodical assessment of parameters of treatment response and adverse events. Acute phase reactants, as CRP and Erythrocyte Sedimentation Rate (ESR) were collected at every visit. Outcome parameters were BASDAI, BASFI, Bath Ankylosing Spondylitis Metrology Index (BASMI), Ankylosing Spondylitis Quality of Life (ASQoL) [24–28].

The analysis of final clinical response was performed in patients receiving anti-TNF therapy at the end of the study. Clinical response was measured according to determined levels of Ankylosing Spondylitis Disease Activity Score (ASDAS) - CRP and ASDAS – ESR [29] and the Ankylosing Spondylitis Disease Activity Score (ASDAS) update of 2018 was used to classify patients according disease activity states as inactive disease (< 1.3) and low disease activity (1.3–2.1) [30].

Treatment for less than 24 weeks or patients that stopped medication due to drug failure, adverse events or multiple switches (i.e. use of the same drug for more than one course) were excluded only from response analysis, at final evaluation and remission predictors.

This study was approved by the Local Ethics Committee on Human Research at the University of São Paulo (CAPPesq). All participants gave written informed consent in compliance with the Helsinki Declaration.

Statistical analysis

The results were presented as mean and standard deviation (SD) for continuous variables (age, disease duration, BASDAI, BASMI, ASQol, ESR, CRP and ASDAS - CRP/ESR) and compared using the T test or Mann-Whitney test when comparing two groups and ANOVA for more than two groups.

Categorical variables (gender, HLA-B27, peripheral arthritis, smoking, use of DMARD, NSAID or prednisone, ASDAS – CRP/ESR) were shown as percentage and evaluated through the Fisher Exact Test or Chi square when indicated.

Multivariate analysis was also performed for possible factors associated with remission and Kaplan-Meier analysis for drug survival on different anti-TNF courses.

Statistical significance was considered when $P < 0.05$. Statistical analyses were performed using SigmaStat version 3.1 (2005) and GraphPad/ Prisma Software.

Results

Baseline demographics

A total of 117 patients treated with TNF inhibitors were identified. Forty-five patients maintained the first agent during the study period; 48 patients switched to a second anti-TNF, due to failure in 58% and adverse effects in 42% of the cases; and 13 patients were treated with a third anti-TNF, 62% due to failure and 38% due to adverse effects (Fig. 1). The most common first anti-TNF was infliximab in 88 patients (75.2%), with adalimumab in 20 (17.1%) and etanercept in 9 patients (7.7%), indicating the drug availability in our country at that moment. Adalimumab was the most frequently used second drug (67%) and etanercept was the common third line treatment (69%). The median of follow-up duration was 41.5 months (0.5 to 116.1 months).

At baseline, demographic data and clinical parameters were similar in switchers and non-switchers (Table 1). There was no difference regarding gender, age, presence of HLA-B27, smoking (current or previous), disease duration and disease parameters. With regard to co-medication, non-switchers used more often DMARD (88.9% vs. 72.9%, $P = 0.023$); among those patients who used concomitant DMARDs, the use of SSZ was also more frequent in patients who maintained the first treatment (37.7% vs. 18.8%, $P = 0.039$), whereas no difference was observed when MTX users were analyzed (18.8% vs. 16.7%, $P = 0.811$). Groups with and without SSZ co-medication presented similar baseline characteristics, as gender ($P = 1.000$), age ($P = 0.869$), smoking ($P = 0.489$), peripheral arthritis ($P = 0.839$), BASDAI ($P = 0.473$) and ASDAS-CRP ($P = 0.923$). The mean dose of SSZ was 2.6 g per day. The concomitant use of conventional DMARDs in the AS patients was quite common due to the high prevalence of peripheral joint involvement (70%) in our patients with axial SpA. Thirty-five patients (29.9%) used more than one DMARD at the introduction of the anti-TNF drug; MTX and SSZ was the main combination. High disease activity was associated with maintenance of combined DMARDs at the study entry as there was no other treatment option at that time.

Disease characteristics at baseline of the second anti-TNF

Switchers' characteristics at baseline of the second anti-TNF were also assessed and compared between patients who remained receiving the second and those who have not responded and switched to the third anti-TNF. Groups were similar with respect to demographic data and characteristics of disease, except for the higher scores of BASDAI at baseline of the 2nd anti-TNF in patients who required the third therapy (6.4 ± 1.7 vs. 4.1 ± 2.5, $P = 0.012$), suggesting worse disease activity in patients who evolved with failure to the second anti-TNF. The choice of the first switch did not influence the maintenance of the second treatment; it was comparable among patients who started and switched to monoclonal antibody (infliximab or adalimumab) and

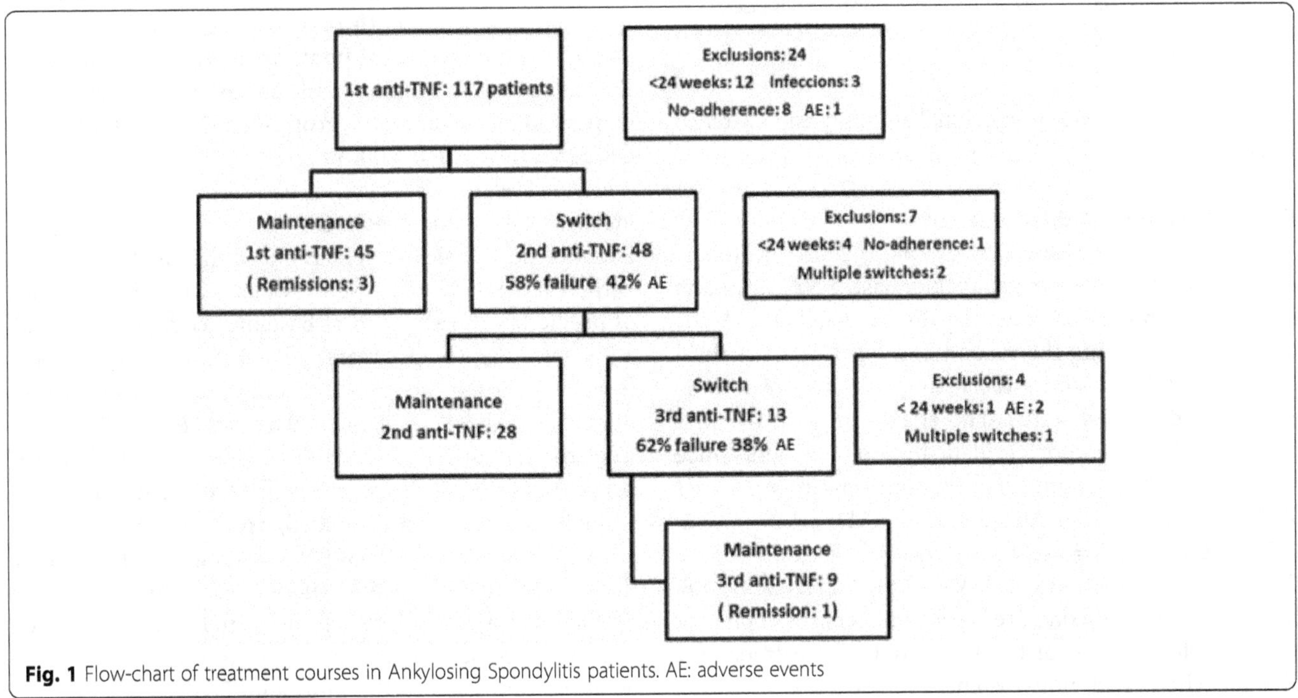

Fig. 1 Flow-chart of treatment courses in Ankylosing Spondylitis patients. AE: adverse events

Table 1 Patients characteristics at baseline

Variable	Non-switchers ($n = 69$)	Switchers ($n = 48$)	*P*
Male gender	61/69 (88.4%)	38/48 (79.2%)	0.199
Age, years	37.3 ± 13.2	38.3 ± 11.2	0.665
HLA-B27 positivity	38/46 (82.6%)	34/40 (85.0%)	1.000
Smoking	17/45 (37.8%)	13/36 (36.1%)	1.000
Disease duration, years	11.4 (6.2, 17.7)	9.2 (5.7, 19.2)	0.840
Peripheral involvement	45/69 (65.2%)	37/48 (77.1%)	0.218
Pure axial involvement	24/69 (34.8%)	11/48 (22.9%)	0.218
BASDAI	5.2 ± 2.0	5.5 ± 2.1	0.482
BASFI	5.2 ± 2.5	5.9 ± 2.4	0.199
BASMI	3.9 ± 2.8	4.5 ± 2.7	0.290
ASQoL	10.4 ± 5.5	12.7 ± 4.7	0.058
CRP, mg/l	21.6 (12.8, 38.0)	20.6 (12.6, 40.0)	0.397
ESR, mm/hr	20.5 (11.0, 34.5)	25.0 (13.1, 48.5)	0.268
ASDAS – CRP	3.8 ± 0.9	3.9 ± 1.0	0.714
ASDAS – ESR	3.3 ± 0.9	3.6 ± 1.0	0.175
Concomitant use of:			
NSAID	50/69 (72.4%)	41/48 (85.4%)	0.117
DMARD	62/69 (88.9%)	35/48 (72.9%)	**0.023***
SSZ only	26/69 (37.7%)	9/48 (18.8%)	**0.039***
MTX only	13/69 (18.8%)	8/48 (16.7%)	0.811
Cyclosporine	1/69 (1.4%)	1/48 (2.1%)	1.000
Leflunomide	7/69 (10.1%)	8/48 (16.7%)	0.400
Prednisone	23/69 (33.3%)	15/48 (31.2%)	0.844

Values are expressed as mean (SD), median (quartile) and percentages. *BASDAI* Bath Ankylosing Spondylitis Disease Activity Index, *BASFI* Bath Ankylosing Spondylitis Functional Index, *BASMI* Bath Ankylosing Spondylitis Metrology Index, *ASQoL* Ankylosing Spondylitis Quality of Life, *CRP* C Reactive Protein, *ESR* Erythrocyte Sedimentation Rate, *ASDAS* Ankylosing Spondylitis Disease Activity Score, *NSAID* Non-steroidal Anti-Inflammatory Drug, *SSZ* Sulfasalazine, *MTX* Methotrexate, *$P < 0.05$

those who started with monoclonal antibody and switched to etanercept (66% vs. 77%, $P = 0.716$).

Final evaluation and disease status

At the end of the study, 78 patients (42 non-switchers and 36 switchers) were using their last TNF inhibitors for more than 6 months; among the 36 switchers, 28 patients were receiving the second and 8 patients the third anti-TNF. Table 2 shows the final parameters of disease activity and clinical status. The effectiveness of the first TNF inhibitor was more evident in non-switchers, since this group had at final evaluation lower scores of BASDAI (1.7 ± 1.6 vs. 2.6 ± 2.0, $P = 0.041$), BASFI (2.8 ± 2.7 vs. 4.2 ± 3.0, $P = 0.034$), ASDAS - CRP (1.5 ± 0.7 vs. 2.0 ± 1.0, $P = 0.012$) and ASDAS - ESR (1.3 ± 0.7 vs. 1.8 ± 1.0, $P = 0.050$) compared to switchers, in spite of comparable duration of the last anti-TNF treatment for the switchers and non-switchers ($P = 0.146$). Of note,

Table 2 Comparison at final evaluation between non-switchers and switchers

	Non-switchers ($n = 42$)	Switchers ($n = 36$)	*P*
BASDAI	1.7 ± 1.6	2.6 ± 2.0	**0.041***
BASFI	2.8 ± 2.7	4.2 ± 3.0	**0.034***
BASMI	2.9 ± 2.2	3.2 ± 2.1	0.635
ASQoL	3.5 (1.0, 8.0)	6.0 (1.5, 10.5)	0.057
CRP, mg/l	2.8 (1.3, 5.0)	4.0 (1.7, 8.6)	0.148
ESR, mm/hr	4.0 (2.0, 8.0)	5.0 (2.0, 15.5)	0.363
ASDAS – CRP	1.5 ± 0.7	2.0 ± 1.0	**0.012***
Last anti-TNF treatment duration, weeks	206.6 (96.9, 287.9)	171.9 (101.6, 210.3)	0.146

Values are expressed as mean (SD) and median (quartile). *ASDAS* Ankylosing Spondylitis Disease Activity Score, *ASQoL* Ankylosing Spondylitis Quality of Life, *BASDAI* Bath Ankylosing Spondylitis Disease Activity Index, *BASFI* Bath Ankylosing Spondylitis Functional Index, *BASMI* Bath Ankylosing Spondylitis Metrology Index, *CRP* C Reactive Protein, *ESR* Erythrocyte Sedimentation Rate, * $P < 0.05$

non-switchers more often achieved inactive/low disease activity (ASDAS< 2.1) by ASDAS - CRP (80.1% vs. 55.9%, $P = 0.024$) and ASDAS - ESR (88.1% vs. 57.6%, $P = 0.003$) and remission (ASDAS < 1.3) by ASDAS - ESR (61.9% vs. 36.4%, $P = 0.037$) and ASDAS - CRP (42.8% vs. 26.5%, $P = 0.156$).

Considering ASDAS - CRP < 1.3, 31 (39%) patients were inactive at the end of the study. Thereby the NNT was 5.57 for non-switchers and 5.33 for second and 13 for the third anti-TNF.

Switchers due to failure or adverse effects were comparable regarding demographic data and baseline characteristics, as disease activity parameters and co-medication. In the final evaluation, 14 switchers due to adverse effects and 14 patients due to lack or loss of efficacy were on treatment with second anti-TNF. Response to treatment and status of disease were comparable between the groups (ASDAS - CRP < 2.1: 64.3% vs. 66.7%, $P = 1.000$).

Inactive disease and predictors

Patients that achieved remission at the final evaluation with ASDAS-CRP < 1.3 were evaluated for the presence of predictors of remission at baseline. Younger age (32.3 ± 9.9 vs. 39.8 ± 11.8 years, $P = 0.004$), non-smoking (smoking: 16.0% vs. 46.3%, $P = 0.016$), shorter disease duration (10.6 ± 9.3 vs. 14.7 ± 9.8 years, $P = 0.047$), more frequent use of SSZ (70.9% vs. 44.9%, $P = 0.037$), lower BASDAI (4.6 ± 2.2 vs. 5.8 ± 2.0, $P = 0.027$), lower BASFI (4.4 ± 2.0 vs. 6.2 ± 2.5, $P = 0.003$) and lower BASMI (3.6 ± 2.8 vs. 5.0 ± 2.7, $P = 0.034$) at the moment of anti-TNF drug introduction were associated with remission (Table 3). Of note, 71% of the patients that achieved remission remained in the first anti-TNF and none achieved remission in the third anti-TNF.

Table 3 Baseline comparison between patients according to inactive disease criteria (ASDAS − CRP < 1.3)

	ASDAS CRP < 1.3 (*n* = 31)	ASDAS CRP ≥ 1.3 (*n* = 49)	*P*
Male gender	27/31 (87.1%)	39/49 (79.6%)	0.548
HLA-B27 positivity	20/27 (74.1%)	37/42 (88.1%)	0.193
Smoking	4/25 (16.0%)	19/41 (46.3%)	**0.016***
Baseline:			
Age, years	32.3 ± 9.9	39.8 ± 11.8	**0.004***
Duration of disease, years	10.6 ± 9.3	14.7 ± 9.8	**0.047***
Co-medication:			
NSAID	23/31 (74.2%)	35/49 (71.4%)	1.000
DMARD	27/31 (87.1%)	37/49 (75.5%)	0.259
MTX	11/31 (35.5%)	21/49 (42.9%)	0.640
SSZ	22/31 (70.9%)	22/49 (44.9%)	**0.037***
BASDAI	4.6 ± 2.2	5.8 ± 2.0	**0.027***
BASFI	4.4 ± 2.0	6.2 ± 2.5	**0.003***
BASMI	3.6 ± 2.8	5.0 ± 2.7	**0.034***
ASQol	10.6 ± 5.6	11.2 ± 4.8	0.669
ASDAS − CRP	3.5 ± 0.9	3.9 ± 1.0	0.126
CRP (mg/L)	20.3 (9.7, 36.7)	24.6 (14.9, 38.9)	0.664
ESR (mm/h)	23.0 (10.3, 32.0)	21.0 (12.5, 36.5)	0.650
1st anti-TNF retention	22/31 (71.0%)	23/49 (46.9%)	**0.040***
Last anti-TNF treatment, weeks	176.9 ± 85.2	182.1 ± 106.2	0.820

Values are expressed as mean (SD), median (quartile) and percentages. *BASDAI* Bath Ankylosing Spondylitis Disease Activity Index, *BASFI* Bath Ankylosing Spondylitis Functional Index, *BASMI* Bath Ankylosing Spondylitis Metrology Index, *ASQoL* Ankylosing Spondylitis Quality of Life, *CRP* C Reactive Protein, *ESR* Erythrocyte Sedimentation Rate, *ASDAS* Ankylosing Spondylitis Disease Activity Score, *DMARD* Disease Modifying Antirheumatic Drug, *NSAID* Non-steroidal Anti-Inflammatory Drug, *SSZ* Sufasalazine, *MTX* Methotrexate, $^{*}P < 0.05$

In the multivariate analysis the variables that remained as predictor of remission were younger age (OR = 0.935; CI 95% 0.886–0.987; $P = 0.016$) and lower BASDAI (OR = 0.725; CI 95% 0.541–0.972; $P = 0.032$) (Table 4).

Further analysis of significant parameters in univariate demonstrated that patients treated with SSZ and anti-TNF achieved more often at the end of the study inactive disease (ASDAS-CRP < 1.3, 47.7% vs. 25.0%, $P = 0.040$) and lower disease activity according to ASDAS − CRP (1.5 ± 0.9 vs. 1.9 ± 0.9, $P = 0.009$) than patients without this co-medication. Non-smokers AS patients also achieved remission more frequently than smoker patients (ASDAS-CRP < 1.3, 48.8% vs. 17.4%, $P = 0.016$) and seemed to present lower disease activity (ASDAS-CRP, 1.5 ± 0.8 vs. 1.9 ± 0.8, $P = 0.056$) at the end of the study.

Table 4 Remission predictors: multivariate analysis

Baseline	OR	CI (95%)		*P*
Age	0.935	0.886	0.987	**0.016***
Sulfasalazine	2.849	0.857	9.472	0.088
BASDAI	0.725	0.541	0.972	**0.032***

BASDAI Bath Ankylosing Spondylitis Disease Activity Index, *OR* Odds Ratio, *CI* confidence interval,$^{*}P < 0.05$

Retention to therapy

The mean anti-TNF drug survival for non-switchers was 5.2 years (95% CI 4.4 to 6.0 years) and for switchers was 1.7 years (95% CI 1.3 to 2.1 years) on first anti-TNF, 4.9 years (95% CI 3.9 to 5.9 years) on second anti-TNF and 3.8 years (95% CI 2.5 to 5.2 years) on third anti-TNF. Retention to therapy was superior for non-switchers when compared to switchers to the second (log rank test $P = 0.007$) and to the third anti-TNF (log rank test $P = 0.02$). The retention to therapy between switchers on the second or third course presented no difference (log rank test $P = 0.07$) (Fig. 2).

Discussion

This is the first long-term study to evaluate AS patients under anti-TNF agents focusing on ASDAS inactive disease, demonstrating an overall 40% remission. We further identified that younger age and lower BASDAI at baseline were predictors of long-term remission.

Switching was a frequent event during long-term anti-TNF therapy in our cohort, occurring in more than a third of our patients and mainly due to treatment failure (lack or loss of efficacy). In the Danish registry (DANBIO) [11], and in a Dutch [31] and a Spanish [32] cohort a high frequency of switching was also observed, mostly associated with lack/loss of effect. In contrast, in the Norwegian registry (NOR-DMARD) [10] and in the Leeds cohort [33] a very low frequency of switching/discontinuation was reported.

We have not identified demographic and baseline disease parameters as relevant predictive factors for switching in our patients opposing to previous report that female gender, MTX use, higher BASFI and BASDAI were associated with the second anti-TNF therapy [11]. Although a previous report has shown that peripheral involvement was a predictive factor of switching [18], it was not observed in this study, probably because that represents a common finding in Brazilian axial SpA patients [43]. With regard to the third anti-TNF, we identified that patients with higher BASDAI at the time of introduction of the second anti-TNF agent were more likely to switch to the third TNF inhibitor, suggesting a refractory disease in these patients.

Although response rates decreased after switching for the second anti-TNF agent, many patients presented satisfactory improvement in the follow-up with a NNT very similar to the first anti-TNF agent. In contrast, the very high

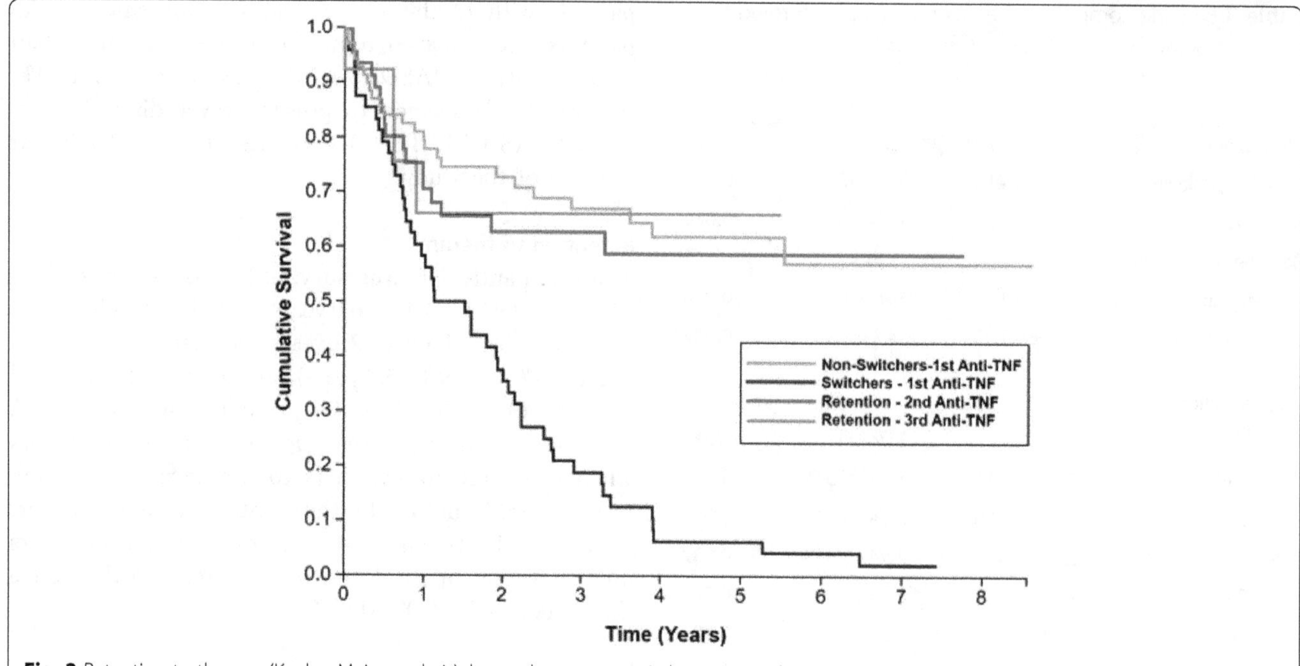

Fig. 2 Retention to therapy (Kaplan-Meier analysis); log-rank test: non-switchers vs switchers - second anti-TNF ($P = 0.007$) and non-switchers vs switchers - third anti-TNF ($P = 0.02$)

NNT for the third TNF blockers and complete absence of remission in this group does not support this switch. At the final evaluation, non-switchers achieved lower levels of BASDAI, BASFI and ASDAS-CRP compared to switchers. Similar trends of reduced response in switchers have been demonstrated [9, 11, 34], but none of these studies considered ASDAS inactive disease as a target. In fact, ASDAS is the only validated and discriminatory instrument for assessing disease activity in AS [29, 30].

The reason for change (lack/loss of efficacy or adverse events) to the second TNF antagonist did not influence anti-TNF response. At the final assessment, both groups presented comparable indexes, including BASDAI, ASDAS-CRP and frequency of ASDAS inactivity/moderate disease activity. Previous studies reported similar results [10, 11, 35, 36]; however, some demonstrated slightly better clinical improvement in switchers due to adverse events [11, 34].

In this study, we presented novel evidence of predictive factors considering ASDAS score as remission criteria. Unlike other studies that considered BASDAI50 or ASAS40 (4–6), ours considered ASDAS-CRP < 1.3 as remission response. Younger age, non-smoking, shorter disease duration, more frequent use of SSZ, lower BASDAI, BASFI and BASMI at the time of anti-TNF drug introduction were identified as possible predictors of remission and only younger age and lower BASDAI at baseline remained significant in the multivariate analysis.

Taking into account that ASDAS considers 3 answers of BASDAI questionnaire plus global assessment of disease and CRP or ESR parameters, we consider that baseline ASDAS index may not have been associated with remission due to similar values of CRP and ESR at baseline between the groups and limited number of patients with ASDAS evaluation at baseline in our cohort, since ASDAS index was published in 2009.

We suggested and extended recent observations that concomitant DMARD use was associated with a better first anti-TNF persistent rate [19, 20, 37]. The non-exclusion of patients who discontinued without switching anti-TNF due to other causes precludes a definitive conclusion about concomitant DMARD use effectiveness in AS in a previous study [37].

Non-smokers AS patients also achieved remission more frequently than smoker patients at the end of the study, in agreement to published data. Previous studies indicate that this factor has a dose-dependent impact on structural damage progression and in worse treatment response of SpA patients [38–41].

The treatment response analysis performed herein was limited to patients under anti-TNF treatment at the final evaluation and with at least 24 weeks of therapy. This strict study design provided novel data demonstrating that SSZ co-medication was more often associated with remission. In the Swiss cohort, a benefit in drug survival was reported, but it was only demonstrated for DMARD on the clinical response in patients treated with infliximab and methotrexate [20].

Baseline disease and activity parameters were alike in patients with and without SSZ minimizing the chance that these factors might have influenced SSZ effect in anti-TNF treatment. In fact, more than 2/3 of our patients have associated peripheral involvement in AS, and the concomitant use of conventional DMARD, as SSZ, is quite common in our daily practice in Brazil [42–44].

Conclusion

This long-term longitudinal study supports that ASDAS-CRP remission is an achievable goal not only for non-switchers but also for the second anti-TNF, particularly in patients with younger age and lower BASDAI at baseline therapy. Co-medication and non-smoker status seems to have a beneficial effect on anti-TNF response in this population.

Abbreviations

AS: Ankylosing spondylitis; ASDAS: Ankylosing Spondylitis Disease Activity Score; ASQoL: Ankylosing Spondylitis Quality of Life; BASDAI: Bath Ankylosing Spondylitis Disease Activity Index; BASFI: Bath Ankylosing Spondylitis Functional Index; BASMI: Bath Ankylosing Spondylitis Metrology Index; CRP: C Reactive Protein; ESR: Erythrocyte Sedimentation Rate; MTX: Methotrexate; NSAID: Non-steroidal Anti-Inflammatory Drug; SpA: Spondyloarthritis; SSZ: Sulfasalazine

Acknowledgements

Not applicable.

Authors' contributions

AYS: study concept and design, assist in subject recruitment, acquisition of subject and data, interpretation of data and drafting the manuscript. CRG: study concept and design, assist in subject recruitment, interpretation of data and revising the manuscript. JCBM: assist in subject recruitment, interpretation of data and revising the manuscript. MGW: assist in subject recruitment and revising the manuscript. ACMR: assist in subject recruitment, interpretation of data and revising the manuscript. PDS: study concept and design, assist in subject recruitment, interpretation of data and drafting the manuscript. CGS: assist in subject recruitment, acquisition of data and revising the manuscript. EB: study concept and design, interpretation of data and drafting the manuscript. CGSS: study concept and design, assist in subject recruitment, interpretation of data and drafting the manuscript. All authors read and approved the final manuscript.

References

1. Braun J, Sieper J. Ankylosing spondylitis. Lancet. 2007;369:1379–90.
2. van der Heijde D, Ramiro S, Landewé R, Baraliakos X, Van den Bosch F, Sepriano A, et al. 2016 update of the ASAS-EULAR management recommendations for axial spondyloarthritis. Ann Rheum Dis. 2017;76(6): 978–991.
3. Sampaio-Barros PD, van der Horst-Bruinsma IE. Adverse effects of TNF inhibitors in SpA: are they different from RA? Best Pract Res Clin Rheumatol. 2014;28:747–63.
4. Arends S, Brouwer E, Efde M, van der Veer E, Bootsma H, Wink F, et al. Long-term drug survival and clinical effectiveness of etanercept treatment in patients with ankylosing spondylitis in daily clinical practice. Clin Exp Rheumatol. 2017;35(1):61–8 Epub 2016 Oct 7.
5. Rudwaleit M, Claudepierre P, Wordsworth P, Cortina EL, Sieper J, Kron M, et al. Effectiveness, safety, and predictors of good clinical response in 1250 patients treated with adalimumab for active ankylosing spondylitis. J Rheumatol. 2009;36:801 8.
6. Glintborg B, Ostergaard M, Krogh NS, Dreyer L, Kristensen HL, Hetland ML. Predictors of treatment response and drug continuation in 842 patients with ankylosing spondylitis treated with anti-tumour necrosis factor: results from 8 years' surveillance in the Danish nationwide DANBIO registry. Ann Rheum Dis. 2010;69:2002–8.
7. Arends S, van der Veer E, Kallenberg CG, Brouwer E, Spoorenberg A. Baseline predictors of response to TNF-α blocking therapy in ankylosing spondylitis. Curr Opin Rheumatol. 2012;24:290–8.
8. Baraliakos X, Braun J. Spondyloarthritides. Best Pract Res Clin Rheumatol. 2011;25:825–42.
9. Cantini F, Niccoli L, Benucci M, Chindamo D, Nannini C, Olivieri I, et al. Switching from infliximab to once-weekly administration of 50 mg etanercept in resistant or intolerant patients with ankylosing spondylitis: results of a fifty-four-week study. Arthritis Rheum. 2006;55:812–6.
10. Lie E, van der Heijde D, Uhlig T, Mikkelsen K, Rødevand E, Koldingsnes W, et al. Effectiveness of switching between TNF inhibitors in ankylosing spondylitis: data from the NOR-DMARD register. Ann Rheum Dis. 2011;70:157–63.
11. Glintborg B, Østergaard M, Krogh NS, Tarp U, Manilo N, Loft AG, et al. Clinical response, drug survival and predictors thereof in 432 ankylosing spondylitis patients after switching tumour necrosis factor α inhibitor therapy: results from the Danish nationwide DANBIO registry. Ann Rheum Dis. 2013;72(7):1149–5.
12. Pradeep DJ, Keat AC, Gaffney K, Brooksby A, Leeder J, Harris C. Switching anti-TNF therapy in ankylosing spondylitis. Rheumatology (Oxford). 2008;47:1726–7.
13. Haberhauer G, Strehblow C, Fasching P. Observational study of switching anti-TNF agents in ankylosing spondylitis and psoriatic arthritis versus rheumatoid arthritis. Wien Med Wochenschr. 2010;160:220–4.
14. de Vries MK, Wolbink GJ, Stapel SO, de Groot ER, Dijkmans BA, Aarden LA, et al. Inefficacy of infliximab in ankylosing spondylitis is correlated with antibody formation. Ann Rheum Dis. 2007;66:133–4.
15. de Vries MK, Brouwer E, van der Horst-Bruinsma IE, Spoorenberg A, van Denderen JC, Jamnitski A, et al. Decreased clinical response to adalimumab in ankylosing spondylitis is associated with antibody formation. Ann Rheum Dis. 2009;68:1787–8.
16. Kristensen LE, Gülfe A, Saxne T, Geborek P. Efficacy and tolerability of anti-tumour necrosis factor therapy in psoriatic arthritis patients: results from the south Swedish arthritis treatment group register. Ann Rheum Dis. 2008;67:364–9.
17. Fagerli KM, Lie E, van der Heijde D, Heiberg MS, Lexberg AS, Rødevand E, et al. The role of methotrexate co-medication in TNF-inhibitor treatment in patients with psoriatic arthritis: results from 440 patients included in the NOR-DMARD study. Ann Rheum Dis. 2014;73:132–7.
18. Kristensen LE, Karlsson JA, Englund M, Petersson IF, Saxne T, Geborek P. Presence of peripheral arthritis and male sex predicting continuation of anti-tumor necrosis factor therapy in ankylosing spondylitis: an observational prospective cohort study from the South Swedish Arthritis Treatment Group Register. Arthritis Care Res (Hoboken). 2010;62:1362–9.
19. Lie E, Kristensen LE, Forsblad-d'Elia H, Zverkova-Sandström T, Askling J, Jacobsson LT, ARTIS Study Group. The effect of co-medication with conventional synthetic disease modifying antirheumatic drugs on TNF inhibitor drug survival in patients with ankylosing spondylitis and undifferentiated spondyloarthritis: results from a nationwide prospective study. Ann Rheum Dis. 2015;74:970–8.
20. Nissen MJ, Ciurea A, Bernhard J, Tamborrini G, Mueller R, Weiss B, et al. The effect of Comedication with a conventional synthetic disease-modifying Antirheumatic drug on drug retention and clinical effectiveness of anti-tumor necrosis factor therapy in patients with axial Spondyloarthritis. Arthritis Rheumatol. 2016;68(9):2141–50.
21. Sepriano A, Ramiro S, van der Heijde D, Ávila-Ribeiro P, Fonseca R, Borges J, et al. Effect of Comedication with conventional synthetic disease-modifying Antirheumatic drugs on retention of tumor necrosis factor inhibitors in patients with Spondyloarthritis: a prospective cohort study. Arthritis Rheumatol. 2016;68(11):2671–9.
22. Fabbroni M, Cantarini L, Caso F, Costa L, Pagano VA, Frediani B, et al. Drug retention rates and treatment discontinuation among anti-TNF-α agents in psoriatic arthritis and ankylosing spondylitis in clinical practice. Mediat Inflamm. 2014;2014:862969.
23. Van der Linden S, Valkenburg HA, Cats A. Evaluation of diagnostic criteria for ankylosing spondylitis. A proposal for modification of the New York criteria. Arthritis Rheum. 1984;27:361–8.

24. Sieper J, Rudwaleit M, Baraliakos X, Brandt J, Braun J, Burgos-Vargas R, et al. The Assessment of Spondyloarthritis international Society (ASAS) handbook: a guide to assess spondyloarthritis. Ann Rheum Dis. 2009;68:ii1–ii44.
25. Garret S, Jenkinson T, Kennedy LG, Whitelock H, Gaisford P, Calin A. A new approach to defining disease status in ankylosing spondylitis: the Bath ankylosing spondylitis disease activity index. J Rheumatol. 1994;21:2286–91.
26. Calin A, Jones SD, Garrett SL, Kennedy LG. Bath ankylosing spondylitis functional index. Br J Rheumatol. 1995;34:793–4.
27. Jenkinson TR, Mallorie PA, Whitelock HC, Kennedy LG, Garrett SL, Calin A. Defining spinal mobility in ankylosing spondylitis (AS). The Bath AS Metrology Index. J Rheumatol. 1994;21:1694–8.
28. Doward LC, Spoorenberg A, Cook A, Whalley D, Helliwell PS, Kay LJ, et al. Development of the ASQol: a quality of life instrument specific to ankylosing spondylitis. Ann Rheum Dis. 2003;63:20–6.
29. Machado P, Landewé R, Lie E, Kvien TK, Braun J, Baker D, et al. Ankylosing spondylitis disease activity score (ASDAS): defining cut-off values for disease activity states and improvement scores. Ann Rheum Dis. 2011;70:47–53.
30. Machado PM, Landewé R, Heijde DV; Assessment of SpondyloArthritis international Society (ASAS). Ankylosing Spondylitis Disease Activity Score (ASDAS): 2018 update of the nomenclature for disease activity states. Ann Rheum Dis. 2018 Feb 16: annrheumdis-2018-213184. [Epub ahead of print].
31. Arends S, Brouwer E, van der Veer E, Groen H, Leijsma MK, Houtman PM, et al. Baseline predictors of response and discontinuation of tumor necrosis factor-alpha blocking therapy in ankylosing spondylitis: a prospective longitudinal observational cohort study. Arthritis Res Ther. 2011;13:R94.
32. Rosales-Alexander JL, Aznar JB, Perez-Vicente S, Magro-Checa C. Drug survival of anti-tumour necrosis factor α therapy: results from the Spanish - AR II study. Rheumatology (Oxford). 2015;54:1459–63.
33. Coates LC, Cawkwell LS, Ng NW, Bennett AN, Bryer DJ, Fraser AD, et al. Real-life experience confirms sustained response to long-term biologics and switching in ankylosing spondylitis. Rheumatology (Oxford). 2008;47:897–900.
34. Rudwaleit M, Van den Bosch F, Kron M, Kary S, Kupper H. Effectiveness and safety of adalimumab in patients with ankylosing spondylitis or psoriatic arthritis and history of anti-tumor necrosis factor therapy. Arthritis Res Ther. 2010;12:R117.
35. Paccou J, Solau-Gervais E, Houvenagel E, Salleron J, Luraschi H, Philippe P, et al. Efficacy in current practice of switching between anti-tumour necrosis factor- α agents in spondyloarthropathies. Rheumatology (Oxford). 2011;50:714–20.
36. Conti F, Ceccarelli F, Marocchi E, Magrini L, Spinelli FR, Spadaro A, et al. Switching tumour necrosis factor alpha antagonists in patients with ankylosing spondylitis and psoriatic arthritis: an observational study over a 5-year period. Ann Rheum Dis. 2007;66:1393–7.
37. Heinonen AV, Aaltonen KJ, Joensuu JT, Lähteenmäki JP, Pertovaara MI, Romu MK, et al. Effectiveness and drug survival of TNF inhibitors in the treatment of ankylosing spondylitis: a prospective cohort study. J Rheumatol. 2015;42(12):2339–46.
38. Villaverde-García V, Cobo-Ibáñez T, Candelas-Rodríguez G, Seoane-Mato D, Campo-Fontecha PDD, Guerra M, et al. The effect of smoking on clinical and structural damage in patients with axial spondyloarthritis: A systematic literature review. Semin Arthritis Rheum. 2016;46(5):569–583.
39. Jones GT, Ratz T, Dean LE, Macfarlane GJ, Atzeni F. In axial spondyloarthritis, never smokers, ex-smokers and current smokers show a gradient of increasing disease severity - results from the Scotland registry for ankylosing spondylitis (SIRAS). Arthritis Care Res (Hoboken). 2017;69(9):1407–1413.
40. Zhao S, Challoner B, Khattak M, Moots RJ, Goodson NJ. Increasing smoking intensity is associated with increased disease activity in axial spondyloarthritis. Rheumatol Int. 2017;37(2):239–44.
41. Glintborg B, Højgaard P, Lund Hetland M, Steen Krogh N, Kollerup G, Jensen J, et al. Impact of tobacco smoking on response to tumour necrosis factor-alpha inhibitor treatment in patients with ankylosing spondylitis: results from the Danish nationwide DANBIO registry. Rheumatology (Oxford). 2016;55(4):659–68.
42. Benegas M, Muñoz-Gomariz E, Font P, Burgos-Vargas R, Chaves J, Palleiro D, et al. RESPONDIA group; ASPECT study group; REGISPONSER study group. Comparison of the clinical expression of patients with ankylosing spondylitis from Europe and Latin America. J Rheumatol. 2012;39:2315–20.
43. Saad CG, Gonçalves CR, Sampaio-Barros PD. Seronegative arthritis in Latin America: a current review. Curr Rheumatol Rep. 2014;16:438.
44. Kohem CL, Bortoluzzo AB, Gonçalves CR, Braga da Silva JA, Ximenes AC, Bértolo MB, et al. Profile of the use of disease modifying drugs in the Brazilian registry of Spondyloartrhritis. Braz J Rheumatol. 2014;54:33–7.

2

Psychoanalytic psychotherapy improves quality of life, depression, anxiety and coping in patients with systemic lupus erythematosus

Céu Tristão Martins Conceição[1], Ivone Minhoto Meinão[1], José Atilio Bombana[2] and Emília Inoue Sato[1*]

Abstract

Background: Systemic Lupus Erythematosus (SLE) is an autoimmune disease which impairs the quality of life. The objective of study was to evaluate the effectiveness of Brief Group Psychoanalytic Psychotherapy to improve quality of life, depression, anxiety and coping strategies in SLE patients.

Methods: In a randomized clinical trial, 80 female SLE patients were allocated into two groups: therapy group ($n = 37$) and control group ($n = 43$). Therapy group (TG) attended weekly psychotherapy sessions for 20 weeks; control group (CG) remained on a waiting list. Both groups received standard medical care. Questionnaires and scales were applied by blinded evaluators at baseline (T1) and after 20 weeks (T2): Socioeconomic Status, SLE International Collaborating Clinic/American College of Rheumatology-Damage Index, SLE International Disease Activity, SLE Specific Symptom Checklist, SLE Quality of life, Hospital Anxiety Depression Scale, Coping Strategies Inventory. Intent to treat intra- and inter-group analysis was performed for all variables in T1 and T2 using Qui-square, t-Student, Mann-Whitney and Wilcoxon tests. Analysis of Variance was used to compare categorical variables over time. $P < 0.05$ was considered significant.

Results: The mean age of patients was 42 years; 54% were white, with mean disease duration of years 12. At baseline, both groups were homogeneous in all variables, including medications. After 20 weeks of psychotherapy TG was significantly different from CG, with lower frequency of symptoms ($p = 0.001$), lower level of anxiety ($p = 0.019$) and depression ($p = 0.022$), better index in five of six domains of quality of life scale ($p \leq 0.005$), including total SLEQOL ($p < 0.001$) and with higher positive planful problem solving strategy ($p = 0.017$). No change in disease activity score was observed in both groups.

Conclusions: Psychoanalytic psychotherapy was effective to improve many domains of quality of life and one positive coping skill and to reduce SLE symptoms, anxiety and depression levels. Brief group psychotherapy can be a useful tool to complement medical care in SLE patients.

Keywords: Systemic lupus erythematosus, Quality of life, Depression, Anxiety, Coping strategies, Psychoanalytic psychotherapy

* Correspondence: eisato@unifesp.edu.br
[1]Rheumatology Division, Escola Paulista de Medicina, Universidade Federal de São Paulo, Rua Botucatu 740 – Disciplina de Reumatologia CEP 04023900, São Paulo, SP, Brazil
Full list of author information is available at the end of the article

Background

Systemic lupus erythematosus (SLE) is an autoimmune disease that can affect several organs and systems. It is more prevalent in females, mainly in the reproductive period of life and has a multifactorial etiology highlighting genetic predisposition, hormonal, environmental and possible infectious factors [1].

The connection between the limbic system, hypothalamic-pituitary-adrenal (HPA) axis and autonomous nervous system has the function to restore body baseline status after exposition to physical or psychological stress [2]. Some authors evaluated the influence of stress as one of the causal factors of SLE and also as a trigger of disease flares [3, 4].

Quality of life (QOL) is considered as being healthy, feeling good and being independent and able to work, according to SLE patient reports [5]. SLE patients have poorer functional status than the general population because specific manifestations of SLE that may decrease quality of life [6, 7]. Feeling of uncertainty about illness, pain and fatigue are important experiences in SLE patients [8], while illness intrusiveness is a stressor that affects QOL [9].

Besides poor QOL in SLE patients, recent studies around the world have shown that anxiety and depression are common symptoms in SLE population. In a systematic review, Palagini et al. found a high variability in the prevalence of depressive disorders in SLE (17–75%) [10]. The incidence of depression in SLE in the Hopkins Lupus Cohort was 29.7 episodes per 1000 person-years [11]. Neuropsychiatric (NP) manifestations occurred in 47.2% and mood disorders in 12.7%, with 38.3% of them attributed to SLE [12]. Ayache and Costa observed prevalence of depression in 65% of SLE patients in Brazil [13].

Coping concept contains a set of strategies to manage stress, reducing its aversive characteristics and increasing the perception of personal control [14]. The development of coping skills to face SLE disease is very important because manifestations of pain and fatigue besides affections in skin and vital organs are stressful events in patient's lives [8, 9]. Coping in SLE patients is usually more passive, with the predominance of acceptance strategies [15].

Haija and Shultz had pointed the necessity of an alternative approach to get more adherence to medical treatment in SLE [16] and psychotherapy has been used to supplement clinical care in several diseases, including cancer [17]. There are few studies evaluating the effectiveness of psychotherapy on autoimmune diseases. These studies have shown improvement in coping, quality of life, depression, anxiety, relationship, self-esteem and general health by psychotherapy and psychosocial support in SLE patients [18–20]. However they presented some weakness like small sample sizes [19, 20], lack of randomization [19] and positive results only in a few domains [18].

The psychotherapy approach performed in our study comes from psychoanalysis, introduced by Freud to alleviate psychic suffering [21–23]. This approach has been modified over time, in relation to the time of analysis (brief duration), number of participants (group therapy) and different types of diseases began to be treated [24–26]. After Alexander's contributions to psychosomatic medicine [27], Pierre Marty developed an influential psychoanalytic theory based on the concept of mentalization which characterizes the psychosomatic functioning [28]. This concept is similar to alexithymia [29] and patients have difficult to express emotions and deal with them. To these patients, the therapy needs to be more directive, only once a week, face-to-face to access body expression, nominate their feelings and unload instinctual excitations [30].

In the Psychiatric Department of *Escola Paulista de Medicina, Universidade Federal de São Paulo,* group psychotherapy has been performed to treat somatoform disorders, adapting the psychoanalytic setting to these patients with good results [31, 32]. We consider that this approach could also help patients with autoimmune diseases.

Until now, there are no studies in Latin America applying psychotherapy techniques in SLE patients. The objective of this study was to evaluate the effectiveness of brief group psychoanalytic psychotherapy (BGPP) to improve quality of life, anxiety, depression and coping skills in Brazilian SLE patients.

Patients and methods

A controlled, randomized clinical trial was registered at clinicaltrials.gov (number NCT01840709).

Participants

Patients were recruited from the Autoimmune Rheumatic Disease outpatient clinic of University Hospital through posters affixed on the outpatient clinic. One hundred and five patients declared interest, however 25 dropped out due to difficulty to fulfill the protocol or presented exclusion criteria. Therefore, a total of 80 female SLE patients were enrolled in the study. Patients were randomized by computer table, receiving an assigned number from 1 to 80 and the secretary informed patients to which group they had been allocated. All patients answered the questionnaires at baseline and after 20 weeks, under the supervision of blind evaluators. The physicians involved in the clinical evaluations were also blinded to the patient allocation group.

Inclusion criteria were: female gender, fulfill American College of Rheumatology (ACR) SLE classification criteria [33], age over 18 years and follow-up at the institution for at least 6 months. All patients signed a consent form approved by the institutional ethics committee (protocol 1655/09).

Exclusion criteria were: illiterate, presence of severe mental diseases (severe cognitive deficit, schizophrenia, bipolar disorder, severe depression), physical conditions that could preclude their weekly participation and patients who were receiving psychological treatment or were participating in other protocols.

Inclusion and exclusion criteria were evaluated by the rheumatologists based on patient's current data and medical records. Only one patient (TG) had a history of psychological treatment many years prior.

The therapy group (TG $n = 37$) was divided into four subgroups, with a maximum of ten patients, according to each patient's preferred schedule (one of four options offered) for psychotherapy attendance. Control group (CG $n = 43$) remained on a waiting list, only receiving standard medical care according to outpatient clinic schedule. The TG was also continuing to receive usual medical treatment throughout the study.

Four patients dropped out of the study (two on CG and two on TG). In CG, one patient died due to SLE activity and one patient was lost to follow-up. In TG, two patients dropped out of the group, reporting difficulty to participate in the weekly meeting. All patients attended at least 15 of 20 sessions (75%), except the two dropouts on TG.

Assessment instruments

Most of the following questionnaires and scales were self-applied with supervision of blinded assessors for some patients with low educational level and difficulty to understand the questions. The clinical evaluations were performed during the medical appointment. Religion and race were self-nominated. All instruments were validated and adapted to the Portuguese language and were applied at baseline (T1) and after 20 weeks (T2), except SLICC score that was applied only at baseline.

1 – ABIPEME Criteria (*Associação Brasileira de Institutos de Pesquisa de Mercado*) - Socioeconomic questionnaire [34].

The education (years of study) and socioeconomic classification (comfort items at home) are presented in categories.

2 – SLICC/ACR-DI (Systemic Lupus International Collaborating Clinic /American College of Rheumatology - Damage Index) [35].

A measure of the irreversible SLE damage index, present for at least 6 months, evaluating 12 organic systems and calculated by a physician.

3 – SLEDAI (Systemic Lupus Erythematosus International Disease Activity) [36].

A measure of the activity of the disease, scoring each variable of the affected system, evaluated by a physician.

4 – SLE-SSC (Systemic Lupus Erythematosus Specific Symptom Checklist) [37, 38].

A self-related SLE symptom checklist with 38 items evaluating the presence and intensity of several symptoms in the last 30 days. Higher scores indicate worse results.

5 – SLEQOL (Systemic Lupus Erythematosus Quality of Life) [37, 39].

A self-related questionnaire with 40 items in 6 domains evaluating the SLE quality of life. The score of each item varies from 0 to 7 and higher scores correspond to poorer quality of life.

6 – HADS (Hospital Anxiety and Depression Scale) [40, 41].

A self-administered questionnaire evaluating the domains of anxiety and depression (7 questions by domain). Higher scores indicate higher severity of symptoms.

7 – CSI (Coping Strategies Inventory) [42, 43].

A self-applied questionnaire evaluating coping strategies to deal stressful events with 66 items in 8 domains. Each item can be scored from 0 to 3. It can measure mature coping, escape/avoidance and aggressiveness strategies.

Intervention

Intervention was performed in 90-min sessions once a week for 20 weeks for each subgroup. The psychological technique (BGPP) was a short-term (20 weeks) therapy derived from psychoanalysis, which is based in long-term therapy that has been used in the Psychiatric Department of *Escola Paulista de Medicina, Universidade Federal de Sao Paulo* to treat psychosomatic patients [31, 32]. This technique works according to Marty's model at the Paris School of Psychosomatics [30] and is similar to supportive expressive treatment [44] and to brief dynamic psychotherapy [45], but applied without a manual. The same facilitators managed all the subgroups in this study to guarantee standardization of treatment.

The sessions were organized to achieve the objective to improve the quality of life, coping strategies and emotional balance by the discussion of elected topics. The group dynamic was free to enable the emergence of important emotional contents, promoting personal integration and increasing relationships in the group. Coping strategies against life stressors, mainly the disease, were trained during the process. All patients in TG did an evaluation about their experience in the group at the end of study. A therapist, an experienced psychologist in this approach (CTMC) and a co-therapist (IMM), who is also a rheumatologist, conducted the intervention. The therapist coordinated and treated the group. The co-therapist was an observer and recorded the group dialogues, behaviors and emotional expressions. A psychoeducational intervention to clarify patients' doubts about the disease was included in the last session.

Statistical analysis

The sample size (80 patients) was calculated considering SLEQOL questionnaire, with power of 80%, significance level of 5% and standard deviation of total SLEQOL of 52 points [37], assuming as significant difference between groups equal to 35 points.

Intra- and inter-group analysis was performed at baseline (T1) and after 20 weeks (T2). Descriptive statistics were used for sample characterization. The proportion of categorical variables was compared using *Chi*-square test. To compare quantitative variables between groups *t*-Student test was used for those with normal distribution and Mann-Whitney or Wilcoxon test for non-normal distribution. Analysis of variance (ANOVA) test was used to compare categorical variables over time (medication). Medians (minimum-maximum) and means (standard deviation) were used to analyze the data with no normal and normal distribution, respectively. Intent to treat statistical analysis was performed. Statistical Package for the Social Sciences (SPSS), version 17.0 (Chicago, USA) was used for all statistical analysis. $P < 0.05$ was considered significant.

Results

Demographic and socioeconomic data, SLICC/ACR-DI score and medication of 80 SLE patients are shown in Table 1. At baseline, there was no difference concerning age, disease duration, race, years of education, economic class and religion between CG and TG. At baseline, the medications used to control lupus and neuropsychiatric symptoms were similar between groups, with a mean prednisone dosage of 10.38 mg/day. These medications did not vary significantly during the study (data not shown). In general, the SLICC/ACR-DI score was low, without difference between groups (Table 1). The SLEDAI scores were also homogeneous in either the intra- or inter-groups analysis. Even if a few patients had presented highly active disease in both groups, the mean level of disease activity was low and comparable between TG and CG at baseline and at the end of the study (Table 2).

At baseline, both groups were comparable concerning SLE-SSC scores, but TG patients showed significant reduction on frequency and intensity of self-related symptoms after psychotherapy, making the score lower in TG than CG at T2 ($p < 0.001$) (Table 3).

At T2 we observed improvement in the quality of life in TG, by positive changes in five of six domains of SLEQOL scores (occupational activity, symptoms, treatment, humor and self-image) and in the total score ($p < 0.001$), with significant difference comparing with the CG (Table 4).

TG patients showed a significant reduction on anxiety ($p = 0.019$) and depression ($p = 0.022$) levels at T2, which was not observed in CG, highlighting a significant difference between groups at end of study (Table 5).

Concerning CSI, the inter-group analysis at T2 showed significant difference in the planful problem solving skill. However, in the intra-group analysis in TG, positive changes were also observed in other domains (confrontive, escape and avoidance, planful problem solving and positive reappraisal) at the end of the study (Table 6).

Discussion

This study aimed to test if BGPP technique could improve quality of life and coping skills, as well, reduce anxiety and depression in SLE female patients attended at a tertiary public service in Brazil. The field of this study is the interface between medicine and psychoanalysis using the psychosomatic concepts and techniques as adjunctive help to patients with physical diseases. Psychotherapeutic treatment can lead patients to better coping with illness and increase the adherence to medical treatment [18–20].

We observed significant improvement in symptoms, quality of life, anxiety, depression and in one positive coping domain. The amount and intensity of symptoms on SLE-SSC scale presented significant reduction in patients after psychoanalytic treatment, improving their quality of life and well-being. After treatment, patients handled their body and disease differently, minimizing the importance of symptoms that were felt before as severe and harmful which interfered in their daily activities. However, this improvement did not reflect in disease activity score, as SLEDAI did not have significant reduction, corroborating previous studies using similar techniques [18–20], concluding that short-time treatment did not have enough power to modify this score.

Patients of the psychotherapy group presented positive changes in quality of life, with improvement in almost all SLEQOL domains: occupational activities, symptoms, humor, self-image and the way to face medical

Table 1 Social, demographic and clinical data of SLE patients in control and therapy groups

Patients ($n = 80$)	Control ($n = 43$)	Therapy ($n = 37$)	P value
Age mean (SD)*	42.7 (11.3)	42.0 (12.3)	0.798
Disease duration mean (SD)**	11.6 (8.2)	12.4 (7.8)	0.511
Education[a] n (%)***			0.625
≤ 3 years	05 (11.6)	03 (8.1)	
4–8 years	16 (37.2)	10 (27.0)	
9–11 years	05 (11.6)	08 (21.6)	
12–15 years	16 (37.2)	14 (37.8)	
≥ 16 years	01 (2.3)	02 (5.4)	
Socioeconomic class[a] n (%)***			0.846
A/B	00 (.0)	00 (.0)	
C	26 (60.5)	20 (54.1)	
D	12 (27.9)	12 (32.4)	
E	05 (11.6)	05 (13.5)	
Race n (%)***			0.642
White	22 (54.2)	17 (45.9)	
Afro descendants	21 (45.8)	20 (54.1)	
Religion n (%)***			0.121
Catholic	17 (39.5)	22 (59.5)	
Evangelic	13 (30.2)	13 (35.1)	
Spiritualist	05 (11.6)	01 (2.7)	
Jehovah witness	04 (9.3)	01 (2.7)	
Buddhist	01 (2.3)	00 (.0)	
No religion	03 (7.0)	00 (.0)	
Lupus medications n (%)***			
Azathioprine	11 (25.6)	09 (24.3)	0.897
Hydroxychloroquine	25 (58.1)	19 (51.4)	0.542
Prednisone	24 (55.8)	21 (56.8)	0.932
Neuropsychiatric medications n (%)***			
Amitriptyline	07 (16.3)	06 (16.2)	0.994
Cyclobenzaprine	03 (7.0)	02 (5.4)	0.770
Fluoxetine	09 (20.9)	07 (18.9)	0.882
SLICC/ACR-DI [b] n (%)***			0.055
Zero	22 (51.2)	11 (29.7)	
1.00	12 (27.9)	17 (45.9)	
2.00	06 (14.0)	02 (5.4)	
3.00	03 (7.0)	04 (10.8)	
4.00	00 (.0)	03 (8.1)	

[a]ABIPEME Criteria - Brazilian Association of Market Research Institutes (1995)
[b]SLICC/ACR-DI - Systemic Lupus International Collaborating Clinics/American College of Rheumatology-Damage Index (Range: 0–46)
**t* -Student test; **Mann-Whitney test; ****Chi*-square test

treatment. These results suggest a strong reduction in negative intrusiveness of the disease in treated patient's life, similar to other studies [18–20]. In CG we observed a change in only one SLEQOL domain with worsening of symptoms that likely occurred by chance.

We also found a significant decrease in depression and anxiety levels evaluated by HADS in TG, whereas CG patients did not change. This data revealed the beneficial effects of psychotherapy in their emotional balance. Treated patients began to feel less tense, worried and

Table 2 Disease activity scores of SLE patients in control and therapy groups over time

Time	Control ($n = 43$) Median (Min-Max)	Therapy ($n = 37$) Median (Min-Max)	Inter-group P*
T1	.0 (.0–22.0)	2.0 (.0–19.0)	0.347
T2	.0 (.0–20.0)	2.0 (.0–21.0)	0.207
Intra-group P**	0.925	0.214	

SLEDAI Systemic Lupus Erythematosus Disease Activity Index (Range: 0–105)
*Mann-Whitney test; **Wilcoxon test

angry. The results are in agreement with Haupt et al. and Navarrete-Navarrete et al. studies [19, 20].

We observed a great improvement in the ability to solve problems but, if we consider the intra-group analyses, changes in four of the eight domains in CSI revealed that psychotherapy improved other coping strategies. These strategies are very important to face daily problems, finding adequate solutions for them and getting enough self-esteem to preserve adequate quality of life. There was a change in the types of coping strategies, trending to face stressors and get emotional balance. Our results are similar to Haupt's study outcomes [19].

At baseline and at the end of the study, the percentage of patients using medications for SLE treatment was similar in both groups and the mean of prednisone dosage used by about 55% of patients was 10.38 mg/day This medication did not vary significantly during the study. Thus, we do not believe there was a significant influence of the use of prednisone in our results.

Medications for co morbidities, including mild anxiety and depressive symptoms, were also similar between groups at baseline and along the study, reducing the possibility that medications may have contributed to the changes observed in the study. Although severe mental diseases had been excluded, we observed that about 40% of patients were taking antidepressant drugs, used for fibromyalgia or for mild anxiety and depression symptoms, which are frequently present in SLE patients [10–13]. The exclusion of patients with mild psychiatric symptoms could make the study unfeasible, considering the high frequency of these symptoms in SLE patients. Furthermore, previous clinical trials also included patients with depressive and anxiety symptoms and with other mild psychological or psychiatric findings [19, 20] and also was using anxiolytic and antidepressant medications [20].

Table 3 Symptom checklist scores of SLE patients in control and therapy groups over time

Time	Control ($n = 43$) Median (Min-Max)	Therapy ($n = 37$) Median (Min-Max)	Inter-group P*
T1	52.0 (7.0–91.0)	51.0 (8.0–119.0)	0.985
T2	53.0 (10.0–99.0)	40.0 (2.0–84.0)	0.001
Intra-group P**	0.101	< 0.001	

SLE-SSC Systemic Lupus Erythematosus Specific Symptom Checklist (Range: 0–152)
*Mann-Whitney test; **Wilcoxon test
$P < 0.05$ significant

In our study, therapeutic intervention helped patients to lead to positive results in psychological measures through the confidence and support atmosphere established in group dynamic. The therapy technique facilitated the patient's integration, increased feeling of willingness to participate and provided social pressure to encourage patients to report symptoms. So, BGPP helped patients to access deep problems and conflicts with the goal of establishing coping strategies to deal with them. During the sessions, patients elected several themes to discuss, such as anxiety and insecurity related to disease, uncertainty about the future, the possibility of death, depressive reactions about life stressors, lack of emotional control, low self-esteem, interpersonal relationship problems, sexual difficulties and reduced quality of life (due to pain and fatigue) beside personal traumatic issues. Thereby, the group functioned as a support to cope with the disease, allowing each patient to handle their anguish and fears and getting more adaptive forms to face stressors improving the quality of life.

Limitations of the study:

1) Low activity and damage scores - As the most of our patients had low SLEDAI and SLICC/ACR-DI scores, these results cannot be generalized to patients with severe disease. For patients with severe disease, it is recommended continued therapy, according to Parth et al. study [46].
2) Additional generalizations - Because of exclusion criteria in our study, we cannot generalize the results to other populations like male gender, illiterate and patients with high education, high socioeconomic status and severe physical and mental diseases. Patients with no personal demand for psychotherapy are also beyond the scope of this study.
3) A restricted choice of coping scales - At the beginning of the study there was only one coping scale translated and validated to the Portuguese language. This questionnaire was considered too complex and long for the majority of our patients.
4) Placebo effect - We consider the possibility of the improvement obtained to be partly due to the general effect of the intervention (more visits to the outpatient clinic to perform the therapy, the special attention of the therapists and the contact with other patients) and not due to specific psychotherapeutic method. This possibility is related to an inherent feature of psychotherapy, which promotes relationships and provides special care for treated patients.

Table 4 Quality of life scores of SLE patients in control and therapy groups over time

Domain	Time	Control ($n = 43$) Median (Min-Max)	Therapy ($n = 37$) Median (Min-Max)	Inter-group P*
Physical function	T1	12.0 (6.0–34.0)	10.0 (2.0–39.0)	0.645
	T2	14.0 (6.0–36.0)	9.0 (6.0–30.0)	0.023
	Intra-group P**	0.245	0.057	
Occupational activity	T1	24.0 (9.0–59.0)	25.0 (1.0–59.0)	0.743
	T2	31.0 (9.0–61.0)	17.0 (9.0–42.0)	0.001
	Intra-group P**	0.055	0.001	
Symptoms	T1	22.0 (8.0–49.0)	23.0 (6.0–51.0)	0.589
	T2	25.0 (8.0–46.0)	14.0 (8.0–37.0)	0.001
	Intra-group P**	0.023	< 0.001	
Treatment	T1	11.0 (4.0–22.0)	10.0 (3.0–19.0)	0.591
	T2	11.0 (4.0–25.0)	8.0 (1.0–20.0)	0.002
	Intra-group P**	0.093	0.008	
Humor	T1	14.0 (4.0–28.0)	15.0 (4.0–28.0)	0.376
	T2	13.0 (4.0–28.0)	9.0 (4.0–26.0)	0.005
	Intra-group P**	0.321	< 0.001	
Self-Image	T1	20.0 (9.0–51.0)	25.0 (9.0–53.0)	0.178
	T2	20.0 (9.0–54.0)	15.0 (9.0–33.0)	0.003
	Intra-group P**	0.764	< 0.001	
Total score	T1	114.0 (40.0–204.0)	109.0 (44.0–226.0)	0.596
	T2	113.0 (45.0–236.0)	71.0 (40.0–153.0)	< 0.001
	Intra-group P**	0.041		

SLEQOL Systemic Lupus Erythematosus Quality of Life (Range: 40–280)
*Mann-Whitney test; **Wilcoxon test
$P < 0.05$ significant

In addition, we have to admit that this type of intervention only works in patients who have personal demand for psychotherapy. In our study, all patients had such a demand and were motivated to accept psychological help. In this case, we believe that psychoanalytic treatment has been able to offer reception and listening to patients' suffering; it has made possible greater self-knowledge for patients and new ways of facing problems arising from the disease.

The psychotherapy technique used in this study did not follow standard manuals because it was similarly conducted by the same therapists in all subgroups. In case of a replication study, we assumed that therapists with similar experience and training in brief group psychoanalytic psychotherapy attendance could reach similar results.

Our single-center sample was smaller than the Canadian multicenter study [18]. However, it was larger than the

Table 5 Anxiety and depression scores of SLE patients in control and therapy groups over time

Domain	Time	Control ($n = 43$) Median (Min-Max)	Therapy ($n = 37$) Median (Min-Max)	Inter-group P*
Anxiety	T1	6.0 (1.0–16.0)	9.0 (.0–20.0)	0.340
	T2	8.0 (1.0–18.0)	6.0 (1.0–16.0)	0.019
	Intra-group P**	0.132	< 0.001	
Depression	T1	5.0 (1.0–16.0)	8.0 (.0–14.0)	0.264
	T2	7.0 (1.0–17.0)	4.0 (.0–14.0)	0.022
	Intra-group P**	0.081	< 0.001	

HADS Hospital Anxiety and Depression Scale (Range: 0–21 by domain)
*Mann-Whitney test; **Wilcoxon test
$P < 0.05$ significant

Table 6 Coping scores of SLE patients in control and therapy groups over time

Domain	Time	Control ($n = 43$) Median (Min-Max)	Therapy ($n = 37$) Median (Min-Max)	Inter-group P*
Confrontive	T1	0.83 (.00–2.33)	1.00 (0.33–2.33)	0.217
	T2	1.00 (.00–2.33)	0.83 (.00–3.00)	0.638
	Intra-group P**	0.490	0.021	
Distancing	T1	1.00 (0.29–2.14)	1.14 (0.14–2.71)	0.698
	T2	0.86 (.00–2.00)	0.86 (.00–2.29)	0.790
	Intra-group P**	0.064	0.073	
Self-controlling	T1	1.40 (0.20–3.00)	1.40 (0.60–3.00)	0.804
	T2	1.20 (.00–2.80)	1.60 (0.60–2.40)	0.186
	Intra-group P**	0.269	0.280	
Seeking social Support	T1	1.67 (0.33–3.00)	1.50 (0.33–2.67)	0.292
	T2	1.50 (.00–3.00)	1.67 (0.17–3.00)	0.520
	Intra-group P**	0.109	0.385	
Accepting responsibility	T1	1.71 (0.14–2.71)	1.43 (0.29–3.00)	0.153
	T2	1.57 (.00–2.71)	1.57 (0.14–2.71)	0.262
	Intra-group P**	0.137	0.099	
Escape and Avoidance	T1	1.50 (.00–3.00)	1.50 (.00–3.00)	0.554
	T2	1.50 (.00–3.00)	1.00 (.00–3.50)	0.124
	Intra-group P**	0.771	0.002	
Planful problem Solving	T1	1.75 (.00–3.00)	1.25 (0.50–3.00)	0.748
	T2	1.50 (.00–3.00)	2.00 (0.75–3.50)	0.017
	Intra-group P**	0.411	< 0.001	
Positive reappraisal	T1	1.89 (.00–2.89)	1.56 (0.22–2.67)	0.218
	T2	1.56 (.00–2.78)	1.78 (0.39–2.67)	0.063
	Intra-group P**	0.061	0.002	

CSI Coping Strategies Inventory (Range: 0–3 by domain)
*Mann-Whitney test; **Wilcoxon test
$P < 0.05$ significant

samples of German and Spanish single-center studies [19, 20] and reached the estimated sample size to achieve the proposed aims. Concerning age and years of disease duration, our patients had means similar to Edworthy et al. and Navarrete-Navarrete et al. studies [18, 20], and all of them had more chronic disease than the patients of Haupt et al. study [19].

We had two drop-outs in each group of the study. The lost patients had the same demographic and clinical characteristics than the long term participants. We believe that, despite the drop-outs, the homogeneity of the groups was maintained. We used intent to treat analysis, repeating the values of the first access.

More psychoanalytic research is needed to clarify the relationship of the immune system and patient's psychological function. Believing that psychological function can be one of the factors that participate as cause and trigger of SLE flares [3, 4], psychotherapeutic support may be useful to supplement clinical and pharmacological treatments in these patients. Psychotherapy group treatment should be offered at specialized centers to treat SLE patients because it can allow cost reduction and emotional benefits for coexistence and exchange of experiences among patients, besides higher effectiveness than individual treatment, according to a systematic review [47].

Conclusion

In conclusion, BGPP was effective to improve quality of life, including occupational activity, treatment, humor and self-image as well as to reduce symptoms, depression and anxiety levels in SLE patients, besides lead to some positive change in coping strategies. Psychoanalytic psychotherapy can help patients to become stronger to deal with the disease and other important life events, relieving their suffering.

Abbreviations

ABIPEME: *Associação Brasileira de Institutos de Pesquisa de Mercado*; ACR: American College of Rheumatology; ANOVA: Analysis of Variance; BGPP: Brief Group Psychoanalytic Psychotherapy; CG: Control Group; CSI: Coping Strategies Inventory; HADS: Hospital Anxiety and Depression Scale; HPA: Hypothalamic-Pituitary-Adrenal; NP: Neuropsychiatric; QOL: Quality Of Life; SLE: Systemic Lupus Erythematosus; SLEDAI: Systemic Lupus Erythematosus International Disease Activity; SLEQOL: Systemic Lupus Erythematosus Quality of Life; SLE-SSC: Systemic Lupus Erythematosus Specific Symptom Checklist; SLICC/ACR-DI: Systemic Lupus International Collaborating Clinic /American College of Rheumatology - Damage Index; SPSS: Statistical Package for the Social Sciences; T1: Baseline; T2: After 20 weeks; TG: Therapy Group

Acknowledgements

Sincere thanks to Prof Dr. Sérgio Blay, Prof Dr. Vanessa Cítero, Prof Dr. Valdecir Marvulle for statistical analysis support and Dr. Edgard Torres Reis Neto for SLEDAI and SLICC scores evaluations. Special thanks to psychologists Ermelinda Rodrigues and Marisa Minhoto for the evaluation of patients.

Authors' contributions

CTMC had the idea of study, performed the therapy, wrote the manuscript, analyzed and interpreted psychological data. IMM helped the intervention, analyzed clinical data and contributed with the recruitment of patients. JAB supervised the therapy and EIS supervised all study and both reviewed the manuscript. All authors read and approved the final manuscript.

Author details

[1]Rheumatology Division, Escola Paulista de Medicina, Universidade Federal de São Paulo, Rua Botucatu 740 – Disciplina de Reumatologia CEP 04023900, São Paulo, SP, Brazil. [2]Department of Psychiatry, Escola Paulista de Medicina, Universidade Federal de São Paulo, São Paulo, Brazil.

References

1. Yazdany J, Dall'Era M. Definitions and classification of lupus and lupus-related disorders. In: Wallace DJ, Hahn BH, editors. Dubois' Lupus Erythematosus and Related Syndromes. 8th ed. Philadelphia: Elsevier Saunders; 2013. p. 1–7.
2. McEwen BS. Protective and damaging effects of stress mediators. N Engl J Med. 1998;338:171–9.
3. Pawlak CR, Witte T, Heiken H, Hundt M, Schubert J, Wiese B, et al. Flares in patients with systemic lupus erythematosus are associated with daily psychological stress. Psychother Psychosom. 2003;72:159–65.
4. Roussou E, Iacovou C, Weerakoon A, Ahmed K. Stress as a trigger of disease flares in SLE. Rheumatol Int. 2013;33:1367–70.
5. Archenholtz B, Burckhardt CS, Segesten K. Quality of life of women with systemic lupus erythematosus or rheumatoid arthritis: domains of importance and dissatisfaction. Qual Life Res. 1999;8:411–6.
6. Thumboo J, Strand V. Health-related quality of life in patients with systemic lupus erythematosus: an update. Ann Acad Med Singap. 2007;36:115–22.
7. Karasz A, Ouellette S. Role strain and psychological well-being in women with systemic lupus erythematosus. Women Health. 1995;23:41–5.
8. Wiginton KL. Illness representations: mapping the experience of lupus. Health Educ Behav. 1999;26:443–53.
9. Devins GM. Illness intrusiveness and the psychosocial impact of lifestyle in chronic life-threatening disease. Adv Ren Repl Ther. 1994;1:251–63.
10. Palagini L, Mosca M, Tani C, Gemignani A, Mauri M, Bombardieri S. Depression and systemic lupus erythematosus: a systematic review. Lupus. 2013;22:409–16.
11. Huang X, Magder LS, Petri M. Predictors of incident depression in systemic lupus erythematosus. J Rheumatol. 2014;41:1823–33.
12. Hanly JG, Su L, Urowitz MB, Romero-Diaz J, Gordon C, Bae SC, et al. Mood disorders in systemic lupus erythematosus. Arthritis Rheumatol. 2015;67: 1837–47.
13. Ayache DC, Costa IP. Personality traits and associated changes in women with lupus. Rev Bras Reumatol. 2009;49:643–57.
14. Lazarus RS, Folkman S. Stress, Appraisal and coping. New York: Springer Publishing Company; 1984.
15. Rinaldi S, Ghisi M, Iaccarino L, Zampieri S, Guirardello A, Sarzi-Puttini P, et al. Influence of Coping Skills on Health-Related Quality of Life in Patients With Systemic Lupus Erythematosus. Arthritis Rheum. 2006;55:427 33.
16. Haija AJ, Schulz SW. The role and effect of complementary and alternative medicine in systemic lupus erythematosus. Rheum Dis Clin N Am. 2011;37:47–62.
17. Spiegel D, Morrow GR, Classen C, Raubertas R, Stott PB, Mudaliar N, et al. Group Psychotherapy for recently diagnosed breast cancer patients: a multicenter feasibility study. Psychooncology. 1999;8:482–93.
18. Edworthy SM, Dobkin PL, Clarke AE, Da Costa D, Dritsa M, Fortin PR, et al. Group Psychotherapy Reduces Illness Intrusiveness in Systemic Lupus Erythematosus. J Rheumatol. 2003;30:1011–6.
19. Haupt M, Millen S, Jänner M, Falagan D, Fischer-Betz R, Schneider M. Improvement of coping abilities in patients with systemic lupus erythematosus: a prospective study. Ann Rheum Dis. 2005;64:1618–23.
20. Navarrete-Navarrete N, Peralta-Ramírez MI, Sabio-Sánchez JM, Coín MA, Robles-Ortega H, Hidalgo-Tenorio C, et al. Efficacy of cognitive behavioural therapy for the treatment of chronic stress in patients with lupus erithematosus: a randomized controlled trial. Psychother Psychosom. 2010;79:107–15.
21. Freud S. The handling of dream interpretation in psychoanalysis. In: Strachey J, editor. Standard Edition, vol. 12. London: Hogarth Press; 1958. p. 89–96.
22. Freud S. The dynamics of transference. In: Strachey J, editor. Standard Edition, vol. 12. London: Hogarth Press; 1958. p. 97–108.
23. Freud S. Observations on transference-love. In: Strachey J, editor. Standard Edition, vol. 12. London: Hogarth Press; 1958. p. 157–71.
24. Ferenczi S. Further contribution to the theory and technique of psychoanalysis. London: Hogarth Press; 1950.
25. Rank O. Will Therapy? An Analysis of the Therapeutic Process in Terms of Relationship. New York: A A Knopf; 1936.
26. Bion WR. Experiences in groups and other papers. London: Tavistock Publications; 1961.
27. Alexander F. Psychosomatic medicine. New York: Norton; 1950.
28. Marty P. Mentalisation et psychosomatic. Paris: Delagrange; 1991.
29. Sifneos PE. The prevalence of alexithymic characteristics in psychosomatics patients. Psychother Psychosom. 1973;22:255–62.
30. Marty P. La psychosomatique de l'adulte. Paris: Puf; 1990.
31. Bombana JA, Leite ALSS, Miranda CT. How to care for somatizers? Description of a program and summarized case reports. Rev Bras Psiquiatr. 2000;22:180–4.
32. Bombana JA, Abud CC, Prado RA. Assistance and teaching of psychotherapy at the program of treatment and studies of somatization (PAES, UNIFESP). Rev Bras Psicot. 2012;14:34–48.
33. Hochberg MC. Updating the American College of Rheumatology revised criteria for the classification of systemic lupus erythematosus. Arthritis Rheum. 1997;40:1725.
34. Jannuzzi PM, Baeninger R. Qualificação socioeconômica e demográfica das classes da escala Abipeme. Rev Administ. 1996;31:82–90.
35. Gladman D, Ginzler E, Goldsmith C, Fortin P, Liang M, Urowitz M, et al. The development and initial validation of the Systemic Lupus International Collaborating Clinics/American College of Rheumatology damage index for Systemic Lupus Erythematosus. Arthritis Rheum. 1996;39:363–9.
36. Bombardier C, Gladman DD, Urowitz MB, Caron D, Chang CH. Derivation of the SLEDAI – A disease activity index for Lupus patients. Arthritis Rheum. 1992;35:630–40.
37. Freire EAM, Bruscato A, Ciconelli RM, Leite DRC, Sousa TTS. Translation into Brazilian Portuguese, cultural adaptation and validatation of the systemic lupus erythematosus quality of life questionnaire (SLEQOL). Acta Reumatol Port. 2010;35:334–9.
38. Grootscholten C, Ligtenberg G, Derksen RH, Schreurs KM, de Glas-Vos JW, Hagen EC, et al. Health-related quality of life in patients with systemic lupus erythematosus: development and validation of a lupus specific symptom checklist. Qual Life Res. 2003;12:635–44.
39. Leong KP, Kong KO, Thong BYH, Koh ET, Lian TY, Teh CL, et al. Development and preliminary validation of a systemic lupus erythematosus-specific quality-of-life instrument (SLEQOL). Rheumatology. 2005;44:1267–76.
40. Botega NJ, Bio MR, Zomignani MA, Garcia C Jr, Pereira WAB. Mood disorders among inpatients in ambulatory and validation of the anxiety and depression scale HAD. Rev Saúde Pública. 1995;29:355–63.
41. Zigmond AS, Sanaith RP. The hospital anxiety and depression scale. Acta Psychiat Scand. 1983;67:361–70.
42. Savoia MG, Santana PR, Mejias NP. The adaptation of coping strategies inventory by Folkman and Lazarus in portuguese. Rev Psicol USP. 1996;7: 183–201.
43. Folkman S, Lazarus RS. If it changes it must be a process: study of emotion and coping during three stages of a college examination. J Pers Soc Psychol. 1985;48:150 70.

44. Luborsky L. Principles of psychoanalytic psychotherapy: a manual for supportive-expressive treatment. New York: Basic Books; 1984.
45. Sifneos PE. Short Term dynamic psychotherapy. Evaluation and Technique. New York: Plenum; 1987.
46. Parth K, Rosar A, Stastka K, Storck T, Loffler-Stastka H. Psychosomatic patients in integrated care: Which treatment mediators do we have to focus on? Bull Menn Clin. 2016;80:326–47.
47. Toseland R, Siporin M. When to recommend group treatment: a review of the clinical and the research literature. Int J Group Psychother. 1986;36:171–201.

3

Association of anti-nucleosome and anti C1q antibodies with lupus nephritis in an Egyptian cohort of patients with systemic lupus erythematosus

Imman Mokhtar Metwally[1], Nahla Naeem Eesa[1*], Mariam Halim Yacoub[2] and Rabab Mahmoud Elsman[3]

Abstract

Introduction: Anti-nucleosome and anti-C1q antibodies demonstrated an association with the development of glomerulonephritis in systemic lupus erythematosus (SLE). Some investigators have proposed that monitoring anti-C1q and anti-nucleosome antibodies might be valuable for making predictions about lupus nephritis (LN) and assessment of disease activity as a non-invasive biological marker of renal disease.

Objectives: The current study was proposed to investigate the presence of anti-C1q and anti-nucleosome antibodies in the sera of Egyptian patients with SLE and their association with LN.

Methods: Eighty patients with SLE were included. Patients were classified into, a LN group including 40 cases with active LN (based on the results of renal biopsy and renal SLEDAI≥4) and a non renal SLE group including 40 patients (with no clinical or laboratory evidence of renal involvement that were attributed in the past or present to SLE). They were subjected to full medical history taking, clinical examination, routine laboratory investigations, measurement of antinuclear antibody (ANA), anti-ds DNA, anti-C1q & anti-nucleosome antibodies.

Results: Anti-C1q antibody showed a statistically significant association with the presence of vasculitis and nephritis while anti-nucleosome antibody didn't show a significant association with the presence of any clinical features. Double positivity of anti-nucleosome and anti-C1q antibodies showed a statistically significant association with the presence of vasculitis and photosensitivity, high ECLAM score, elevated ESR, low serum albumin and low C3 levels.

Conclusion: Serum anti-C1q antibody has a significant association with LN while double positive antibodies have a significant association with vasculitis and low C3 levels in Egyptian patients with SLE.

Keywords: Systemic lupus erythematosus, Lupus nephritis, Anti-C1q antibody, Anti-nucleosome antibody

Introduction

Renal involvement in systemic lupus erythematosus (SLE), known as lupus nephritis (LN), is a common and serious complication and a major predictor of poor outcome with reports of 5-year survival with treatment ranging from 46 to 95% [1]. Early diagnosis and initiation of immunosuppressive treatment is critical to improve outcome of patients with LN and hence long-term survival in SLE [2]. However, the insidious onset and fluctuating nature of LN can make early detection and follow-up very difficult [3, 4]. Being an invasive, painful and risky procedure, the utility of renal biopsy as the first approach to patients with suspected LN is still controversial [5]. Renal biopsy remains the gold standard for the evaluation of LN disease activity. Renal biopsy is important to define the nature of renal involvement. Mechanisms other than immune-complex mediated glomerulonephritis can result in renal injury and require a different approach to management [6]. A more comprehensive picture of kidney pathology may be desirable as therapy of LN develops beyond the currently available non-targeted immunosuppressives to interventions that

* Correspondence: nahlanaeem@gmail.com; nahla.ali@kasralainy.edu.eg
[1]Rheumatology and Rehabilitation Department, Faculty of Medicine, Cairo University, Cairo, Egypt
Full list of author information is available at the end of the article

focus on specific immune pathways [7]. Up to date, the available literature does not allow us to state that omitting renal biopsy in the diagnostic and therapeutic routine brings more advantages than threats [5]. A reliable clinical biomarker that can forecast LN well before thresholds of proteinuria, renal function and urine sediment that signal clinical flare are reached would be a valuable tool [8, 9]. There are several autoantibodies that required attention in LN, including their use in diagnosis and monitoring, and their role in the pathogenesis [10]. Anti-nucleosome and anti-C1q antibodies demonstrated an association with the development of glomerulonephritis in SLE [11]. It has been suggested that autoantibodies to C1q were found to be elevated in the sera of SLE patients and are closely associated with renal involvement [12]. Some investigators have proposed that monitoring anti-C1q might be valuable for the clinical management of SLE patients as a non-invasive biological marker of renal disease [13]. A Brazilian study on SLE patients confirmed the association of anti-C1q antibodies with nephritis and disease activity [14]. Another autoantibody that has been proposed to be linked to the occurrence of glomerulonephritis in lupus is antinucleosome antibody [15]. Nucleosomes are generated during cell apoptosis by cleavage of the chromatin by endonucleases. Studies have shown that the clearance of apoptotic cells by macrophages in patients with SLE is impaired. This leads to decreased clearance of nucleosome [16]. Anti-nucleosome antibodies could be a useful parameter for early diagnosis and follow-up of SLE with nephritis [17]. The current work was carried out to investigate the association of both anti-nucleosome and anti-C1q antibodies with the occurrence of lupus nephritis.

Patients and methods

Study population

This study was conducted on eighty patients with SLE diagnosed according to the American College of Rheumatology (ACR) 1997 revised criteria for the classification of SLE [18]. Subjects were recruited from the Rheumatology and Rehabilitation Department, Faculty of Medicine, Cairo University hospitals and Rheumatology clinic of Helwan University Hospital from December 2016 to December 2017. An Informed consent was obtained from all patients and the study was approved by the local ethics committee.

Patients were classified into two groups, group (I) which included 40 cases with active LN [based on the results of kidney biopsy and renal systemic lupus erythematosus disease activity index (rSLEDAI) ≥4] and group (II) which included 40 age matched SLE patients without LN [with no evidence of major renal manifestations that were attributed in the past or present to SLE disease and with normal serum creatinine and urine sediment].

Methods

All SLE patients were subjected to full history taking, general examination, cardio pulmonary, abdominal, neurological and locomotor systems examination. Peripheral blood was obtained within 3 days before renal biopsy for measurement of autoantibodies, complete blood count (CBC), complement C3 and C4 levels, erythrocyte sedimentation rate (ESR), blood urea nitrogen (BUN), serum albumin, and creatinine. Urine analysis and protein quantification in 24 h urine samples were performed for all patients. ANA were determined by indirect immunofluorescence (Hemagen Diagnostics, USA), titres of 1:160 were taken as a cut off value. Anti-dsDNA were done by *Crithidia Luciliae* indirect immunofluorescence test (CLIFT). Serum C3 and C4 levels by nephelometry (Beckman, USA). Anti C1q and antinucleosome IgG antibodies were tested in sera using Enzyme Linked Immunosorbent Assay (ELISA) [19, 20]. (According to the manufacturers' instructions from Orgentic Diagnostika GmbH). Cut off values were ≥ 10 u/ml for Anti C1q and ≥ 20 u/ml for antinucleosome antibodies.

Renal pathology was classified according to the revised International Society of Nephrology and Renal Pathology Society (ISN/RPS) classification [21].

Assessment of disease activity

Disease activity was assessed using The European Consensus Lupus Activity Measurement (ECLAM) [22]. A global activity score which assesses disease activity within the past month. It comprises 15 weighted clinical and serological items with a theoretically possible range of 0–10, with 0 being no disease activity.

Statistical analysis

Data was collected, tabulated and statistically analyzed using Statistical package for social science (SPSS) software version 15. Measurement of data consistent with normal distribution was expressed as mean ± SD. Measurement of categorical variables was expressed using the odds ratio and 95% confidence interval. Statistical differences between groups were tested using Chi Square test for qualitative variables, Student's T test between 2 groups for quantitative normally distributed variables while Nonparametric Mann–Whitney test and Kruskal–Wallis test were used for quantitative variables which are not normally distributed. Correlations were done to test for linear relations between variables. *P*-values less than 0.05 were considered statistically significant.

Results

Clinical and laboratory features among patient groups

Eighty Egyptian patients with SLE, 40 with LN (group I) and 40 without (group II) were included in this study. Active LN patients were receiving pulse methylprednisolone, cyclophosphamide and mycophenolate mofetil while those without LN were maintained on oral prednisolone, hydroxychloroquine and azathioprine. Clinical features did not show a significant difference between the two groups. However statistically significant differences were found between both groups in the following variables: ECLAM score, serum albumin, serum creatinine, low C3 & C4 and anti-C1q antibody positivity. Detailed comparisons between groups are presented in Table 1.

Relationship between anti-nucleosome antibodies and other disease parameters among study groups

Anti-nucleosome antibody was positive in 49 (61.25%) patients of the 80 SLE patients. 24 (60%) patients in group I and in 25 (62.5%) patients in group II. Clinical features, activity assessment by ECLAM and renal histopathology did not show a significant difference between patients with positive and those with negative anti-nucleosome antibody. However serum creatinine was statistically significantly lower among patients with positive anti-nucleosome antibody ($t = 2.11$, $P < 0.05$). (Tables 2 and 3).

Table 1 Comparison between both SLE groups (with and without LN) regarding demographic, laboratory and clinical characteristics

Parameter mean ± SD or n (%)		Group I (*n* = 40)	Group II (*n* = 40)	t/x²	*P* value
Demographic features	Age (year)	29.0 ± 7.2	32.5 ± 9.4	1.756	0.083
	Disease duration (year)	4.4 ± 3.7	6.8 ± 5.6	2.280	0.025
	Male/ Female	6 (15) /34 (85)	1 (2.5) /39 (97.5)	3.914	0.048
Clinical features	Arthritis	34 (85.0)	38 (95.0)	2.200	0.136
	Malar rash	25 (62.5)	25 (62.5)	0.00	1.000
	Fever	22 (55.0)	17 (42.5)	1.251	0.263
	Pleurisy	21 (52.5)	21 (52.5)	0.000	1.000
	Oral ulcers	17 (42.5)	21 (52.5)	0.802	0.370
	Alopecia	17 (42.5)	17 (42.5)	0.000	1.000
	Photosensitivity	13 (32.5)	18 (45.0)	1.317	0.251
	Vasculitis	10 (25.0)	4 (10.0)	3.117	0.077
	APS	10 (25.0)	9 (22.5)	0.069	0.793
	Neurological manifestations	9 (22.5)	11 (27.5)	0.267	0.606
	Pericarditis	6 (15.0)	4 (10.0)	0.457	0.499
	Discoid rash	2 (5.0)	4 (10.0)	0.721	0.396
	Myositis	1 (2.5)	0 (0.0)	1.013	0.314
ECLAM		4.7 ± 2.3	2.9 ± 1.4	4.326	<0.001
Laboratory features	ESR (mm/1st hour)	54.6 ± 32.4	41.7 ± 26.9	1.942	0.056
	Serum creatinine (μmol/L)	1.0 ± 0.7	0.6 ± 0.2	2.79	0.008
	Serum albumin (g/dl)	3.6 ± 0.6	4.1 ± 0.7	3.895	< 0.001
	24 h urinary proteins (g/24 h)	2 ± 1.7			
	Low C3 < 90	26 (65.0)	10 (25.0)	12.929	< 0.001
	Low C4 < 10	17 (42.5)	2 (5.0)	15.531	< 0.001
	Anti-nucleosome antibody positivity	24 (60.0)	25 (62.5)	0.053	0.818
	Anti-C1q antibody positivity	23 (57.5)	11 (27.5)	7.366	0.007
Renal biopsy	Lupus nephritis class I	0 (0)	–	–	–
	Lupus nephritis class II	5 (12.5)	–	–	–
	Lupus nephritis class III	13 (32.5)	–	–	–
	Lupus nephritis class IV	11 (27.5)	–	–	–
	Lupus nephritis class V	3 (7.5)	–	–	–
	Lupus nephritis class II- III	6 (15)	–	–	–
	Lupus nephritis class II & V	2 (5)	–	–	–

APS Antiphospholipid syndrome, *ESR* Erythrocyte sedimentation rate, *ECLAM* European Consensus Lupus Activity Measurement

Table 2 Relationship between anti-nucleosome antibody and other disease parameters among patients under study

Variable n (%) or mean ± SD		Positive Anti-nucleosome (*n* = 49)	Negative Anti-nucleosome (*n* = 31)	t/x²	*P* value
Clinical features	Arthritis	42 (85.7)	30 (96.8)	2.581	0.108
	Pleurisy	28 (57.1)	14 (45.2)	1.093	0.296
	Fever	27 (55.1)	12 (38.7)	2.042	0.153
	Malar rash	27 (55.1)	23 (74.2)	2.953	0.086
	Oral ulcers	24 (49.0)	14 (45.2)	0.111	0.739
	Alopecia	22 (44.9)	12 (38.7)	0.298	0.585
	Photosensitivity	15 (30.6)	16 (51.6)	3.528	0.060
	Neurologic manifestations	13 (26.5)	7 (22.6)	0.158	0.691
	APS	12 (24.5)	7 (22.6)	0.038	0.845
	Vasculitis	11 (22.4)	3 (9.7)	2.145	0.143
	Pericarditis	8 (16.3)	2 (6.5)	1.693	0.193
	Discoid rash	4 (8.2)	2 (6.5)	0.080	0.777
	Myositis	1 (2.0)	0 (0.0)	0.641	0.423
	Nephritis	24 (49%)	16 (51.6)	2.937	0.230
ECLAM		4.1 ± 2.2	3.3 ± 1.8	1.805	0.075
Laboratory features	ESR (mm/1st hour)	51.0 ± 30.7	43.7 ± 29.7	1.051	0.296
	Serum creatinine (μmol/L)	0.7 ± 0.3	1.0 ± 0.8	2.110	0.038
	Serum albumin (g/dl)	3.8 ± 0.7	4.0 ± 0.7	1.207	0.232
	Low C3 < 90 (mg/dl)	25 (51.0)	11 (35.5)	1.852	0.174
	Low C4 < 10 (mg/dl)	11 (22.4)	8 (25.8)	0.118	0.731

APS: Antiphospholipid syndrome, *ESR*: Erythrocyte sedimentation rate, ECLAM: European Consensus Lupus Activity Measurement

Relationship between anti-C1q antibodies and other disease parameters among study groups

Anti-C1q antibody was positive in 34 (42.5%) of the 80 SLE patients. 23 (57.5%) patients in group I and in 11 (27.5%) patients in group II. Positivity of anti-C1q antibody showed a statistically significant association with the presence of vasculitis and nephritis, elevated ESR, low serum albumin and low C3 and C4 levels. However, activity assessment by ECLAM and renal histopathology did not show a significant difference between patients with positive and those with negative anti-C1q antibody. (Tables 4 & 5).

Double positivity of anti-nucleosome and anti-C1q antibodies

Both anti-nucleosome and anti-C1q antibodies were positive in 22 (27.5%) patients. 15 (37.5%) patients in group I and 7 (17.5%) patients in group II. However both antibodies were negative in 19 (23.75%) patients. 8 (20%) patients in group I and 11 (27.5%) patients in group II. Double positivity of anti-nucleosome and anti-C1q antibodies anti-C1q antibody showed a statistically significant association with the presence of vasculitis and photosensitivity, high ECLAM score, elevated ESR, low serum albumin and low C3 levels. However,

Table 3 Relationship between anti-nucleosome antibody and renal histopathology in patients with LN.

Renal biopsy, *n* (%)	Positive anti-nucleosome antibody (*N* = 24)	Negative anti-nucleosome antibody (*N* = 16)	x²	*P* value
Lupus nephritis class I	0	0 (0)	0.000	0.000
Lupus nephritis class II	2 (8.3)	3 (18.8)	0.952	0.329
Lupus nephritis class III	5 (20.8)	8 (50)	2.401	0.121
Lupus nephritis class II –III	5 (20.8)	1 (6.3)	1.601	0.206
Lupus nephritis class IV	9 (37.5)	2 (12.5)	3.009	0.083
Lupus nephritis class V	2 (8.3)	1 (6.3)	0.060	0.806
Lupus nephritis class II & V	1 (4.2)	1 (6.3)	0.088	0.767

Table 4 Relationship between anti-C1q antibody and other disease parameters among patients under study

Variable n (%) or mean ± SD		Positive Anti-C1q (*n* = 34)	Negative Anti-C1q (*n* = 46)	t/x^2	*P* value
Clinical features	Arthritis	31 (91.2)	41 (89.1)	0.091	0.763
	Pleurisy	15 (35.7)	27 (58.7)	1.666	0.197
	Fever	19 (55.9)	20 (43.5)	1.204	0.273
	Malar rash	20 (58.8)	30 (65.2)	0.341	0.559
	Oral ulcers	17 (50.0)	21 (45.7)	0.148	0.700
	Alopecia	13 (38.2)	21 (61.8)	0.440	0.507
	Photosensitivity	11 (32.4)	20 (43.5)	1.020	0.313
	Neurologic manifestations	6 (17.6)	14 (30.4)	1.705	0.192
	APS	6 (17.6)	13 (28.3)	1.216	0.270
	Vasculitis	10 (29.4)	4 (8.7)	5.811	0.016
	Pericarditis	5 (14.7)	5 (10.9)	0.263	0.608
	Discoid rash	4 (11.8)	2 (4.3)	1.550	0.213
	Myositis	0 (0.0)	1 (2.2)	0.748	0.387
	Nephritis	23 (67.6)	17 (37.0)	7.366	0.007
ECLAM		4.2 ± 1.9	3.5 ± 2.2	1.572	0.120
Laboratory features	ESR (mm/1st hour)	57.7 ± 32.5	41.1 ± 26.8	2.500	0.015
	Serum creatinine (μmol/L)	0.9 ± 0.7	0.8 ± 0.3	0.643	0.500
	Serum albumin (g/dl)	3.6 ± 0.5	4.0 ± 0.8	2.677	0.009
	Low C3 < 90 (mg/dl)	20 (58.8)	16 (34.8)	4.565	0.033
	Low C4 < 10 (mg/dl)	12 (35.3)	7 (15.2)	4.351	0.037

APS Antiphospholipid syndrome, *ESR* Erythrocyte sedimentation rate, *ECLAM* European Consensus Lupus Activity Measurement

renal histopathology did not show a significant difference between patients with double positive and those with double negative antibodies. (Table 6).

Predictors of lupus nephritis

Multivariate analysis demonstrated that a low C4 complement level was most highly predictive of the presence of lupus nephritis, with a relative risk of 14.04 and a *P* value of < 0.001. A low C3 complement level was the next most significant factor, with a relative risk of 5.57 and a P value of < 0.001. In addition, the presence of anti-C1q antibody provided a significant predictive value with a relative risk of 3.60 and a *P* value of 0.007 (Table 7).

Discussion

There is a prevailing need for validated biomarkers that can diagnose active organ involvement during SLE disease flares. Lupus nephritis (LN) is a common major organ manifestation and a main cause of morbidity and mortality. The diagnosis of LN has an important clinical implication in guiding treatment of SLE [23]. Some investigators have proposed that monitoring anti-C1q and anti-nucleosome antibodies might be valuable for making predictions about lupus nephritis and assessment of

Table 5 Relationship between anti-C1q antibody and renal histopathology in patients with LN

Renal biopsy, n (%)	Positive anti-C1q (*N* = 23)	Negative anti-C1q (*N* = 17)	x^2	*P* value
Lupus nephritis class I	0 (0)	0 (0)	0.000	0.000
Lupus nephritis class II	2 (8.7)	3 (17.6)	0.716	0.397
Lupus nephritis class III	9 (39.1)	4 (23.5)	0.589	0.443
Lupus nephritis class II- III	5 (21.7)	1 (5.9)	1.928	0.165
Lupus nephritis class IV	4 (17.4)	7 (41.2)	2.774	0.096
Lupus nephritis class V	3 (13)	0 (0)	2.397	0.122
Lupus nephritis class II & V	0 (0)	2 (11.8)	2.848	0.091

Table 6 Relationship between double positivity of anti-nuclesome and anti-C1q antibodies and other disease parameters among patients under study

Variable n (%) or mean±SD		Double Positive (*n*=22)	Double Negative (*n*=19)	t/x²	*P* value
Clinical features	Arthritis	19 (86.4)	18 (94.7)	0.812	0.368
	Pleurisy	14 (63.6)	13 (68.4)	0.104	0.747
	Fever	14 (63.6)	7 (36.8)	2.930	0.087
	Malar rash	11 (50.0)	14 (73.7)	2.403	0.121
	Oral ulcers	12 (54.5)	9 (47.4)	0.21	0.647
	Alopecia	10 (45.5)	9 (47.4)	0.015	0.902
	Photosensitivity	6 (27.3)	11 (57.9)	3.939	0.047
	Neurologic manifestations	5 (22.7)	6 (31.6)	0.407	0.524
	APS	5 (22.7)	6 (31.6)	0.407	0.524
	Vasculitis	8 (36.4)	1 (5.3)	5.756	0.016
	Pericarditis	5 (22.7)	2 (10.5)	1.072	0.301
	Discoid rash	3 (13.6)	1 (5.3)	0.812	0.368
	Myositis	0 (0.0)	0 (0.0)	--	--
	Nephritis	15 (68.18)	8 (42.1)	3.051	0.217
ECLAM		4.6±2.1	3.1±2.1	2.254	0.030
Laboratory features	ESR (mm/1st hour)	59.6±32.3	37.0±25.1	2.471	0.018
	Serum creatinine (μmol/L)	0.7±0.3	0.9±0.4	1.443	0.157
	Serum albumin (g/dl)	3.6±0.5	4.2±0.8	2.960	0.005
	Low C3 < 90 (mg/dl)	14 (63.6)	5 (26.3)	5.711	0.017
	Low C4 < 10 (mg/dl)	7 (31.8)	5 (15.8)	1.420	0.233
	24 hours urinary proteins (gm/24hrs)	2.1±2.0	1.6±1.5	0.606	0.551

APS: Antiphospholipid syndrome, *ESR*: Erythrocyte sedimentation rate, ECLAM: European Consensus Lupus Activity Measurement

disease activity as a non-invasive biological marker of renal disease [13].

In this study we investigated the association of anti-nucleosome and anti-C1q antibodies with the development of lupus nephritis. Our study enrolled 80 SLE patients with and without LN. Anti-nucleosome antibodies were elicited in 49 (61.25%) patients, 24 (60%) in group I and in 25 (62.5%) in group II ($p = 0.818$) with a non-statistically significant difference between both groups. Although, some investigators suggest that anti-nucleosome antibodies are more likely to be detected in patients with nephritis and may serve as a useful biomarker in the diagnosis of active LN [24–26], our study was unable to confirm this association. In agreement with our findings, several authors showed that anti-nucleosome antibodies have a limited value in distinguishing SLE patients with or without active nephritis [15, 17, 27–29]. Furthermore, data from a meta-analysis conducted on 26 articles showed that anti-nucleosome antibody didn't correlate with kidney involvement in SLE, but was significantly associated with disease activity measured by the international score systems [30]. Identification of patients with active SLE is anchored on the presence of clinical symptoms, with compatible serological abnormalities reinforcing the clinical impression. Several reports have addressed the utility of anti-nucleosome antibodies to monitor disease activity with varying findings. In our study, disease activity as assessed by ECLAM score was not mirrored by the presence of anti-nucleosome antibody. Furthermore, anti-nucleosome antibodies were not associated with laboratory features that signify active disease as elevated ESR, low C3, low C4, & low albumin. This conclusion was consistent with other studies [15, 31–34].

Our study was able to support the association of anti-C1q antibody and the development of LN. Anti-C1q antibody was detected in 34 (42.5%) patients,

Table 7 Multivariate analysis of factors associated with lupus nephritis

Risk Factors	Relative Risk		*P* value
	OR	CI (95%)	
Low C4	14.04	(2.97-66.43)	<0.001
Low C3	5.57	(2.12-14.65)	<0.001
Anti-C1q antibody	3.60	(1.40-9.10)	0.007
Anti-nucleosome antibody	0.90	(0.37-2.21)	0.818

OR: Odds ratio, *CI*: Confidence interval

23 (67.6%) were in group I and 11 (62.5%) in group II and this difference was statistically significant (p<0.001). After a multivariate analysis in our patients, positive anti-C1q antibody has been isolated as a statistically significant risk factor for developing lupus nephritis (OR = 3.60, p = 0.007). Anti-C1q antibodies were also associated laboratory markers of active disease as elevated ESR (p = 0.015), low serum albumin (p = 0.009) and low levels of C3 (p = 0.033) and C4 (p = 0.037). Several studies demonstrate a strong correlation between the presence of anti-C1q antibodies and lupus nephritis, and suggest that anti-C1q determination may serve as a noninvasive biomarker to monitor renal involvement and/or predict renal flares [11–13, 35]. On the other hand, Katsumata and colleagues demonstrated that antibodies to C1q were associated with global activity of SLE but not specifically with active LN [36]. In a review of 28 studies measuring anti-C1q antibodies to detect a history of LN in SLE patients and 9 studies in which anti-C1q was measured to distinguish between active and inactive LN, they suggested that the measurement of anti-C1q auto-antibodies as a 'stand-alone' biomarker is not diagnostically useful [37] The variability reported in different studies for anti-C1q antibody could be in part attributed to differences in classes of nephropathy, the time of serum sample and methodological differences in the commercial ELISA kits used.

In spite of a growing number of reports on the study of anti-nucleosome and anti-C1q antibodies, only few studies focus on the simultaneous presence of both antibodies. In the current study, double positivity of anti-nucleosome and anti-C1q antibodies was found in 22 (27.5%) patients. In an effort to explore the relationship between double positive antibodies and different disease manifestations, a statistically significant association was found with vasculitis (p = 0.016). To date, no studies have investigated the association between double positive antibodies (anti-nucleosome and anti-C1q) and clinical features in SLE patients. Regarding the relationship between double positive antibodies and laboratory findings, our study showed that patients with double positive antibodies have a significantly higher disease activity as assessed by ECLAM score, elevated ESR, lower serum albumin and low C3 levels. Our findings parallel those of other authors [38, 39].

As this study did not investigate the relationship between longitudinal changes in disease activity and autoantibody titres in individual patients, detection of alterations in antibodies with clinically significant changes might have been masked by a predominance of individuals with no change in disease activity or a balance between individuals with flaring and remitting disease. We suggest that longitudinal tracking of biomarkers and disease activity may be more useful for updating clinical decisions at the time of assessment than forecasting flares.

Conclusions

In conclusion, presence of anti-C1q antibody is associated with the risk of developing LN; however, further, larger prospective studies are warranted to clarify and evaluate the specificity and predictive value of anti-C1q antibodies as a non-invasive biomarker of active LN to help in early identification of patients at risk whom would be eligible for early intense immunosuppressive treatment.

Authors' contributions

IMMetwally Study design; Elaboration of the article and critical review; Data analysis and interpretation. NNEesa Elaboration of the article and critical revision; Data analysis and interpretation. MHYacoub Laboratory workup. RMElsman; Study design; Data collection; Data analysis and interpretation; Manuscript preparation. All authors read and approved the final manuscript to be published.

Author details

[1]Rheumatology and Rehabilitation Department, Faculty of Medicine, Cairo University, Cairo, Egypt. [2]Clinical and Chemical Pathology Department, Faculty of Medicine, Cairo University, Cairo, Egypt. [3]Rheumatology Department, Helwan University Hospital, Helwan, Egypt.

References

1. Korbet SM, Lewis EJ, SchwartzMM. Factors predictive of outcome in severe lupus nephritis Lupus Nephritis Collaborative Study Group. Am J Kidney Dis 2000; 35:904–914.
2. Esdaile JM, Joseph L, MacKenzie T, Kashgarian M, Hayslett JP. The benefit of early treatment with immunosuppressive agents in lupus nephritis. J Rheumatol. 1994;21:2046–51.
3. Illei GG, Tackey E, Lapteva L, Lipsky PE. Biomarkers in systemic lupus erythematosus: II. Markers of disease activity. Arthritis Rheum. 2004;50:2048–65.
4. Schwartz N, Michaelson JS, Putterman C. Lipocalin-2, TWEAK, and other cytokines as urinary biomarkers for lupus nephritis. Ann N Y Acad Sci. 2007; 1109:265–74.
5. Haładyj E, Cervera R. Do we still need renal biopsy in lupus nephritis? Reumatologia. 2016;54(2):61–6.
6. Song D, Wu LH, Wang FM, Yang XW, Zhu D, Chen M, et al. The spectrum of renal thrombotic microangiopathy in lupus nephritis. Arthritis Res Ther. 2013;15(1):R12.
7. Salem A, Alexa M, Brad HR. Update on lupus nephritis. CJASN. 2017;12:825–35.
8. Fiehn C, Hajjar Y, Mueller K, Waldherr R, Ho AD, Andrassy K. Improved clinical outcome of lupus nephritis during the past decade: importance of early diagnosis and treatment. Ann Rheum Dis. 2003;62:435–9.
9. Houssiau FA, Vasconcelos C, D'Cruz D, Sebastiani GD, Garrido ER, Danieli MG, et al. Early response to immunosuppressive therapy predicts good renal outcome in lupus nephritis. Arthritis Rheum. 2004;50:3934–40.
10. Karim Y, Yong F, Cruz P. Importance of autoantibodies in lupus nephritis. Expert Rev Clin Immunol. 2007;3(6):937–47.
11. Bock M, Heijnen I, Trendelenburg M. Anti-C1q antibodies as a follow-up marker in SLE patients. PLoS One 2015;16: 10(4): e0123572.
12. Trendelenburg M. Antibodies against C1q in patients with systemic lupus erythematosus. Springer Semin Immunopathol. 2005;27:276–85.
13. Siegert CE, Daha MR, Tseng CM, Coremans IE, van Es LA, Breedveld FC. Predictive value of IgG autoantibodies against C1q for nephritis in systemic lupus erythematosus. Ann Rheum Dis. 1993;52(12):851–6.
14. Moura CG, Lima I, Barbosa L, Athanazio D, Reis E, Reis M, et al. Anti-C1q antibodies: association with nephritis and disease activity in systemic lupus erythematosus. J Clin Lab Anal. 2009;23(1):19–23.
15. Saigal R, Goyal L, Agrawal A, Mehta A, Mittal P, Yadav R, et al. Anti-nucleosome antibodies in patients with systemic lupus erythematosus :

potential utility as a diagnostic tool and disease activity marker and its comparison with anti-dsDNA antibody. J Assoc Physicians India. 2013;61(6): 372–7.
16. Shao WH, Cohen PL. Disturbances of apoptotic cell clearance in systemic lupus erythematosus. Arthritis Res Ther. 2011;13(1):202.
17. Bigler C, Lopez-Trascasa M, Potlukova E, Moll S, Danner D, Schaller M. Antinucleosome antibodies as a marker of active proliferative lupus nephritis. Am J Kidney Dis. 2008;51:624–9.
18. Hochberg MC. Updating the American College of Rheumatology revised criteria for the classification of systemic lupus erythematosus. Arthritis Rheum. 1997;40(9):1725.
19. Walport J, Davies A, Botto M. C1q and systemic lupus erythematosus. Immunobiology. 1998;199:265–85.
20. Amital H, Shoenfeld Y, Nucleosomes DNA. SLE: where is the starting point? Clin Exp Rheumatol. 1996;14(5):475–7.
21. Weening JJ, D'Agati VD, Schwartz MM, Seshan SV, Alpers CE, Appel GB, et al. International Society of Nephrology Working Group on the classification of lupus nephritis and Renal Pathology Society working group on the classification of lupus nephritis: classification of glomerulonephritis in systemic lupus erythematosus revised. Kidney Int. 2004;65(5):521–30.
22. Vitali C, Bencivelli W, Isenberg D, Smolen J, Snaith M, Sciuto M, et al. Disease activity in systemic lupus erythematosus: report of the consensus study Group of the European Workshop for rheumatology research. II. Identification of the variables indicative of disease activity and their use in the development of an activity score. Clin Exp Rheuma. 1992;10(5):541–7.
23. Moroni G, Quaglini S, Radice A, Trezzi B, Raffiotta F, Messa P, et al. The value of a panel of autoantibodies for predicting the activity of lupus nephritis at time of renal biopsy. J Immunol Res. 2015;2015:8.
24. Cervera R, Vinas O, Ramos-Casals M, Font J, Garcia-Carrasco M, Siso A. Anti-chromatin antibodies in systemic lupus erythematosus: a useful marker for lupus nephropathy. Ann Rheum Dis. 2003;62(5):431–4.
25. Gutierrez-Adrianzen O, Koutouzov S, Mota R, das Chagas Medeiros M, Bach J, de Holanda Campos H. Diagnostic value of anti-nucleosome antibodies in the assessment of disease activity of systemic lupus erythematosus: a prospective study comparing anti-nucleosome with anti-dsDNA antibodies. J Rheumatol. 2006;33:1538–44.
26. Haddouk S, Ben Ayed M, Baklouti S, Hachicha J, Bahloul Z, Masmoudi H. Clinical significance of anti-nucleosome antibodies in Tunisian systemic lupus erythematosus patients. Clin Rheumatol. 2005;24:219–22.
27. Liu C, Kao A, Manzi S, Ahearn J. Biomarkers in systemic lupus erythematosus: challenges and prospects for the future. Ther Adv Musculoskelet Dis. 2013;5(4):210–33.
28. Quattrocchi P, Barrile A, Bonanno D, Giannetto L, Patafi M, Tigano V, et al. Anti-nucleosome antibodies in SLE. Reumatismo. 2005;57:109–13.
29. Bose N, Wang X, Gupta M, Yao Q. The clinical utility of anti-chromatin antibodies as measured by BioPlex 2200 in the diagnosis of systemic lupus erythematosus versus other rheumatic diseases. Int J Clin Exp Med. 2012;5: 316–20.
30. Bizzaro N, Villalta D, Giavarina D, Tozzoli R. Are anti-nucleosome antibodies a better diagnostic marker than anti-dsDNA antibodies for systemic lupus erythematosus? A systematic review and a study of metanalysis. Autoimmun Rev. 2012;12(2):97–106.
31. El Desouky S, El-Gazzar I, Rashed L, Salama N. Correlation between various clinical parameters of systemic lupus erythematosus and levels of anti-histone and anti-chromatin antibodies. The Egyptian Rheumatologist. 2015; 37:97–104.
32. Su Y, Jia R, Han L, Li Z. Role of anti-nucleosome antibodyin the diagnosis of systemic lupus erythematosus. Clin Immunol. 2007;122(1):115–20.
33. Sardeto G, Simas L, Skare T, Nishiara R, Utiyama S. Antinucleosome in systemic lupus erythematosus. A study in a Brazilian population. Clin Rheumatol. 2012;31:553–6.
34. Manson J, Ma A, Rogers P, Berden H, van der Vlag J, D'Cruz P, et al. Relationship between anti-dsDNA, anti-nucleosome and anti-alpha-actinin antibodies and markers of renal disease in patients with lupus nephritis: a prospective longitudinal study. Arthritis Res Ther. 2009;11(5):154.
35. Sinico R, Rimoldi L, Radice A, Bianchi L, Gallelli B, Moroni G. Anti-C1q autoantibodies in lupus nephritis. Ann N Y Acad Sci. 2009;1173:47–51.
36. Katsumata Y, Miyake K, Kawaguchi Y, Okamoto Y, Kawamoto M, Gono T, et al. Anti-C1q antibodies are associated with systemic lupus erythematosus global activity but not specifically with nephritis: a controlled study of 126 consecutive patients. Arthritis Rheum. 2011;63(8):2436–44.
37. Eggleton P, Ukoumunne OC, Cottrell I, Khan A, Maqsood S, Thornes J, et al. Autoantibodies against C1q as a diagnostic measure of lupus nephritis: systematic review and meta-analysis. J Clin Cell Immunol. 2014;5(2):210.
38. Chen Z, Wang G, Wang G, Li X. Anti-C1q antibody is a valuable biological marker for prediction of renal pathological characteristics in lupus nephritis. Clin Rheumatol. 2012;31:1323–9.
39. Živković V, Aleksandra Stanković1, Tatjana Cvetković2, Branka Mitić2, Svetislav Kostić2, Jovan Nedović1, et al. Anti-dsDNA, anti-nucleosome and anti-C1q antibodies as disease activity markers in patients with systemic lupus erythematosus. Srp Arh Celok Lek 2014; 142 (7–8): 431–436.

4

$CD4^+CD69^+$ T cells and $CD4^+CD25^+FoxP3^+$ Treg cells imbalance in peripheral blood, spleen and peritoneal lavage from pristane-induced systemic lupus erythematosus (SLE) mice

Tatiana Vasconcelos Peixoto[1*], Solange Carrasco[1], Domingos Alexandre Ciccone Botte[1], Sergio Catanozi[2], Edwin Roger Parra[3], Thaís Martins Lima[4], Natasha Ugriumov[1], Francisco Garcia Soriano[4], Suzana Beatriz Verissímo de Mello[1], Caio Manzano Rodrigues[5] and Cláudia Goldenstein-Schainberg[6]

Abstract

Background: Adaptive immune cells, including $CD4^+CD69^+$ and $CD4^+CD25^+FoxP3^+$ regulatory T (Treg) cells, are important for maintaining immunological tolerance. In human systemic lupus erythematosus (SLE), $CD4^+CD25^+FoxP3^+$ Treg cells are reduced, whereas CD69 expression is increased, resulting in a homeostatic immune imbalance that may intensify autoreactive T cell activity. To analyze the mechanisms implicated in autotolerance failure, we evaluated $CD4^+CD69^+$ and $CD4^+CD25^+FoxP3^+$ T cells and interleukin profiles in a pristane-induced SLE experimental model.

Methods: For lupus induction, 26 female Balb/c mice received a single intraperitoneal 0.5 ml dose of pristane, and 16 mice received the same dose of saline. Blood and spleen samples were collected from euthanized mice 90 and 120 days after pristane or saline inoculation. Mononuclear cells from peripheral blood (PBMC), peritoneal lavage (PL) and splenocytes were obtained by erythrocyte lysis and cryopreserved for further evaluation by flow cytometry using the GuavaEasyCyte TM HT. After thawing, cells were washed and stained with monoclonal antibodies against CD3, CD4, CD8, CD25, CD28, CD69, FoxP3, CD14 and Ly6C (BD Pharmingen TM). Interleukins were quantified using Multiplex® MAP. The Mann-Whitney test and the Pearson coefficient were used for statistical analysis, and $p < 0.05$ considered significant.

Results: Compared with the controls, SLE-induced animals presented increased numbers of $CD4^+CD69^+$ T cells in the blood on T90 and T120 ($p = 0.022$ and $p = 0.008$) and in the spleen on T120 ($p = 0.049$), but there were decreased numbers in the PL ($p = 0.049$) on T120. The percentage of Treg was lower in blood ($p < 0.005$ and $p < 0.012$) on T90 and T120, in spleen ($p = 0.043$) on T120 and in PL ($p = 0.001$) on T90. Increased numbers of CD4 + CD69+ T cells in the PL were positively associated with high IL-2 ($p = 0.486$) and IFN-γ ($p = 0.017$) levels, whereas reduced Treg cells in the blood were negatively correlated with TNFα levels ($p = 0.043$) and positively correlated with TGFβ1 ($p = 0.038$).

Conclusion: Increased numbers of $CD4^+CD69^+$ T cells and reduced numbers of $CD4^+CD25^+FoxP3^+$ Treg cells with an altered interleukin profile suggests loss of autotolerance in pristane-induced lupus mice, which is similar to human lupus. Therefore, this model is useful in evaluating mechanisms of cellular activation, peripheral tolerance and homeostatic immune imbalance involved in human SLE.

* Correspondence: tatianavasconceloss@gmail.com
[1]Laboratório de Imunologia Celular (LIM-17) - Faculdade de Medicina FMUSP, Universidade de Sao Paulo, Sao Paulo, SP, Brazil
Full list of author information is available at the end of the article

Introduction

Systemic lupus erythematosus (SLE) is a complex multifactorial disease characterized by loss of autotolerance, autoreactive T cell activation and production of inflammatory mediators and auto-antibodies. Immune tolerance is the state of unresponsiveness of the immune system to substances or tissues that have the potential to induce an immune response and comprises central and peripheral mechanisms [1]. Central tolerance is the primary response that allows immune system to discriminate self from non-self [2] [3], and it is centered in the thymus, bone marrow and spleen; however, peripheral tolerance controls self-reactive immune cells and prevents overreactive immune responses to various environmental factors [3], and it takes place in tissues and lymph nodes after lymphocyte maturation.

The balance between adaptive immune cells such as $CD4^{+}CD69^{+}$ effector T cells and $CD4^{+}CD25^{+}FoxP3^{+}$ suppressor/regulatory T (Treg) cells is important for the maintenance of immunological tolerance [4] [5] [6]. In a normal immune response, the CD69 receptor is a protective inducible activation marker expressed on effectors T cells [7]. Because Treg cells can suppress the activation and proliferation of those effector T cells, Treg cells play a key role in the pathogenesis of inflammatory conditions [7]. If this process fails, the loss of tolerance may result in autoimmune disorders, including SLE [3]. Dysregulation of both adaptive and innate immune systems mechanisms are marked in SLE, culminating with tissue and organ damage induced by chronic inflammation and a variety of clinical manifestations [8] [9] [10].

Abnormal T cell activation and signaling problems appear to contribute to chronic disease activity in patients with SLE. Increased expression of the CD69 activation receptor [8] [11] [12] may enhance the activity of autoreactive T cells associated with disease severity [8] [6] [13] [14] [15]. Additionally, Treg cell numbers are reduced in SLE patients [16] [17] [18] and may explain the increased activity and autoreactivity of CD4 T cells [18] [19], which results in a homeostatic immune imbalance [20]. The mechanisms implicated in autotolerance failure during SLE development, maintenance and chronicity remain unknown, highlighting the importance of studies using experimental disease models [21] [22] [23]. Several genetic lupus mouse models are available, however the high cost of developing and maintaining these modified mouse lines prompts the need for studies using induced disease murine models [3], such as pristane-induced lupus mice. Pristane is a mineral oil that is injected intraperitoneally and is capable of generating clinical and laboratory abnormalities similar to those observed in human SLE, including the production of autoantibodies and inflammatory mediators and the development of arthritis [20] [24] [22, 25]. Therefore, to determine some aspects involved in immune dysregulation in murine lupus, we analyzed the expressions of $CD4^{+}CD69^{+}$ T cells and Treg cells and some interleukin profiles in pristane-induced Balb/c mice.

Materials and methods

Mice

Six-to-eight-week-old (18–22 g) female wild-type Balb/c mice were purchased from the Centro Multidisciplinar para Investigação Biológica – CEMIB/UNICAMP (Campinas, Brazil) and housed in the animal facility of the Rheumatology Division of the University of São Paulo School of Medicine (São Paulo, Brazil). All animal protocols were approved by the Institutional Animal Care and Research Advisory Committee (CAPPesq HC-USP Protocol # 009/11 - Comissão de Ética para Análise de Projetos de Pesquisa do Hospital das Clínicas da Faculdade de Medicina da USP) and were strictly conducted according to the U.S. National Institutes of Health (NIH) Guide for the Care and Use of Laboratory Animals. Mice were maintained in a conventional animal facility at 22 ± 2 °C with a 12-h light/dark cycle and fed a pelleted commercial chow ad libitum (Nuvilab CR1, São Paulo, Brazil) with free access to drinking water.

SLE induction by pristane in Balb/c mice

Twenty-six mice received a single intraperitoneal (i.p.) injection of 0.5 ml pristane (2,6,10,14 tetramethylpentadecane, Sigma Chemical Co., St. Louis, MO, USA) for SLE induction. Before injection, pristane was filtered through a 0.22-µm filter (Millipore, Billerica, MA, USA). Sixteen control mice received i.p. injections of 0.5 ml 0.9% saline. At 90 and 120 days following SLE induction (T90, T120), 13 SLE-induced animals and 8 controls were euthanized with CO_2 to obtain peripheral blood, spleen and PL samples. The time points of 90 and 120 days were chosen for euthanasia and experimental procedures based on previous reports that described autoantibody production observed after 2 weeks [20] [22] [26] [27] [28] [29] and the development of arthritis 3 months [24] [30] [28] [31] after pristane induction, indicating the beginning of the inflammatory SLE process. In addition, we conducted a pilot experiment in which these periods were shown to be the most important for assessing the beginning and perpetuation of the lupus inflammatory processes, such as autoantibody production, arthritis development, cellular imbalance and inflammatory mediator alterations [32].

SLE induced in Balb/c mice

A) Clinical characteristics: lipogranulomas, splenomegaly and arthritis in front and back paws were evaluated by visualization. The presence and severity of arthritis was graded visually using the scoring system described by Patten (2004) [31].

B) Histopathological features: the spleens of all SLE-induced and control mice were removed, fixed in paraformaldehyde (4%), and embedded in paraffin; 5-μm spleen sections were then stained with H&E. Histopathological features were examined by an independent and experienced pathologist blinded to the study protocol using Panoramic Viewer software (3DHistech, Budapest, Hungary).

C) Plasma and peritoneal lavage evaluation: antinuclear Abs (ANAs) were detected by indirect immunofluorescence using Hep2 cell slides (NOVA Lite™ IFA) with 1:40 diluted plasma and peritoneal lavage, followed by staining with FITC antibody anti-.

IgG-conjugated at a dilution of 1:50 (Southern Biotechnology, Birmingham, AL). Anti-dsDNA, anti-Sm and anti-RNP Abs were measured by ELISA (1:250 dillution of plasma and peritoneal lavage) according to the manufacturer's instructions (ALPHA DIAGNOSTICS and eBioscience). Levels of interleukin (IL)-1, IL-2, IL-10, interferon I (IFN-I) and transforming growth factor (TGF) $_{\beta 1}$, $TGF_{\beta 2}$ and $TGF_{\beta 3}$ were quantified using Multiplex® MAP (multi-analyte panels) according to the manufacturer's instructions (Luminex® Technology, Millipore, Minneapolis, NM, USA) and using Analyst Milliplex software (Millipore).

D) Total and differential leucocyte counts: total peripheral leukocytes in the blood, spleen and peritoneal lavage (PL) were counted in a Neubauer chamber using blue methylene (1:1), and the differential counts of polymorphonuclear cells (PMNs), monocytes and lymphocytes were realized by smears of blood, spleen and PL.

Obtaining peripheral blood mononuclear cells (PBMCs) and blood plasma

Peripheral blood (200 μl) was collected from the caudal veins of all animals 90 days after induction of SLE. The samples were centrifuged (1200 rpm for 10 min at 4 °C) for plasma separation and frozen (− 80 °C) until further laboratory analyses. Red blood cells (RBC) were then lysed in whole blood by incubating the samples in FACS™ Lysing Solution (Becton Dickinson). The cell solution was centrifuged and washed several times and resuspended in RPMI (*Roswell Park Memorial Institute*) medium 1640. PBMCs obtained from the pellet were cryopreserved with DMSO (dimethyl sulfoxide) and fetal bovine serum (FBS) (1:4) and frozen in liquid nitrogen for at most 2 weeks until flow cytometry experiments.

Obtaining peritoneal lavage mononuclear cells (PLMCs) and peritoneal lavage supernatants

Cell suspensions were collected from the peritoneal cavities of all euthanized mice after local asepsis with 70% ethanol, inoculation with 2 ml RPMI medium 1640 and abdominal incision. PLMCs obtained were centrifuged to separate supernatants, washed with RPMI medium 1640, and cryopreserved in DMSO and FBS until flow cytometry experiments.

Extracting the spleen and obtaining splenocytes

Spleens were removed, weighed for evaluation of splenomegaly, chopped with a sterile scalpel and crushed in a mortar with a sterile pestle using a fine mesh metal sieve in a petri plate with RPMI medium 1640. The cell suspension was transferred to a Falcon tube and allowed to stand for approximately 2 min to allow precipitation of larger tissue blocks. The supernatant was transferred to another Falcon tube and centrifuged (800 g for 10 min at 4 °C). The pellet containing splenocytes were washed twice with RPMI medium 1640 and cryopreserved with DMSO and FBS for at most 2 weeks until further evaluation by flow cytometry.

Flow cytometry

To perform the flow cytometry experiments, PBMCs, splenocytes and PLMCs were unfrozen, resuspended with RPMI medium 1640 at room temperature, washed and centrifuged (1500 rpm for 10 min at 4 °C) twice and resuspended with PBS and FBS. All samples were stained for one hour in the dark at 4–8 °C with a variety of anti-mouse monoclonal Abs (BD Biosciences): CD3; CD4; CD8; CD25; CD28; CD69; FoxP3; CD14; and-Ly6C. Cells were permeabilized with permeabilization buffer (Biolegend) at a dilution of 1:10 to stain for intracellular Foxp3.

After incubation with each of above monoclonal Abs, the samples were centrifuged and washed with PBS and then fixed in 4% paraformaldehyde. Flow cytometry analysis was conducted using a Guava EasyCyteTM HT (Millipore), and analyses was conducted with InCyte software (Millipore).

Statistical analysis

Data are expressed as the mean ± SD of percentages of positive cells to monoclonal antibodies tested. The chi-square test was used in qualitative analyses, and the Mann-Whitney test was used to analyze quantitative differences between both SLE-induced and control groups. The Pearson coefficient was used to evaluate correlation. *P* values ≤0.05 were considered statistically significant.

Results

SLE-induced experimental model

a) **Clinical characteristics (Fig. 1).** All 26 SLE-induced mice presented lupus clinical alterations compared to controls (A, D and F) on both T90 and T120 evaluations. SLE-induced animals were heavier than controls on T90 (28 g ± 2 vs. 26 g ± 2, $p < 0.001$) and on T120 (29 g ± 3 vs. 27 g ± 2, $p < 0.001$). Lipogranulomas (B and C) and splenomegaly (E) developed in the peritoneal cavity, and greater

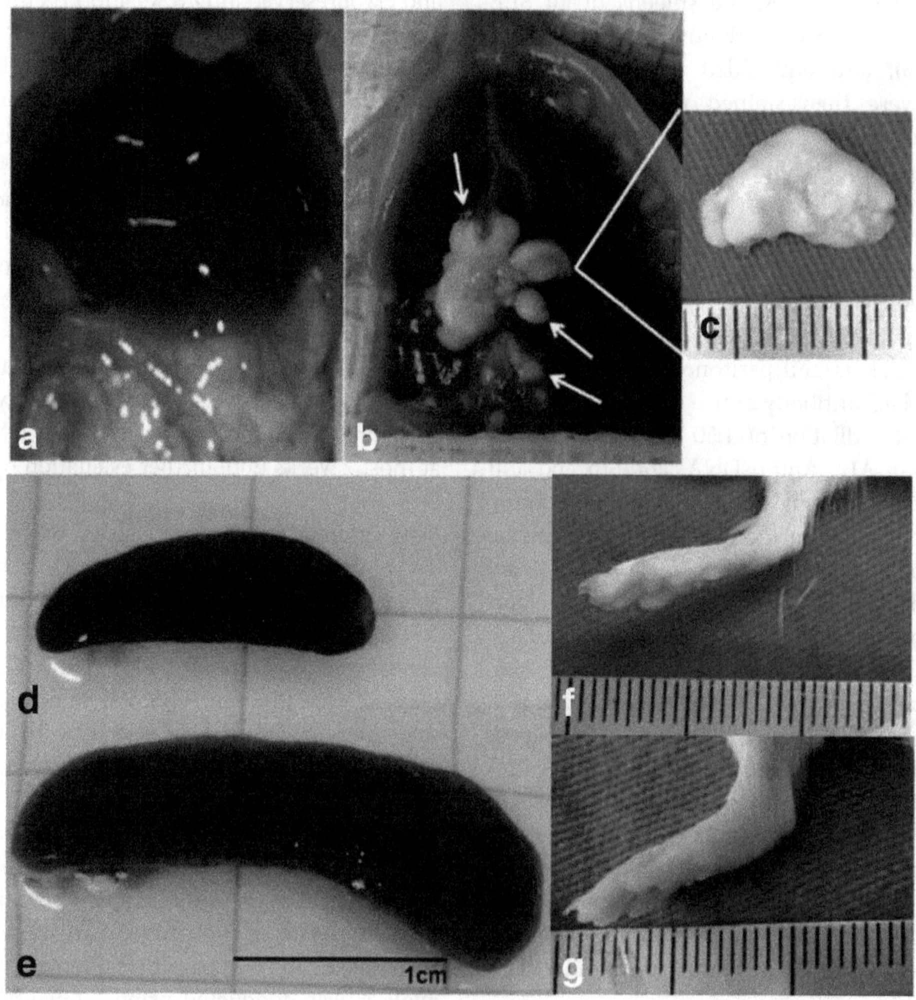

Fig. 1 Peritoneal cavity of a control animal (**a**) and of a SLE induced animal (**b**) with lipogranulomas on liver and spleen surface (arrows). Lipogranuloma's detail in (**c**). Spleen of control (**d**) and SLE induced mice (**e**) showing splenomegaly. Later members of normal (**f**) and of SLE induced animal (**g**) showing joints affect by arthritis.

spleen weights were demonstrated in the SLE-induced mice compared to controls (0.25 g ± 0.07 vs. 0.12 g ± 0.03, $p < 0.001$ on T90 and 0.11 g ± 0.01 vs. 0.30 g ± 0.04, $p < 0.001$ on T120). Arthritis was observed in 7 of 13 mice on T90 (53%, score of 0.9 ± 0.9) and in all 13 mice on T120 (100%, score of 1.8 ± 0.6), whereas no control mice had this manifestation.

b) Histological characteristics. Fig. 2 shows spleens from control group animals with preserved capsules of dense connective tissue and splenic parenchyma consisting of red and white pulp with preserved architecture (A and B). On the other hand, spleens from SLE-induced animals showed rarefaction of the white pulp and loss of lymph node architecture (C and D, arrow), randomly distributed deposits of greasy material (Fig. 1 D, tip of arrow), and increased inflammatory cells, primarily neutrophils, suggesting a greater inflammatory process in this organ. These alterations were intensified on T120 (Fig. 1 D, tip of arrow).

Plasma and peritoneal lavage characteristics of the SLE-induced experimental model

a) Antinuclear (ANA), anti-dsDNA, anti-Sm and anti-RNP autoantibodies. Prior to SLE induction, ANA, anti-dsDNA, anti-RNP and anti-Sm autoantibodies were negative in plasma and PL from all 42 animals. Following induction, control mice remained negative for these autoantibodies, whereas 13 SLE-induced mice presented at least one autoantibody: 9 ANA (69%), 5 anti-dsDNA (38%), 4 anti-Sm (31%) and 4 (31%) anti-RNP in plasma and 6 (46%), 9 (69%), 3 (23%) and 4 (31%) were positive for the same antibodies in the PL on T90; 11 (85%), 7 (54%), 3 (23%) and 5 (38%) mice had ANA, anti-dsDNA, anti-Sm and anti-RNP antibodies in plasma and 6 (46%), 8 (62%), 7 (54%) and 2 (15%) were positive for the same antibodies in the PL on T120. Interestingly, all 4 autoantibody negative SLE-induced mice on T90 also had no signs of arthritis but showed large percentages of $CD4^{+}CD69^{+}$ T cells, mainly in the blood and PL. In

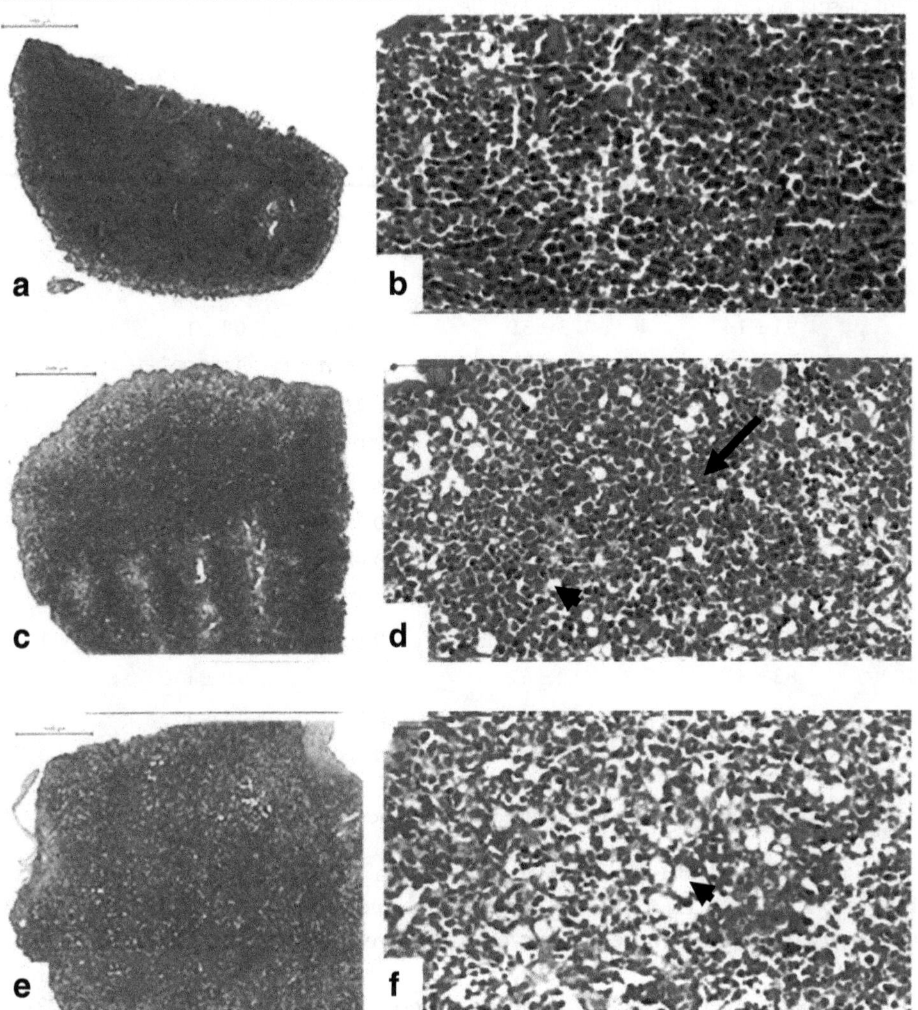

Fig. 2 Panoramic histological cut of spleen from control group animal and SLE induced animal. **a**) Spleen of control animal showing preserved capsule of dense connective tissue and septa dividing the interior tissue of the organ in lobules interconnected. **b**) splenic parenchyma consisting of red pulp rich in sinusoids capillaries and splenic tissue cords constituted by macrophages, plasma cells, reticular cells and blood cells within the standards of normality. It is observed still rare megakaryocytes cells. The white pulp is constituted by lymphatic nodes characterized by lymphocyte cells arranged around the arterial branches with preserved architecture. **c**) Spleen of a SLE induced animal revealing rarefaction of white pulp characterized by loss of architecture of lymphatic nodes (**d**, arrow) which is characterized by replacement of lymphatic nodes by deposits of greasy material distributed diffusely (tips of arrows). These alterations are intensified on T120 (**e** and **f**, tips of arrows) Original magnification X2 and X40.

contrast, on T120, although 2 SLE-induced animals were ANA negative, they had signs of arthritis and increased percentage of $CD4^{+}CD69^{+}$ T cells in blood and spleen, but not in the PL.

b) Interleukins (Table 1). The production of plasma TNFα (12.3 ± 3.9 vs. 9.1 ± 1.4, $p < 0.048$, T90 10.2 ± 6.2 vs. 6.0 ± 2.2, $p < 0.001$, T120); $TGF_{\beta1}$ (2780.0 ± 1050.0 vs. 1255.0 ± 821.4, $p < 0.010$, T90); and $TGF_{\beta2}$ (79.3 ± 28.6 vs. 38.7 ± 31.9, $p < 0.027$, T90, and 169.6 ± 68.0 vs. 125.8 ± 64.9, $p = 0.031$, T120) was higher in SLE-induced animals compared to controls. In contrast, SLE-induced and control animals had similar IL-2, IL-10 and IFN-γ levels. In the PL, a similar interleukin profile was observed on T90. However, on T120, SLE-induced animals had higher $TGF_{\beta1}$ (525.0 ± 110.3 vs. 318.1 ± 223.6, $p = 0.039$) and lower IL-2 and IL-10 secretions (0.4 ± 0.3 vs. 2.1 ± 1.8, $p = 0.007$ and 0.9 ± 0.6 vs. 7.8 ± 10.0, $p = 0.007$, respectively) compared to controls.

Cellular characteristics of the SLE-induced experimental model

a) Quantification of polymorphonuclear, monocytes and lymphocytes in blood, spleen and peritoneal lavage. The peritoneal blood from SLE-induced mice had higher PMN numbers on T90 and T120 (14.7 ± 15.2 vs. 4.3 ± 3.2, $p = 0.049$; 7.5 ± 3.6 vs. 2.8 ± 1.8, $p = 0.002$) and fewer lymphocytes on T120 (13.5 ± 7.6 vs. 33.53 ± 14.2, $p = 0.003$) compared to controls, whereas the number of monocytes and total leucocytes were similar in both groups. In the spleen, SLE-induced animals had more

Table 1 Data represent plasma and PL levels (mean ± standard deviation) of interleukins in SLE induced and control mice on both periods T90 and T120

Interleukins	Periods (days)	Blood			PL		
		Control $n = 8$	SLE-induced $n = 13$	p	Control n = 8	SLE-induced n = 13	p
IL-1	T90	74.6 ± 136.6	45.4 ± 20.7	0.289	5.7 ± 9.9	71.9 ± 45.6	0.114
	T120	223.4 ± 154.0	236.1 ± 239.5	1.000	8.9 ± 8.8	2.3 ± 2.2	0.450
IL-2	T90	3.3 ± 1.2	2.9 ± 1.4	0.616	0.9 ± 0.4	2.5 ± 0.9	0.057
	T120	7.5 ± 9.2	3.2 ± 1.9	0.817	2.1 ± 1.8	0.4 ± 0.3	**0.007**
TNFa	T90	9.1 ± 1.4	12.3 ± 3.9	**< 0.048**	0.8 ± 1.2	18.4 ± 11.8	0.057
	T120	6.0 ± 2.2	10.2 ± 6.2	**< 0.001**	3.1 ± 6.2	2.4 ± 3.2	0.314
$TGF_{\beta 1}$	T90	1255.0 ± 821.4	2780.0 ± 1050.0	**< 0.010**	759.3 ± 1186.0	516.3 ± 337.8	1.000
	T120	4514.0 ± 2653.0	5498.0 ± 2184.0	0.415	318.1 ± 223.6	525.0 ± 110.3	**0.039**
$TGF_{\beta 2}$	T90	38.7 ± 31.9	79.3 ± 28.6	**< 0.027**	376.3 ± 205.4	204.3 ± 102.1	0.228
	T120	125.8 ± 64.9	169.6 ± 68.0	**0.031**	294.4 ± 171.1	258.2 ± 98.1	0.451
TGFβ3	T90	6.4 ± 2.0	7.1 ± 1.5	0.404	16.3 ± 3.8	13.0 ± 6.2	0.400
	T120	6.9 ± 0.7	8.0 ± 2.4	0.400	16.7 ± 5.2	13.7 ± 5.9	0.291
IL-10	T90	10.7 ± 5.3	17.6 ± 25.9	0.923	3.7 ± 5.7	17.3 ± 10.6	0.114
	T120	8.3 ± 4.1	11.2 ± 6.2	0.379	7.8 ± 10.0	0.9 ± 0.6	**0.007**
IFNg	T90	3.7 ± 1.0	3.0 ± 1.1	0.245	1.1 ± 1.1	3.4 ± 2.6	0.229
	T120	85.8 ± 163.5	3.3 ± 3.3	0.239	1.3 ± 1.1	0.3 ± 0.1	0.119

$p < 0.05$ are set in bold
IL = interleukin; *IFN* = interferon; *TNF* = tumor necrosis factor; *TGF* = transforming growth factor

total leucocytes (76.7 ± 36.4 vs. 43.3 ± 20.5, $p = 0.048$, T90), more PMNs (8.3 ± 8.0 vs. 1.9 ± 2.6, $p = 0.009$; 11.6 ± 6.4 vs. 1.0 ± 0.8, $p < 0.001$) and more monocytes (126.2 ± 448.8 vs. 0.3 ± 0.5, $p = 0.036$; 4.2 ± 3.0 vs. 0.3 ± 0.8, $p = 0.001$) in both periods, T90 and T120, respectively, than control animals, and the numbers of lymphocytes were similar in both groups. In turn, SLE-induced animals had more PMNs (8.6 ± 7.2 vs. 0.8 ± 1.4, $p = 0.003$; 3.2 ± 2.4 vs. 0.5 ± 0.4, $p = 0.001$) and more monocytes (1.5 ± 1.5 vs. 0.4 ± 0.4, $p = 0.019$, T90) in the PL compared to controls.

Flow cytometry

a) Monocytes $CD14^+Ly6C^{high}$. The expression of $CD14^+Ly6C^{high}$ on monocytes from SLE-induced mice was significantly higher in both periods, T90 and T120, respectively, in the blood (7.8 ± 3.4 vs. 4.0 ± 1.9, $p = 0.031$; 12.1 ± 3.0 vs. 8.1 ± 1.7, $p = 0.001$) and in the PL (26.7 ± 12.2 vs. 9.0 ± 1.5, $p = 0.031$; 5,4 ± 2.3 vs. 13.1 ± 6.5, $p < 0.005$) compared to controls, but it was similar in the spleen (8.0 ± 4.3 vs. 8.8 ± 2.7, $p = 0.203$; 7.8 ± 8.0 vs. 17.7 ± 12.6, $p = 0.068$). There was a positive correlation between PL monocytes $CD14^+Ly6C^{high}$ and the proinflammatory cytokines IFN-γ ($p < 0.0001$), TNFα ($p = 0.010$) and IL-1 ($p < 0.0001$) as shown in Fig. 3.

b) $CD4^+$ T cells and $CD8^+$ T cells. The expression of $CD4^+$ T cells was similar in the blood (80.7 ± 4.6 vs. 83.9 ± 1.6, $p = 0.933$), PL (89.6 ± 2.3 vs. 85.0 ± 2.5, $p = 0.324$) and spleen (89.6 ± 2.3 vs. 91.0 ± 2.7, $p = 0.511$) between SLE-induced and control animals. The same trend was observed with respect to $CD8^+$ T cells, which had similar expression levels in both groups: 12.7 ± 3.9 vs. 11.2 ± 3.8 ($p = 0.412$) in blood, 1.8 ± 1.5 vs. 1.6 ± 1.0 ($p = 0.373$) in PL and 2.9 ± 1.1 vs. 3.7 ± 2.0 ($p = 0.968$) in spleen.

c) $CD69^+$ expression on $CD4^+$ T cells (Fig. 4). At T90, SLE-induced animals had higher expression of $CD4^+CD69^+$ T cells in the blood (16.4 ± 8.3 vs. 7.0 ± 2.6 $p < 0.022$) compared to controls, whereas in both the spleen and PL, the expression levels of these cells were similar (22.6 ± 10.9 vs. 15.1 ± 4.3, $p > 0.05$ and 18.0 ± 11.4 vs. 18.3 ± 5.0, $p > 0.05$, respectively). However, 120 days after SLE induction, the expression of $CD4^+CD69^+$ T cells was higher in the blood (18.3 ± 6.9 vs. 10.1 ± 2.7, $p = 0.008$) and spleen (23.8 ± 6.3 vs. 19.0 ± 4.9, $p = 0.049$) but lower in the PL (8.2 ± 3.9 vs. 15.0 ± 5.0, $p = 0.001$) compared to controls. Increased percentages of $CD4^+CD69^+$ T cells in the PL were positively associated with higher levels of IL-2 ($p = 0.486$) and IFN-γ ($p = 0.017$).

d) Coexpression of $CD28^+$ and $CD69^+$ on $CD4^+$ T cells. At T90, SLE-induced animals had increased coexpression of $CD28^+$ and $CD69^+$ on $CD4^+$ T cells in blood (9.7 ± 4.5 vs. 3.5 ± 3.8, $p < 0.05$) compared to control animals, although expression was similar in the PL (13.2 ± 6.6 vs. 12.6 ± 3.1, $p > 0.999$) and in the spleen (9.0 ± 6.3 vs. 4.1 ± 0.8, $p = 0.405$). At T120, $CD28^+$ and $CD69^+$ coexpression remained enhanced in the blood

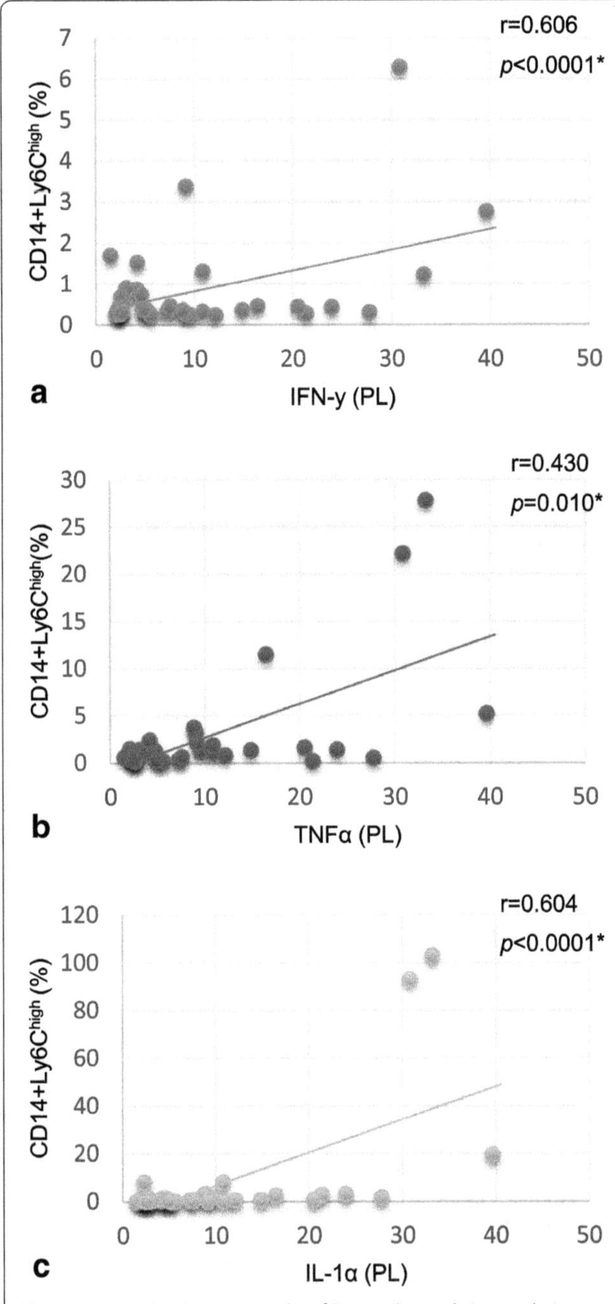

Fig. 3 Scatter plot showing results of Pearson's correlation analysis. Positive correlation between CD14+Ly6Chigh monocytes in PL of SLE-induced animals and (**a**) IFN-y ($r=0.606$, $p<0.0001$), (**b**) TNF-α ($r=0.430$, $p=0.001$) and (**c**) IL-1α ($r=0.604$, $p=0.0001$). *$p=0.005$.

(9.2 ± 5.9 vs. 3.8 ± 1.9, $p = 0.020$), whereas in the PL, it was significantly reduced (6.9 ± 2.9 vs. 11.9 ± 5.6, $p = 0.031$).

e) Expression of CD4^{+}CD25^{+}FoxP3^{+} Treg cells. Figs. 5 demonstrates that the expression of CD4^{+}CD25^{+}FoxP3^{+} Treg cells was lower in SLE-induced mice compared to controls in blood at T90 and T120, respectively (2.6 ± 1.8 vs. 5.1 ± 2.4, $p < 0.005$, 3.5 ± 1.2 vs. 5.7 ± 1.8, $p = 0.012$), but in the PL, this same trend occurred only at T90 (3.2 ± 3.0 vs. 7.0 ± 4.3, $p = 0.001$). At T120, these cells were also increased in the spleen (2.6 ± 1.5 vs. 4.6 ± 0.7, $p = 0.018$). In addition, in the blood, Treg cells were negatively correlated with TNFα production ($p = 0.043$) and positively correlated with $TGF_{\beta1}$ levels ($p = 0.038$).

Discussion

This study shows for the first time, that in pristane-induced SLE Balb/c mice, there is an imbalance of CD4^{+}CD69^{+} T cell and CD4^{+}CD25^{+}FoxP3^{+} Treg expressions in blood, spleen and PL. This alteration might be involved in the breakdown of immune autotolerance contributing to lupus development and chronicity.

All of our SLE-induced mice developed lupus clinical characteristics with great amounts of lipogranulomas in the peritoneal cavity, especially in the diaphragm and the surfaces of the liver and spleen; they also developed splenomegaly and arthritis similar to previous studies in this model performed by Utbonaviciute et al. (2013), Bossaller et al. (2013) and Leiss et al. (2013) [33] [33] [34] [35] [33] [30] [36]. Spleen histomorphology changes, such as hyperplasia of the red pulp and reduction of the white pulp, increased infiltration of inflammatory cells (especially neutrophils), and random oil deposits were observed in all SLE-induced animals as described in the studies by Leiss et al. (2013) [30] and Zhuand et al. (2014) [37]. Likewise, in human SLE [38], atrophic changes with lower volume and numbers of splenic corpuscles (lymphatic nodes or follicles) were also evidenced. These histological findings suggest that pristane-induced murine SLE model is more similar to human SLE than other commonly used models of this disease such as B/WF1 mice, in which only slight inflammatory cell infiltration [39] is observed.

Previous reports have detected ANAs in the pristane SLE model following the first two weeks after induction [40] [30] [29] [36] [35]. We also found ANAs in plasma and/or in PL from most of our SLE-induced mice. Interestingly, at T90, 4 SLE-induced (30%) mice were ANA negative and had no signs of arthritis but had higher percentages of CD4^{+}CD69^{+} T cells in the blood and PL, suggesting the beginning of the inflammatory process. Remarkably, at T120, only 2 SLE-induced animals (15%) were ANA negative and had arthritis and increased percentages of CD4^{+}CD69^{+} T cells in the blood and spleen although not in PL, suggesting a possible migration of these activated inflammatory cells from the LP to other sites such as the blood and spleen. These data may indicate that by T90, the inflammatory process is in the very early stages when sufficient apoptotic cells are not yet present to trigger ANA production. Hence, we have demonstrated that, according to the postinduction period evaluated, different cellular and clinical alterations were observed during disease development and progression.

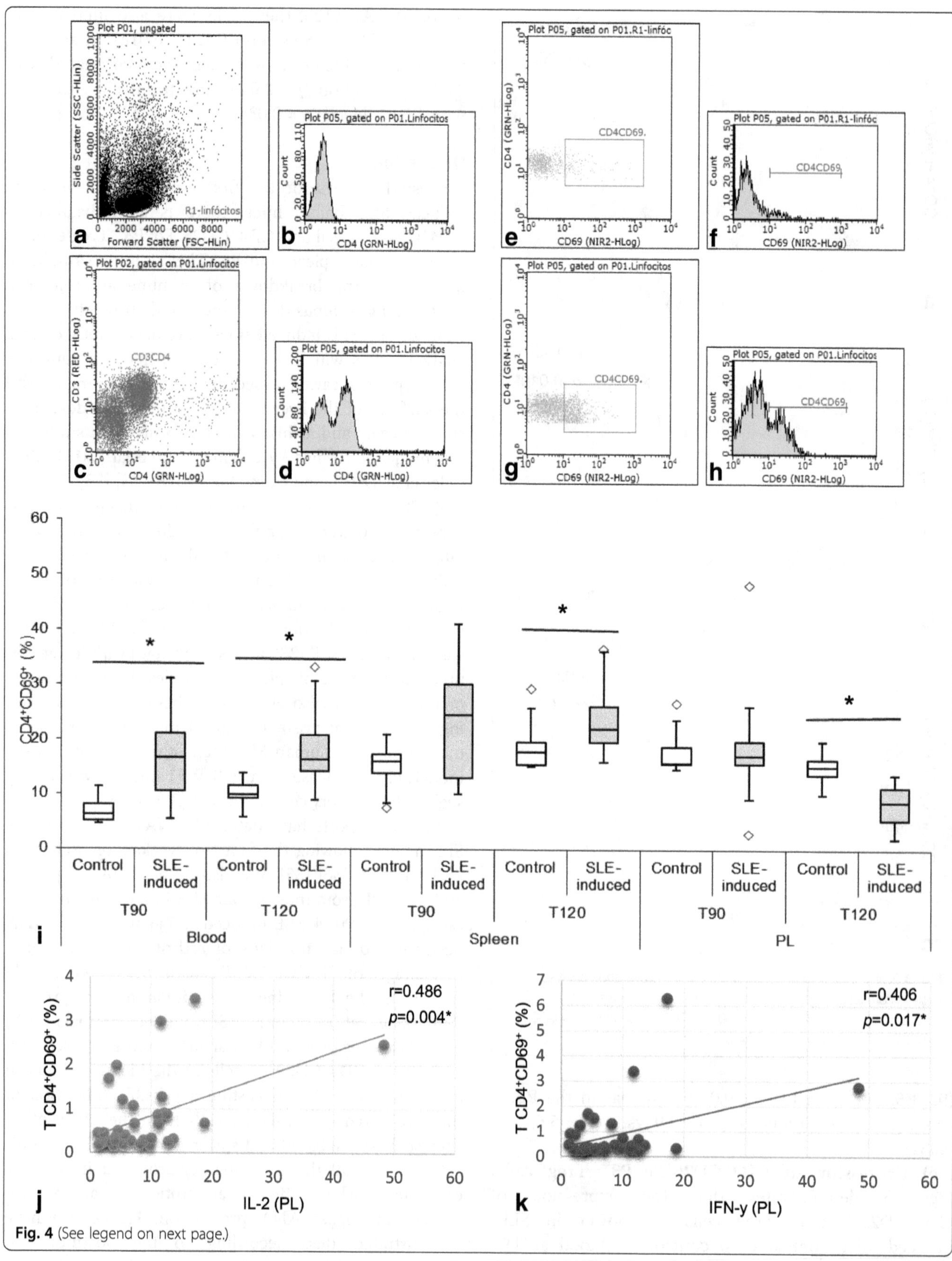

Fig. 4 (See legend on next page.)

(See figure on previous page.)

Fig. 4 Dot-plot and histograms of lymphocytes separated by size and granularity (**a** and **b**) and the subpopulation of CD4 T cells (**c** and **d**) which express CD69, highlighted in the central quadrant, from a control (**e** and **f**) and a SLE induced animal (**g** e **h**). **i**: Expression of CD69 in CD4+ T cells in blood, spleen and PL of SLE induced animals (dark bars) and controls (light bars) on D90 and D120. Results expressed as mean ± SD. Mann-Whitney Test, *p=0.005. Scatter plot showing results of Pearson's correlation analysis. Positive correlation between CD4+CD69+ T cells in PL of SLE-induced animals and (**j**) IL-2 (r=0.606, p<0.0001) and (**k**) IFN-γ (r=0.604, p=0.0001). *p=0.005.

Interestingly, the interleukin profile was different between the two groups of induced and controlled animals. In fact, we have shown increased TNFα, $TGF_{\beta1}$ and $TGF_{\beta2}$ levels in plasma from SLE-induced animals while IL-1, IL-2, IL-10, $TGF_{\beta3}$ and IFN-γ levels were similar in both induced and control animals. In contrast, in PL, IL-2 e IL-10 levels were reduced and $TGF_{\beta1}$ was increased 120 days after induction, while IL-1, TNFα, $TGF_{\beta1}$, $TGF_{\beta2}$ e IFN-γ were similar on both groups. Therefore, SLE-induced animals had increased production of pro inflammatory plasmatic TNFα. In human SLE, TNFα is increased in plasma [41] and influences the regulation of INF-γ production [42] involved in inflammation and in apoptosis [43]. Despite increased TNFα in our SLE-induced mice, INF-γ production was not altered, similar to the study by Mizutani et al. (2015) [22]. However, Xu et al. (2015) noted increased INF-γ only 6 months after pristane SLE induction that returned to basal levels after this period [42]. In humans and B/WF1 mice, IL-2 is reduced [44] and IL-10 is usually increased [45] [46] [47]. Lower production of IL-2 in human SLE suggests diminished T helper cell function and an imbalance in Th1 and Th2 cells [48], whereas IL-10 may be related to B cell proliferation and apoptosis [49] and is linked to disease severity [50]. Interestingly, similar levels of plasma IL-2 and IL-10 were detected in our SLE-induced animals compared to controls; in contrast, in the PL, both cytokines were reduced on T120 suggesting that the inflammatory process is not maintained in the peritoneal cavity. $TGF_{\beta1}$ and $TGF_{\beta3}$ have important roles in controlling cytotoxic T cell proliferation and differentiation [51]. In human SLE, they down regulate chronic lymphocyte hyper responsiveness, despite decreased production [52]. In our SLE-induced animals, the production of plasma $TGF_{\beta1}$ and $TGF_{\beta3}$ was significantly higher, suggesting an attempt to regulate immune homeostasis during the inflammatory process; in fact, TGF_{β} can inhibit the proliferation of naive but not activated T cells [53] and therefore promotes high plasmocytic activity [51].

White cell count was higher in the spleens from SLE-induced animals at T90, suggesting more pronounced inflammatory activity during this period. CPMN number was higher in the blood, spleen and PL of SLE-induced mice at T90 and T120, and monocyte numbers were increased in the spleen (T90 and T120) and PL (T90). On the other hand, lymphocyte numbers were higher only in the blood (T120) and similar in the spleen and PL between both groups. The presence of pristane in the peritoneal cavity months after inoculation could cause lymphocyte and dendritic cell apoptosis, as evaluated by Calvani et al. (2005) [26], and explain the increase in CPMN and monocytes, which are professional phagocytes.

Increased numbers of activated $CD14^{+}Ly6C^{high}$ monocytes were observed in the blood and PL from SLE-induced mice on T90 and T120, suggesting a possible role of these cells in the beginning and perpetuation of the inflammatory process observed in this model. In a similar way, Lee et al. (2008b) [54] and Bossaller et al. (2013) [33] also observed increases in these cells two weeks after induction accompanied by high expression of INF-I [54]. Furthermore, in the PL, there was a positive correlation between high numbers of $CD14^{+}Ly6C^{high}$ monocytes and the production of IFN-γ, TNFα and IL-1. In fact, monocytes play a fundamental role in the production of proinflammatory cytokines present in the peritoneal cavity and plasma from SLE-induced mice [54]. IFN-γ and TNFα [28] contribute to the great influx of CD4 T cells towards the peritoneal cavity in the first months after induction [55], whereas IL-1 has been considered a biomarker of disease activity or organ involvement in humans [56] [57].

The percentages of CD4 and CD8 T cells from SLE-induced and control animals were similar in all sites evaluated. In human lupus, a variety of changes in CD4 and CD8 numbers and proportions have been described [6] [7] [15] [11] [12], but the role of these cells in the development and maintenance of disease activity is still controversial.

SLE-induced mice had increased activated $CD4^{+}CD69^{+}$ T cells similar to human SLE [17] [18] [7], suggesting peripheral auto tolerance breakdown [58] [59] [60] [7]; this alteration may be even greater in patients with active disease [58] [60] [7]. We have also shown increased activated CD4 T cells expressing CD69 in the spleen only 120 days after induction possibly due to migration of immune cells from LP to other regions and consequent increases in inflammatory infiltrates in the spleen. In contrast, in B/WF1 mice, $CD4^{+}CD69^{+}$ T cells are increased in the spleen [13] [61] [20] [22] [62] [63] and lymph nodes but not in the peripheral blood, indicating continuous activation of CD4 T cells in lymphoid organs [6] [13] [20] [22]. In MRL animals as well, $CD4^{+}CD69^{+}$ T cell expression in the blood and peripheral lymphoid organs are similar to those of normal Balb/c [64]. Therefore, the behavior of $CD4^{+}CD69^{+}$ T cell expression in our pristane induced

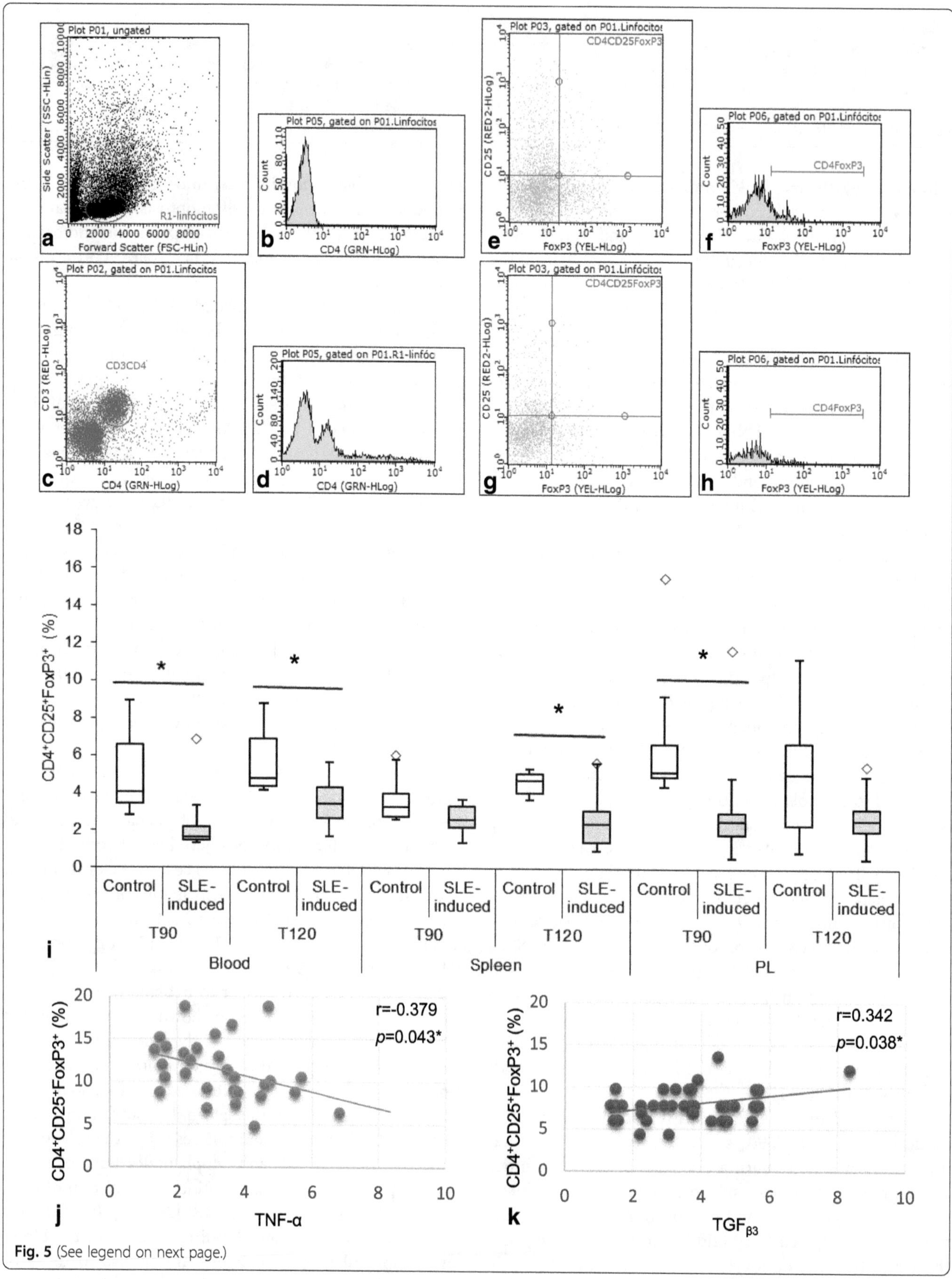

Fig. 5 (See legend on next page.)

(See figure on previous page.)

Fig. 5 Dot-plot and histograms of lymphocytes separated by size and granularity (**a** and **b**) and the subpopulation of CD4 T cells (**c** and **d**) which expresses CD25 and FoxP3, highlighted in the larger quadrant, of a control (**e** and **f**) and a SLE induced animal (**g** and **h**). **i**: Expression of Treg CD4+CD25+FoxP3+ cells in blood (**a**). spleen (**b**) and PL (**c**) from SLE induced animals (dark bars) and controls (light bars) on T90 and T120. The results are expressed by mean ± SD. Mann-Whitney Test. *$p<0.005$. Scatter plot showing results of Pearson's correlation analysis. Positive correlation between Treg cells in blood of SLE-induced animals and (**j**) TNF-α (r=0.379, $p<0.043$) and (**k**) TGFβ3 (r=0.342, $p=0.038$). *$p=0.005$.

mice is similar to human disease in contrast to B/WF1 and MRL mice models, indicating that our model may be a better experimental murine model for the study of inflammatory process involved in lupus. Remarkably, in the PL from our mouse model, the increase in $CD4^+CD69^+$ T cells was directly correlated with high IL-2 and IFN-γ levels. This reinforces the concept that IL-2, which is primarily produced by T cells, can exert stimulatory effects on immune responses by expanding effector T cells populations [65] and thus promoting positive feedback in this model. Interestingly, $CD4^+CD69^+$ T cells [13] and IFN-γ levels were strongly associated with disease activity [13] [66]; in fact, IFN-γ was recently described as a potential biomarker in human SLE [66]. In contrast, there was no correlation between $CD4^+CD69^+$ T cells and IL-10 levels, and actually, a pathogenic role for IL-10 in human SLE remains controversial. Even though IL-10 is mainly produced by Treg cells and acts as a regulator of the immune response, paradoxically, it also improves B cells proliferation and Ig class switching, thus increasing antibody secretion [67].

We further demonstrated that SLE-induced animals had increased CD4 T cells coexpressing CD69 and CD28, suggesting amplified proliferation of activated CD4 T cells. Yang et al. (2008) proposed that CD69 is necessary but not sufficient for activation of CD4 T cells [68]. The stimulation of CD28, continuously expressed in CD4 T cells [69], in the presence of CD69 intensively increases the proliferation of CD4 T cells [26], as well as the production and secretion of IL-2 [70]. The reduction in CD4 + CD25 + FoxP3+ Treg cells in peripheral blood from our pristane SLE-induced animals suggests the loss of peripheral autotolerance and a homeostatic immune imbalance [71] [34] [10]. This alteration was also observed in the spleen (T120) and PL (T90), suggesting that Treg cells play an important role in the development of autoimmunity in this model. Moreover, the initial reduction of Treg cells in LP and in spleen suggests that the inflammatory process may starts in the peritoneum and is followed by Treg cell migration to inflammatory sites such as joins, kidneys and lungs [24] [32] [72]. Therefore, the current study cannot completely rule out possible causes of the differences in cell numbers found in PL and spleen which may result from a variety of possibilities such as cell migration, destruction, impaired production, etc. In fact, we have previously shown that pristane induced lupus animals exhibited increased mesangial cell proliferation in glomerulus, increased IgG levels and proteinuria [24], reproducing lupus nephritis. Moreover, Kluger (2016) observed multipotent Treg cells expressing FoxP3 with proinflammatory properties in the peritoneum of SLE-induced mice 3 weeks after induction, indicating the participation of these cells at the beginning of lipogranuloma formation [35]. Similarly, in lupus patients, the number of $CD4^+CD25^+FoxP3^+$ peripheral Treg cells is also reduced, showing dysregulation of peripheral tolerance [73] [19] [74] [40] [60] [10]. In addition, some studies have revealed that the reduction in these cells may be inversely correlated with disease activity, although correlation with SLEDAI was not significant [18]. In the B/WF1 murine model, the percentage of $CD4^+CD25^+FoxP3^+$ Treg cells in peripheral blood, spleen and lymph nodes [73] [68] [20] [39] [62] is reduced with time compared to Balb/c [68] [27]. In MRL mice, the expression of Treg cells in the blood and peripheral lymphoid organs is similar to that in Balb/c [64] and its suppressive capacity is normal. Interestingly, in our model, the percentage of Treg cells in the blood was negatively correlated with TNFα and positively correlated with $TGF_{β1}$; no correlation between Treg cells and IL-2 and IL-10 was observed. Thus, higher titers of TNFα [57] may play an important role in SLE development and could be responsible for an increased proinflammatory response especially in active disease [57] [75]. $TGF_{β1}$ promotes the development of peripheral Treg cells, and curiously, IL-2, produced by activated T cells [72], may regulate Treg proliferation that contributes to homeostasis and maintenance of Treg suppressive capacity [65], which suggests a negative feedback. While IL-2 is generally considered to promote T-cell proliferation and enhance effector T-cell function, recent studies have demonstrated that treatments that utilize low-dose IL-2 unexpectedly induce immune tolerance and promote Treg development [76]. However, that capture of IL-2 was dispensable for the control of CD4+ T cells but was important for limiting the activation of CD8+ T cells [72]. This may explain our data, however, overall, our findings may not have power enough to rule out such hypothesis.

Additional experiments including immunohistochemical, immunophenotyping and functional assays in order to evaluate Treg cells suppressor activity and migration of are currently being conducted for better understanding about the mouse model capabilities and deficiencies.

Conclusion

In conclusion, our study has shown for the first time, higher expression of $CD4^+CD69^+$ T cells and reductions in $CD4^+CD25^+FoxP3^+$ Treg cells with altered interleukin profiles in pristane-induced SLE mice peripheral blood, spleen and PL, suggesting loss of autotolerance and a homeostatic immune imbalance similar to human SLE. Therefore, this easily reproducible experimental low cost model may help to generate new knowledge concerning cellular immune defects related to human lupus as well as the study of future therapies capable of reestablishing the immune homeostatic balance.

Abbreviations

Ab: Antibody; ANA: Anti-nuclear antibody; BALB/c: a mouse strain; CD: "Cluster of differentiation"; DMSO: dimethyl sulfoxide; ELISA: enzyme-linked immunosorbent assay; FACS: fluorescence-activated cell sorter; FBS: fetal bovine serum; h: hour; H&E: hematoxylin and eosin; i.p: intraperitoneal; IFN: interferon (e.g., IFN-γ); IL: interleukin (e.g., IL-2); mAb: monoclonal Ab; min: minute; PBMC: peripheral blood mononuclear cell; PL: peritoneal lavage; PLMC: peritoneal lavage mononuclear cell; PMN: polymorphonuclear cell; rpm: revolutions per minute; RPMI: (usually RPMI 1640); SD: standard deviation; SLE: Systemic Lupus Erythematosus; TGF: transforming growth factor; TNF: tumor necrosis factor; wk: week; µg: microgram; µl: microliter

Acknowledgments

The authors acknowledge Eloisa S. Dutra de Oliveira Bonfá, Rosa Maria Rodrigues Pereira, Walcy Rosolia Teodoro, Maria Aurora Gomes da Silva, Maria de Fátima de Almeida, Vilma dos Santos Trindade Viana, Margarete Borges Galhardo Vendramini, Cleonice Bueno and Antônio dos Santos Filho.

Authors' contributions

TV P conceived the presented idea, designed and carried out the experiments, interpreting the results and writing the manuscript with input from all authors, who pro provided critical feedback and helped shape the research. SC carried out the experiments and aided in interpreting the results, working and commenting on the manuscript. DA C Botte aided in interpreting the results, working and commenting on the manuscript. SC, TM L and NU carried out the experiments. ERP, pathologist involved in the interpretation of histological slide results. FGS and SBV de M were involved in planning and supervising the work. CM. Rodrigues proofread the manuscript. CG-S contributed to the interpretations of the results and supervised this work.

Author details

[1]Laboratório de Imunologia Celular (LIM-17) - Faculdade de Medicina FMUSP, Universidade de Sao Paulo, Sao Paulo, SP, Brazil. [2]Laboratório de Lípides (LIM-10) - Faculdade de Medicina FMUSP, Universidade de Sao Paulo, Sao Paulo, SP, Brazil. [3]Departamento de Patologia Clínica - Faculdade de Medicina FMUSP, Universidade de Sao Paulo, Sao Paulo, SP, Brazil. [4]Laboratório de Emergências Clínicas (LIM-51) - Faculdade de Medicina FMUSP, Universidade de Sao Paulo, Sao Paulo, SP, Brazil. [5]Faculdade de Medicina de Botucatu (FMB), Universidade Estadual Paulista Júlio de Mesquita Filho (Unesp), Botucatu, SP, Brazil. [6]Laboratório de Imunologia Celular (LIM-17) – Hospital das Clínicas HCFMUSP, Faculdade de Medicina, Universidade de Sao Paulo, Sao Paulo, SP, Brazil.

References

1. *Immune Tolerance.* [https://www.nature.com/subjects/immune-tolerance] 2019.
2. Ichinohe T, et al. Next-generation immune repertoire sequencing as a clue to elucidate the landscape of immune modulation by host-gut microbiome interactions. Front Immunol. 2018;9:668.
3. Zhang P, et al. Genetic and epigenetic influences on the loss of tolerance in autoimmunity. Cellular & Molecular Immunology. 2018;5:137.
4. Nagarkatti P. Tolerance and autoimmunity associate dean for basic science and health sciences distinguished professor. Medical Microbiology:6–17.
5. Abbas A. Imunologia Básica: Funções e Distúrbios do Sistema Imunológico. San Francisco: Elsevier/Medicina Nacionais; 2013.
6. Bonelli M, et al. Quantitative and qualitative deficiencies of regulatory T cells in patients with Sistemic lupus erythematosus. Int Immunol. 2008;20:861–8.
7. Vitales-noyola M, et al. Patients with systemic lupus erythematosus show increased levels and defective function of CD69+ T regulatory cells. Mediat Inflamm. 2017;9.
8. Mak A, et al. The pathology of T cells in systemic lupus erythematosus. J Immunol Res. 2014;8.
9. Bartels C, et al. Systemic lupus erythematosus (SLE) clinical presentation: Drugs & Diseases; 2017. https://emedicine.medscape.com/article/332244-clinical
10. Ebrahimiyan H, et al. Survivin and autoimmunity; the ins ando uts. Immunol Lett. 2018:14–24.
11. Chavez-rueda K, et al. Prolactine effect on CD69 and CD154 expression by CD4+ cells from systemic lupus erythematosus patients. Clin Exp Rheumatol. 2005;23:769–77.
12. STARSKA K, et al. The role of tumor cells in the modification of T lymphocytes activity—the expression of the early CD69+, CD71+ and the late CD25+, CD26+, HLA/DR+ activation markers on T CD4+ and CD8+ cells in squamous cell laryngeal carcinoma. Part I. Folia Histochemica et Cytobiologica. 2011;4:579–92.
13. Fujii R, et al. Genetic control of the spontaneous activation of CD4+ Th cells in systemic lupus erythematosus-prone (NZBXNZW) F1 mice. Genes Immun. 2006;7:647–54.
14. Lee J-H, et al. Inverse correlation between CD4+ regulatory T cell population and autoantibody levels in pediatric patients with systemic lupus erythematosus. Immunology. 2006;177:280–6.
15. Bonelli M, et al. Foxp3 expression in CD4+ T cells of patients with systemic lupus erythematosus: a comparative phenotypic analysis. Ann Rheum Dis. 2008;67:664–71.
16. Hu S, et al. Regulatory T cells and their molecular markers in peripheral blood of the patients with systemic lupus erythematosus. Journal of Huazhong University of Science and Technology (Medical Sciences). 2008;28:549–52.
17. Liu MF, et al. Decreased CD4+CD25+ T cells in peripheral blood of patients with systemic lupus erythematosus. Scand J Immunol. 2004;59:198–202.
18. Barreto M, et al. Low frequency of CD4+CD25+ Treg in SLE patients: a heritabletra it associated with CTLA-4 and TGFb gene variants. BMC Immunol. 2009;10:14.
19. VALENCIA X, et al. Deficient CD4+CD25high T regulatory cell function in patients with active systemic lupus erythematosus. J Immunol. 2007;178: 2579–88.
20. Humrich JY, et al. Homeostatic imbalance of regulatory and effector T cells due to Il-2 deprivation amplifies murine lupus. PNAS. 2010;107:204–9.
21. Gunawan M, et al. A novel human systemic lupus erythematosus model in humanised mice. Sci Rep. 2017;7:11.
22. Mizutani A, et al. Pristane-induced autoimmunity in germ-free mice. Clin Immunol. 2005;114:110–8.
23. Reeves WH, et al. Induction of autoimmunity by pristine and other naturally occurring hydrocarbons. Trends Immunol. 2009;30:455–64.
24. Botte DA, et al. Alpha-melanocyte stimulating hormone ameliorates disease activity in na induce murine lupus-like model. Clinical & Experimental Immunology. 2014;177(2):381–90.
25. Dimitrova I, et al. Target silencing of disease-associated Blymphocytes by chimeric molecules in SCID model off pristane-induced autoimmunity. Lupus. 2010;0:1–11.
26. Calvani N, et al. Induction of apoptosis by the hydrocarbon oil pristane: implications for pristane-induced lupus. J Immunol. 2005;175:4777–82.
27. Zhuang H, et al. Autoimmunity. In: Essencial Clinical Immunology. Nova York: Cambridge University Press; 2009.
28. Satoh M, et al. Induction of lupus autoantibodies by adjuvants. J Autoimmun. 2003;21:1–9.
29. SATOH M, et al. Widespread susceptibility among inbred mouse strains to the induction of lupus autoantibodies by pristane. Clin Exp Immunol. Detroit;2008;121:399–405.
30. Leiss H, et al. Pristane-induced lupus as a model of human lupus arthritis: evolvement of autoantibodies, internal organ and joint inflammation. Lupus. 2013;22:778–92.

31. Patten C, et al. Characterization of Pristane-induced arthritis, a murine model of chronic disease. Arthritis & Rheumatism. 2004;50:3334–45.
32. Peixoto TV. Aumento de células T CD4+CD69+ e redução de células T reguladoras CD4+CD25+FoxP3+ em camundongos com Lúpus Eritematoso Sistêmico (LES) induzido por pristane. Tese Biblioteca Digital USP. São Paulo; 2015. http://www.teses.usp.br/teses/disponiveis/5/5165/tde-14122 015-152214/pt-br.php
33. Bossaller L, et al. Overexpression of membrane-bound Fas ligand (CD95L) exacerbates autoimmune disease and renal pathology in pristane-induced lupus. J Immunol. 2013;191:2104–14.
34. Urbonaviciute V, et al. Toll-like receptor 2 is required for autoantibody production and development of renal disease in pristane-induced lupus. Arthritis & Rheumatism. 2013;65:1612–23.
35. Kluger MA, et al. RORγt expression in Tregs promotes systemic lupus erythematosus via IL-17 secretion, alteration of Treg phenotype and suppression of Th2 responses. Clinical & Experimental Immunology. 2017;188:63–78.
36. Richard ML, et al. Mouse models of lupus: what they tell us and what they don't. Lupus Science & Medicine. 2018;5:7.
37. Zhuang H, et al. Toll-like receptor 7-stimulated tumor necrosis factor a causes bone marrow damage in systemic lupus erythematosus. Arthritis & Rheumatology. 2014;66:140–51.
38. Li N, et al. Pathologic diagnosis of spontaneuous splenic rupture in systemic lupus erythematosus. Int J Clin Exp Pathol. 2013;6:273–80.
39. Gleisner MA, et al. Dendritic and stromal cells from the spleen of lupic mice present phenotypic and functional abnormalities. Mol Immunol. 2013;54:423–34.
40. Shaheen VM, et al. Immunopathogenesis of environmentally induced lupus in mice. Environ Health Perspect. 1999;107:723–7.
41. Zickert AP, et al. IL-17 and IL-23 in lupus nephritis – association to histopathology and response to treatment. BMC Immunol. 2015;16:7.
42. XU Y, et al. Mechanisms of tumor necrosis factor a antagonist-induced lupus in a murine model. Arthritis & Rheumatology. 2015;67:225–37.
43. Ivanova W, et al. Differential immune-reactivity to genomic DNA, RNA and mitochondrial DNA is associated with auto-immunity. Cell Physiol Biochem. 2014;34:2200–8.
44. Horwitz DA. The clinical significance of decreased T cell interkeukin-2 production in systemic lupus erythematosus: connecting historical dots. Arthritis & Rheumatism. 2010;62:2185–7.
45. Sun Z, et al. Serum IL-10 from systemic lupus erythematosus patients suppresses the differentiation and function of monocyte-derived dendritic cells. J Biomed Res. 2012;26:456–66.
46. Theofilopoulos AN, et al. The rolo of IFN-gamma in systemic lupus erythematosus: a challenge to the Th1/Th2 paradigm in autoimmunity. Arthritis Research & Therapy. 2001;3:136–41.
47. Sullivan, K. E. Genetics of systemic lupus erythematosus. Clinical implications. Rheumatic diseases clinics of North America. 2000;26:229–56.
48. Bermas BL, et al. T helper cell dysfunction in systemic lupus erythematosus (SLE): relation to disease activity. J Clin Immunol. 1994;14:169–77.
49. Georgescu L, et al. Interleukin-10 promotes activation-induced cell death of SLE lymphocytes mediated by Fas ligand. J Clin Invest. 1997;100:2622–33.
50. LIORENTE L, et al. The rolo of interleukin-10 in systemic lupus erythematosus. J Autoimmun. 2003;20:287–9.
51. Fernandez T. S. et al. disruption of transforming growth factor b signaling by a novel ligand-dependent mechanism. J Exp Med. 2002;195:1247–55.
52. Lahita RG. Systemic lupus erythematosus. Toronto: Academic Press; 2004.
53. Sanjabi S. Regulation of the immune response by TGR-b: from conception to autoimmunity and infection. Cold Spring Harb Perspect Biol. 2019.
54. Lee PY, et al. A novel type I IFN-producing cell subset in murine lupus. J Immunol. 2008;180:5101–8.
55. Mcdonald AH, et al. Pristane induces an indomethacin inhibitable inflammatory influx of CD4+ T cells and IFNγ production in plasmacytoma-susceptible Balb/cAnPt mice. Cell Immunol. 1993;146:157–70.
56. Liu CC, et al. Biomarkers in systemic lupus erythematosus: challenges and prospects for the future. Therapeutic Advances in Musculoskeletal Disease. 2013;5:210–33.
57. Italiani P. IL-1 family cytokines and soluble receptors in systemic lupus erythematosus. Arthritis Research & Therapy. 2018;20.
58. Loissis S-NC, et al. Sustemic Lupus Erythematosus In. Principles of Molecular Rheumatology. 2000.
59. Alvarado-Sánchez B, et al. Regulatory T cells in patients with systemic lupus erythematosus. J Autoimmun. 2006;27:110–8.
60. Male D, et al. Immunology. [S.l.]: Elsevier; 2006.
61. Miyara M, et al. Global natural regulatory T cell depletion in active systemic lupus erythematosus. J Immunol. 2005;175:8392–0.
62. Scalapino KJ, et al. Suppression of disease in new Zeland black/new Zeland white lupus-prone mice byu adoptive transfer of ex vivo expanded regulatory T cells. J Immunol. 2006;177:1451–9.
63. Sasidhar MV, et al. The XX sex chromosome complement in mice is associated with increased spontaneous lupus compared with XY. 2012. Ann Rheum Dis. 2012;71:1418–22.
64. Monk CR, et al. MRL/Mp CD4+, CD25- T cells show reduced sensitivity to suppression by CD4+, CD25+ regulatory T cells in vitro. A novel defect of T cell regulation in systemic lupus erythematosus. Arthritis & Rheumatism. 2005;52:1180–4.
65. Heiler S, et al. Prophylactic and therapeutic effects os interleukin-2 (IL-2) /anti-IL-2 complexes in systemic lupus erythematosus-like chronic graft-versus-host disease. Front Immunol. 2018.
66. Wen S, et al. IFN-y, CXCL16, uPAR: potential biomarkers for systemic lupus erythematosus. Clin Exp Rheumatol. 2017:36.
67. Rojas M, et al. Cytokines and inflammatory mediators in systemic lupus erythematosus. Rheumatology. 2018.
68. Yang C-H, et al. Immunological mechanisms and clinical implications of regulatory T cell deficiency in a systemic autoimmune disorder: roles of IL-2 versus IL-15. Eur J Immunol. 2008;38:1664–76.
69. Satoh M, et al. Induction of hypergammaglobulinemia and macrophage activation by silicone gels and oils in female a.SW mice. Clin Diagn Lab Immunol. 2000;7:366–70.
70. Parietti V, et al. Functions of CD4+CD25+ Tregcells in MRL/lpr mice is compromised by intrinsic defects in antigen-presentin cells and effector T cells. Arthritis & Rheumatism. 2008;58:1751–61.
71. Crispin JC, et al. Quantification of regulatory T cells in patients with systemic lupus erythematosus. Journal of Autoimmunology. 2003;21:273–6.
72. Chinen T, et al. An essential role for the IL-2 receptor in Treg function. Nat Immunol. 2016;17(11):1322–33.
73. Wood P. Understanding Immunology. Pearson Education Limited: England; 2006.
74. Wallace DJ, et al. Dubois' lupus erythematosus. Philadelphia: Lippincott Williams & Wilkin; 2007.
75. Talaat R, et al. Th1/Th2/Th17/Treg cytokine imbalance in systemic lupus erythematosus (SLE) patients: correlation with disease activity. Cytokine. 2015;72.
76. Ye C. Targeting IL-2: an unexpected effect in treating immunological diseases. Signal Transduction and Targeted Therapy. 2018;3(2):1–10.

5

Comparison among ACR1997, SLICC and the new EULAR/ACR classification criteria in childhood-onset systemic lupus erythematosus

Adriana Rodrigues Fonseca[1*], Marta Cristine Felix Rodrigues[1], Flavio Roberto Sztajnbok[1], Marcelo Gerardin Poirot Land[2†] and Sheila Knupp Feitosa de Oliveira[1†]

Abstract

Background: To date there are no specific classification criteria for childhood-onset systemic lupus erythematosus (cSLE). This study aims to compare the performance among the American College of Rheumatology (ACR) 1997, the Systemic Lupus International Collaborating Clinics criteria (SLICC) and the new European League Against Rheumatism (EULAR)/ACR criteria, in a cSLE cohort.

Methods: We conducted a medical chart review study of cSLE cases and controls with defined rheumatic diseases, both ANA positive, to establish each ACR1997, SLICC and EULAR/ACR criterion fulfilled, at first visit and 1-year-follow-up.

Results: Study population included 122 cSLE cases and 89 controls. At first visit, SLICC criteria had higher sensitivity than ACR 1997 (89.3% versus 70.5%, $p < 0.001$), but similar specificity (80.9% versus 83.2%, $p = 0.791$), however performance was not statistically different at 1-year-follow-up. SLICC better scored in specificity compared to EULAR/ACR score ≥ 10 at first visit (80.9% versus 67.4%, $p = 0.008$) and at 1-year (76.4% versus 58.4%, $p = 0.001$), although sensitivities were similar. EULAR/ACR criteria score ≥ 10 exhibited higher sensitivity than ACR 1997 (87.7% versus 70.5%, $p < 0.001$) at first visit, but comparable at 1-year, whereas specificity was lower at first visit (67.4% versus 83.2%, $p = 0.004$) and 1-year (58.4% versus 76.4%, $p = 0.002$). A EULAR/ACR score ≥ 13 against a score ≥ 10, resulted in higher specificity, positive predictive value, and cut-off point accuracy. Compared to SLICC, a EULAR/ACR score ≥ 13 resulted in lower sensitivity at first visit (76.2% versus 89.3%, $p < 0.001$) and 1-year (91% versus 97.5%, $p = 0.008$), but similar specificities at both assessments. When compared to ACR 1997, a EULAR/ACR total score ≥ 13, resulted in no differences in sensitivity and specificity at both observation periods.

Conclusions: In this cSLE population, SLICC criteria better scored at first visit and 1-year-follow-up. The adoption of a EULAR/ACR total score ≥ 13 in this study, against the initially proposed ≥10 score, was most appropriate to classify cSLE. Further studies are necessary to address if SLICC criteria might allow fulfillment of cSLE classification earlier in disease course and may be more inclusive of cSLE subjects for clinical studies.

Keywords: Systemic lupus erythematosus, Childhood, Adolescence, Classification criteria

* Correspondence: adrirfonseca@gmail.com; drcarlosoliver@yahoo.com.br
†Marcelo Gerardin Poirot Land and Sheila Knupp Feitosa de Oliveira contributed equally to this work.
[1]Pediatric Rheumatology Unit, Instituto de Puericultura e Pediatria Martagão Gesteira, Universidade Federal do Rio de Janeiro (UFRJ), Rua Bruno Lobo, 50– Cidade Universitária, Rio de Janeiro, Brazil
Full list of author information is available at the end of the article

Background

Systemic lupus erythematosus (SLE) is a chronic autoimmune disease, with a broad spectrum of clinical patterns. SLE affects women predominantly at reproductive age but may present at any age [1]. Childhood-onset SLE (cSLE) represents approximately 20% of SLE cases [2] and displays a higher frequency of atypical manifestations, more severe presentation and course, higher rates of disease activity and cumulative damage, than that reported for adult-onset disease [3, 4].

As the purpose of classification criteria is to identify a well-defined patient population suitable for research, specificity thus generally outweighs sensitivity in determining classification performance.

The SLE classification criteria set most commonly used is the one established by the American College of Rheumatology (ACR) [5]. Besides the development in adult-onset SLE and scarce validation in cSLE, concerns arose about the redundancy of photosensitivity with skin rashes, non inclusion of several clinically relevant integument and nervous system lupus manifestations, as well as hypocomplementemia, inadequate quantification of urine protein by dipstick, and, classification as SLE for patients without positive autoantibodies [6].

Alternative methods for SLE classification have been developed predominantly in adults, such as the SLICC (Systemic Lupus International Collaborating Clinics) criteria [7] and the new EULAR/ACR criteria [8–12].

The main changes proposed in SLICC criteria were the expansion of cutaneous and neurological criteria, allocation of cytopenias and autoantibodies in individual criterion, inclusion of alopecia and hypocomplementemia, and the classification for patients with only documented lupus nephritis with ANA or anti-dsDNA [7]. SLICC criteria yielded higher sensitivity (97% versus 83%) but lower specificity (84% versus 96%) than ACR 1997 criteria in the original validation set [7]. In subsequent studies in adult and cSLE, SLICC higher sensitivity was also found, especially for early SLE, however, results were conflicting regarding specificity [13–20]. The SLICC criteria have also been criticized because they were derived comparing the expert's decision ("gold standard") with a standardized group of manifestations [6]. Moreover, as SLICC criteria emphasize immunological and hematological events, it might be possible that subjects classified through SLICC criteria may exhibit less clinically significant multisystem involvement compared with subjects classified through ACR criteria [6].

In 2017, the EULAR and ACR joined in a four-phase project to develop more sensitive (especially for initial classification) and more specific SLE classification criteria [8–12]. The first phase of this project was designed to gather potential candidate items broadly, through an SLE expert Delphi exercise and an international early SLE cohort study. The second phase consisted of item reduction by nominal group technique. The third phase was for item definition (literature based) and weighting (multiparameter decision analysis) and the fourth phase for item testing and validation against ACR 1997 and SLICC [10]. These criteria rely on a scoring system for clinical and laboratory domains [21], and a positivity of antinuclear antibody (ANA) at a titer 1:80 or higher by immunofluorescence (IFA) as an entry criterion [22]. The patient is classified as SLE if the total score is equal to or greater than 10 [10, 11]. EULAR/ACR criteria were tested, simplified and validated in a large (n = 2.218) international cohort. Performance characteristics found a sensitivity similar to the SLICC criteria (98% versus 95% for SLICC and 85% for ACR 1997) while maintaining the specificity of the ACR 1997 criteria (97% versus 95% for ACR 1997 and 90% for SLICC) [10]. Limitations indicated by the authors were the possible misclassification of patients with overlapping syndromes and the non-inclusion of new biomarkers [10, 19]. Other authors pointed out that the lack of extensive data on the longitudinal expression of ANA could affect the application of classification criteria in which ANA expression is the entry point [23].

This study aims to compare the performance of ACR 1997, SLICC criteria and the new EULAR/ACR criteria, to identify patients with cSLE at first visit and 1-year-follow-up.

Methods

Inclusion criteria

Children and adolescents, with cSLE (cases) or other defined rheumatic diseases (controls), with ANA reactivity at ≥1:80 serum dilution, followed-up at the Pediatric Rheumatology Unit of our University Hospital, from 2000 to 2017, were consecutively selected, from the number of patients evaluated in the clinic during the inclusion period.

To be included, cases and controls patients needed to have a well-established clinical diagnosis, performed and confirmed by three highly experienced pediatric rheumatologists, with over than 20 years experience in pediatric rheumatology and cSLE, of the medical staff of the outpatient clinic. All baseline and evolutionary information (physical examination, laboratory parameters, and imaging), was routinely discussed and re-evaluated at each visit, by attending pediatric rheumatologists, which established the diagnosis based on continuous follow-up of all patients and total agreement about diagnosis, supported by internationally accepted criteria [24–29].

Exclusion criteria

Patients with overlapping syndromes or undifferentiated disease and those patients followed-up for less than 1 year were excluded.

Data collection

We performed a medical chart review for all eligible patients, and information collected in a standardized file. Data collection was retrospective, extracted by two of the authors and reviewed by the other three authors before classification sets scoring. Discrepancies were solved by team discussion. Finally, all patient's files (from cSLE cases and controls) were rated for each ACR 1997, SLICC and EULAR/ACR criterion that was or was not met, as laid out by the respective classification rule, at first visit, and at 1-year-follow-up. Cases and controls were classified as SLE if met ≥4 criteria for ACR 1997, ≥ 4 criteria or documented lupus nephritis with ANA, anti-dsDNA or both for SLICC and ≥ 10 or ≥ 13 total score for EULAR/ACR.

Baseline/first visit data were those obtained from the clinical history, physical examination and laboratory tests requested by attending pediatric rheumatologists at first visit. The immunologic assessments evaluated for cSLE and control patients were antinuclear antibody (ANA), anti-dsDNA, anti-Sm, anticardiolipin IgM and IgG, lupus anticoagulant, anti- β2-glycoprotein-I IgM and IgG (for patients who started follow-up after the year of 2012), direct Coombs test, levels of complement proteins C3 and C4, and VDRL (*Venereal Disease Research Laboratory).*

Criteria definitions

Definitions for each clinical or laboratory criterion were those provided by the respective criteria set. 1) ANA by indirect immunofluorescence, on human cell epithelioma (HEp-2) cells substrate, defined as positive if staining reactivity at ≥1:80; 2) Anti-dsDNA by indirect immunofluorescence, on *Crithidia lucilae* substrate, described as positive if staining reactivity at > 1:10 serum dilution; 3) Anti-Sm by enzyme-linked immunosorbent assay (ELISA), considered positive if above kit manufacturer cut-off value. 4) Anticardiolipin (aCL) IgM and IgG by ELISA, a cut-off value of 20 MPL or GPL for ACR1997 and SLICC criteria, and a cut-off value of 40 MPL or GPL for EULAR/ACR criteria set.

EULAR/ACR criteria: A positivity of antinuclear antibody (ANA) at a titer 1:80 or higher by immunofluorescence (IFA) is required as an entry criterion [22]. These criteria rely on weighted additive criteria divided into seven clinical domains and three immunological domains, for which attribution to SLE is critical [21]. For each domain, only the individual criterion of highest value is considered for the total score [10, 11]. Clinical domains include: 1) unexplained fever; 2) arthritis; 3) serositis (pleural or pericardial effusion, acute pericarditis); 4) mucocutaneous (acute cutaneous lupus, subacute/discoid lupus, alopecia, oral ulcers); 5) central nervous system involvement (seizures, psychosis and delirium); 6) hematological involvement (autoimmune hemolytic anemia, thrombocytopenia and leukopenia); 7) nephritis (proteinuria > 0.5 g/d, nephritis class III/IV, nephritis class II/V). Lupus nephritis class II/IV over class II/V gain the highest weight. Immunological domains consist of 1) autoantibodies (anti-dsDNA, anti-Sm); 2) low complement (both C3 and C4 OR only C3 or C4); 3) Antiphospholipid antibodies (anticardiolipin IgG ≥ 40 GPL or anti-β2 glycoprotein I IgG ≥ 40 GPL or lupus anticoagulant). The patient is classified as SLE if the total score is equal to or greater than 10, in the presence of at least one clinical criterion, and each criterion may occur serially or simultaneously and on at least one occasion [10, 11].

Statistical analysis

The Statistical Package for the Social Sciences (SPSS) 20.0 for *Windows* (IBM, Armonk, NY, USA) was used. Data were shown in median (range, IQR) for continuous variables, and further comparisons between groups were conducted using Student's t-test. Differences between proportions or categorical variables were analyzed by Fisher exact test. We performed the calculation of two types of accuracy: global accuracy and cut-off point accuracy [30]. The global accuracy was calculated for all three criteria sets, through the area under the ROC curve (AUC), to estimate how high is the discriminative power of each criteria set. However, as the AUC tell us nothing about individual cut-off points, we calculated the cut-off point accuracy for ACR 1997 ≥ 4 criteria, for SLICC ≥4 criteria and EULAR/ACR total score (total score ≥ 10, ≥11 and ≥ 13), through two-by-two contingency tables. McNemar's test was applied to assess differences in sensitivity and specificity between ACR1997, SLICC and EULAR/ACR classification sets. A $p <$ 0.05 value was regarded as significant, and all analyses were two-tailed.

Ethics

The local Research Ethics Committee approved the study protocol before study commencement, under Number 2.421.080, on December 7th, 2017.

Results

Sample description

133 cSLE and 96 controls fulfilled inclusion criteria, but there were 11 (9.0%) losses for cases group and 7 (8.2%) for control group due to missing information about some variables in medical charts. Study population included 122 cases with a well-established clinical diagnosis of cSLE (82.8% female, median onset age of 10.32 years (2.8–17.1) and median follow-up time of 6.0 years) and 89 controls (75.3% female, median onset age of 9.0 years and median follow-up time of 6.0 years), see Table 1.

Controls had the following diagnoses: 8 systemic-onset juvenile idiopathic arthritis (SoJIA), 34 juvenile

Table 1 General characteristics of case and control groups

	Cases ($N = 122$)	Controls ($N = 89$)	P value
Sex ratio (female: male)	101:21	67:22	0.226
Median onset age, years	10.32	9.00	< 0.001
(range)	(2.8–17.1)	(1.1–15.8)	
Interquartile range (years)	3.2	6.3	
Median age at diagnosis, years	10.63	9.5	0.024
(range)	(4.1–17.3)	(1.9–17.8)	
Interquartile range (years)	3.0	7.0	
Median time to diagnosis, months	3.00	9.00	< 0.001
(range)	0–60	1–68	
Interquartile range (years)	4.0	18.5	
Median follow-up time, years	6.00	6.00	0.91
(range)	1–13	2–16	
Interquartile range (years)	4.0	4.0	

Cases were patients with a well-established clinical diagnosis of childhood-onset SLE (cSLE). Controls had systemic-onset juvenile idiopathic arthritis, *JDM* juvenile dermatomyositis, *JSS* juvenile systemic sclerosis, *MCTD* mixed connective tissue disease, *SS* Sjögren syndrome, *APS* primary antiphospholipid syndrome, or primary vasculitis (Behçet, polyarteritis nodosa, Takayasu's arteritis and granulomatosis with polyangiitis)

dermatomyositis (JDM), 10 juvenile systemic sclerosis (JSS), 14 mixed connective tissue disease (MCTD), 12 Sjögren syndrome (SS), 3 primary antiphospholipid syndromes (APS), 8 primary vasculitides.

ACR 1997 criteria

The most commonly observed ACR criteria in cSLE cases, both at the first visit and at 1-year-follow-up, respectively, were: arthritis (77 and 86.1%), immunologic (59 and 76.2%), hematologic (59 and 73.8%) and malar rash (36.9 and 52.5%). Arthritis (64 and 70.8%), malar rash (19.1 and 29.2%), and hematological (18 and 21.3%) were the most observed criteria in the control group.

At first visit, the mean number of ACR criteria was 4.54 ± 0.16 for cases and 2.52 ± 0.12 for controls ($p < 0.001$). At 1-year-follow-up, this average was 5.71 ± 0.14 for cases and 2.82 ± 0.12 for controls ($p < 0.001$).

Fifteen controls were misclassified as JSLE at first visit: 1 SoJIA, 8 JDM, 1 JSS, 4 MCTD, and 1 SS. Six additional controls were misclassified at 1-year-follow-up: 1 JDM and 5 MTCD.

SLICC criteria

The most frequent SLICC criteria in cSLE, both at first visit and at 1-year-follow-up, were, respectively: arthritis (78.7 and 87.7%), hypocomplementemia (56.6 and 60.7%), acute cutaneous lupus (49.2 and 65.6%), alopecia (42.6 and 44.3%) and anti-dsDNA (37.7 and 53.3%). At first visit, cSLE cases fulfilled a mean of 6.07 ± 0.21 and controls 2.69 ± 0.13 SLICC criteria ($p < 0.001$). At 1-year-follow-up, cases had a mean of 7.42 ± 0.20 and controls 3.00 ± 0.14 ($p = 0.012$) SLICC criteria.

Seventeen controls were misclassified as cSLE at first visit: one SoJIA, 2 JDM, 2 JSS, 9 MCTD, 1 primary APS, one SS, and one primary vasculitis. Four additional controls were misclassified at 1-year-follow-up: 2 JDM and 2 MCTD.

Table 2 presents the prevalence of SLICC criteria in cSLE cases and controls at baseline/first visit and 1-year-follow-up.

EULAR/ACR criteria

To better evaluate the use of EULAR/ACR criteria in our cSLE population, we searched through ROC curve analysis, the total score cut-off that might optimize sensitivity and specificity, and we noticed that a total score ≥ 13, against the initially proposed ≥10 score, was more suitable for our cSLE patients. Besides, we also decided to perform a sensitivity analysis for different cut-off points of EULAR/ACR total score.

At first visit, if a EULAR/ACR total score ≥ 13 is adopted, a lower sensitivity (76.2% versus 87.7% for score ≥ 10, $p < 0.0001$) but a higher specificity (87.6% versus 67.4% for score ≥ 10, $p < 0.0001$), higher positive predictive value (89.4% versus 78.7% for score ≥ 10) and higher cut-off point accuracy would result.

At 1-year-follow-up, if an EULAR/ACR total score ≥ 13 is adopted, a similar sensitivity (91.0% versus 95.1% for score ≥ 10, $p = 0.063$), but again a higher specificity (83.2% versus 58.4% for score ≥ 10, $p < 0.0001$), higher positive predictive value (88.1% versus 75.8% for score ≥ 10) and higher cut-off point accuracy would result.

At first visit, cSLE cases achieved a mean EULAR/ACR total score of 19.64 ± 0.78 and controls 7.93 ± 0.54 ($p = 0.002$). At 1-year-follow-up, cases had a mean total score of 24.42 ± 0.74 and controls 9.19 ± 0.57 ($p = 0.038$).

Twenty-nine controls were misclassified as cSLE at first visit if total score ≥ 10 (3 SoJIA, 10 JDM, 2 JSS, 8 MCTD, 1 primary APS, 4 SS and 1 primary vasculitis), against eleven misclassified controls, if total score ≥ 13 (2 SoJIA, 1 JDM, 1 JSS, 6 MCTD, and 1 SS). Eight additional controls were misclassified at 1-year-follow-up if score ≥ 10 (4 JDM, 1 MCTD, 2 SS and 1 primary vasculitis), against 4 other controls if score ≥ 13 (2 JDM and 2 MCTD).

Table 3 displays the global accuracy for each criteria set.

First visit - ACR 1997 versus SLICC criteria

SLICC criteria exhibited higher sensitivity (89.3% versus 70.5%, $p < 0.001$), but similar specificity (80.9% versus 83.2% ACR 1997, $p = 0.791$). SLICC criteria resulted in less misclassifications (30 versus 51, $p < 0.001$).

First visit - ACR 1997 versus EULAR/ACR total score ≥ 10

EULAR/ACR criteria total score ≥ 10 exhibited higher sensitivity than ACR 1997 (87.7% versus 70.5%, $p < 0.001$).

Table 2 Prevalence of clinical and immunological criterion of Systemic Lupus International Collaborating Clinics (SLICC) Classification Criteria in 122 cSLE cases and 89 controls, at baseline/first visit and 1-year-follow-up

Criterion	Cases Baseline/First visit n (%)	Controls Baseline/First visit n (%)	*P* value	Cases 1-year follow-up n (%)	Controls 1-year follow-up n (%)	*P* value
Acute cutaneous lupus	60 (49.2)	22 (24.7)	< 0.001	80 (65.6)	30 (33.7)	< 0.001
Malar rash	45 (36.9)	17 (19.1)	0.006	64 (52.5)	26 (29.2)	0.001
Photosensitive lupus rash	29 (23.8)	14 (15.7)	0.169	34 (27.9)	16 (18.0)	0.104
Subacute cutaneous lupus	18 (14.8)	1 (1.1)	< 0.001	21 (17.2)	1 (1.1)	< 0.001
Chronic cutaneous lupus	13 (10.7)	1 (1.1)	0.005	16 (13.1)	1 (1.1)	0.001
Discoid rash	13 (10.7)	1 (1.1)	0.005	15 (12.3)	1 (1.1)	0.003
Oral ulcers	44 (36.1)	11 (12.4)	< 0.001	64 (52.5)	12 (13.5)	< 0.001
Alopecia	52 (42.6)	12 (6.8)	< 0.001	54 (44.3)	14 (9.1)	< 0.001
Synovitis	96 (78.7)	59 (66.3)	0.058	107 (87.7)	65 (73.0)	0.011
Serositis	30 (24.6)	3 (3.4)	< 0.001	41 (33.6)	4 (4.5)	< 0.001
Pleuritis	22 (18.0)	2 (2.3)	< 0.001	32 (26.2)	3 (3.4)	< 0.001
Pericarditis	8 (6.6)	0	0.022	9 (7.4)	2 (2.3)	0.124
Renal disorder	33 (27.0)	1 (1.1)	< 0.001	49 (40.2)	2 (2.3)	< 0.001
Proteinuria	33 (27.0)	1 (1.1)	< 0.001	49 (40.2)	2 (2.3)	< 0.001
Red blood cell casts	10 (8.2)	0	< 0.001	15 (12.3)	1 (1.1)	< 0.001
Neuropsychiatric	10 (8.2)	1 (1.1)	0.027	23 (18.9)	1 (1.1)	< 0.001
Seizures	5 (4.1)	0	0.075	17 (13.9)	0	< 0.001
Psychosis	2 (1.6)	0	0.510	6 (4.9)	0	0.041
Myelitis	1 (0.8)	0	0.999	3 (2.5)	0	0.265
Confusional state	1 (0.8)	0	0.999	1 (0.8)	0	0.999
Hemolytic anemia	44 (36.1)	4 (4.5)	< 0.001	61 (50.0)	4 (4.5)	< 0.001
Leukopenia/lymphopenia	39 (32.0)	(10.1)	< 0.001	53 (43.4)	11 (12.4)	< 0.001
Thrombocytopenia	18 (14.8)	4 (4.5)	0.021	20 (16.4)	4 (4.5)	0.008
Anti-dsDNA	46 (37.7)	4 (4.5)	< 0.001	65 (53.3)	5 (5.6)	< 0.001
Anti-Sm	29 (23.8)	5 (5.6)	< 0.001	38 (31.1)	5 (5.6)	< 0.001
Antiphospholipid	30 (24.6)	5 (5.6)	< 0.001	38 (31.1)	4 (4.5)	< 0.001
Anticardiolipin IgM	11 (9.0)	2 (2.3)	0.047	12 (9.8)	2 (2.3)	0.046
Anticardiolipin IgG	23 (18.9)	2 (2.3)	< 0.001	27 (22.1)	3 (2.5)	< 0.001
Lupus anticoagulant	6 (4.9)	5 (5.6)	0.999	8 (6.6)	5 (5.6)	0.999
Anti-β2 GPI I IgM	3/61 (4.9)	1/42 (2.4)	0.644	3/61(4.9)	1/42(2.4)	0.644
Anti- β2 GPI I IgG	3/61 (4.9)	2/42 (4.9)	0.999	3/61(4.9)	2/42(4.9)	0.999
False-positive VDRL	4 (3.3)	1 (1.1)	0.4	4 (3.3)	1 (1.1)	0.4
Low complement	69 (56.6)	4 (4.5)	< 0.001	74 (60.7)	5 (5.6)	< 0.001
Direct Coombs test	34 (27.9)	6 (6.7)	< 0.001	38 (31.1)	6 (6.7)	< 0.001

The Pearson chi-square test analyzed differences between proportions, and the difference was regarded as statistically significant when $p < 0.05$
No patients had toxic epidermal necrolysis, hypertrophic lupus, mucosal lupus, lupus tumidus, and chilblains lupus. One cSLE case had bullous lupus, another one cSLE had panniculitis, and one control had mononeuritis multiplex at 1-year-follow-up. Anti-β2 glycoprotein-I IgM and IgG were tested in 61/122 (50%) cSLE cases and 42/89 (47.2%) controls, at baseline/first visit and 1-year-follow-up

However, ACR 1997 specificity was higher at first visit (83.2% versus 67.4%, p = 0.004). The number of misclassified patients was similar (44 for EULAR/ACR versus 51 for ACR 1997, $p = 0.15$).

First visit - ACR 1997 versus EULAR/ACR total score ≥ 13

An EULAR/ACR total score ≥ 13, resulted in no statistically significant difference in sensitivity (76.2% versus 70.5% for ACR 1997, $p = 0.189$); and specificity (87.6%

Table 3 Global accuracy for ACR 1997, SLICC and the new EULAR/ACR criteria, at baseline/first visit and 1-year-follow-up

Classification System	Follow-up time	Global accuracy (IC 95%)
ACR 1997	Baseline/First visit	0.830 (0.776–0.884)
	1-year-follow-up	0.933 (0.896–0.969)
EULAR/ACR	Baseline/First visit	0.874 (0.827–0.921)
	1-year-follow-up	0.929 (0.894–0.964)
SLICC	Baseline/First visit	0.910 (0.870–0.949)
	1-year-follow-up	0.952 (0.923–0.982)

Global accuracy was measured through the area under the ROC curve
IC 95–95% confidence interval, *ACR* American College of Rheumatology, *SLICC* Systemic Lupus International Collaborating Clinics criteria, *EULAR/ACR* European League Against Rheumatism (EULAR)/ACR

versus 83.2% for ACR 1997,$p = 0.424$. EULAR/ACR ≥13 resulted in less misclassifications (40 versus 51, $p = 0.023$).

First visit - SLICC versus EULAR/ACR total score ≥ 10
Sensitivities were similar at first visit (89.3% for SLICC versus 89.3%, $p = 0.687$). However, SLICC specificity was higher at first visit (80.9% versus 67.4%, $p = 0.008$), with less misclassifications (30 versus 44, $p = 0.003$).

First visit - SLICC versus EULAR/ACR total score ≥ 13
The higher SLICC sensitivity persisted (89.3% versus 76.2%, $p < 0.001$). There were no differences in specificity (87.6% versus 80.9% for SLICC, $p = 0.109$). There were less misclassifications for SLICC (30 versus 40, $p = 0.032$).

1-year-follow-up - ACR 1997 versus SLICC criteria
Sensitivity (97.5% versus 95.1%, $p = 0.250$), and specificity (76.4% both, $p = 0{,}999$) were similar, as well as the number of misclassifications (24 versus 27, $p = 0.48$).

Global accuracy and cut-off point accuracy were higher for SLICC criteria at both observation periods.

1-year-follow-up - ACR 1997 versus EULAR/ACR total score ≥ 10
EULAR/ACR criteria total score ≥ 10 had similar sensitivity (95.1% for both, $p = 0.999$). However, ACR 1997 specificity again was higher (76.4% versus 58.4%, $p = 0.002$), with less misclassifications (43 versus 27, $p = 0.006$).

1-year-follow-up - ACR 1997 versus EULAR/ACR total score ≥ 13
An EULAR/ACR total score ≥ 13, displayed no statistical significant difference in sensitivity (91.0% versus 95.1% for ACR 1997, $p = 0.063$), or specificity (83.2% versus 76.4% for ACR 1997, $p = 0.146$), or in the number of misdiagnosis (26 versus 27, $p = 0.816$).

1-year-follow-up - SLICC versus EULAR/ACR total score ≥ 10
Sensitivities were similar (97.5% for SLICC versus 95.1%, $p = 0.250$). However, SLICC specificity was higher (76.4% versus 58.4%, $p = 0.001$). There were less misclassifications for SLICC (24 versus 43, $p < 0.001$).

1-year-follow-up-SLICC versus EULAR/ACR total score ≥ 13
The higher SLICC sensitivity persisted (97.5% versus 91.0%, $p = 0.008$). There were no differences in specificity (83.2% versus 76.4% for SLICC, $p = 0.146$) and misclassifications (24 versus 26, $p = 0.636$).

Table 4 (first visit), Table 5 (1-year follow-up) and Additional file 1: Tables S1-S5 summarizes comparative performance measures of the three classification criteria sets.

Discussion

Recently it was published that the new EULAR/ACR could be more sensitive and specific for adult SLE classification (especially for initial classification) than previous criteria sets. Concerning the need for more specific criteria for cSLE classification, we compared three available classification criteria sets. To the best of our knowledge, this is the first study regarding the assessment of performance among three classification systems (ACR 1997, SLICC and especially the new EULAR/ACR criteria) applied exclusively to cSLE patients, in two different observation periods (first visit and 1-year-follow-up).

Few studies have evaluated the performance of different SLE classification criteria in cSLE, showing variables results. For cSLE, three studies demonstrated that SLICC criteria classify patients earlier than ACR 1997 [18–20]. In the multicentre European study by Sag and colleagues, the sensitivity of SLICC was higher (98.7% versus 85.3%, $p < 0.001$) but specificity was lower (76.6% versus 93.4%, $p < 0.001$) compared to ACR 1997, at time of diagnosis [18]. The lower specificity of SLICC criteria was mainly attributed to the fulfillment by controls with hemolytic-uremic syndrome or JDM [18]. Our group has previously assessed ACR 1997 versus SLICC classification at first visit and 1-year-follow-up, in a Brazilian single center cSLE cohort. Sensitivity for SLICC was higher than ACR 1997, 82.7% versus 58.0% at first visit ($p < 0.001$), but similar at 1-year (96.3% versus 91.3%, $p = 0.125$). Specificity was not significantly different [19]. The UK juvenile SLE cohort evaluated only sensitivity, and SLICC also were more sensitive than ACR 1997, both at diagnosis (92.9% versus 84.1%, $p < 0.001$) and at last visit (100% versus 92%, $p < 0.001$) [20].

Hartman and colleagues [17] conducted a systematic literature review for studies comparing ACR 1997 and SLICC criteria with clinical diagnosis in adult SLE and cSLE patients with disease duration up to 5 years. A meta-analysis estimated the sensitivity and specificity of these criteria sets and their variables. Four cSLE studies

Table 4 Performance measures for ACR 1997, SLICC and new EULAR/ACR criteria, at baseline/first visit

Classification System	Cut-off point	Sensitivity (IC 95%)	Specificity (IC 95%)	PPV (%)	NPV (%)	Cut-off point accuracy (IC 95%)
ACR 1997	≥ 4	70.5%	83.2%	85.2%	67.3%	75.8
	criteria	(61.6–78.4)	(73.7–90.3)			(69.5–81.4)
EULAR/ACR	Total	87.7	67.4	78.7	80.0	79.2
	score ≥ 10	(80.5–93.0)	(56.7–77.0)			(73.0–84.4)
	Total	76.2	87.6	89.4	72.9	81.0
	score ≥ 13	(67.9–83.5)	(79.0–93.7)			(75.1–86.1)
SLICC	≥ 4	89.3	80.9	86.5	84.7	85.8
	criteria	(82.5–94.2)	(71.2–88.5)			(80.3–90.2)

IC 95–95% confidence interval, *PPV* positive predictive value, *NPV* negative predictive value, *ACR* American College of Rheumatology, *SLICC* Systemic Lupus International Collaborating Clinics criteria, *EULAR/ACR* European League Against Rheumatism (EULAR)/ACR

(568 cSLE patients, 339 controls), including our group previous study [19], were included, showing a higher sensitivity for early classification with SLICC criteria (99.9% versus 84.3%), but lower specificity than ACR 1997 (82.0% versus 94.1%).

In this present study, the lower SLICC specificity was not found, in contrast with most previous studies. Some reasons to explain why SLICC specificity was comparable to ACR1997 and higher than EULAR/ACR ≥ 10 in our study might be a different control group composition, the assessment of performance in distinct observation periods and especially the cut-off point for total EULAR/ACR score derived from our data.

SLICC criteria also exhibited the highest sensitivity for earlier classification (at first visit), in comparison to ACR 1997 ($p < 0.001$) and EULAR/ACR ≥ 13 ($p < 0.001$), but similar to EULAR/ACR proposed total score ≥ 10 (89.3% versus 87.7%, $p = 0.687$).

EULAR/ACR total score cut-off point influenced its performance measures. The selection of a EULAR/ACR total score ≥ 13, as determined by ROC curve analysis, against the initially proposed ≥10 score, resulted in higher specificity, positive predictive value, and accuracy. SLICC criteria exhibited higher global accuracy at both observation periods. Concerning the EULAR/ACR total score cut-off point being compared (whether ≥10 or ≥ 13), application of SLICC criteria still better scored in cut-off point accuracy both at first visit and at 1-year-follow-up, in our cSLE population.

The expanded scope of clinical (especially cutaneous and CNS manifestations) and immunologic manifestations included in SLICC criteria, besides the allocation of cytopenias and antibodies into separate criterion might have allowed a higher sensitivity, especially earlier in the disease course. The SLICC rule to classify only patients that have at least one immunologic criterion, preventing SLE classification based solely on clinical manifestations, and the ending of the "double counting" of photosensitive malar rash as two criteria (as in ACR 1997), may have increased SLICC specificity.

The differences in performance among those three sets of classification criteria might be due to changes either in the definition of organ involvement, to cut-off points for positive autoantibodies or to the form in which several clinical manifestations and laboratory parameters are gathered within each criteria set.

We are aware that this study is limited by the retrospective design and the relatively small number of patients and controls included. However, the extraction and collection of data by two authors, and the confirmation by the other three authors, before criteria set scoring, minimized this methodological limitation.

Table 5 Performance measures for ACR 1997, SLICC and new EULAR/ACR criteria, at 1-year-follow-up

Classification System	Cut-off point	Sensitivity (IC 95%)	Specificity (IC 95%)	PPV (%)	NPV (%)	Cut-off point accuracy (IC 95%)
ACR 1997	≥ 4 criteria	95.1	76.4	84.7	91.9	87.2
		(89.6–98.2)	(66.2–84.8)			(81.9–91.4)
EULAR/ACR	Total score ≥ 10	95.1	58.4	75.8	89.7	79.6
		(89.6–98.2)	(47.5–68.8)			(73.6–84.8)
	Total score ≥ 13	91.0	83.2	88.1	87.1	87.7
		(84.4–95.4)	(73.7–90.3)			(82.5–91.8)
SLICC	≥ 4 criteria	97.5	76.4	85.0	95.8	88.6
		(93.0–99.5)	(66.2–84.8)			(83.6–92.6)

IC 95–95% confidence interval, *PPV* positive predictive value, *NPV* negative predictive value, *ACR* American College of Rheumatology, *SLICC* Systemic Lupus International Collaborating Clinics criteria, *EULAR/ACR* European League Against Rheumatism (EULAR)/ACR

Second, a structural problem in designing and validating classification criteria, and thereby in interpreting our study, is an inherent lack of an objective diagnosis as the standard of reference other than clinical diagnosis, so that the treating physician's diagnosis, is still adopted by most studies. We also decided to use as our standard of reference, the diagnosis consolidated during continuous follow-up of all patients by a group of highly experienced pediatric rheumatologists. It may be argued that this could lead to inconsistency; yet, it does allow evaluation of classification criteria in a real-world setting. Finally, we decided to compose our control group with rheumatic diseases that impose difficult differential diagnosis with JSLE, simulating the daily clinical practice; however, we did not include controls with undifferentiated disease or overlapping syndromes.

Considering the peculiarities of cSLE (more severe presentation and course, higher rates of disease activity and cumulative damage, higher frequency of atypical and constitutional manifestations) and taking into account that these three sets of criteria were developed in adult SLE, it should be considered modifications to increase early sensitivity and specificity for cSLE classification.

Conclusion

In this cSLE population, SLICC criteria better scored at first visit and 1-year-follow-up. The adoption of a EULAR/ACR total score ≥ 13 in this study, against the initially proposed ≥10 score, was most appropriate to classify cSLE. Further studies are necessary to address if SLICC criteria might allow fulfillment of cSLE classification earlier in disease course and may be more inclusive of cSLE subjects for clinical studies.

Additional file

Additional file 1: Table S1. Comparison among ACR 1997 and SLICC criteria. **Table S2.** Comparison among ACR 1997 and EULAR/ACR criteria (total score ≥ 10). **Table S3.** Comparison among ACR 1997 and EULAR/ACR criteria (total score ≥ 13). **Table S4.** Comparison among EULAR/ACR (total score ≥10) and SLICC criteria. **Table S5.** Comparison among EULAR/ACR (total score ≥13) and SLICC criteria.

Abbreviations

APS: Antiphospholipid syndrome; JDM: Juvenile dermatomyositis; JSS: Juvenile systemic scleroderma; MCTD: Mixed connective tissue disease; SoJIA: Systemic onset juvenile idiopathic arthritis; SS: Sjögren syndrome

Acknowledgements

We acknowledge Dr. Mariana Aires M.D. PhD and Dr. Elaine Sobral M.D. PhD, for helpful inputs.

Authors' contributions

ARF, MCFR, FRS, MGPL and SKFO contributed to the conception and design of study. ARF, MCFR, FRS, MGPL and SKFO contributed to acquisition of data. ARF and MGPL contributed to analysis of data and with the interpretations of data. ARF and MGPL were the major contributors in writing the manuscript. All authors revised the manuscript critically for intellectual content. All authors read and approved the final manuscript and the listing of authors.

Author details

[1]Pediatric Rheumatology Unit, Instituto de Puericultura e Pediatria Martagão Gesteira, Universidade Federal do Rio de Janeiro (UFRJ), Rua Bruno Lobo, 50- Cidade Universitária, Rio de Janeiro, Brazil. [2]Internal Medicine Post-graduation Program, Faculty of Medicine, Universidade Federal do Rio de Janeiro (UFRJ), Rio de Janeiro, Brazil.

References

1. Hedrich CM, Smith EMD, Beresford MW. Juvenile-onset systemic lupus erythematosus (jSLE)-Pathophysiological concepts and treatment options. Best Pract Res Clin Rheumatol. 2017;31:488–504.
2. Harry O, Yasin S, Brunner H. Childhood-Onset Systemic Lupus Erythematosus: A Review and Update. J Pediatr. 2018;196:22–30 e2.
3. Brunner HI, Gladman DD, Ibanez D, Urowitz MD, Silverman ED. Difference in disease features between childhood-onset and adult-onset systemic lupus erythematosus. Arthritis Rheum. 2008;58:556–62.
4. Bundhun PK, Kumari A, Huang F. Differences in clinical features observed between childhood-onset versus adult-onset systemic lupus erythematosus: A systematic review and meta-analysis. Medicine (Baltimore). 2017;96:e8086.
5. Hochberg MC. Updating the American College of Rheumatology revised criteria for the classification of systemic lupus erythematosus. Arthritis Rheum. 1997;40:1725.
6. Larosa M, Iaccarino L, Gatoo M, Punzi L, Doria A. Advances in the diagnosis and classification of systemic lupus erythematosus. Expert Rev Clin Immunol. 2016;12:1309–20.
7. Petri M, Orbai AM, Alarcon GS, Gordon C, Merrill JT, Fortin PR, et al. Derivation and validation of the systemic lupus international collaborating clinics classification criteria for systemic lupus erythematosus. Arthritis Rheum. 2012;64:2677–86.
8. Aringer M, Dörner T, Leuchten N, Johnson SR. Toward new criteria for systemic lupus erythematosus—a standpoint. Lupus. 2016;25:805–11.
9. Tedeschi SK, Johnson SR, Boumpas DA, Daikh D, Dörner T, Jayne D, et al. Developing and refining new candidate criteria for SLE classification: an international collaboration. Arthritis Care Res (Hoboken). 2018;70:571–81.
10. Aringer M, Costenbader KH, Brinks R, Boumpas D, Daikh D, Jayne D, et al. Validation of New Systemic Lupus Erythematosus Classification Criteria. In: 2018 ACR/AHRP annual meeting. Chicago; 2018. https://acrabstracts.org. Accessed 24 Oct 2018.
11. Aringer M, Dörner T. Systemic Lupus Erythematosus (SLE) - New Classification Criteria [in German]. Dtsch Med Wochenschr. 2018;143:811–4.
12. Mosca M, Costenbader KH, Johnson SR, Lorenzoni V, Sebastiani GD, Hoyer BF, et al. How do patients with newly diagnosed systemic lupus erythematosus present? A multicenter cohort of early systemic lupus erythematosus to inform the development of new classification criteria. Arthritis Rheumatol. 2019;71(1):91–8.
13. Amezcua-Guerra LM, Higuera-Ortiz V, Arteaga-García U, Gallegos-Nava S, Hübbe-Tena C. Performance of the 2012 SLICC and the 1997 ACR classification criteria for systemic lupus erythematosus in a real-life scenario. Arthritis Care Res (Hoboken). 2015;67:437–41.
14. Inês L, Silva C, Galindo M, López-Longo FJ, Terroso G, Romão VC, et al. Classification of Systemic Lupus Erythematosus: Systemic Lupus International Collaborating Clinics versus American College of Rheumatology Criteria. A Comparative Study of 2.055 patients from a real-life, international systemic lupus erythematosus cohort. Arthritis Care Res (Hoboken). 2015;67:1180–5.
15. Ighe A, Dahlström O, Skogh T, Sjöwall C. Application of the 2012 Systemic Lupus International Collaborating Clinics classification criteria to patients in a regional Swedish systemic lupus erythematosus register. Arthritis Res Ther. 2015;17:3.
16. Oku K, Atsumi T, Akiyama Y, Amano H, Azuma N, Bohgaki T, et al. Evaluation of the alternative classification criteria of systemic lupus erythematosus established by systemic lupus international collaborating clinics (SLICC). Mod Rheumatol. 2018;28:642–8.
17. Hartman EAR, Van Royen-Kerkhof A, Jacobs JWG, Welsing PMJ, Fritsch-Stork RDE. Performance of the 2012 systemic lupus international collaborating clinics classification criteria versus the 1997 American College of Rheumatology Classification Criteria in adult and juvenile systemic lupus

erythematosus. A systematic review and meta-analysis. Autoimmun Rev. 2018;17:316–22.

18. Sag E, Tartaglione A, Batu ED, Ravelli A, Khalil SM, Marks SD, Ozen S, et al. Performance of the new SLICC classification criteria in childhood systemic lupus erythematosus: a multicentre study. Clin Exp Rheumatol. 2014;32:440–4.
19. Fonseca AR, Gaspar-Elsas MIC, Land MGP, de Oliveira SKF. Comparison between three systems of classification criteria in juvenile systemic lupus erythematous. Rheumatology (Oxford). 2015;54:241–7.
20. Lythgoe H, Morgan T, Heaf E, Lloyd O, Al-Abadi E, Armon K, et al. Evaluation of the ACR and SLICC classification criteria in juvenile-onset systemic lupus erythematosus: a longitudinal analysis. Lupus. 2017;26:1285–90.
21. Schmajuk G, Hoyer BF, Aringer M, Johnson SR, Daikh DI, Dörner T. Multicenter Delphi Exercise Reveals Important Key Items for Classifying Systemic Lupus Erythematosus. Arthritis Care Res (Hoboken). 2018;70:1488–94.
22. Leuchten N, Hoyer A, Brinks R, Schoels M, Schneider M, Smolen J, et al. Performance of anti-nuclear antibodies for classifying systemic lupus erythematosus: a systematic literature review and meta-regression of diagnostic data. Arthritis Care Res (Hoboken). 2018;70:428–38.
23. Pisetsky DS, Lipsky PE. The Role of ANA Determinations in Classification Criteria for SLE. Arthritis Care Res (Hoboken). 2018. https://doi.org/10.1002/acr.23559.
24. Petty RE, Southwood TR, Manners P, Baum J, Glass DN, Goldenberg J, et al. International league of associations for rheumatology classification of juvenile idiopathic arthritis: second revision, Edmonton, 2001. J Rheumatol. 2004;31:390–2.
25. Bohan A, Peter JB. Polymyositis and dermatomyositis (first of two parts). N Engl J Med. 1975;292:344–7.
26. Zulian F, Woo P, Athreya BH, Laxer RM, Medsger TA Jr, Lehman TJ, et al. The Pediatric Rheumatology European Society/American College of Rheumatology/European League against Rheumatism provisional classification criteria for juvenile systemic sclerosis. Arthritis Rheum. 2007;57: 203–12.
27. Bartunkova J, Sediva A, Vencovsky J, Tesar V. Primary Sjögren's syndrome in children and adolescents: proposal for diagnostic criteria. Clin Exp Rheumatol. 1999;17:381–6.
28. Miyakis S, Lockshin MD, Atsumi T, Branch DW, Brey RL, Cervera R, et al. International consensus statement on an update of the classification criteria for definite antiphospholipid syndrome. J Thromb Haemost. 2006;4:295–306.
29. Kasukawa R, Tojo T, Miyawaki S. Preliminary diagnostic criteria for classification of mixed connective tissue disease. In: Kasukawa R, Sharp GC, editors. Mixed connective tissue disease and antinuclear antibodies. Amsterdam: Elsevier; 1987. p. 41–7.
30. Šimundić AM. Measures of Diagnostic Accuracy: Basic Definitions. EJIFCC. 2009;20(19):203–11.

6

Risk factors for cytomegalovirus disease in systemic lupus erythematosus (SLE)

Hui Min Charlotte Choo[1,4*†], Wen Qi Cher[1†], Yu Heng Kwan[2] and Warren Weng Seng Fong[3]

Abstract

Background: Cytomegalovirus (CMV) is an opportunistic pathogen causing reactivation and disease in Systemic Lupus Erythematosus (SLE) patients. This study aims to systematically review the literature for risk factors associated with CMV disease in SLE patients, in order to identify those more susceptible to CMV infection during their treatment.

Methods: A systematic review was conducted on 4 different search engines and via hand search until May 2017. Studies were included after quality assessment via the Standard Quality Assessment Criteria for Evaluating Primary Research Papers from a Variety of Fields (HTA KMET).

Results: Two studies on CMV disease were included. Elevated CMV viral load, higher steroid doses, use of immunosuppressants and disease duration were the most commonly associated risk factors for CMV disease.

Conclusion: High CMV viral loads, longer SLE disease duration and higher steroid doses were associated with CMV disease. Further studies studying the risk of treatment drugs and role of interventions in the development of CMV infection are needed.

Keywords: Risk factors, Cytomegalovirus infection, Systemic lupus erythematosus (SLE), Systematic review

Introduction

Human cytomegalovirus (CMV), under the class of beta-herpesvirus, stays latent in an infected host throughout its life and is rarely reactivated to cause clinical illness. However, it is an important opportunistic pathogen causing morbidity and mortality in immunocompromised patients [1]. Across the world, the overall prevalence of CMV ranges from 40 to 100% [2], and seropositivity for CMV is shown to be higher in SLE compared to the general population [3].

CMV can manifest in various ways. CMV may remain undetected as a latent infection in immunocompetent hosts, or persist as asymptomatic low level CMV viremia. CMV dissemination and disease may present subtly with fever and lethargy, or a myriad of atypical manifestations, most commonly with respiratory or gastrointestinal symptoms and SLE flare-like presentations [4]. CMV disease subsequently leads to damage of multiple organ systems such as lung, liver, gastrointestinal tract and retina [5]. Greater CMV viral loads has been shown to correlate with increased risk of developing CMV disease in Human-immunodeficiency Virus (HIV) and transplant patients [6, 7], but this has not been demonstrated conclusively in autoimmune disease patients.

Several studies and case reports have highlighted CMV reactivation, resulting in CMV antigenemia or disease, as a concern during treatment of rheumatic diseases, particularly SLE [8–11]. This occurs as the treatment of SLE and autoimmune disease often involves chronic use of immunosuppressive therapy [12], which is a potential risk factor for CMV infection and disease [8, 13–15]. This is of significant concern as aside from developing end-organ CMV disease as reported in aforementioned case reports, it can also lead to significant mortality. In a recently

* Correspondence: choo.charlotte@gmail.com
†Hui Min Charlotte Choo and Wen Qi Cher are contributed equally to this work
[1]Yong Loo Lin School of Medicine, National University of Singapore, Singapore, Singapore
[4]Department of Internal Medicine, Singapore General Hospital, Academia Building, Level 4, 20 College Road, Singapore 169856, Singapore
Full list of author information is available at the end of the article

published retrospective 26-year review of death causes and pathogen analysis of SLE, infections, including cytomegalovirus, was amongst the top three most frequent causes of death in SLE patients [16].

While there are few studies which looked at the clinical characteristics of CMV infection in patients with rheumatic diseases, there is no systematic review till date which comprehensively studies the risk factors of CMV disease in the SLE population. Our study thus aims to systematically review the literature for risk factors associated with CMV disease in patients with SLE.

Methods

Study design

A systematic review was conducted using the Preferred Reporting Items for Systematic Review and Meta-Analysis (PRISMA).

Studies in our review included patients diagnosed with SLE using the 1997 or 1982 American College of Rheumatology criteria [17, 18]. CMV disease was defined as positive CMV antigenemia assay with associated CMV clinical syndromes, with or without biopsy-proven CMV in organ tissue samples, either via a positive CMV culture or immunohistochemical staining, or a bronchoalveolar lavage fluid specimen with a positive CMV immunohistochemical staining or detection of CMV DNA via PCR [19]. We included primary studies which fulfilled the above definition of CMV disease [20].

Identification and selection of studies

Literature search was conducted on PubMed®, Embase®, Cochrane Library and Web of Science®. The search was restricted to articles in English and in humans. The search strategy included MeSH terms and free text of related terms relating to risk factors (clinical characteristic, rate, association, burden), SLE (lupus, systemic lupus erythematosus), CMV (cytomegalovirus), disease and infection (reactivation, infection, transmission). Further hand searches were conducted using references of related articles. The start date of the search was unrestricted and end date was till May 2017. Two authors, Kwan YH and Cher WQ independently reviewed the articles and applied the inclusion criteria. Disagreements were resolved through discussion or by a third reviewer (Choo HMC) if necessary.

Inclusion and exclusion

This systematic review included peer-reviewed publications of both randomized controlled trials and observational data. Observational data included quantitative epidemiological studies and all forms of cohort, case control and cross-sectional studies.

We excluded studies not written in English, not concerned with human subjects, case reports, case series ($N \leq 10$), systematic reviews and meta-analyses and grey literature such as opinion pieces, editorial letters, abstracts, comments, conference proceedings and reviews that were not systematic.

Data extraction

Evidence related to cytomegalovirus disease in SLE patients were included. Relevant data including author, year of publication, type of study, country, duration, study size, patient demographics, type of medications (steroids and immuno-suppressants), duration and severity of autoimmune disease were extracted.

Methodological data quality assessment

The quality of the studies included was appraised by two independent reviewers (Cher WQ, Choo HMC) using the criteria proposed by the HTA KMET (Standard Quality Assessment Criteria for Evaluating Primary Research Papers from a Variety of Fields) [21]. This tool was chosen because it captures the range in methodological quality and risk of bias across both qualitative and quantitative studies. The two reviewers applied a 14-item checklist for quantitative studies and a 10-item checklist for qualitative studies to assess study quality. The score helps to objectively quantify the quality of each study by taking the observed agreement score between two independent reviewers with maximum score of 1.0 (100%) with higher scores given to studies with better study design and accuracy of data. We did not exclude any studies from our review based on quality.

Results

We reviewed 344 distinct titles and excluded 110 based on title screening. We assessed 234 potentially relevant abstracts and downloaded 126 full text articles. 2 studies were included in qualitative synthesis (Fig. 1). Reasons for exclusion of reviewed articles were included in Additional file 1: Table S1.

Among the total of 90 SLE patients across the primary studies, most were females (range from 77.7 to 81%), age ranging from 31.7 to 52.0 years. Both were cross-sectional studies. W. P Tsai (2012)'s study included 38 SLE patients while Yu and Li et al. (2016)'s study included patients with different rheumatological diseases, of which 52 out of 142 (37%) were SLE patients.

Reporting of study quality

Both primary studies had a quality score of more than 0.75 (Table 1). Inter-rater agreement for the primary studies were largely similar and discrepancies were discussed between the two reviewers until consensus was reached.

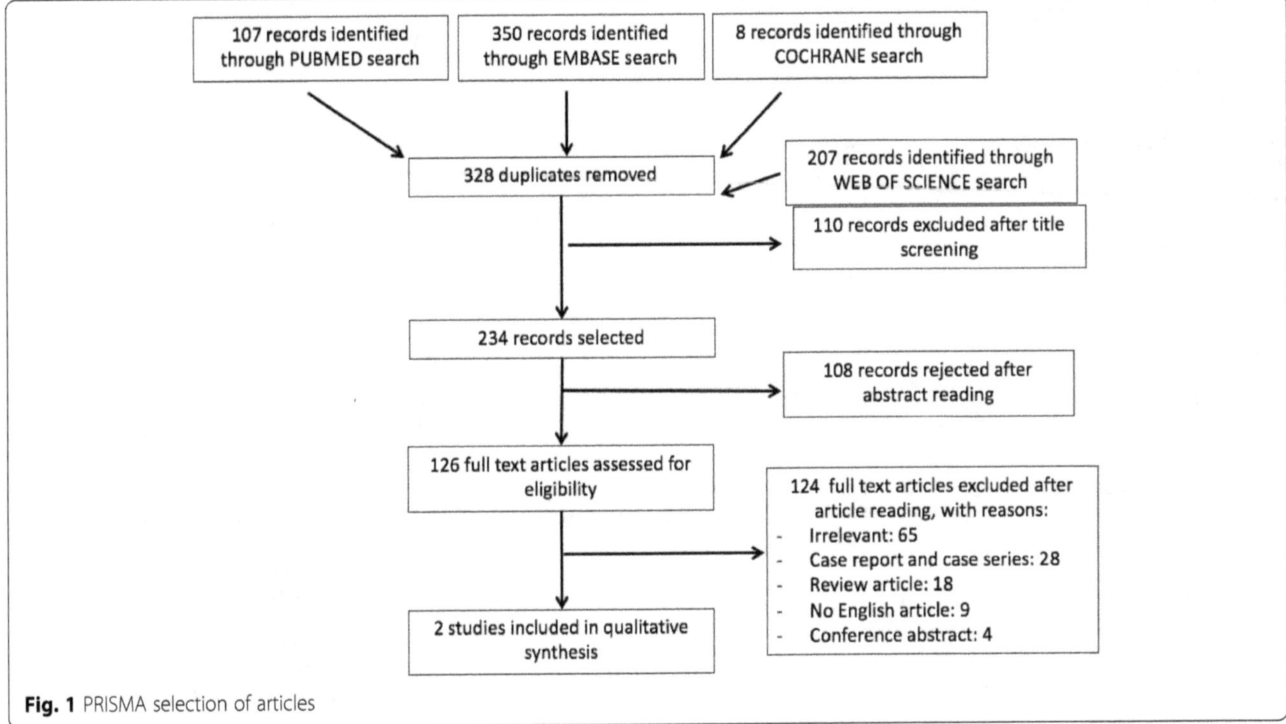

Fig. 1 PRISMA selection of articles

Predictors for CMV disease

The risk factors for CMV disease in rheumatic disease patients are reported in Table 2.

Lymphopenia

Yu and Li et al. (2016) found that 73 patients with CMV pneumonia had a lower lymphocyte count compared to 69 asymptomatic patients [median (range) 0.6 (0.1–4.0) × 10^9/L vs 1.2 (0.1–5.7) × 10^9/L respectively, $p < 0.05$] [22]. Receiver Operating Characteristic (ROC) curve analysis indicated that when CD^{4+} T cell count was < 0.39 × 10^9/L, patients with rheumatic diseases were at high risk for symptomatic CMV infection, with a sensitivity of 77.5% and specificity of 87.5%.

On the other hand, lymphocyte count was not significantly associated with CMV disease in W.P. Tsai et al. (2012)'s study. Lymphocyte count was not statistically different between patients with CMV disease compared to those without CMV disease [mean (S.D.) 743 (615) mm^3 vs 1062 (767) mm^3, respectively, $p = 0.175$] [23].

Elevated CMV viral loads

Yu and Li et al. (2016) found that the mean (S.D.) CMV DNA value was higher in the patients with CMV pneumonia compared to asymptomatic patients [3.68 (1.90) × 10^4 copies/ml vs 0.60 (0.35) × 10^4 copies/ml, respectively, $p < 0.01$] [22]. ROC curve analysis showed that a level of 1.75 × 10^4 copies/ml was the optimal threshold for prediction of CMV-associated symptoms, with a sensitivity of 84.9% and specificity of 98.6% [22].

Treatment drugs

Both studies consistently reported higher corticosteroid doses being related with CMV disease. Yu and Li et al. (2016) noted that higher corticosteroid doses were correlated with CMV pneumonia [22]. The prednisolone dose was higher in the CMV pneumonia group compared to the asymptomatic group [median (range) 32(4–100) mg/day vs 20(1–50) mg/day, respectively, $p < 0.010$]. Similarly, the total prednisolone dose in the recent three months prior to diagnosis was higher in the CMV pneumonia group compared to the asymptomatic group [median (range) 2.8(0.1–9.0) g vs 1.8 (0.1–4.6) g, respectively, $p < 0.01$]. Likewise, in W.P. Tsai et al. (2012)'s study of 38 SLE patients, the CMV disease group received a higher prednisolone dose than the non-CMV disease group [mean (S.D.) 25.9 (17.1) mg/day vs 9.0 (4.1) mg/day, respectively, $p = 0.006$] [23].

Apart from steroids, the use of other immunosuppressants were also associated with CMV disease. W.P. Tsai et al. (2012) noted a higher percentage of Azathioprine use 1 month prior to admission in the CMV disease group than the non-CMV disease group (7/20 cases vs 1/18, respectively, $p = 0.045$) [23].

Similarly, Yu and Li et al. (2016) found that use of immunosuppressants was more common in the CMV pneumonia group than the asymptomatic group (79% vs 58%, $p < 0.010$). For instance, MMF and Cyclosporine A were more frequently used in patients who

Table 1 Characteristics of studies looking at risk factors for CMV disease in SLE patients

	Yu Xue (2016) [29]	W.P Tsai (2012) [22]
Number of SLE patients with CMV disease (n and %)	Not known	38/38 (100%)
Number of SLE patients in study population (*n* and %)	52/142 (36.6%)	20/38 (52.5%) SLE patients are CMV positive
Study type	CS	CS
Study Duration (years)	8	Not stated
Quality review	0.82	0.75
Country	China	Taiwan
Gender (% females)	81%	77.7%
Age (years)	Mean (SD): Asymptomatic: 52.0 (14.7) Symptomatic: 48.5 (16.7)	CMV SLE group: 35.6 (12.0 SD) Non-CMV SLE group: 31.7 (11.0 SD)
How CMV disease was diagnosed	Positive CMV DNA PCR AND CMV pneumonia: clinical and radiological findings	Positive CMV antigenemia (CMV pp65 antigenemia or CMV IgM) assay and any of the following: fever, malaise, leukopenia, Diarrhea, retinitis, pneumonia, or hepatitis, a tissue biopsy specimen with a CMV-positive culture or immunohisto-chemical staining, or a bronchoalveolar lavage (BAL) fluid specimen (6 out of 21 patients) with a positive CMV shell vial culture or the detection of CMV DNA by the polymerase chain reaction (PCR)
Significant risk factors	- Male gender - SLE disease duration - Bacteria pneumonia - BUN - CD4+ T cell count - Co-infection - Creatinine - Elevated ALP, ALT - Fungal infection - Lymphocyte count - γ-GT - Cyclophosphamide - Cyclosporine - Immunosuppressants - Mycophenolate mofetil - Prednisolone average dose - Prednisolone use for recent 3 months	- Prednisolone (mg/day) - Azathioprine (50-100 mg/day) use
Non-significant factors	- Age - CD8+ T cell count - AST - Leukocyte count - Neutrophil count - Duration of prednisolone therapy (months)	- Age - Age of disease onset - Disease duration - Lymphocyte count - SLEDAI score on admission - Positive bacterial culture in blood or sputum

CS Cross sectional, *CMV* Cytomegalovirus, *SLE* Systemic Lupus Erythematosus Disease, *SLEDAI* Systemic Lupus Erythematosus Disease Activity Index, *BUN* Blood urea nitrogen, *ALP* Alanine Phosphatase, *ALT* Alanine transaminase, *AST* Aspartate transaminase, *γ-GT* Gamma-Glutamyl Transferase (GGT)

developed CMV pneumonia than asymptomatic patients ($p < 0.050$) [22].

SLE disease characteristics

Yu and Li et al. (2016) found a positive correlation between SLE disease duration and CMV disease. Patients with CMV pneumonia had a longer SLE disease duration compared to patients without disease [median (range) 8 (0.03–360) months vs 3 (0.25–156) months, respectively, $p < 0.05$] [22].

Discussion

SLE is a chronic autoimmune disease which can be complicated by cytomegalovirus disease during its course but little attention has been given to investigate the factors that predispose SLE patients to this opportunistic infection. To the best of our knowledge, this is the first systematic review to explore the risk factors of developing CMV disease in SLE patients.

Elevated CMV viral loads has found to highly correlate with CMV disease. The presence of CMV antigen positive cells in bloodstream may reflect dissemination of

Table 2 Risk factors associated with CMV disease in the SLE population (2 studies)

RISK FACTOR	Positive correlation with CMV disease		Negative correlation with CMV disease		Neutral correlation with CMV disease	
	No. of supporting studies	Type of studies	No. of supporting studies	Type of studies	No. of supporting studies	Type of studies
1. Demographics						
Age					I II	CS CS
Age of disease onset					II	CS
Gender – Male			I	CS		
2. Clinical features including autoimmune disease characteristics						
SLE disease duration	I	CS			II	CS
SLE disease score/severity					II	CS
3. Laboratory characteristics						
Bacterial pneumonia	I	CS				
BUN	I	CS				
CD4 count			I	CS		
CD8 count					I	CS
Co-infection	I	CS				
Creatinine			I	CS		
Elevated ALP	I	CS				
Elevated ALT	I	CS				
Elevated AST					I	CS
Elevated CMV viral load	I	CS				
Elevated CMV IgG levels	II	CS				
Fungal infection	I	CS				
LDH	I	CS				
Leukopenia					I	CS
Lymphopenia	I	CS			II	CS
Neutropenia					I	CS
Positive blood/sputum bacterial culture					II	CS
γ-GT	I	CS				
4. Treatment						
Azathioprine	II	CS				
Cyclosporine	I	CS				
Cyclophosphamide	I	CS				
Mycophenolate	I	CS				
Immunosuppressants	I	CS				
Prednisolone	II	CS				
Duration of prednisolone use					I	CS
Prednisolone dose in last 3 months			II	CS		
Glucocorticoid dose	I	CS				

CS Cross sectional, *BUN* Blood urea nitrogen, *ALP* Alanine Phosphatase, *ALT* Alanine transaminase, *AST* Aspartate transaminase
γ-GT Gamma-Glutamyl Transferase (GGT)

CMV in host system, leading to potential CMV end-organ disease. In a study in bone marrow transplant patients, multivariate logistic regression analysis found that only elevated viral load remained a significant risk factor for CMV disease [24]. Similarly, in patients with Acquired-immune deficiency syndrome (AIDS), elevated levels of CMV antigenemia during follow-up was found to be associated with CMV disease [7]. In a cross-sectional study of 74 SLE patients, Takizawa Y. (2008) found that CMV viral load was higher in those with CMV disease (n = 117) compared to asymptomatic patients (n = 34) [median (range), 10.1 (0.0–2998.0)/105 PMNs vs 4.0 (1.3–1144.4)/105 PMNs, respectively, p = 0.001] [25]. A higher median (range) CMV antigenemia count of 5.6 (1.3–1144.4)/10^5 PMNs by ROC curve analysis predicted that patients have a higher risk of developing CMV disease with a higher mortality rate [25]. Future research with larger sample size can be useful to determine a cut-off CMV antigenemia level that predicts development of CMV disease in SLE patients and this can subsequently guide management on use of prophylactic therapy against CMV disease based on CMV antigenemia levels. This practice of pre-emptive therapy has been adopted as standard of care in patients following hematopoietic stem cell transplantation cases with CMV antigenemia or CMV seropositivity [26].

There are studies which have also looked at risk factors leading to elevated CMV viral load. In Fujimoto D. (2013)'s cross-sectional study on patients with autoimmune diseases, a multi-variate analysis conducted found that lymphopenia < 700 mm^3, (OR 34.44, 95% CI 7.82–151.66, p = 0.001), SLE (OR 6.71, 95% CI 1.23–36.49, p = 0.028) and Polymyositis/Dermatomyositis (OR 10.62, 95% CI 1.41–79.77, p = 0.022) were significantly associated with elevated CMV viral load [27].

Lymphocytes play a role in host cellular immune response against CMV, as seen in previous studies looking at human immunodeficiency virus (HIV) patients and stem cell transplant patients [28, 29]. Lymphopenia could thus suggest CMV reactivation, as CMV can lead to bone marrow suppression [19].

The mechanism of action of SLE treatment drugs can also explain the process of CMV disease in SLE patients [30]. Cyclophosphamide suppresses lymphocyte proliferation and function, thus increasing the risk of CMV reactivation. Cyclophosphamide use was found to be a risk factor for the reactivation of CMV in glomerulonephritis patients [31]. While the mechanism of action of these immunosuppressive drugs used in treatment of SLE makes development of CMV infection highly probable, other considerations such as the immunosuppression dose, duration of treatment and combination therapy with other immunosuppressive drugs may play a bigger role in the pathogenesis of CMV infection and disease in SLE patients. These factors were not sufficiently explored in the primary studies, thus it remains inconclusive.

Of note, two studies which looked into use of mycophenolate mofetil (MMF) as a risk factor for CMV antigenaemia consistently reported positive association [22, 32]. In a recent small case series, 3 out of the 4 SLE patients with disseminated CMV infection had prior treatment with 3 g of MMF daily in addition to concurrent use of other immunosuppressive drugs [9]. In another randomized controlled trial comparing Everolimus to MMF in renal transplant patients found that viral infections, particularly CMV infection increased in the MMF group (20% in MMF group compared to 6–7% in Everolimus group, p = 0.0001) [33]. This shows that use of MMF can be associated with higher incidence of CMV infection, and care should be taken to monitor for CMV disease when using MMF.

Our systematic review has its limitations due to the intrinsic nature of the primary studies. Firstly, there are only a small number of studies relevant to our research question. The two primary studies were conducted in Taiwan and China, thus limiting the scope to Asian patients. Secondly, the studies did not consistently analyze all of the same factors and stopped at univariable analysis and did not proceed with a multi-variable logistic regression. Thirdly, the baseline characteristics of SLE patients were variable across studies, and one of the two studies grouped SLE patients together with other rheumatic diseases patients in its analysis. This is a limitation as certain rheumatic diseases may be more predisposed to development of CMV disease than others. Lastly, treatment regimens and drugs doses were not standardized across studies, due to the heterogenous mix of different rheumatological disease patients, thus it was difficult to draw meaningful conclusions about treatment drugs and their implication on development of CMV disease. Both studies are also cross-sectional studies, thus it only captures data at one time-point and we are unable to know if the SLE subjects in the study subsequently developed CMV disease at a later time point.

Conclusion

This systematic review identified high CMV viral loads, lymphopenia and and higher corticosteroid doses to be associated with development of CMV disease in patients with SLE. Overall quality of studies ranged from 0.75 to 0.82. As reflected from our systemic review, there are few studies that have looked into the risk factors of developing CMV disease in SLE patients despite its prevalence in the SLE population. Studies on the risk of different treatment drugs and regimes on development of CMV disease are also lacking and is a potential for future research. These will be needed before guidelines on surveillance and pre-emptive treatment of CMV infection in SLE patients can be developed.

Additional file

Additional file 1: Table S1. Reasons for exclusion of reviewed articles

Acknowledgements

We would like to acknowledge Pang Jie Kie for her assistance in the formatting process of this manuscript. Both authors (Hui Min Charlotte CHOO and Wen Qi CHER) had equal contribution.

Authors' contribution

WF is the principal investigator of the study while WQC, CHMC and YHK are co-investigators. WQC and CHMC contributed equally to the study. They are responsible for the study. design, reviewing of articles and preparation of the manuscript. YHK and WF mentored the entire data collection, processing and manuscript preparation. All authors revised the draft critically for important intellectual content. All authors read and approved the final manuscript.

Author details

[1]Yong Loo Lin School of Medicine, National University of Singapore, Singapore, Singapore. [2]Program in Health Services and Systems Research, Duke-NUS Medical School, Singapore, Singapore. [3]Department of Rheumatology and Immunology, Singapore General Hospital, Singapore, Singapore. [4]Department of Internal Medicine, Singapore General Hospital, Academia Building, Level 4, 20 College Road, Singapore 169856, Singapore.

References

1. Boeckh M, Leisenring W, Riddell SR, Bowden RA, Huang ML, Myerson D, Stevens-Ayers T, Flowers ME, Cunningham T, Corey L. Late cytomegalovirus disease and mortality in recipients of allogeneic hematopoietic stem cell transplants: importance of viral load and T-cell immunity. Blood. 2003;101: 407–14.
2. Krech U. Complement-fixing antibodies against cytomegalovirus in different parts of the world. Bull World Health Organ. 1973;49:103–6.
3. Barber C, Gold WL, Fortin PR. Infections in the lupus patient: perspectives on prevention. Curr Opin Rheumatol. 2011;23:358–65.
4. Ramos-Casals M, Cuadrado MJ, Alba P, Sanna G, Brito-Zeron P, Bertolaccini L, Babini A, Moreno A, D'Cruz D, Khamashta MA. Acute viral infections in patients with systemic lupus erythematosus: description of 23 cases and review of the literature. Medicine (Baltimore). 2008;87:311–8.
5. Ramanan P, Razonable RR. Cytomegalovirus infections in solid organ transplantation: a review. Infect Chemother. 2013;45(3):260–71.
6. Strippoli GF, Hodson EM, Jones CJ, Craig JC. Pre-emptive treatment for cytomegalovirus viraemia to prevent cytomegalovirus disease in solid organ transplant recipients. Cochrane Database Syst Rev. 2006. https://doi.org/10.1002/14651858.CD005133.pub3.
7. Chevret S, Scieux C, Garrait V, Dahel L, Morinet F, Modai J, Decazes JM, Molina JM. Usefulness of the cytomegalovirus (CMV) antigenemia assay for predicting the occurrence of CMV disease and death in patients with AIDS. Clin Infect Dis. 1999;28:758–63.
8. Mori T, Kameda H, Ogawa H, Iizuka A, Sekiguchi N, Takei H, Nagasawa H, Tokuhira M, Tanaka T, Saito Y, et al. Incidence of cytomegalovirus reactivation in patients with inflammatory connective tissue diseases who are under immunosuppressive therapy. J Rheumatol. 2004;31:1349–51.
9. Berman N, Belmont HM. Disseminated cytomegalovirus infection complicating active treatment of systemic lupus erythematosus: an emerging problem. Lupus. 2016;26. https://doi.org/10.1177/0961203316671817.
10. Ikura Y, Matsuo T, Fau - Ogami M, Ogami M, Fau - Yamazaki S, Yamazaki S, Fau - Okamura M, Okamura M, Fau - Yoshikawa J, Yoshikawa J, Fau - Ueda M, Ueda M. Cytomegalovirus associated pancreatitis in a patient with systemic lupus erythematosus. J Rheumatol. 2000;27:2715–7.
11. Rozenblyum EV, Allen UD, Silverman ED, Levy DM. Cytomegalovirus infection in childhood-onset systemic lupus erythematosus. Int J Clin Rheumatol. 2013;8(1):137–46.
12. Bertsias G. Ioannidis Jp Fau - Boletis J, Boletis J Fau - Bombardieri S, Bombardieri S Fau - Cervera R, Cervera R Fau - Dostal C, Dostal C Fau - font J, font J Fau - Gilboe IM, Gilboe Im Fau - Houssiau F, Houssiau F Fau - Huizinga T, Huizinga T Fau - Isenberg D, et al: EULAR recommendations for the management of systemic lupus erythematosus. Report of a task force of the EULAR standing committee for international clinical studies including therapeutics. Ann Rheum Dis. 2008;67:195–205.
13. Hanaoka R, Kurasawa K, Maezawa R, Kumano K, Arai S, Fukuda T. Reactivation of cytomegalovirus predicts poor prognosis in patients on intensive immunosuppressive treatment for collagen-vascular diseases. Mod Rheumatol. 2012;22:438–45.
14. Tamm M, Traenkle P, Grilli B, Soler M, Bolliger CT, Dalquen P, Cathomas G. Pulmonary cytomegalovirus infection in immunocompromised patients. Chest. 2001;119:838–43.
15. Yoon KH, Fong Ky Fau - Tambyah PA, Tambyah PA. Fatal cytomegalovirus infection in two patients with systemic lupus erythematosus undergoing intensive immunosuppressive therapy: role for cytomegalovirus vigilance and prophylaxis? JCR Journal of Clinical Rheumatology. 8:217–22. https://doi.org/10.1097/01.RHU.0000022543.49406.24.
16. Fei Y, Shi X, Gan F, Li X, Zhang W, Li M, Hou Y, Zhang X, Zhao Y, Zeng X, Zhang F. Death causes and pathogens analysis of systemic lupus erythematosus during the past 26 years. Clin Rheumatol. 2014;33:57–63.
17. Hochberg MC. Updating the American College of Rheumatology revised criteria for the classification of systemic lupus erythematosus. Arthritis Rheum. 1997;40:1725.
18. Tan EM, Cohen AS, Fries JF, Masi AT, McShane DJ, Rothfield NF, Schaller JG, Talal N, Winchester RJ. The 1982 revised criteria for the classification of systemic lupus erythematosus. Arthritis & Rheumatism. 1982;25:1271–7.
19. Ljungman P, Boeckh M, Hirsch HH, Josephson F, Lundgren J, Nichols G, Pikis A, Razonable RR, Miller V, Griffiths PD. Definitions of cytomegalovirus infection and disease in transplant patients for use in clinical trials. Clin Infect Dis. 2017;64:87–91.
20. Francisci D, Tosti A, Fau - Baldelli F, Baldelli F, Fau - Stagni G, Stagni G, Fau - Pauluzzi S, Pauluzzi S. The pp65 antigenaemia test as a predictor of cytomegalovirus-induced end-organ disease in patients with AIDS. AIDS (London, England). 1997;11:1341–5. https://doi.org/10.1097/00002030-199711000-00007.
21. Leanne M. Kmet, Robert C. Lee, Linda S. Cook,: Standard Quality Assessment Criteria For Evaluating Primary Research Papers From A Variety Of Fields. Edmonton: Alberta Heritage Foundation for Medical Research (AHFMR) 2004. AHFMR - HTA Initiative #13.
22. Xue Y, Jiang L, Wan WG, Chen YM, Zhang J, Zhang ZC. Cytomegalovirus pneumonia in patients with rheumatic diseases after immunosuppressive therapy: a single center study in China. Chin Med J. 2016;129:267–73.
23. Tsai WP, Chen MH, Lee MH, Yu KH, Wu MW, Liou LB. Cytomegalovirus infection causes morbidity and mortality in patients with autoimmune diseases, particularly systemic lupus: in a Chinese population in Taiwan. Rheumatol Int. 2012;32:2901–8.
24. Gor D, Sabin C, Prentice HG, Vyas N, Man S, Griffiths PD, Emery VC. Longitudinal fluctuations in cytomegalovirus load in bone marrow transplant patients: relationship between peak virus load, donor/recipient serostatus, acute GVHD and CMV disease. Bone Marrow Transplant. 1998;21:597–605.
25. Takizawa Y, Inokuma S, Tanaka Y, Saito K, Atsumi T, Hirakata M, Kameda H, Hirohata S, Kondo H, Kumagai S, Tanaka Y. Clinical characteristics of cytomegalovirus infection in rheumatic diseases: multicentre survey in a large patient population. Rheumatology (Oxford). 2008;47:1373–8.
26. Chan ST, Logan AC. The clinical impact of cytomegalovirus infection following allogeneic hematopoietic cell transplantation: why the quest for meaningful prophylaxis still matters. Blood Rev. 2017;31:173–83.
27. Fujimoto D, Matsushima A, Nagao M, Takakura S, Ichiyama S. Risk factors associated with elevated blood cytomegalovirus pp65 antigen levels in patients with autoimmune diseases. Mod Rheumatol. 2013;23:345–50.
28. Boeckh M, Leisenring W, Riddell SR, Bowden RA, Huang ML, Myerson D, Stevens-Ayers T, Flowers MED, Cunningham T, Corey L. Late cytomegalovirus disease and mortality in recipients of allogeneic hematopoietic stem cell transplants: importance of viral load and T-cell immunity. Blood. 2003;101:407–14.
29. Salmon-Ceron D, Mazeron MC, Chaput S, Boukli N, Senechal B, Houhou N, Katlama C, Matheron S, Fillet AM, Gozlan J, et al. Plasma cytomegalovirus DNA, pp65 antigenaemia and a low CD4 cell count remain risk factors for cytomegalovirus disease in patients receiving highly active antiretroviral therapy. Aids. 2000;14:1041–9.
30. Ho M. Observations from transplantation contributing to the understanding of pathogenesis of CMV infection. Transplant Proc. 1991;23:104–8 discussion 108-109.
31. Lim CC, Tung YT, Tan BH, Lee PH, Mok IY, Oon L, Chan KP, Choo JC. Epidemiology and risk factors for cytomegalovirus infection in glomerular diseases treated with immunosuppressive therapy. Nephrology. 2018;23(7): 676–81.
32. Su BY, Su CY, Yu SF, Chen CJ. Incidental discovery of high systemic lupus erythematosus disease activity associated with cytomegalovirus viral activity. Med Microbiol Immunol. 2007;196:165–70.
33. Vitko S, Margreiter R, Weimar W, Dantal J, Kuypers D, Winkler M, Oyen O, Viljoen HG, Filiptsev P, Sadek S, et al. Three-year efficacy and safety results from a study of everolimus versus mycophenolate mofetil in de novo renal transplant patients. Am J Transplant. 2005;5:2521–30.

7

The diagnostic benefit of antibodies against ribosomal proteins in systemic lupus erythematosus

Zhen-rui Shi[1], Yan-fang Han[1], Jing Yin[2], Yu-ping Zhang[1,3], Ze-xin Jiang[1,4], Lin Zheng[1], Guo-zhen Tan[1*] and Liangchun Wang[1*]

Abstract

Background: Anti-ribosomal P (anti-Rib-P) antibody is a specific serological marker for systemic lupus erythematosus (SLE) and routinely tested by targeting the common epitope of three ribosomal proteins of P0, P1 and P2. This study aimed to investigate if testing antibodies against individual ribosomal protein, but not the common epitope, is required to achieve the best diagnostic benefit in SLE.

Methods: The study included 82 patients with SLE and 22 healthy donors. Serum antibodies were determined by ELISA and immunoblot.

Results: The prevalence of each antibody determined by ELISA was 35.4% (anti-Rib-P), 45.1% (anti-Rib-P0), 32.9% (anti-Rib-P1) and 40.2% (anti-Rib-P2) at 99% specificity, respectively. Of 53 patients with negative anti-Rib-P antibody, 21 (39.6%) were positive for anti-Rib-P0, 9 (17.0%) for anti-Rib-P1 and 12 (22.6%) for anti-Rib-P2 antibody. The positive rate of anti-Rib-P antibody detected by ELISA was close to the results by immunoblot (33.4%). Patients with any of these antibodies were featured by higher disease activity and prevalence of skin rashes than those with negative antibodies. Moreover, each antibody was particularly related to some clinical and laboratory disorders. The distribution of subclasses of IgG1–4 was varied with each antibody. Anti-Rib-P0 IgG1 and IgG3 were strongly correlated with disease activity and lower serum complement components 3 and 4.

Conclusions: Anti-Rib-P antibody is not adequate to predict the existence of antibodies against ribosomal P0, P1 and P2 protein. The examination of antibodies against each ribosomal protein is required to achieve additional diagnostic benefit and to evaluate the association with clinical and serological disorders as well.

Keywords: Systemic lupus erythematosus, Diagnosis, Anti-ribosomal P antibodies

Introduction

A broad spectrum of autoantibodies was detected in systematic lupus erythematosus (SLE). Of them, anti-nuclear (ANA), anti-Smith (anti-Sm) and anti-double-stranded DNA (anti-dsDNA) antibodies are included in the American College of Rheumatology (ACR) classification criteria for SLE [1]. Anti-ribosomal P (anti-Rib-P) antibody is not listed in the criteria, but specifically detected in SLE patients instead of the other autoimmune diseases and healthy subjects [2, 3]. It was suggested to be an additional biomarker for SLE, especially for those with negative anti-dsDNA or anti-Sm antibodies to fulfill the ACR criteria [4, 5]. The prevalence of anti-Rib-P antibody is about 15–40% in SLE patients and varies with the ethnicity, disease activity and detection method [6]. It is highly associated with facial erythema, arthritis, lymphopenia, neuropsychiatric symptoms, lupus nephritis, liver involvement and juvenile SLE [7, 8].

Anti-Rib-P antibody routinely tested in SLE targets a homologous 22-amino acid C-terminal (C-22) sequence

* Correspondence: guozhentan1@hotmail.com; wliangch@mail.sysu.edu.cn
[1]Department of Dermatology, Sun Yat-sen Memorial Hospital, Sun Yat-sen University, 107 Yanjiang Rd W, Guangzhou 510120, China
Full list of author information is available at the end of the article

shared by three ribosomal phosphoproteins known as P0, P1, and P2 (with molecular mass of 38, 19, and 17 kDa, respectively) [9]. Normally, the three proteins are organized in a pentameric complex containing one P0 monomer and two P1/P2 dimers in the 60S subunit of ribosomes [10]. Beyond the main immunodominant epitope of C-22, several other epitopes were described, but rarely used as immunoreactive domains [11]. Lately, anti-Rib-P antibody test using common epitopes of the three P proteins as substrate was challenged by two studies. The results were partially controversial regarding the antibody prevalence against each ribosomal P proteins, but nevertheless both studies found that the sensitivity and specificity of anti-Rib-P antibody were significantly different from that of anti-Rib-P0, –P1, and -P2 antibodies determined by each recombinant ribosomal P protein [12, 13]. Moreover, our previous study suggested that anti-Rib-P0, but not anti-Rib-P1/P2 antibodies were pathogenic antibodies that were particularly involved in the development of SLE skin damage [7, 14].

Thus, in this study we evaluated the necessity of testing each antibody against ribosomal proteins in SLE by determining the sensitivity and specificity of anti-Rib-P, –P0, –P1, –P2 antibody, investigating the association of each antibody with clinical and laboratory disorders and characterizing the four subclasses of Immunoglobulin G (IgG1–4) of each antibody as well.

Material and methods

Patients

Serum samples were collected from 82 SLE patients consecutively visiting our department. All patients were diagnosed with SLE according to the ACR revised criteria [1]. The disease activity was measured by the SLE disease activity index (SLEDAI) score [15]. The clinical examination and routine laboratory test were performed at the time of enrollment. Serum was collected and kept at – 80 °C until used. Healthy controls were 22 sex- and age-matched blood donors. The study was approved by the research ethic board of Sun Yat-sen Memorial Hospital and informed consent was obtained from all subjects (No. 2016–155).

Measurement of antibodies

Enzyme-linked immunosorbent assay (ELISA) was performed as described previously [16]. Briefly, microtiter plates were coated with 50 µl (1 µg/ml diluted in PBS) full-length recombinant ribosomal protein P0 (Prospec, Israel), P1 (Abnova, Taipei, Taiwan) or P2 (Prospec, Israel) overnight at 4 °C. For detection of serum IgG, antigen was incubated with serum samples diluted in 1: 2000 and sequentially with HRP-conjugated anti-human-IgG (Santa Cruz, Dallas, TX, USA). For detection of the subclasses of IgG, serum samples were diluted in 1:2000 for IgG1, 1:800 for IgG2, 1:800 for IgG3 and 1:25 for IgG4, respectively. Bound antibodies were detected using peroxidase conjugated mouse anti-human IgG1 (Abcam, UK), IgG2 (Invitrogen, Carlsbad, CA, USA), IgG3 (Invitrogen, Carlsbad, CA, USA) and IgG4 (Abcam, UK). The color was developed with 3,3′,5,5′-tetramethylbenzidine dihydrochloride (TMB) and measured in a plate reader at 450 nm (SpectraMax M5, Molecular Devices, USA).

Antibody against ribosomal P proteins was determined both by ELISA (anti-Rib-P_{ELISA}) and immunoblot kit (anti-Rib-P_{BLOT}). According to the manufacturer, the ribosomal P proteins in both kits are purified by affinity chromatography from calf thymus. The major immunoreactive epitope is localized to the carboxy terminus of all 3 proteins (P0, P1, and P2) and consists of an identical sequence of 17 amino acids. Anti-dsDNA antibodies were determined by indirect immunofluorescence. Anti-Sm and other anti-ENA antibodies (anti-nucleosomes, anti-Histones, anti-U1snRNP, anti-SSA/Ro60, anti-SSA/Ro52, anti-SSB/La) were determined by immunoblot kit. All commercially available assays are purchased from EUROIMMIUN (Luebeck, Germany). The detection was performed according to the manufacturers' instructions.

Statistical analysis

Statistical analysis was performed using GraphPad Prism5 software (GraphPad Software, La Jolla, CA, USA). Receiver operating characteristics (ROC) curve analysis was used for the evaluation of diagnostic accuracy, selection of cut-off values and determination of the characteristics at predefined specificities. The Mann-Whitney U test (for measurement data), Fisher's exact test (for categorical data) and Spearman's rank test (for correlation) were used to determine the associations. p value below 0.05 was considered statistical significant.

Results

Measurement of serum autoantibodies against ribosomal proteins by ELISA

Serum antibodies against Rib-P_{ELISA}, recombinant Rib-P0, –P1 and -P2 proteins were examined by ELISA. The diagnostic significance was determined using ROC curve. According to the area under the curve (AUC) value and the maximum sum of sensitivity and specificity, the most efficient protein in determining antibody-positive and -negative serum was Rib-P_{ELISA}, followed by Rib-P0, –P2, and -P1 protein (Table 1). In a cohort of 82 SLE patients, the sensitivity of anti-Rib-P0, –P2, –PELISA and -P1 antibodies was 45.1% (n = 37), 40.2% (n = 33), 35.4% (n = 29) and 32.9% (n = 27) at a predefined specificity of 99%, respectively (Fig. 1, Table 1). The mean of the 99th percentile of each antibody was used as a cut-off value to define antibody positive and negative serum in the following

Table 1 Overall Test Characteristics of Anti-Rib Proteins by ELISA in ROC Curve Analysis

	Anti-Rib-P_{ELISA} [a]	Anti-Rib-P0	Anti-Rib-P1	Anti-Rib-P2
Area under the curve (AUC) with 95% confidence interval (CI)	0.778 (0.683–0.872)	0.724 (0.625–0.822)	0.677(0.576–0.778)	0 .686 (0.587–0.785)
Maximal sum of sensitivity and specificity[c]	153% (22.10)	145% (1.04)	143% (0.67)	146% (0.421)
Sensitivity at 95% specificity cut-off [b]	36.6% (17.69)	47.6% (0.98)	47.6% (0.70)	46.3% (0.49)
Sensitivity at 99% specificity cut-off [b]	35.4% (23.8)	45.1% (1.04)	32.9% (0.92)	40.2% (0.597)

[a]Anti-Rib-P_{ELISA} means antibodies directly against native ribosomal P heterocomplex determined by ELISA
[b]Cut-off values are presented in relative units/ml for anti-Rib-P_{ELISA}, and in optical densities (OD450) for anti-Rib-P0, anti-Rib-P1, and anti-Rib-P2 antibodies
[c] Numbers in the parentheses refer to the relative-units or OD value to achieve the Maximal sum of sensitivity and specificity

study. Notably, the cut-off value of anti-Rib-P_{ELISA} antibody optimized by the analysis of ROC curve is 23.8 RU/ml in this study, very close to the level (20 RU/ml) recommended by the manufacturer.

Diagnostic benefit of autoantibodies against each ribosomal protein

Anti-Sm and anti-dsDNA antibodies possess a high specificity as a serum diagnostic marker for SLE. In our study, antibodies against Sm and dsDNA were found in 14/75 (18.7%) and 60/81 (74.0%) of enrolled SLE patients, respectively, and not detected in17/75 (22.7%) of them. To investigate whether antibodies against ribosomal P proteins were able to serve as an additional diagnostic marker, we examined the positivity rates of these antibodies in SLE patients who were tested negative for solitary anti-Sm and anti-dsDNA antibody, or for both. Antibodies against Rib-P_{ELISA}, –P0, –P1 and -P2 were found in 21 (34.4%), 21 (34.4%), 16 (26.2%), and 20 (32.8%) of the 61 cases with negative anti-Sm antibody and in 4 (19.0%), 5 (23.8%), 1 (4.8%), and 2 (9.5%) of the 21 cases with negative anti-dsDNA antibody. Of 17 patients negative for both anti-Sm and anti-dsDNA antibodies, 4 (23.5%), 4 (23.5%), 1 (5.9%) and 2 (11.8%) cases presented antibodies against Rib-P_{ELISA}, –P0, –P1, and -P2, respectively (Table 2). Therefore, these findings suggest that autoantibodies against each ribosomal protein, especially anti-Rib-P_{ELISA} and -P0 antibodies could serve as a supplementary diagnostic marker for SLE in those patients negative for anti-dsDNA and anti-Sm antibody.

Frequencies of anti-rib-P0, –P1 and -P2 antibodies in anti-rib-P negative lupus patients

We further investigated whether patients with negative anti-Rib-P_{ELISA} and anti-Rib-P_{BLOT} antibody were positive for anti-Rib-P0, –P1 or -P2 antibody. Of 53 patients

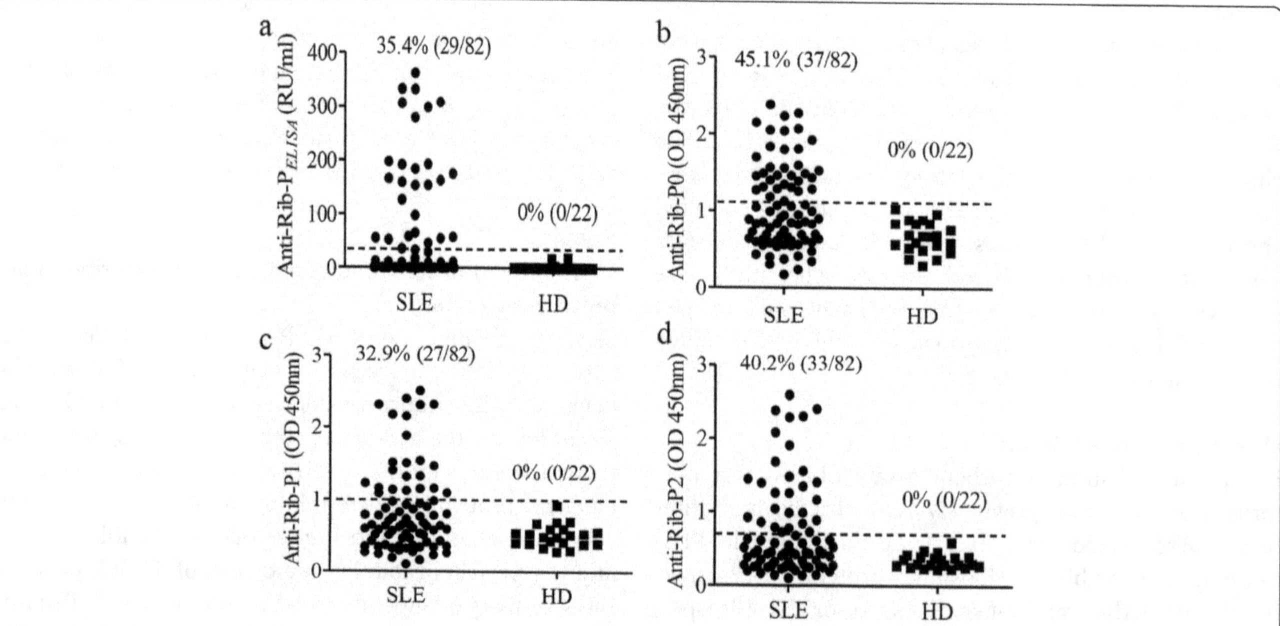

Fig. 1 Serum levels of autoantibodies against ribosomal proteins in SLE and healthy donors. Autoantibodies directly against native ribosomal P heterocomplex (Rib-P_{ELISA}) (**a**), recombinant ribosomal P0 protein (Rib-P0) (**b**), recombinant ribosomal P1 (Rib-P2) (**c**) and recombinant ribosomal P2 protein (Rib-P2) (**d**) were measured by enzyme-linked immunosorbent assay. Dotted lines represent the distinct cut-offs based on ROC curve analysis at the specificities of 99%. The prevalence of antibodies are indicated in percentage for each cohort. Numbers in brackets represent serum positive and total cases, respectively. Data represent at least three independent experiments

Table 2 Diagnostic benefit of autoantibodies against ribosomal P proteins

	Positive N (%)	Anti-Rib-P_{ELISA} [a]	Anti-Rib-P0	Anti-Rib-P1	Anti-Rib-P2
Anti-Sm (–)	61	21 (34.4)	21 (34.4)	16 (26.2)	20 (32.8)
Anti-Sm (+)	14	8 (57.1)	12 (85.7)	8 (57.1)	10 (71.4)
Anti-dsDNA (–)	21	4 (19.0)	5 (23.8)	1 (4.8)	2 (9.5)
Anti-dsDNA (+)	60	25 (41.7)	32 (53.3)	26 (43.3)	31 (51.7)
Anti-Sm and dsDNA (–)	17	4 (23.5)	4 (23.5)	1 (5.9)	2 (11.8)

N number of patients
[a]Anti-Rib-P_{ELISA} means antibodies directly against native ribosomal P heterocomplex determined by ELISA

with negative anti-Rib-P_{ELISA} antibody, 21 (39.6%) were positive for anti-Rib-P0, 9 (17.0%) for anti-Rib-P1 and 12 (22.6%) for anti-Rib-P2 antibody. Notably, of 21 patients with positive anti-Rib-P0 but negative anti-Rib-P_{ELISA} antibody, 9 were exclusively reactive to Rib-P0, but not to -P1 and -P2 proteins (Fig. 2). Of 75 patients, 26 were determined anti-Rib-P_{BLOT} positive by immunoblot. The detective rate (34.6%) is close to the result examined by ELISA (35.4%). There were 5 patients with reactivity exclusively against anti-Rib-P by ELISA and 2 patients against anti-Rib-P by immunoblot. Serum levels of anti-Rib-P_{ELISA}, anti-Rib-P1 and anti-Rib-P2 antibodies were significantly lower in anti-Rib-P_{BLOT} negative than in positive group, whereas anti-Rib-P0 antibodies had no association with the presence and absence of anti-Rib-P_{BLOT} antibody, which is consistent with the result of the comparison of the frequency of antibody positivity listed in Supplementary Table 1.

Thus, these findings suggest that anti-Rib-P antibody is not adequate to predict the presence and serum level of each antibody against ribosomal P0, P1 and P2 protein.

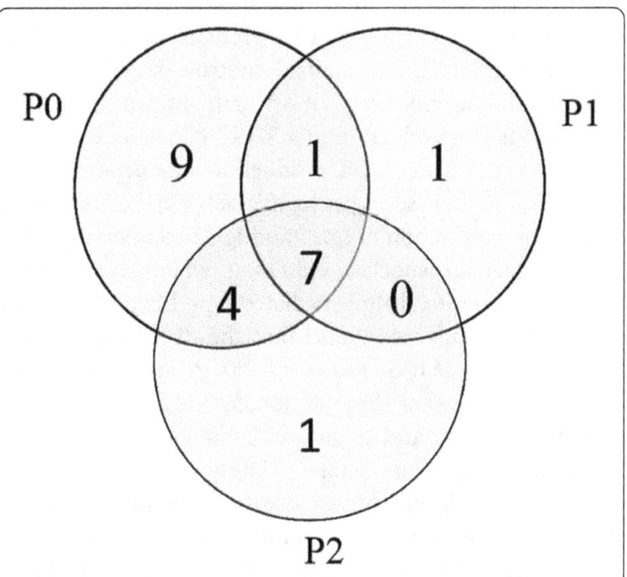

Fig. 2 Prevalence of anti-Rib-P0, anti-Rib-P1, and anti-Rib-P2 antibodies in 53 SLE patients with negative anti-Rib-P_{ELISA} antibody

Correlation of anti-ribosomal P antibodies with SLE disease features

Patients were divided into antibody-positive and -negative groups based on the results of ELISA tests. The demographic information and the clinical and laboratory examinations were listed in Supplementary Table 1.

Patients with positive antibody against any of ribosomal proteins showed higher clinical disease activity and prevalence of skin rashes. Patients with positive anti-Rib-P_{ELISA} were more often with photosensitivity ($p = 0.001$) and alopecia ($p = 0.003$). Cutaneous vasculitis was associated with the presence of anti-Rib-P0 ($P = 0.0075$), –P1 ($p = 0.0005$) and -P2 ($p = 0.0001$) antibodies, while arthritis was only related to anti-Rib-P2 antibody ($p = 0.027$). There was no significant difference in the presences of oral ulcers, serositis, neuropsychiatric SLE (NPSLE), renal and hematologic disorders between antibody-positive and -negative groups in each antibody category.

As for laboratory examination, lymphocytopenia was related to the presence of anti-Rib-P0 ($p = 0.043$) and -P1 ($p = 0.044$) antibodies. Erythrocyte sedimentation rate (ESR) was higher in patients with the tested autoantibodies except anti-Rib-P0 antibody. Serum complement component 3 (C3) was significantly lower in patients with positive any of examined antibodies than those with negative antibodies. Serum IgG was higher in patients with anti-Rib-P0 ($P = 0.01$) and -P2 antibodies ($P = 0.02$), but not associated with the presence of anti-Rib-P_{ELISA} and -P1 antibodies. Regarding lupus-related autoantibodies, anti-dsDNA antibody was closely related to the presence of anti-Rib-P0 ($P = 0.003$), –P1 ($P < 0.0001$) and -P2 ($P = 0.0002$) antibodies, whereas anti-Sm antibody was only related to anti-Rib-P0 ($P = 0.0007$) and -P2 antibody ($P = 0.014$). To further investigate how anti-ribosomal P antibodies behave among active SLE patients, we made a subgroup analysis of all anti-rib P antibodies using patients exclusively with SLEDAI> 6. As shown in Supplemental Table 2, the data from cohorts of all SLE patients and active SLE patients showed a similar pattern regarding the clinical and laboratory association. Overall, these findings demonstrate that each antibody against individual ribosomal protein is specifically related to some clinical and laboratory disorders in SLE.

Association of the subclasses of IgG antibody against recombinant ribosomal proteins with SLE disease features

Therefore, to facilitate the understanding of autoantibody against each ribosomal protein, we characterized the distribution and the associations of four subclasses of IgG with clinical and laboratory features of SLE.

Regarding anti-Rib-P0 antibody, IgG1 was nearly 4 folds higher, while IgG2, IgG3 and IgG4 was only 1.19, 1.54 and 1.63 folds higher in SLE than it in healthy controls. Moreover, Anti-Rib-P0 IgG1 and IgG3 were strongly clustered with SLEDAI score ($r = 0.46$, $p = 0.004$; $r = 0.47$, $p = 0.004$) and negatively correlated with serum levels of C3 ($r = -0.38$, $p = 0.024$; $r = -0.52$, $p = 0.014$) and C4 ($r = -0.48$, $p = 0.003$; $r = -0.39$, $p = 0.018$). In addition, anti-Rib-P0 IgG1 was significantly associated with ESR ($r = 0.37$, $p = 0.029$) (Supplementary Table 3). As for anti-Rib-P1 antibodies, IgG1 and IgG2 was five and four folds higher in SLE, respectively, while IgG3 and IgG4 was 2 folds higher. However, all subclasses of anti-Rib-P1 IgG were not correlated with the clinical and laboratory disorders examined in this study (Supplementary Table 3). The four subclasses of anti-Rib-P2 IgG were about 2 to 3 folds higher than those in healthy donors. Anti-Rib-P2 IgG1 was negatively correlated with serum C3 ($r = -0.45$, $p = 0.011$) and C4 ($r = -0.40$, $p = 0.022$) (Supplementary Table 3). Collectively, the distribution and the association of IgG subclasses against ribosomal proteins were antigen-related in SLE.

Discussion

In the current study, we evaluated the diagnostic efficiency, the clinical and laboratory significances of antibody against native ribosomal heterocomplex, and of IgG antibody and its subclasses of IgG1–4 against recombinant protein P0, P1 and P2 in SLE patients. The results suggest that anti-Rib-P is not adequate to predict the presence of antibody against each ribosomal protein, and that each antibody may be involved in SLE-related tissue and organ damages independently.

Our results showed that the prevalence of anti-Rib-P antibody ranged from 32.9% (anti-Rib-P1) to 45.1% (anti-Rib-P0) at 99% specificity, which is in line with data from an Asian group (28–42%), but higher than those from other ethnic populations (6–35%) [17]. In addition, our data established that anti-Rib-P0 presented the best diagnostic value with a more positive rate at high specificity. Interestingly, this finding is more consistent with data shown by a Caucasian cohorts with a sequential sensitivity of anti-Rib-P0 > anti-Rib-P2 > anti-Rib-P > anti-Rib-P1 antibody [13], but not by a Chinese SLE cohorts (anti-Rib-P1 > anti-Rib-P2 > anti-Rib-P0 > anti-Rib-P) [12]. Therefore, the discrepancy of studies should not be simply explained as ethnic differences. The disease activity, features of patient cohorts and the methods of antibody detection should be considered in interpreting the results.

In lines with previous studies [3, 5], the sensitivity of anti-ribosomal P antibodies was superior to that of anti-Sm (18.7%), but inferior to that of anti-DNA (74.0%). Importantly, among 19 SLE patients lacking anti-dsDNA and anti-Sm, 8 (42%)patients was showed positive for at least one of the investigated anti-Rib-P antibodies, suggesting that antibodies against ribosomal P proteins are important complementary parameters to anti-dsDNA and anti-Sm, and should be considered for inclusion in the classification criteria for SLE. Another striking finding is the differential clinical and laboratory association among anti-Rib-P antibody and each subsets (anti-Rib-P0, –P1, and -P2 antibodies). For example, the positivity of anti-Rib-P0 antibodies was closely related with the presence of skin rash and vasculitis whilst such clinical association was not observed in terms of anti-Rib-P antibody. Therefore, testing additional anti-P subsets could be beneficial for bringing additional laboratory information.

A considerable percentage of patients with negative anti-Rib-P antibody presented at least one antibody against Rib-P0, P1 or P2, with anti-Rib-P0 antibody as the most frequent one. Thus, the negativity of anti-Rib-P antibody does not automatically imply the negativity of the other antibodies, especially anti-Rib-P0 antibody. It could attribute to the fact that ribosomal P0 protein facilitates antibody detection by providing more accessible epitopes than Rib-P does [13]. Thus, anti-Rib-P0 would provide additional diagnostic benefit, especially in those with negative anti-Rib-P antibody.

The four IgG subclasses present considerable different bioactivities, including the abilities to fix complements (IgG3 > IgG1 > IgG2 > IgG4) and to bind to Fc receptors [18]. Several studies found that IgG1 and IgG3 in SLE were elevated, IgG4 was not different from it in healthy control, whereas IgG2 remained controversial [19]. In the context of autoimmunity, most autoantigens stimulate IgG1 and IgG3 production in a T cell-dependent manner, while few stimulate IgG2 production independent of T cells [20]. As for subtypes of T cell, Th1 cells mainly induce the production of IgG1 and IgG3 by releasing cytokines to regulate subclass switching, while Th2 cells are essential for mast cell/IgE-mediated type I hypersensitivity [21]. In this study, we found that the distribution of the four subclasses of IgG against Rib-P0, P1 and P2 were different, implying that these antibodies could be driven by distinct pathways and might contribute to SLE development separately. For instance, IgG1 was the dominant anti-Rib-P0 IgG, and highly related to SLEDAI, C3, C4 and ESR. Thus, anti-Rib-P0 antibody could be driven by autoantigen with T cell involvement and potentially holds substantial pathogenicity in SLE, although further researches are required to prove the hypothesis.

Some limitations should be considered in the current study. First, the sample size of our study is limited and may not allow an accurate sub-analysis of the less frequent clinical manifestations like serositis and NPSLE. Second, our study uses healthy donors as the only control group. Rib-P protein and anti-Rib-P antibodies have been detected in several conditions like Sjogren's Syndrome (pSS) [22],Chagas disease [23], viral hepatitis [24] and so on. Moreover, the ratio of SLE patients and healthy control is unequal. Further studies are warranted to enlarge the sample size and add other disease groups to develop more accurate cutoffs for the in-house ELISAs.

Conclusion

In summary, autoantibodies against Rib-P, ribosomal protein P0, P1 and P2 should be examined individually in order to achieve additional diagnostic benefit, especially in suspected SLE patients with negative anti-dsDNA or anti-Sm antibody.

Supplementary information

Additional file 1: Table S1. Associations of autoantibodies against ribosomal proteins with the clinical and laboratory disorders of SLE. **Table S2.** Associations of autoantibodies against ribosomal proteins with the clinical and laboratory disorders in active SLE patients (SLEDAI> 6). **Table S3.** Correlation of IgG subclasses of antibodies against ribosomal proteins with SLE disease features †.

Acknowledgements

Not applicable.

Authors' contributions

Zhen-rui Shi, Yan-fang Han: conception and design, writing and revision of the manuscript, figure creation, data acquisition and interpretation, statistical analysis. Jing Yin, Yu-ping Zhang, Ze-xin Jiang and Lin Zheng: design of study, drafting the article and data acquisition. Liangchun Wang and Guozhen Tan: study design and supervision, revision of the manuscript and approval of the final version. The author(s) read and approved the final manuscript.

Author details

[1]Department of Dermatology, Sun Yat-sen Memorial Hospital, Sun Yat-sen University, 107 Yanjiang Rd W, Guangzhou 510120, China. [2]Affiliated Hospital of Shandong Academy of Medical Sciences, Jinan, China. [3]Department of Dermatology, Zhongshan People's Hospital, No.2 Sunwen East Road, Zhongshan 528403, Guangdong, China. [4]Department of Dermatology, The First People's Hospital of Foshan, Foshan 528000, China.

References

1. Hochberg MC. Updating the American College of Rheumatology revised criteria for the classification of systemic lupus erythematosus. Arthritis Rheum. 1997;40(9):1725.
2. Ghirardello A, Doria A, Zampieri S, Gambari PF, Todesco S. Autoantibodies to ribosomal P proteins in systemic lupus erythematosus. Isr Med Assoc J. 2001;3(11):854–7.
3. Carmona-Fernandes D, Santos MJ, Canhao H, Fonseca JE. Anti-ribosomal P protein IgG autoantibodies in patients with systemic lupus erythematosus: diagnostic performance and clinical profile. BMC Med. 2013;11:98.
4. Toubi E, Shoenfeld Y. Clinical and biological aspects of anti-P-ribosomal protein autoantibodies. Autoimmun Rev. 2007;6(3):119–25.
5. Hirohata S, Kasama T, Kawahito Y, Takabayashi K. Efficacy of anti-ribosomal P protein antibody testing for diagnosis of systemic lupus erythematosus. Mod Rheumatol. 2014;24(6):939–44.
6. Mahler M, Kessenbrock K, Raats J, Fritzler MJ. Technical and clinical evaluation of anti-ribosomal P protein immunoassays. J Clin Lab Anal. 2004; 18(4):215–23.
7. Shi ZR, Cao CX, Tan GZ, Wang L. The association of serum anti-ribosomal P antibody with clinical and serological disorders in systemic lupus erythematosus: a systematic review and meta-analysis. Lupus. 2015;24(6): 588–96.
8. Valoes CC, Molinari BC, Pitta AC, Gormezano NW, Farhat SC, Kozu K, et al. Anti-ribosomal P antibody: a multicenter study in childhood-onset systemic lupus erythematosus patients. Lupus. 2017;26(5):484–9.
9. Mahler M, Kessenbrock K, Raats J, Williams R, Fritzler MJ, Bluthner M. Characterization of the human autoimmune response to the major C-terminal epitope of the ribosomal P proteins. J Mol Med (Berl). 2003;81(3): 194–204.
10. Kiss E, Shoenfeld Y. Are anti-ribosomal P protein antibodies relevant in systemic lupus erythematosus? Clin Rev Allergy Immunol. 2007;32(1):37–46.
11. Lin JL, Dubljevic V, Fritzler MJ, Toh BH. Major immunoreactive domains of human ribosomal P proteins lie N-terminal to a homologous C-22 sequence: application to a novel ELISA for systemic lupus erythematosus. Clin Exp Immunol. 2005;141(1):155–64.
12. Li J, Shen Y, He J, Jia R, Wang X, Chen X, et al. Significance of antibodies against the native ribosomal P protein complex and recombinant P0, P1, and P2 proteins in the diagnosis of Chinese patients with systemic lupus erythematosus. J Clin Lab Anal. 2013;27(2):87–95.
13. Barkhudarova F, Dahnrich C, Rosemann A, Schneider U, Stocker W, Burmester GR, et al. Diagnostic value and clinical laboratory associations of antibodies against recombinant ribosomal P0, P1 and P2 proteins and their native heterocomplex in a Caucasian cohort with systemic lupus erythematosus. Arthritis Res Ther. 2011;13(1):R20.
14. Shi ZR, Tan GZ, Meng Z, Yu M, Li KW, Yin J, et al. Association of anti-acidic ribosomal protein P0 and anti-galectin 3 antibodies with the development of skin lesions in systemic lupus erythematosus. Arthritis Rheum. 2015;67(1): 193–203.
15. Bombardier C, Gladman DD, Urowitz MB, Caron D, Chang CH. Derivation of the SLEDAI. A disease activity index for lupus patients. The committee on prognosis studies in SLE. Arthritis Rheum. 1992;35(6):630–40.
16. Meng Z, Shi ZR, Tan GZ, Yin J, Wu J, Mi XB, et al. The association of anti-annexin1 antibodies with the occurrence of skin lesions in systemic lupus erythematosus. Lupus. 2014;23(2):183–7.
17. Mahler M, Kessenbrock K, Szmyrka M, Takasaki Y, Garcia-De La Torre I, Shoenfeld Y, et al. International multicenter evaluation of autoantibodies to ribosomal P proteins. Clin Vaccine Immunol. 2006;13(1):77–83.
18. Fang QY, Yu F, Tan Y, Xu LX, Wu LH, Liu G, et al. Anti-C1q antibodies and IgG subclass distribution in sera from Chinese patients with lupus nephritis. Nephrol Dial Transplant. 2009;24(1):172–8.
19. Zhang H, Li P, Wu D, Xu D, Hou Y, Wang Q, et al. Serum IgG subclasses in autoimmune diseases. Medicine (Baltimore). 2015;94(2):e387.
20. Loizou S, Cofiner C, Weetman AP, Walport MJ. Immunoglobulin class and IgG subclass distribution of anticardiolipin antibodies in patients with systemic lupus erythematosus and associated disorders. Clin Exp Immunol. 1992;90(3):434–9.
21. Kawasaki Y, Suzuki J, Sakai N, Isome M, Nozawa R, Tanji M, et al. Evaluation of T helper-1/−2 balance on the basis of IgG subclasses and serum cytokines in children with glomerulonephritis. Am J Kidney Dis. 2004;44(1):42–9.
22. Mei YJ, Wang P, Jiang C, Wang T, Chen LJ, Li ZJ, et al. Clinical and serological associations of anti-ribosomal P0 protein antibodies in systemic lupus erythematosus. Clin Rheumatol. 2018;37(3):703–7.

23. Skeiky YA, Benson DR, Parsons M, Elkon KB, Reed SG. Cloning and expression of Trypanosoma cruzi ribosomal protein P0 and epitope analysis of anti-P0 autoantibodies in Chagas' disease patients. J Exp Med. 1992; 176(1):201–11.
24. Wang YX, Luo C, Zhao D, Beck J, Nassal M. Extensive mutagenesis of the conserved box E motif in duck hepatitis B virus P protein reveals multiple functions in replication and a common structure with the primer grip in HIV-1 reverse transcriptase. J Virol. 2012;86(12):6394–407.

8

Machine learning techniques for computer-aided classification of active inflammatory sacroiliitis in magnetic resonance imaging

Matheus Calil Faleiros[1], Marcello Henrique Nogueira-Barbosa[2,3,4,5*], Vitor Faeda Dalto[4], José Raniery Ferreira Júnior[2,3], Ariane Priscilla Magalhães Tenório[2], Rodrigo Luppino-Assad[2], Paulo Louzada-Junior[2], Rangaraj Mandayam Rangayyan[6] and Paulo Mazzoncini de Azevedo-Marques[2,3]

Abstract

Background: Currently, magnetic resonance imaging (MRI) is used to evaluate active inflammatory sacroiliitis related to axial spondyloarthritis (axSpA). The qualitative and semiquantitative diagnosis performed by expert radiologists and rheumatologists remains subject to significant intrapersonal and interpersonal variation. This encouraged us to use machine-learning methods for this task.

Methods: In this retrospective study including 56 sacroiliac joint MRI exams, 24 patients had positive and 32 had negative findings for inflammatory sacroiliitis according to the ASAS group criteria. The dataset was randomly split with ~ 80% (46 samples, 20 positive and 26 negative) as training and ~ 20% as external test (10 samples, 4 positive and 6 negative). After manual segmentation of the images by a musculoskeletal radiologist, multiple features were extracted. The classifiers used were the Support Vector Machine, the Multilayer Perceptron (MLP), and the Instance-Based Algorithm, combined with the Relief and Wrapper methods for feature selection.

Results: Based on 10-fold cross-validation using the training dataset, the MLP classifier obtained the best performance with sensitivity = 100%, specificity = 95.6% and accuracy = 84.7%, using 6 features selected by the Wrapper method. Using the test dataset (external validation) the same MLP classifier obtained sensitivity = 100%, specificity = 66.7% and accuracy = 80%.

Conclusions: Our results show the potential of machine learning methods to identify SIJ subchondral bone marrow edema in axSpA patients and are promising to aid in the detection of active inflammatory sacroiliitis on MRI STIR sequences. Multilayer Perceptron (MLP) achieved the best results.

Keywords: Magnetic resonance imaging, Sacroiliac joint inflammation, Spondyloarthritis, Machine learning, Artificial intelligence, Computer-assisted diagnosis

* Correspondence: marcello@fmrp.usp.br
[2]Ribeirão Preto Medical School, University of São Paulo, Ribeirão Preto, SP, Brazil
[3]MAInLab Medical Artificial Intelligence Laboratory, Ribeirão Preto Medical School, Ribeirão Preto, Brazil
Full list of author information is available at the end of the article

Introduction

The term spondyloarthritis (SpA) encompasses a group of diseases characterized by inflammation in the spine and in the peripheral joints, as well as other clinical features. The current concept of the spectrum of SpA comprises axial spondyloarthritis (axSpA) and peripheral spondyloarthritis. In recent years, there has been tremendous progress in understanding the natural history and pathogenetic mechanisms underlying SpA, leading to the development of effective treatments. It has become imperative to identify the disease early and accurately, to offer patients effective treatment in a safe manner [1]. SpA usually starts in the young adult age. Its progression frequently contributes to significant physical disability and decreased quality of life if early diagnosis and early treatment are not achieved. This group of diseases presents with high prevalence and incidence in early age causing great socioeconomic impact, because of both the associated clinical characteristics and treatment [2].

AxSpA involves primarily the entheses of the sacroiliac joints (SIJs) and the spine, which are the most frequently compromised anatomic regions due to this disease. The SIJs are considered to be the most important sites of impairment and magnetic resonance imaging (MRI) is recognized as the most sensitive technique for early diagnosis of inflammatory sacroiliitis due to its great textural contrast resolution, by revealing subchondral bone marrow edema [3].

The Assessment of SpondyloArthritis International Society (ASAS) group recommends T2-weighted MRI sequence sensitive for free water, such as short tau inversion recovery (STIR) or T2 fat saturation (fat-sat), to detect SIJ active inflammation [3]. The MRI characteristics of SIJ related to active inflammation include high-intensity gray levels close to the joint surface, in the subchondral bone, and the depth of that intensity. Figure 1 shows examples of a positive and a negative case for active inflammatory sacroiliitis.

Despite efforts to standardize the evaluation, the qualitative and semiquantitative diagnosis performed by expert radiologists and rheumatologists still remains subject to significant intrapersonal and interpersonal variation [4]. Therefore, this is an important field for potential application of computer-assisted methods using artificial intelligence or machine learning techniques to achieve reliable and early diagnosis.

Machine learning is a branch of artificial intelligence, which allows the extraction of meaningful patterns from examples [5, 6]. The artificial intelligence approach has been widely used in medical image classification tasks, such as melanoma [7], discrimination of smoking status based on deep learning with MRI [8], classification of dermatological ulcers [9], evaluation of breast cancer [10], lung diseases [11, 12], and vertebral compression fractures [13, 14]. Computer-assisted analysis can be based on different approaches, such as statistical methods, instance-based analysis, decision trees, and artificial neural networks (ANNs). However, machine-learning models could have some limitations, for instance, bias to the majority class with imbalanced datasets and overfitting due to high feature-vector dimensionality. Therefore, it is required to evaluate the performance of machine learning techniques for each specific application.

In this context, our proposal was to evaluate the applicability of classical machine learning models and feature selection methods for the classification of active inflammatory sacroiliitis in magnetic resonance images.

Material and methods

This retrospective study was approved by the Institutional Review Board (IRB) at the University Hospital. IRB waived the requirement to obtain informed consent of patients.

Image acquisition and preprocessing

Images from SIJ MRI exams of 56 patients were retrospectively recovered from the Picture Archiving and

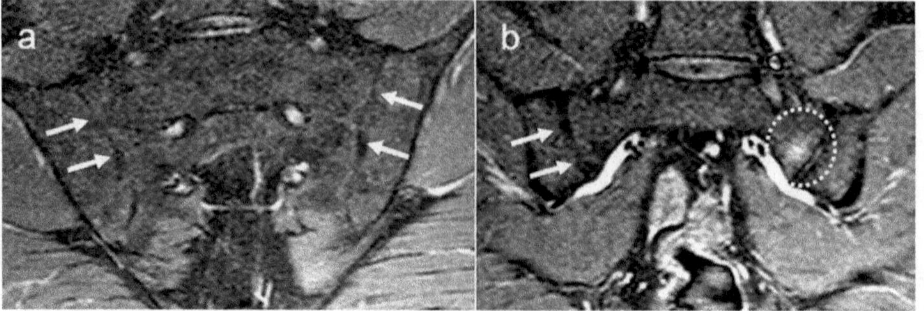

Fig. 1 a. Negative case for active inflammatory sacroiliitis on MRI illustrated with one of its coronal STIR images. There are no hyperintense foci at the subchondral bone adjacent to the articular surfaces (white arrowheads). **b**. A positive example of bone marrow edema related to active sacroiliitis on MRI. The subchondral bone marrow edema is characterized by ill-defined foci of hyperintensity and is shown inside the dotted white circle. White arrowheads indicate the right sacroiliac joint surface

Communication System (PACS) of the University Hospital. Exams were acquired with a 1.5 T scanner (Achieva, Philips Medical Systems), using the spine coil, with the acquisition of coronal STIR sequences. From each MRI exam, a musculoskeletal radiologist selected six images as being the most representative images of the SIJs of the patient, resulting in a total of 336 images.

Patients whose MRIs were included in this study were all initially investigated for suspected inflammatory sacroiliitis. Some of them finally had the diagnosis of spondyloarthritis, and others did not. At the end of 2 years of follow-up, all patients in the positive group (SIJ active inflammation) were diagnosed with spondyloarthritis according to clinical and laboratory criteria. In the negative group (SIJ without active inflammation), half of the patients (13 individuals) did not meet the clinical and laboratorial criteria for spondyloarthritis, and received other diagnosis, such as osteoarthritis, fibromyalgia, gout, or psychiatric disorder. The other half of patients in the negative group, despite having the final diagnosis of spondyloarthritis during follow-up, did not present active inflammation at the time of the MRI examination.

All images were anonymized and manually segmented by the same musculoskeletal radiologist. The segmentation was performed using Adobe Photoshop CC version 14.1 x 64. Two musculoskeletal radiologists classified, in consensus, each MRI exam as positive or negative for active inflammation. One of the radiologists had, at the time of this study, 2 years of experience after a clinical fellowship in musculoskeletal radiology, and the other was a senior radiologist with 18 years of clinical experience. MRI exams were categorized by the radiologists as a positive or a negative test for inflammatory sacroiliitis for each patient according to the ASAS criteria [3]. The MRI criteria used to define positivity of SIJ inflammation correspond to foci of subchondral edema seen at two different sites or at the same site in at least two consecutive images [3].

The radiologists' classification defined 24 patients as positive and 32 as negative for inflammatory sacroiliitis, and this classification was used as the reference standard to calculate sensitivity, specificity, and the area under the receiver operating characteristic curve (AUC). The dataset was randomly split with ~ 80% (46 samples, 20 positive and 26 negative) for training and ~ 20% for external test (10 samples, 4 positive and 6 negative).

Each original image has the spatial resolution of 256 × 256 pixels and contrast resolution of 256 Gy levels. The SIJ region of interest (ROI) was placed on a black background during the process of manual segmentation. However, this background could cause noise and artifacts in the feature extraction step (described in Section 2.2), such as high frequencies present in the transition between the ROI and the background. To minimize high-frequency noise, a preprocessing method based on the warp perspective transform, including a polynomial transformation [15], was used to expand the ROI and cover all of the background (Fig. 2).

Feature extraction and selection

Statistical analysis was performed based on features extracted from the histograms of the preprocessed ROIs with 256 bins. The features derived included the Mean, Variance, Standard Deviation, Kurtosis, Coefficient of Variation, Skewness, and Maximum Pixel Value.

Texture analysis was based on the features proposed by Haralick et al. [16] using the gray-level cooccurrence matrix, and the features proposed by Tamura et al. [17] extracted from image gray levels. Haralick's features were calculated using a cooccurrence matrix with distance 1 and are listed as follows: Second Angular Momentum, Contrast, Correlation, Variance, Moment of Inverse Difference, Mean Sum, Sum Entropy, Sum of

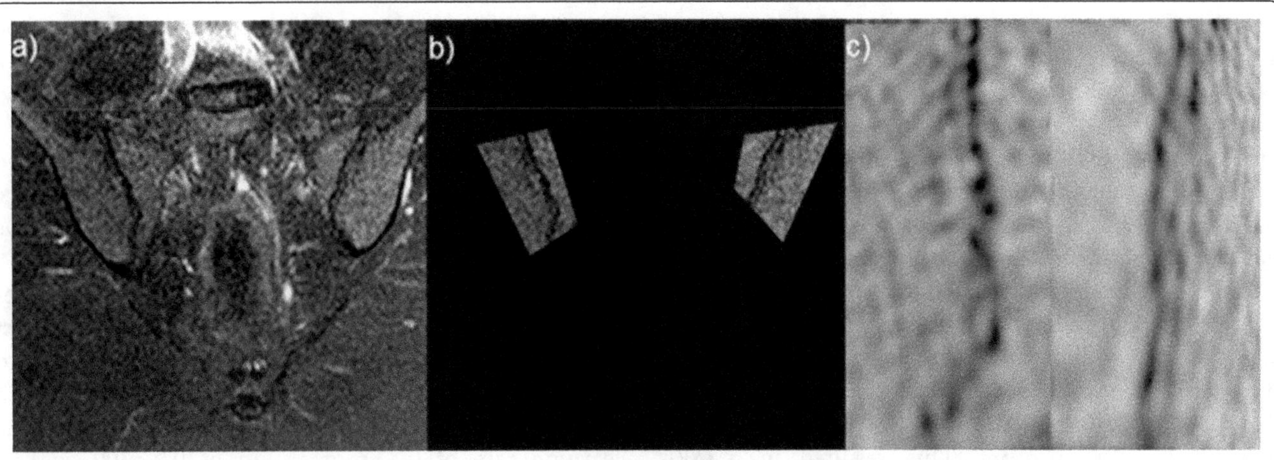

Fig. 2 **a** MRI slice selected. **b** ROI manually segmented and placed on a black background. **c** ROI after the warp transform

Variance, Difference of Variance, Difference of Entropy, two Measures of Information Correlation, and Maximum Correlation Coefficient. Tamura's features were Contrast, Granularity, and Directionality, computed in 16 directions, for a total of 18 features. All of these features were computed using the open-source Java library JFeatureLib [18].

The fast Fourier transform (FFT) was applied to the warped images to obtain the power spectrum using the open-source library ImageJ [19]. The attributes extracted from the two-dimensional rectangular power spectrum were called Fourier features, which include the Mean, Variance, Standard Deviation, Asymmetry, Kurtosis, Coefficient of Variation, and Maximum Pixel Value. The statistics of the power spectrum summarize the frequency intensities, which may be a simple and intuitive way to discriminate instances using frequency features.

The Haar wavelet transform [20] was applied to decompose each image into subimages to obtain the energy in the low-frequency band (LL) and high-frequency bands (HH, HL, LH) in levels 2 and 3. The Haar wavelet is defined as a noncontinuous function and its application to an image results in subimages with vertical, horizontal, and diagonal details from the original image. The energy of each subimage was defined as the sum of all pixel values. The Haar wavelet was implemented using the Fractional Wavelet Module in ImageJ [19].

Gabor filters were applied to each image to obtain the energy in each frequency band, capturing local frequency features [21] in five scales and six orientations. Gabor filters are defined as continuous functions that can detect features in various directions, but have an implicit assumption that all of the images are captured in the same orientation. For each filter output, the mean and standard deviation were calculated, resulting in 60 Gabor features. Gabor filters were implemented using the open-source Java library JFeatureLib [18].

The estimation of fractal dimension was implemented using the box counting method. This approach uses boxes of different sizes and counts the number of occurrences of a specified pattern in the image. Square boxes with width from 6 to 24 pixels were used; boxes with inside pixel values of 50, 100, 150, and 200 were counted; and the mean values of such counts were obtained. The fractal dimension was then estimated as the slope of the line when the logarithm of the mean number of boxes is plotted on the Y axis against the size of the boxes on the X axis. The fractal dimension estimation results in one feature.

The final feature vector for each patient was created using the mean and standard deviation of each feature across the six warped MRI ROIs, because the inflammatory pattern may not be presented in all images of a given exam. This resulted in a 230-dimension feature vector for each patient's MRI exam. Before classification, all features were normalized to the interval [0,1].

The large dimension of the feature vector defined as above may result in poor performance by the classifiers used in machine learning, a problem known as the curse of dimensionality; therefore, we used two feature selection methods to remove irrelevant or redundant features and reduce the vector dimensionality: ReliefF and Wrapper. The ReliefF method assigns a probability of relevance to each feature based on its individual values between multiple nearest instances [22]. The ReliefF algorithm used in this work was implemented with the Weka machine learning platform [23] using 10 nearest neighbors and a search method based on the Ranker algorithm. The Ranker algorithm sorts the feature list from the highest probability to the lowest.

The Wrapper method uses a learning scheme to select features. The idea behind the Wrapper method is to run the chosen classifier with subsets of the feature vector, evaluate the classifier, and choose the feature set with the highest performance [24]. The classifiers used to select features in this work are the Support Vector Machine (SVM), the Multilayer Perceptron (MLP), and the Instance-Based Algorithm (IBA), which will be explained in Section 2.3. The methods were trained and validated using 10-fold cross-validation and the training dataset (46 samples). A feature was considered to be relevant in the training step if it appeared as relevant in at least two folds. The trained model with the best performance was then tested (external validation) using the test dataset (10 samples). Figure 3 shows a flowchart representation of the experiments carried out.

Machine learning

Three machine learning models were used to evaluate the capability of the features to classify SIJ cases.

The SVM is a method that uses hyperplanes to separate the samples provided in an optimal way, such that the margin of separation between the classes (Positive and Negative) will be the maximum possible. The method transforms a multisolution problem to a problem with a unique solution [25]. The equations used to create the hyperplanes were specified to be linear in this work.

IBAs derived from k-nearest neighbors (kNN), referred to as IBk, support robust learning with noisy data, storage reduction during the learning process, and are intuitive [26]. The k values used in this work were 1, 3, and 5.

The MLP is a fully connected ANN which uses backpropagation as the learning scheme. It is a robust model which adjusts synaptic weights according to the error gradient calculated from each training epoch [27]. The MLP model used in this work has the learning rate of 0.3, momentum of 0.2, 500 epochs, and one hidden layer with 231 neurons. The

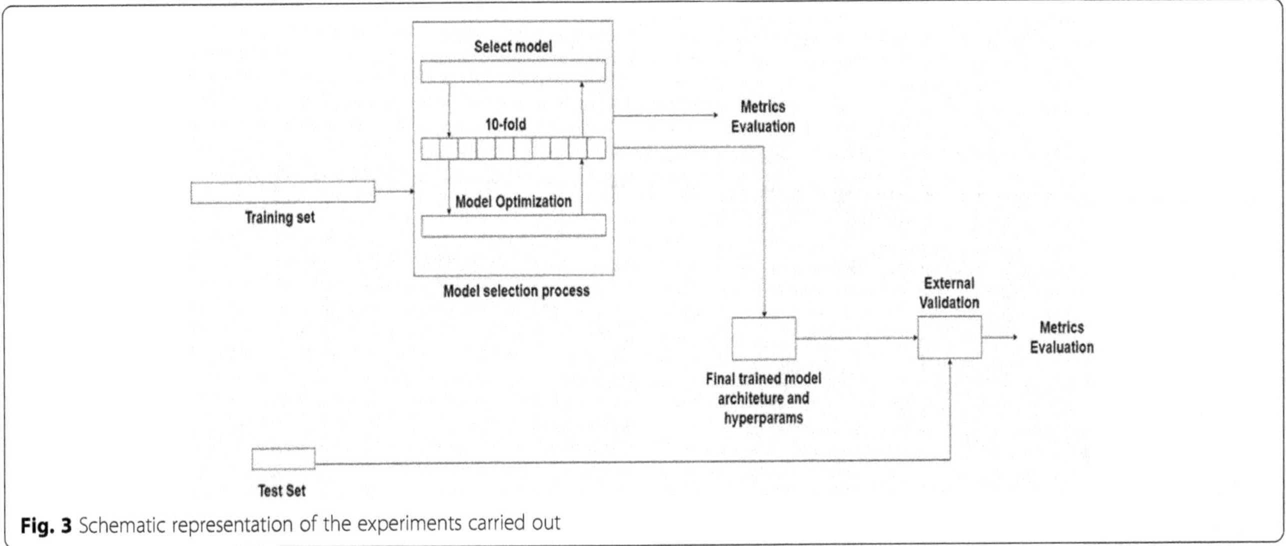

Fig. 3 Schematic representation of the experiments carried out

classifiers were implemented using the open-source library Weka [23].

Results

Initial evaluation of the methods was performed using the training dataset and features ranked by ReliefF and Wrapper, which means that we classified the images using N features for each evaluation, where $0 < N < 231$. The results are presented in Figs. 4, 5 and 6 for AUC, sensitivity (true-positive rate), and specificity (true-negative rate), respectively. Table 1 summarizes the best performance of each classifier. Table 2 shows the classification performance using each of the feature vectors selected by the wrapper method for each classifier. Table 3 shows the MLP classifier's best performance using six features selected by the Wrapper method for the training dataset (10-fold cross-validation, 46 samples) and for the test dataset (external validation, 10 samples).

MLP obtained the best results when all patients categorized as positive for SIJ active inflammation were correctly identified (sensitivity = 1). Of the 26 negative

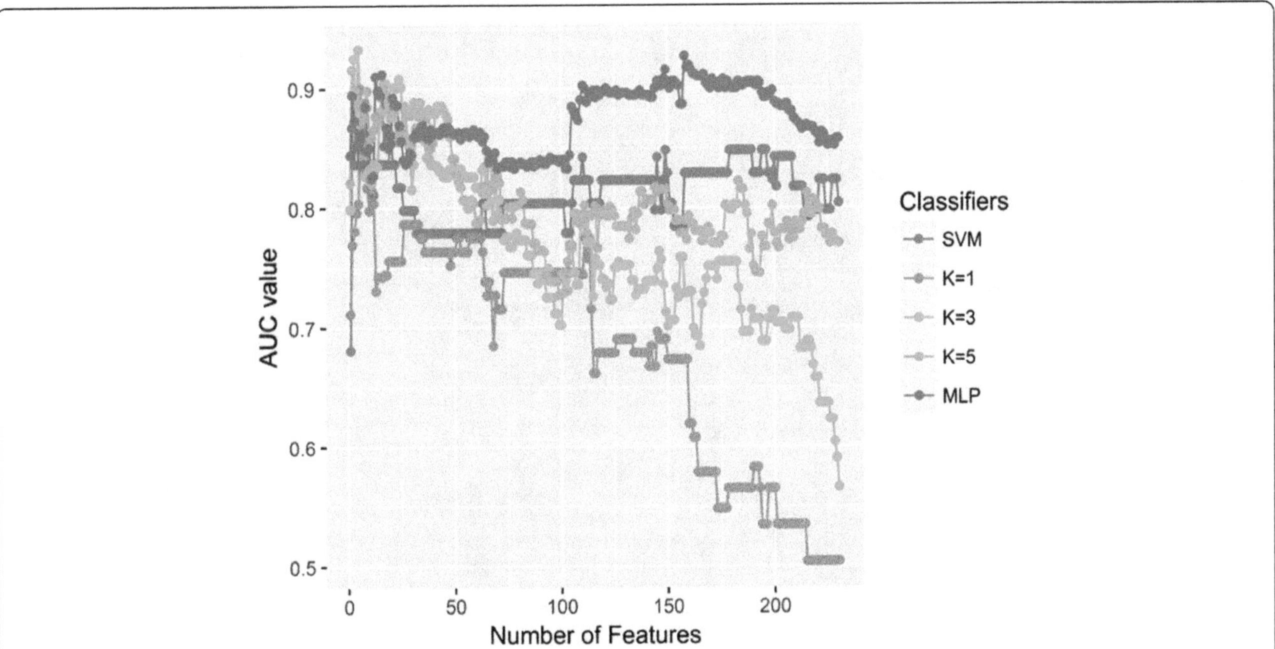

Fig. 4 AUC obtained with different numbers of features for the various classifiers studied to classify negative and positive active inflammatory sacroiliitis on MRI using the training dataset. SVM = Support Vector Machine; MLP = Multilayer Perceptron; Instance-Based Algorithm (IBA) derived from k-nearest neighbors (IBk) (k = 1, k = 3, k = 5)

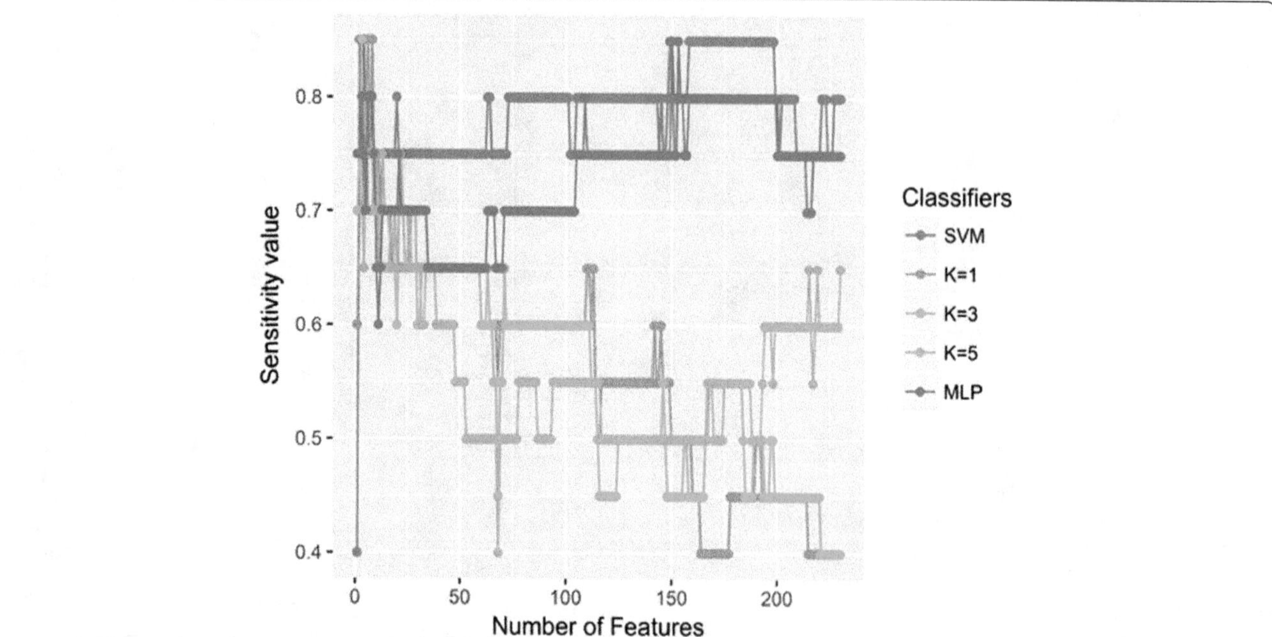

Fig. 5 Sensitivity obtained with different numbers of features for the various classifiers studied to classify negative and positive active inflammatory sacroiliitis on MRI using the training dataset. SVM = Support Vector Machine; MLP = Multilayer Perceptron; Instance-Based Algorithm (IBA) derived from k-nearest neighbors (IBk) (k = 1, k = 3, k = 5)

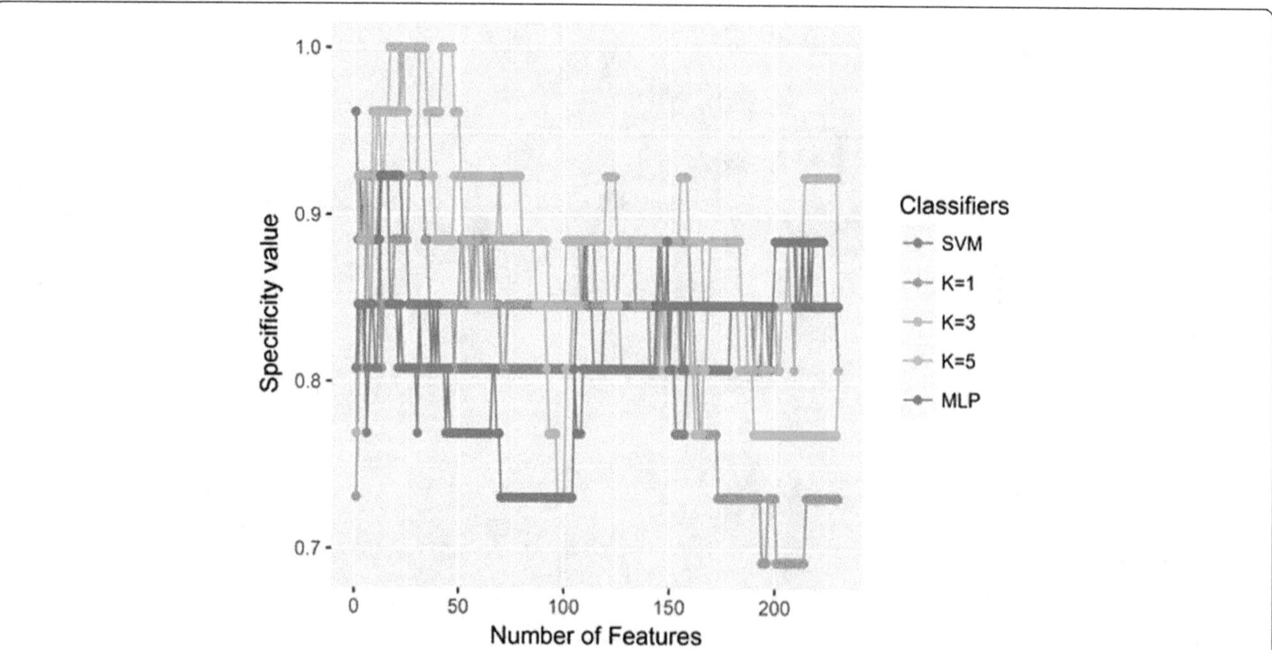

Fig. 6 Specificity obtained with different numbers of features for the various classifiers studied to classify negative and positive active inflammatory sacroiliitis on MRI using the training dataset. SVM = Support Vector Machine; MLP = Multilayer Perceptron; Instance-Based Algorithm (IBA) derived from k-nearest neighbors (IBk) (k = 1, k = 3, k = 5)

Table 1 Best performance for each classifier and number of features used to yield the same result. SVM = Support Vector Machine; MLP = Multilayer Perceptron; Instance-Based Algorithm (IBA) derived from k-nearest neighbors (IBk) (k = 1, k = 3, k = 5); AUC = Area under the ROC curve

Classifier	Metric name	Metric value	Number of features
SVM	AUC	0.867	2
	Sensitivity	0.850	2
	Specificity	0.960	1
IBk with k = 1	AUC	0.900	6
	Sensitivity	0.850	6
	Specificity	0.923	6
IBk with k = 3	AUC	0.932	5
	Sensitivity	0.850	3
	Specificity	1.000	24
IBk with k = 5	AUC	0.915	2
	Sensitivity	0.800	5
	Specificity	1.000	17
MLP	AUC	0.926	158
	Sensitivity	0.85	150
	Specificity	0.923	16

cases, only 2 cases were erroneously classified by the algorithm as positive (specificity = 0.923). Therefore, the final agreement between the radiologists and the algorithm reached 95.6% (Accuracy) in this scenario.

Discussion

Recent literature dedicated to musculoskeletal radiology shows increasing interest in the application of machine learning and other computer techniques, for example, in the analysis of benign and malignant vertebral compression fractures [28], skeletal maturity [29], and differentiation between benign and malignant cartilaginous bone tumors [30]. However, to our best knowledge, there is no previous study dedicated to SpA SIJ inflammation.

Our study examined the use of machine learning models to aid in the classification of MRI of SIJs as positive or negative for active inflammation. The visual diagnosis of sacroiliitis in clinical practice consists of the detection of changes in the gray levels in the tissues close to the SIJ surfaces by a medical specialist, with high signal intensity of subchondral bone indicating active inflammation. Based on this and related observations, we performed statistical, textural, spectral, and fractal analyses to extract features and characterize SIJs for classification.

In general, classifiers provided their best performance with low-dimension feature vectors obtained using ReliefF or Wrapper methods.

ReliefF provides a classifier-independent list of relevant features. Table 1 shows that kNN with k = 3 reached the highest AUC using only 5 features selected by ReliefF. These five features are the mean of the energy of Haar wavelet for LH on level 2, mean of the maximum value of pixel, standard deviation of the energy of Haar wavelet for HH on level 2, standard deviation for the maximum value of pixel, and standard deviation of the energy of Haar wavelet for LH on level 2.

The high-frequency filters detect abrupt transitions between gray levels. As shown by the results, the maximum value of pixel discriminates between positive and negative instances, indicating that the maximum values are probably causing some high-frequency components in the SIJ ROIs.

For the Wrapper method using 10 folds, kNN with k = 5 reached the highest performance with 9 features. The Wrapper method provides a classifier-based list of relevant features, which are the standard deviation of 6° directionality of Tamura (relevant on 2 folds), standard deviation of 13° directionality of Tamura (relevant on 3 folds), mean of Tamura correlation (relevant on 4 folds), mean of maximum correlation coefficient of Haralick (relevant on 2 folds), mean of the maximum pixel value (relevant on 2 folds), mean of skewness of the Fourier power spectrum (relevant on 3 folds), mean of Haar wavelet from LL on level 2 (relevant on 2 folds), mean of Haar wavelet of LH on level 2 (relevant on 8 folds), and mean of fractal dimension (relevant on 2 folds).

Again, the maximum pixel value and Haar wavelet from LH on level 2 were selected as relevant, implying that these features are, in fact, discriminative. High-frequency components are caused by large changes in

Table 2 - Performance of each classifier using the features selected by the wrapper method. SVM = Support Vector Machine; MLP = Multilayer Perceptron; Instance-Based Algorithm (IBA) derived from k-nearest neighbors (IBk) (k = 1, k = 3, k = 5); AUC = Area under the ROC curve

Classifier	AUC	Sensitivity	Specificity	Accuracy (%)	Number of Features
SVM	0.842	0.800	0.885	87.8	15
IBk with k = 1	0.798	0.800	0.769	78.2	13
IBk with k = 3	0.867	0.750	0.885	82.6	14
IBk with k = 5	0.969	0.750	0.962	86.9	9
MLP	0.965	1.000	0.923	95.6	6

Table 3 - Multilayer perceptron (MLP) classifier selected model performance using 10-fold cross-validation on training samples (46 samples) and external validation on test set (10 samples)

	10-Fold			Test set		
Model	Sensitivity	Specificity	Accuracy (%)	Sensitivity	Specificity	Accuracy (%)
MLP	1	0.923	95.6%	1	0.667	80%

gray levels across small distances in the image. However, not all frequency features were selected, which is probably due to correlation between those features, a characteristic that is detected by the Wrapper method.

The classifier that reached the highest AUC, kNN, has a performance problem in prediction because it always needs to calculate the distance between the predicted instance and all other instances, which is not scalable. If scalability is important, the MLP may be the better choice of classifier using the Wrapper method. The features selected by the MLP are the mean of the 1° directionality of Tamura (relevant on 2 folds), standard deviation of the 13° directionality of Tamura (relevant on 2 folds), mean of sum variance from the gray levels (relevant on 4 folds), mean of maximum pixel value (relevant on 2 folds), mean of second Gabor directionality (relevant on 5 folds), and mean of Haar wavelet from LH on level 2 (relevant on 10 folds).

An important observation is that, always, the maximum pixel value and Haar wavelet from LH on level 2 were selected as relevant by both feature selection methods, asserting that these features are important to discriminate instances. The maximum pixel value is intuitive to be important because inflammation manifests as high-intensity of gray level around the SIJ. Gabor directionality measures are probably selected due to the directionality change caused by the depth of inflammation in SIJ.

We have used the STIR sequence in the coronal plane to apply the machine learning methods, but in clinical practice, radiologists may have access to other fluid-sensitive fat-saturated MRI sequences with images acquired also in the axial and sagittal planes. We chose to use the STIR sequence because this is one of the recommended sequences by the ASAS guidelines [3]. Recently, two different studies have shown that other fluid-sensitive fat-saturated MRI techniques may be equally sensitive and accurate in the diagnosis of inflammatory sacroiliitis [31, 32]. Therefore, it could be interesting to investigate in the future if different fluid-sensitive fat-saturated MRI techniques could provide and support similar results using the machine learning approach. We also encourage future studies exploring the potential of radiomics [33, 34] in the evaluation of inflammatory sacroiliitis, with the potential impact of deriving new diagnostic and prognostic information.

We did not investigate the potential of artificial intelligence techniques to identify postinflammatory structural damage on the SIJ surface and subchondral bone, because the aim was to classify active inflammation. However, the identification of such abnormalities may be important for the diagnosis of SpA and future studies should use T1-weighted sequences for this assessment, since these sequences provide a greater conspicuity of such findings.

As expected, in the external validation test the accuracy fell down from 95.6 to 80.0 and specificity from 0.923 to 0.667 (Table 3). We believe that our results are still encouraging, and we suggest new studies to improve AI techniques to investigate inflammatory sacroiliitis and SpA.

Some limitations of this study need mentioning. First, the study was retrospective. In addition, the number of patients was relatively small, which usually precludes the use of deep learning methods [35]. We used the segmentation performed by only one musculoskeletal radiologist as the ground truth, but even experienced specialists may show interpersonal variability, and the inclusion of more radiologists would be desirable to validate future artificial intelligence algorithms. Besides, to use the methods described in our study, it is necessary that a musculoskeletal radiologist or an experienced rheumatologist choose the most representative images of the synovial SIJ region on the coronal plane. The development of a semiautomatic or automatic segmentation tool would be desirable to obviate this workload. Finally, although the database was divided into training and testing sets, which made it possible to make an independent evaluation of the generalization of the validated classifier model obtained during the training phase (10-fold cross-validation), our study enrolled cases from only one institution. Future validation with cases from another institution is required before one can generalize our results for potential clinical application.

Conclusion

Our results show the potential of machine learning methods to identify SIJ subchondral bone marrow edema in axSpA patients and are promising to aid in the detection of active inflammatory sacroiliitis on MRI STIR sequences. Multilayer Perceptron (MLP) achieved the best results.

Acknowledgments
Coordenação de Aperfeiçoamento de Pessoal de Nível Superior - Brasil (CAPES).

Authors' contributions
MCF and PMAM conceived and designed the experiments; MCF, APMT, VFD, RLA analyzed the data, MCF and MHN-B drafted the manuscript; MCF, JRFJ performed experiments and acquired data; MCF, VFD and RLA collected samples; MCF, PMAM, RMR, PL-J, MHN-B interpreted data and critically revised the manuscript. All authors read and approved the final version of the manuscript.

Author details
[1]São Carlos School of Engineering, University of São Paulo, São Carlos, SP, Brazil. [2]Ribeirão Preto Medical School, University of São Paulo, Ribeirão Preto, SP, Brazil. [3]MAInLab Medical Artificial Intelligence Laboratory, Ribeirão Preto Medical School, Ribeirão Preto, Brazil. [4]Ribeirão Preto Medical School Musculoskeletal Imaging Research Laboratory, Ribeirão Preto, Brazil. [5]Radiology Division / CCIFM, Ribeirão Preto Medical School, Av. Bandeirantes, 3900, Ribeirão Preto, SP CEP 14048-900, Brazil. [6]Electrical and Computer Engineering Schulich School of Engineering University of Calgary, Calgary, Alberta, Canada.

References

1. Garg N, van der Bosh F, Deodhar A. The concept of Spondyloarthritis: where are we now? Best Pract Res Clin Rheumatol. 2014;28:663–72.
2. Boonen A. Socioeconomic consequences of ankylosing spondylitis. Clin Exp Rheumatol. 2002;20:S23–6.
3. Lambert RGW, Bakker PAC, van der Heijde D, Weber U, Rudwaleit M, et al. Defining active sacroiliitis on MRI for classification of axial spondyloarthritis: update by the ASAS MRI working group. Ann Rheum Dis. 2016;75:1958–63.
4. Maksymowych WP, Inman RD, Salonen D, Dhillon SS, Wiliians M, Stone M, Conner-Spady B, Palsat J, Lambert RGW. Spondyloarthritis research consortium of Canada magnetic resonance imaging index for assessment of sacroiliac joint inflammation in Ankylosing spondylitis. Arthritis Rheumatism. 2005;53:703–9.
5. Erickson BF, Korfiatis P, Akkus Z, Kline TL. Machine learning for medical imaging. RadioGraphics. 2017;37:505–15.
6. Chartrand G, Cheng PM, Vorontsov E, Drozdzal M, Turcotte S, Pal CJ, Kadoury S, Tang A. Deep learning: a primer for radiologists. Radiographics. 2017;37:2113–31.
7. Nasr-Esfahani E, Samavi S, Karimi N, Soroushmehr SMR, Jafari MH, Ward K, Najarian K. Melanoma detection by analysis of clinical images using convolutional neural network. Conf Proc IEEE Eng Med Biol Soc. 2016;2016: 1373–6.
8. Wang S, Zhang R, Deng Y, Chen K, Xiao D, Peng P, Jiang T. Discrimination of smoking status by MRI based on deep learning method. Quant Imaging Med Surg. 2018;8:1113–20.
9. Pereira SM, Frade MAC, Rangayyan RM, Azevedo-Marques PM. Classification of color images of dermatological ulcers. IEEE Journal of Biomedical and Health Informatics. 2013;17:136–42.
10. Azevedo-Marques PM, Rosa NA, Traina AJM, Traina Junior C, Kinoshita SK, Rangayyan RM. Reducing the semantic gap in content-based image retrieval in mammography with relevance feedback and inclusion of expert knowledge. Int J Comput Assist Radiol Surg. 2008;3:123–30.
11. Ferreira Junior JR, Koenigkam-Santos M, Cipriano FER, Fabro AT, Azevedo-Marques PM. Radiomics-based features for pattern recognition of lung cancer histopathology and metastases. Comput Methods Prog Biomed. 2018;159:23–30.
12. Allende-Cid H, Rangayyan RM, Azevedo-Marques PM, Almeida E, Frery A, Cardoso I, Ramos H. Analysis of machine learning algorithms for diagnosis of diffuse lung diseases. Methods Inf Med. 2018;57:272–9.
13. Azevedo-Marques PM, Spagnoli HF, Frighetto-Pereira L, Reis RM, Metzner GA, Rangayyan RM, Nogueira-Barbosa MH. Classification of vertebral compression fractures in magnetic resonance images using spectral and fractal analysis. Conf Proc IEEE Eng Med Biol Soc. 2015;2015:723 6.
14. Casti P, Mencattini A, Nogueira-Barbosa MH, Frighetto-Pereira L, Azevedo-Marques PM, Martinelli E, Di Natale C. Cooperative strategy for a dynamic ensemble of classification models in clinical applications: the case of MRI vertebral compression fractures. Int J Comput Assist Radiol Surg. 2017;12:1971–83.
15. Faleiros MC, Zavala EJR, Ferreira-Junior JR, Dalto VF, Assad RL, Louzada Junior P, Nogueira-Barbosa MH, Azevedo-Marques PM. Computer-aided classification of inflammatory sacroiliitis in magnetic resonance imaging. Int J Comput Assist Radiol Surg. 2017 Jun;12(Suppl 1):154–5.
16. Haralick RM, Shanmugam K, Dinstein I. Textural features for image classification. IEEE Transactions on Systems man and cybernetics. 1973;SMC-3:610–523.
17. Tamura H, Mori S, Yamawaki T. Textural features corresponding to visual perception. IEEE Transactions on Systems, Man, & Cybernetics. 1978;8:460–73.
18. Keuschnig M & Penz C. JFeatureLib open source project. 2008. Available in http://github.com/locked-fg/JFeatureLib. Acessed 1 May 2020.
19. Schneider CA, Rasband WS, Eliceiri KW. NIH image to ImageJ: 25 years of image analysis. Nat Methods. 2012;9:671–5.
20. Haar A. Zur Theorie der orthogonalen Funktionensysteme. Math Ann. 1910;69:331–71.
21. Zhang D, Wong A, Indrawan M, Lu G. Content-based image retrieval using Gabor texture features. University of Sydney: IEEE Pacific-Rim Conference on Multimedia; 2000.
22. Kononenko I. Estimating attributes: analysis and extensions of relief. European Conference of Machine Learning; 1994.
23. Frank E, Hall MA, Witten I. In: Kaufmann M, editor. The WEKA Workbench. Online Appendix for "Data Mining: Practical Machine Learning Tools and Techniques". 4th ed; 2016.
24. Kohavi R, John GH. Wrappers for feature subset selection. Artif Intell. 1997;97:273–324.
25. Hearst MA, Dumais ST, Osuna E, Platt J, Scholkopf B. Support vector machines. IEEE Intelligent Systems and their Appl. 1998;13:18–28.
26. Aha DW, Kibler D, Albert MK. Instance-based learning algorithms. Mach Learn. 1991;6:37–66.
27. Haykin S. Neural networks - a comprehensive foundation second edition, Pearson education; 1999.
28. Frighetto-Pereira L, Rangayyan RM, Metzner GA, Azevedo-Marques PM, Nogueira-Barbosa MH. Shape, texture and statistical features for classification of benign and malignant vertebral compression fractures in magnetic resonance images. Comput Biol Med. 2016;73:147–56.
29. Larson DB, Chen MC, Lungren MP, Halabi SS, Stence NV, Langlotz CP. Performance of a deep-learning neural network model in assessing skeletal maturity on pediatric hand radiographs. Radiology. 2018;287:313–22.
30. Lisson CS, Lisson CG, Flosdorf K, Mayer-Steinacker R, Schultheiss M, von Baer A, Barth TFE, Beer AJ, Baumhauer M, Meier R, Beer M, Schmidt SA. Diagnostic value of MRI-based 3D texture analysis for tissue characterisation and discrimination of low-grade chondrosarcoma from enchondroma: a pilot study. Eur Radiol. 2018;28:468–77.
31. Dalto VF, Assad RL, Crema MD, Louzada-Junior P, Nogueira-Barbosa MH. MRI assessment of bone marrow oedema in the sacroiliac joints of patients with spondyloarthritis: is the SPAIR T2w technique comparable to STIR? Eur Radiol. 2017;27:3669–76.
32. Sung S, Kim HS, Kwon JW. MRI assessment of sacroiliitis for the diagnosis of axial spondyloarthropathy: comparison of fat-saturated T2, STIR and contrast-enhanced sequences. Br J Radiol. 2017;90(1078):20170090.
33. Gillies RJ, Kinahan PE, Hricak H. Radiomics: images are more than pictures, they are data. Radiology. 2016;278:563–77.
34. Hou Z, Yang Y, Li S, Yan J, Ren W, Liu J, Wang K, Liu B, Wan S. Radiomic analysis using contrast-enhanced CT: predict treatment response to pulsed low dose rate radiotherapy in gastric carcinoma with abdominal cavity metastasis. Quant Imaging Med Surg. 2018;8:410–20.
35. Lecun Y, Bengio Y, Hinton G. Deep learning. Nature. 2015;28:436–44.

9

Comparison of lupus patients with early and late onset nephritis: A study in 71 patients from a single referral center

Juliana Delfino*, Thiago Alberto F. G. dos Santos and Thelma L. Skare

Abstract

Background: Nephritis occurs frequently in systemic lupus erythematosus (SLE) and may worsen disease morbidity and mortality. Knowing all characteristics of this manifestation helps to a prompt recognition and treatment.

Aim: To compare the differences in clinical data, serological profile and treatment response of nephritis of early and late onset.

Methods: Retrospective study of 71 SLE patients with biopsy proven nephritis divided in early nephritis group (diagnosis of nephritis in the first 5 years of the disease) and late nephritis (diagnosis of nephritis after 5 years). Epidemiological, serological, clinical and treatment data were collected from charts and compared.

Results: In this sample, 70. 4% had early onset nephritis and 29.6% had late onset. No differences were noted in epidemiological, clinical, serological profile, SLICC and SLEDAI, except that late onset nephritis patients were older at nephritis diagnosis ($p = 0.01$). Regarding renal biopsy classification, C3 and C4 levels, serum creatinine, 24 h proteinuria and response rate to treatment the two groups were similar (p = NS). Patients with early onset had lower levels of hemoglobin at nephritis onset than those of late onset ($p = 0.02$).

Conclusions: Most of SLE patients had nephritis in the first 5 years of disease. No major differences were noted when disease profile or treatment outcome of early and late onset nephritis were compared.

Keywords: Systemic lupus Erythematosus, Nephritis, Treatment, Prognosis

Introduction

Renal involvement in systemic lupus erythematosus (SLE) is one of most common and feared manifestations of this disease as it is related to high morbidity and increased rate of mortality [1]. It has been estimated that almost half of adults and 80–90% of children with systemic lupus will develop kidney involvement [2] and that 10% of them will go into renal failure [3, 4].

Several factors may affect the prognosis in this context. Ethnic background is one of them; nephritis is more common and more severe in African, Asian and Latin American individuals [5]. Early age at lupus onset and male gender are other factors [6].

Lupus nephritis is more frequent in those with anti-dsDNA [7] and it is less common in those with discoid manifestations [8] and positivity for rheumatoid factor [9]. It usually occurs within the first years after diagnosis [10] although some patients do develop this complication later on. Few studies [11, 12] address to the characteristics of patients with late onset of nephritis that could allow an early identification and treatment.

Herein we studied systemic lupus patients with nephritis to see if there are differences in clinical, serologic profile and treatment response in patients to analyze those who develop this manifestation early (within the first 5 years) or later in the disease course.

Methods

This study was approved by the local Committee of Ethics in Research. It was a retrospective study that included patients with lupus nephritis from a single rheumatology outpatient clinic that attended for regular consultation during the period of 10 years. To be included patients should have SLE diagnosis after 16 years

* Correspondence: juliana.delfino@live.com
Mackenzie Evangelical University Hospital, Curitiba, PR, Brazil

of age, nephritis proved by renal biopsy and received standard treatment for the renal involvement: induction with glucocorticoid, intravenous cyclophosphamide (0.5 to 1.0 g/m2/month for 6 months) or mophetyl mycophenolate (MMF) (2-3g/day - 6 months) and maintenance for at least 2 years with either azathioprine or MMF. Pregnant patients, those who did not complete the treatment and that received any other immunosuppressants were excluded. Clinical and serological data were collected from the charts. The clinical profile was considered in a cumulative manner and collected following the definition of the 1997 American College of Rheumatology revised criteria for the classification of Systemic Lupus Erythematosus [13]; secondary APS (antiphospholipid antibody syndrome) followed the 2006 modified APS criteria [14]. The autoantibodies tested in the serological profile were: anti-Ro/SS-A, anti-La/SS-B, anti-RNP, anti-Sm, anti-dsDNA, anticardiolipin (aCl) IgG, aCl IgM, LA (lupus anticoagulant), direct Coombs and rheumatoid factor (RF). Anti-Ro/SS-A, anti-La/SS-B, anti-RNP, anti-Sm, aCl-IgG, aCl-IgM were tested by ELISA (using ALKA and Orgentec Kits); anti-dsDNA, by immunofluorescence technique (IFT); the lupus anticoagulant, by screening test, the dRVVT (dilute Russell viper venom test) and confirmed by RVVT. Latex agglutination test (BioSystems) was used to search IgM RF and monoclonal anti human globulin Fresenius-Kabi-Brasil was used for the direct Coombs test.

Data on nephritis included: renal biopsy classification according to ISN/RPS (International Society of Nephrology/ Renal Pathology Society) [15], 24 h proteinuria, creatinine levels, creatinine clearance, values of serum complement fractions C3 and C4, anti-dsDNA positivity and hemoglobin (hb) levels just prior to induction treatment, and after 2 years of treatment. The time from the end of treatment until the first nephritis relapse was also collected.

To be considered as treatment responder patient should have had stabilization or improvement of renal function and reduction of proteinuria to less than 0.5 g / day and /or normal clearence or increase of only up to 10% without active sediment. To be considered as partially responders, they should show reduction of 50% of proteinuria with < 3 g / day and normal clearance or with alteration of up to 10% of the previous value [16]. Non-responders were those with deterioration of renal function after excluding causes such as sepsis, drugs, dehydration and renal vein thrombosis and / or increased proteinuria or non-reduction of proteinuria in order to fall into partial or total remission.

SLEDAI (Systemic Lupus Erythematosus disease activity) [17] and SLICC/ACR DI (Systemic Lupus International Collaborating Clinics/ American College of Rheumatology Damage Index) [18] were calculated in the beginning of the treatment and after 2 years.

Patients were divided in two groups, for comparison: (1) those with nephritis that initiated within the first 5 years after SLE diagnosis and classified as early nephritis group; (2) those with nephritis diagnosed more than 5 years after SLE diagnosis and classified as late nephritis group.

Data was collected in frequency and contingency tables. Data distribution was tested by the Shapiro Wilk test. Central tendency was expressed in mean and standard deviation or median and interquartile range (IQR) according to the distribution of studied data. Nominal data were compared by Fisher and chi-squared tests and the numeric, by U-Mann-Whitney and unpaired t tes, respectively. The software Medcalc 10.0 was used for calculations. The adopted significance was of 5%.

Results

a) **Description of studied sample and comparison of clinical and serological data:**
Seventy-one patients met the inclusion criteria: 50 (70. 4%) of them had early onset of nephritis and 21 (29.6%) had late onset. Table 1 shows the main characteristics of this group and the comparison between early and late onset nephritis groups.
b) **Comparison of renal involvement in early and late onset nephritis.**

The comparison between early and late onset nephritis is on Table 2. In this table it is possible to see that patients from the late nephritis group had a better hemoglobin level in the initial evaluation, showed tendency to recur earlier and had a positive anti-dsDNA more frequently than those in the early nephritis group. Otherwise the two groups had similar results.

We performed a logistic regression - with group of early or late onset as the dependent variable taking into account age, SLICC, SLEDAI and patients age and GNF class. We could not obtain any significance.

Studying only class III and class IV glomerulonephritis, no differences were noted in the remission rate at 1 year ($p = 0.72$) neither at 2 years ($p = 0.30$).

Discussion

Our results showed that almost 2/ 3 of lupus patients developed nephritis in the first 5 years after the diagnosis. This preference for early development of nephritis was already highlighted by Cameron [19] that emphasized that 25 to 50% of unselected patients with lupus have abnormalities of urine or renal function early in the course of disease. Also, in juvenile lupus up to 80% of patients developing lupus nephritis do it within the first 5 years from diagnosis [20]. The present sample had only adult SLE patients and the age at SLE diagnosis was similar in both groups, but patients in the early nephritis

Table 1 Comparative analysis of clinical and serological data in 71 patients with Systemic Lupus Erythematosus (SLE) with early and late onset nephritis

	Total sample N = 71	Early nephritis N = 50 (70. 4%)	Late nephritis N = 21 (29.6%)	P [a]
Ethnic background [b]	Caucasians 27 Afrodescendants 44	Caucasians 16 Afrodescendants 34	Caucasians 11 Afrodescendants 10	0.64
Median age at SLE diagnosis (years) (IQR)	26.0 (21.0–38.0)	27 (21-40.2)	26 (21.0–37.0)	0.67
Median age at nephritis diagnosis (years) (IQR)	30.0 (23.0–42.0)	27.5 (21. 7-41.0)	35 (29. 5-43.5)	0.01
Female gender	62 (87. 3%)	43 (84. 3%)	19 (90. 4%)	0.71
Tobaco exposure	8 (11.2%)	4 (9%)	4 (19.0%)	0.22
Malar rash	30 (42.2%)	20 (40%)	10 (47.6%)	0.55
Discoid lesions	2 (2.8%)	0	2 (9.5%)	0.08
Photossensitivity	48 (67.6%)	32 (64%)	16 (76.1%)	0.72
Oral ulcers	35 (49.2%)	24 (48%)	11 (52. 3%)	0.73
Articular involvement	60 (84.5%)	40 (80%)	20 (95.2%)	0.15
Serositis	18 (25. 3%)	15 (30%)	3 (14.2%)	0.23
Psychosis	1 (1. 4%)	0	1 (4.7%)	0.29
Convulsions	6 (8. 4%)	6 (12%)	0	0.16
Hemolytic anemia	8 (11. 4%)	7 (14.2%)	1 (4.7%)	0.42
Leukopenia	25 (35.2%)	15 (30%)	10 (47.6%)	0.15
Lymphocytopenia	15 (21.1%)	11 (22%)	4 (19.0%)	1.00
Thrombocytopenia	2 (2.8%)	1 (2%)	1 (4.7%)	0.50
Anti-Ro (SS-A)	26 (36.6%)	19 (38%)	7 (33. 3%)	0.70
Anti-La (SS-B)	10 (14.0%)	7 (14%)	3 (14.2%)	1.00
Anti-RNP	13 (18. 3%)	7 (14%)	6 (28.5%)	0.14
Anti-Sm	13 (18. 3%)	8 (16%)	5 (23.8%)	0.50
Positive Coombs	6 (8. 4%)	5 (10%)	1 (4.7%)	0.66
Rheumatoid factor	6 (8. 4%)	6 (12%)	0	0.16
Anticardiolipin IgG	1 (1. 4%)	1 (2%)	0	1.00
Anticardiolipin IgM	2 (2.8%)	2 (4%)	0	1.00
Lupus anticoagulante	5 (7.0%)	3 (6%)	2 (9.5%)	0.62
Antiphospholipid antibody syndrome	5 (7.0%)	3 (6%)	2 (9.5%)	0.62

[a] refers to early onset versus late onset; [b]- auto declared; *IQR* interquartile range, *n* number

group were younger at nephritis diagnosis. Unfortunately, no other clinical or serological differences could be noted between the two groups that could be associated to the nephritis onset. However our sample was small and may not have had enough strength to demonstrate any differences. It is worthwhile to note that in this sample there were 61.9% of class IV nephritis in the late onset compared to 50% in the early onset group and this data should be take into account to explain the tendency for early relapse in the late onset group. Relapse rate in class IV nephritis is more common [21].

Renal involvement in SLE is recognized as a major cause of high morbidity and mortality [22] and its prompt recognition and treatment is associated with better prognosis [23].

Regarding treatment, the rate of response was similar in both groups, although a tendency to early relapse was noticed in the late onset nephritis group, with no significance (Table 2). Considering this, patients with late onset nephritis should be treated as aggressively as those of early onset in order to prevent renal damage.

Contrary to our findings, Varela et al. [12] associated the delayed onset nephritis with the presence of antiphospholipid antibody syndrome (AAF). Our sample had only few cases of AAF that precluded a good observation of this aspect.

This study has some limitations: its retrospective design and the follow up of only 2 years. Another is that nephritis remission was judged only on clinical grounds. It is well known that lupus patients with nephritis may

Table 2 Comparative analysis of main characteristics and treatment response in Systemic Lupus Erythematosus (SLE) patients with early and late onset nephritis

	Early onset *N* = 50	Late onset *N* = 21	P
Glomerulonephritis classification			
Class II	5 (10%)	3 (14.2%)	0.79
Class III	10 (20%)	3 (14.2%)	
Class III+ V	2 (4%)	0	
Class IV	25 (50%)	13 (61.9%)	
Class IV+ V	1 (2%)	0	
Class V	7 (14%)	2 (9.5%)	
Induction treatment			
Cyclophosphamide	44 (88%)	20 (95.2%)	0.66
MMF	6 (12%)	1 (4.7%)	
Maintenance treatment			
Azathioprine	31 (62%)	14 (66.6%)	1.00
MMF	18 (36%)	7 (33. 3%)	
Treatment response in 2 years			
Total remission	30 (60%)	12 (57.1%)	0.35
Partial remission	10 (20%)	2 (9.5%)	
Treatment failure	10 (20%)	7 (33. 3%)	
Median creatinine (IQR)- mg/dL			
Initial	0.98 (0. 6-1. 3)	0.97 (0. 7-1. 3)	0.94
After 2 years	0.80 (0. 7-1.1)	0.74 (0. 6-1.0)	0.45
Creatinine clearence (mL/min)			
Initial (median;IQR)	83.5 (52. 3–120.6)	82. 3 (52. 7-89.0)	0.60
After 2 years (mean ± SD)	94.7 ± 38.7	97.0 ± 37.8	0.81
Positive anti-ds-DNA			
Initial	20 (40%)	13 (61.9%)	0.09
After 2 years	14 (28%)	9 (42.8%)	0.22
Median 24 h proteinuria (g/L) (IQR)			
Initial	2.9 (1. 7-5. 4)	2.0 (1. 2-5.1)	0.17
After 2 years	0.36 (0. 1-1.1)	0.35 (0. 1-1.0)	0.48
C3 (mg/dL)			
Initial (median; IQR)	72.5 (46. 5-99.6)	85.7 (56. 4–104.5)	0.22
After 2 years (mean ± SD)	109. 4±29. 4	103. 3±36. 3	0.45
Median C4 (IQR) (mg/dL)			
Initial	11.9 (7. 9-21.8)	12.0 (7.0–23.2)	0.93
After 2 years	19.0 (13. 9-26.9)	23.0 (13. 7-28.5)	0.68
Hemoglobine (g/dL)			
Initial (mean ± SD)	11.6 ± 2.2	12.8 ± 1.5	0.02
After 2 years (median;IQR)	13.0 (12.0–14.1)	12.6 (12.0–13.8)	0.58
SLEDAI			
Initial (mean ± SD)	14.8 ± 5. 4	13.2 ± 6.1	0.28
After 2 years (mean ± SD)	5.8± 4.6	6. 4± 4.8	0.59
Median SLICC/ACR DI (IQR)			
Initial	0 (0–1)	0 (0–1)	0.93
After 2 years	0 (0–2)	1.0 (0–2)	0.41
Interval (years) until first recurrence – median (IQR)	4.5 (2. 2-6.7)	3.0 (1.0–5.0)	0.07

N number, *IQR* interquartile range, *SD* standard deviation, *MMF* mophetyl mycophenolate, *SLEDAI* Systemic lupus erythematosus disease activity index, *SLICC/ACR DI* Systemic Lupus International Collaborating Clinics/ American College of Rheumatology Damage Index

have silent activity only disclosed by repeated biopsy [24]. However, repeated renal biopsy is an aggressive approach not well accepted by all patients. Nevertheless, this study highlights the fact that late and early nephritis have similar outcomes and should not be treated differently.

Conclusion

Our results have shown that nephritis onset is more common in the first 5 years after SLE diagnosis and that lupus patients with early and late onset nephritis share same clinical and serological characteristics. It also shows that these two situations had similar outcomes.

Acknowledgements
Not applicable.

Authors' contributions
JD, M.D.; project; bibliographic revision; date a collection; Mackenzie Evangelical Hospital, Curitiba, PR, Brazil. TAS, MD; paper draft; bibliographic revision; Mackenzie Evangelical Hospital, Curitiba, PR, Brazil. E-mail: thiagoalbertofgs@gmail.com. TLS, MD, PhD. statistical analyzis; paper review; Mackenzie Evangelical Hospital, Curitiba, PR, Brazil. Email: tskare@onda.com.br. All the authors have read the final paper in agreed with it. All authors give consent for publication if accepted. All authors read and approved the final manuscript.

References

1. Clark MR, Trotter K, Chang A. The pathogenesis and therapeutic implications of tubulointerstitial inflammation in human lupus nephritis. Semin Nephrol. 2015;35:455–64.
2. Brunner HI, Gladman DD, Ibañez D, Urowitz MD, Silverman ED. Difference in disease features between childhood-onset and adult-onset systemic lupus erythematosus. Arthritis Rheum. 2008;58:556–62.
3. Hanly JG, O'Keeffe AG, Su L, Urowitz MB, Romero-Diaz J, Gordon C, et al. The frequency and outcome of lupus nephritis: results from an international inception cohort study. Rheumatology. 2016;55:252–62.
4. Ribeiro FM, Fabris CL, Bendet I, Lugon JR. Survival of lupus patients on dialysis: a Brazilian cohort. Rheumatol. 2013;52:494–500.
5. Isenberg D, Appel GB, Contreras G, Dooley MA, Ginzler EM, Jayne D, et al. Influence of race/ethnicity on response to lupus nephritis treatment: the ALMS study. Rheumatology (Oxford). 2010;49:128–40.
6. Pons-Estel GJ, Ugarte-Gil MF, Alarcón GS. Epidemiology of systemic lupus erythematosus. Expert Rev Clin Immunol. 2017;13:799–814.
7. Hsieh SC, Tsai CY, Yu CL. Potential serum and urine biomarkers in patients with lupus nephritis and the unsolved problems. Open Access Rheumatol. 2016;8:81–91 eCollection 2016.

8. Skare TL, Stadler B, Weingraber E, De Paula DF. Prognosis of patients with systemic lupus erythematosus and discoid lesions. An Bras Dermatol. 2013; 88:755–8.
9. Fedrigo A, Dos Santos TAF, Nisihara R, Skare T. The lupus patient with positive rheumatoid factor. Lupus. 2018;27(8):1368–73.
10. Ortega LM, Schultz DR, Lenz O, Pardo V, Contreras GN. Lupus nephritis: pathologic features, epidemiology and a guide to therapeutic decisions. Lupus. 2010;19:557–74.
11. Ugolini-Lopes MR, Santos LPS, Stagnaro C, Seguro LPC, Mosca M, Bonfá E. Late-onset biopsy-proven lupus nephritis without other associated autoimmune diseases: severity and long-term outcome. Lupus. 2019;28:123–8.
12. Varela DC, Quintana G, Somers EC, Rojas-Villarraga A, Espinosa G, Hincapie ME, et al. Delayed lupus nephritis. Ann Rheum Dis. 2008;67:1044–6.
13. Hochberg MC. Updating the American College of Rheumatology revised criteria for the classification of systemic lupus erythematosus [letter]. Arthritis Rheum. 1997;40:1725.
14. Miyakis S, Lockshin MD, Atsumi T, Branch DW, Brey RL, Cervera R, et al. International consensus statement on an update of the classification criteria for definite antiphospholipid syndrome (APS). J Thromb Haemost. 2006;4: 295–306.
15. Weening JJ, D'Agati VD, Schwartz MM, Seshan SV, Alpers CE, Appel GB, et al. The classification of glomerulonephritis in systemic lupus erythematosus revisited. Kidney Int. 2004;65:521–30.
16. Bertsias GK, Tektonidou M, Amoura Z, Aringer M, Bajema I, Berden JH, et al. Joint European league against rheumatism and European renal association-European Dialysis and transplant association (EULAR/ERA-EDTA) recommendations for the management of adult and paediatric lupus nephritis. Ann Rheum Dis. 2012;71:1771–82.
17. Buyon JP, Petri MA, Kim MY, Kalunian KC, Grossman J, Hahn BH, et al. The effect of combined estrogen and progesterone hormone replacement therapy on disease activity in systemic lupus erythematosus: a randomized trial. Ann Intern Med. 2005;142:953–62.
18. Gladman D, Ginzler E, Goldsmith C, Fortin P, Liang M, Urowitz M, Bacon P, et al. The development and initial validation of the systemic lupus international collaborating clinics/American College of Rheumatology damage index for systemic lupus erythematosus. Arthritis Rheum. 1996;39: 363–9.
19. Cameron JS. Lupus nephritis. J Am Soc Nephrol. 1999;10:413–24.
20. Smith EM, Yin P, Jorgensen AL, Beresford MW. Clinical predictors of active LN development in children - evidence from the UK JSLE cohort study. Lupus. 2018;27:2020–8.
21. Illei GG, Takada K, Parkin D, Austin HA, Crane M, Yarboro CH, et al. Renal flares are common in patients with severe proliferative lupus nephritis treated with pulse immunosuppressive therapy: long-term followup of a cohort of 145 patients participating in randomized controlled studies. Arthritis Rheum. 2002;46:995–1002.
22. Mok CC, Kwok RC, Yip PS. Effect of renal disease on the standardized mortality ratio and life expectancy of patients with systemic lupus erythematosus. Arthritis Rheum. 2013;65:2154–60.
23. Houssiau FA, Vasconcelos C, D'Cruz D, Sebastiani GD, de Ramon GE, Danieli MG, et al. Early response to immunosuppressive therapy predicts good renal outcome in lupus nephritis: lessons from long-term follow up of patients in the euro- lupus nephritis trial. Arthritis Rheum. 2004;50:3934–40.
24. Ishizaki J, Saito K, Nawata M, Mizuno Y, Tokunaga M, Sawamukai N, et al. Low complements and high titer of anti-Sm antibody as predictors of histopathologically proven silent lupus nephritis without abnormal urinalysis in patients with systemic lupus erythematosus. Rheumatology (Oxford). 2015;54:405–12.

10

Impact of *C4*, *C4A* and *C4B* gene copy number variation in the susceptibility, phenotype and progression of systemic lupus erythematosus

Kaline Medeiros Costa Pereira[1], Sandro Perazzio[1], Atila Granado A. Faria[1], Eloisa Sa Moreira[2], Viviane C. Santos[1], Marcelle Grecco[1], Neusa Pereira da Silva[1] and Luis Eduardo Coelho Andrade[1*]

Abstract

Background: Complement component 4 (C4) gene copy number (GCN) affects the susceptibility to systemic lupus erythematosus (SLE) in different populations, however the possible phenotype significance remains to be determined. This study aimed to associate *C4A*, *C4B* and total *C4* GCN and SLE, focusing on the clinical phenotype and disease progression.

Methods: *C4*, *C4A* and *C4B* GCN were determined by real-time PCR in 427 SLE patients and 301 healthy controls, which underwent a detailed clinical evaluation according to a pre-established protocol.

Results: The risk of developing SLE was 2.62 times higher in subjects with low total *C4* GCN (< 4 copies, OR = 2.62, CI = 1.77 to 3.87, $p < 0.001$) and 3.59 times higher in subjects with low *C4A* GCN (< 2 copies; OR = 3.59, CI = 2.15 to 5.99, $p < 0.001$) compared to those subjects with normal or high GCN of total *C4* (≥4) and *C4A* (≥2), respectively. An increased risk was also observed regarding low *C4B* GCN, albeit to a lesser degree (OR = 1.46, CI = 1.03 to 2.08, $p = 0.03$). Furthermore, subjects with low *C4A* GCN had higher permanent disease damage as assessed by the Systemic Lupus International Collaborating Clinics – Damage Index (SLICC-DI; median = 1.5, 95% CI = 1.2–1.9) than patients with normal or high copy number of *C4A* (median = 1.0, 95% CI = 0.8–1.1; $p = 0.004$). There was a negative association between low *C4A* GCN and serositis ($p = 0.02$) as well as between low *C4B* GCN and arthritis ($p = 0.02$).

Conclusions: This study confirms the association between low *C4* GCN and SLE susceptibility, and originally demonstrates an association between low *C4A* GCN and disease severity.

Keywords: Complement C4, C4A, C4B, Gene copy number variation, Systemic lupus erythematosus

Background

Human *C4* is one of the most striking examples of genetic diversity, due to the great variation in number and size of genes between subjects, as well as some intrinsic polymorphisms. *C4* is the only component of complement that displays two different isotypes encoded by two different genes: *C4A* and *C4B*. These genes differ in only five nucleotides, but the proteins encoded by them have different functions. While *C4A* protein is more reactive against targets containing amino groups and has greater ability to covalently bind immune complexes, *C4B* has greater affinity for hydroxyl groups and exhibit a hemolytic potential at least four times higher than *C4A* [1].

Genes encoding the C4 protein are located in the MHC class III region, in the short arm of chromosome 6, and form, together with three neighboring genes (serine-threonine kinase, steroid 21-hydroxylase and tenascin-X), a genetic unit called RCCX module [2]. Theoretically, each chromosome 6 can harbor zero to four copies of these modules, determining wide gene copy number variation of *C4*.

* Correspondence: luis.andrade@unifesp.br
[1]Disciplina de Reumatologia, Universidade Federal de São Paulo, Rua Botucatu 740, 3o andar, São Paulo, SP ZIP: 04023-062, Brazil
Full list of author information is available at the end of the article

Around 80% of the Caucasians from United States and Europe have three or four *C4* copies, 20% have five or six, and less than 2% have only two copies in a diploid genome [3]. Complete deficiency of components *C4A* and *C4B* is extremely rare in healthy controls [3]. *C4A* or *C4B* homozygous deficiency occurs in 0.5–1% Caucasians, while the presence of a single *C4A* or *C4B* gene occurs in approximately 20% [4, 5]. *C4A* deficiency has been linked to systemic autoimmune diseases, especially systemic lupus erythematosus (SLE) [6–9]; the complete absence of *C4A* appears in 10–15% of patients [10, 11] and the heterozygous deficiency appears in 40–60% of SLE patients in several ethnic groups [12–14]. The association with certain clinical manifestations, however, is still not clear as different studies show different associations [7, 15–17].

The significant association of *C4A* deficiency with SLE in different ethnic groups suggests that *C4A* deficiency is a risk factor for this disease. There are several potential mechanisms for this association, such as the role of C4 in humoral immune response [18] and in the clearance of immune complexes and apoptotic cells [19, 20]. Interestingly, patients with SLE in Spain have an increased frequency of *C4B* deficiency and not *C4A*, which highlights the importance of both *C4A* and *C4B* in autoimmunity control in other ethnic groups [21].

Most epidemiologic studies of C4 in SLE, however, do not consider Copy Number Variation (CNV) of both *C4A* and *C4B*. In fact, there are few studies demonstrating that a low copy number of *C4A* and *C4B* increases the susceptibility to SLE [7–9, 17]. In the present study, we originally investigated the association of *C4*, *C4A* and *C4B* GCN variation with SLE in a large cohort of Brazilian adult patients and healthy controls, as well as a possible association with the disease phenotype and severity.

Methods

Study subjects

This observational cross-sectional study included 427 patients with SLE and 301 healthy controls. SLE patients were recruited consecutively from the Autoimmune Rheumatic Diseases Out-patient Clinic of the University Hospital, and fulfilled four or more classification criteria for SLE from the American College of Rheumatology [22]. Patients underwent a detailed clinical evaluation, with emphasis on SLE clinical manifestations, recurrent infections, current and previous medications, age at SLE onset, presence of other autoimmune diseases, and determination of Systemic Lupus International Collaborating Clinics – Damage Index (SLICC-DI) [23]. All subjects were at least 18 years old and signed the informed consent. This study was approved by the hospital ethics committee (protocol CEP#0330/09). The healthy volunteers answered a questionnaire, emphasizing signs and symptoms of autoimmune diseases and recurrent infections, which could be related to deficiency of some component of Complement. In this study, recurrent infections was defined according to the criteria suggested by Modell et al. [24], i.e., two or more upper respiratory infections (otitis or sinusitis, in the absence of the allergy) or pneumonias in one year (for more than one year), recurrent viral infections (herpes, warts), persistent fungal infections or tuberculosis. All data collected were used to analyze possible associations with the configuration of the complex gene *C4A*/*C4B*. Subjects with changes detected in any of the items in the questionnaire or a family history of SLE or other autoimmune rheumatic disease were excluded from the control group.

Determination of GCN of *C4A*, *C4B* and total *C4*

Genomic DNA was extracted from peripheral blood using the FlexiGene DNA purification kit (Qiagen). GCN was determined by real time PCR (qPCR) using TaqMan probes conjugated with a minor groove binder (MGB), as described in the study of Szilagyi et al. [5]. In both reactions to determine *C4A* and *C4B* GCN, we used 250 nM of forward *C4* primer (5′-GCAGGAGA-CATCTAACTGGCTTCT-3′) and 500 nM of reverse (5′-CCGCACCTGCATGCTCCT-3′), 250 nM of the TaqMan probe specific for *C4A* (5′-FAM-ACCC CTGTCCAGTGTTAG-MGB-3′) or *C4B* (5'FAM-ACCT CTCTCCAGTGATAC-MGB-3′), 1x TaqMan Universal Master Mix with UNG (Applied Biosystems, Foster City, CA) and 30 ng of genomic DNA in a total volume of 25 μL. Reactions targeting *RNase P*, which was our single-copy reference gene, contained the mix of primers and TaqMan probe labeled with VIC for this gene (Applied Biosystems Foster City, CA), 30 ng of genomic DNA and 1x TaqMan Universal Master Mix with UNG (Applied Biosystems),

Triplicates of each reaction were amplified and read on the Rotor Gene 3000 (Corbett, Sidney) using the following conditions (50 °C for 2 min, 95 °C for 10 min, 45 cycles of 95 °C for 15 s and 60 °C for 1 min). The results were analyzed by Rotor Gene 3000 software. For the relative quantification of the number of alleles *C4A* and *C4B*, we used control DNA samples with previously defined *C4A* and *C4B* GCN, kindly provided by Szilagyi et al. [5]. The *RNase P* constitutive gene was used as a control for the amplification reaction. The calculation of GCN was made using the ΔΔCT method [25].

Statistical analysis

Continuous variables with normal distribution were analyzed with the Student's t test and those with non-parametric distribution were analyzed with the Mann-

Whitney test. Qualitative parameters were analyzed by the Chi-square test and the Fisher's exact test when appropriate. Multiparametric analyses were performed with the one-way ANOVA test with Bonferroni's test as a post-hoc test when appropriate. Correlation analysis was performed by the Spearman's correlation method. To calculate the risk of developing disease (OR + 95% CI), we performed a binary logistic regression analysis. Statistical analysis was performed with the Statistical Package for the Social Sciences (SPSS) version 17.0 (SPSS Inc., 2008). Statistical inference level was set at 0.05.

Results

Study subjects

The female to male ratio was 286:15 in the healthy control group and 406 to 21 in the SLE group, with ages varying from 18 to 61 years old (35.1 ± 11.1) and 17 to 77 years old (39.9 ± 12.2), respectively. Patients and controls did not differ regarding gender distribution, although patients were significantly older ($p < 0.001$). Patients presented more recurrent infections ($n = 60$; 14.05%) compared to healthy controls ($n = 10$; 3.33%; $p < 0.001$). The clinical characteristics of SLE patients are depicted in Table 1.

Gene copy number of total *C4*, *C4A* and *C4B* in SLE patients and healthy controls

Total *C4* GCN ranged from two to eight in controls and from one to eight in SLE patients. *C4A* GCN varied from zero to six in patients and in controls, while *C4B* GCN varied from zero to five in both groups. SLE patients presented lower mean GCN for total *C4* and *C4A* compared to healthy controls (Table 2).

Table 1 Clinical characteristics of systemic lupus erythematosus patients ($n = 427$)

Clinical characteristics/organ involvement	*n* (%)
Cutaneous manifestations	394 (92.3)
Oral ulcers	64 (21.3)[a]
Arthritis or arthralgia	373 (87.4)
Kidney involvement	246 (57.6)
Hematologic manifestations	294 (68.8)
Serositis	111 (26.0)
CNS involvement	95 (22.2)
Disease duration in years (median/min – max)	9/0–53
SLICC-DI (median/min – max)	1/0–7
SLEDAI (median/min – max)	0/0–14

[a]Information available only for 300 patients

CNS central nervous system, *SLICC-DI* Systemic Lupus International Collaborating Clinics - Damage Index, *SLEDAI* Systemic Lupus Erythematosus Disease Activity Index

Table 2 Gene copy number of total *C4*, *C4A* and *C4B* in SLE and controls

C4 isotype	Number of copies (mean ± SD)		
	Controls ($n = 301$)	SLE ($n = 427$)	*p*-value
Total *C4*	4.17 ± 0.83	3.87 ± 0.96	< 0.001
C4A	2.24 ± 0.73	2.06 ± 0.86	0.001
C4B	1.95 ± 0.71	1.87 ± 0.77	0.192

Accordingly, patients had a higher frequency of low GCN for total *C4* and *C4A* compared to healthy controls (Fig. 1a-b). Comparing to healthy controls, the SLE group showed higher frequency of subjects with two (SLE = 7% vs controls = 1%, $p < 0.001$) and three copies of total *C4* (SLE = 22% vs controls = 12.6%, $p = 0.001$). On the other hand, a higher number of controls with four copies of total *C4* was observed compared to patients (SLE = 52.5% vs controls = 63.1%, $p < 0.01$) (Fig. 1a; Table 3).

Regarding *C4A* GCN, there was a higher frequency of SLE patients with only one copy (SLE = 18.3% vs controls = 6.3%, $p < 0.001$), while there was a greater proportion of controls with two copies of *C4A* (SLE = 58.3% vs controls = 69.4%, $p < 0.01$) (Table 3). There was a trend toward higher frequency of total absence of *C4A* genes (*C4A* = 0) in SLE patients (2.1%) compared to controls (0.3%; $p = 0.053$) (Fig. 1b). Although there was no significant difference of the *C4B* GCN between the two studied groups ($p = 0.192$), the distribution of subjects according to the GCN resembled the distribution curve for total *C4* and *C4A* (Fig. 1c). Interestingly, a lower percentage of patients with two copies of *C4B* compared to controls was observed (SLE = 57.4% vs controls = 65.8%; $p = 0.025$) (Table 3).

There was a higher frequency of SLE patients in the group of subjects with low GCN (total *C4* < 4, *C4A* or *C4B* < 2) than in the group of subjects with normal or high GCN (total *C4* ≥ 4, *C4A* or *C4B* ≥ 2) (Table 4). The risk of developing SLE was 2.62 times higher in subjects with low total *C4* GCN and 3.59 times higher in subjects with low *C4A* GCN compared to those with normal or high *C4* and *C4A* GCN. The same was observed regarding *C4B*, albeit to a lesser degree (OR = 1.46).

Total *C4*, *C4A* and *C4B* GCN impacts in SLE progression and clinical phenotype

The clinical phenotype analysis showed no association between low GCN for *C4*, *C4A* or *C4B* and a specific clinical manifestation. On the contrary, a higher frequency of articular involvement was seen in SLE patients with high *C4B* GCN compared to those with low GCN ($p = 0.022$; Table 5). Furthermore, there was higher frequency of serositis in patients with high *C4A* copy number compared to those with low copy number ($p = 0.019$).

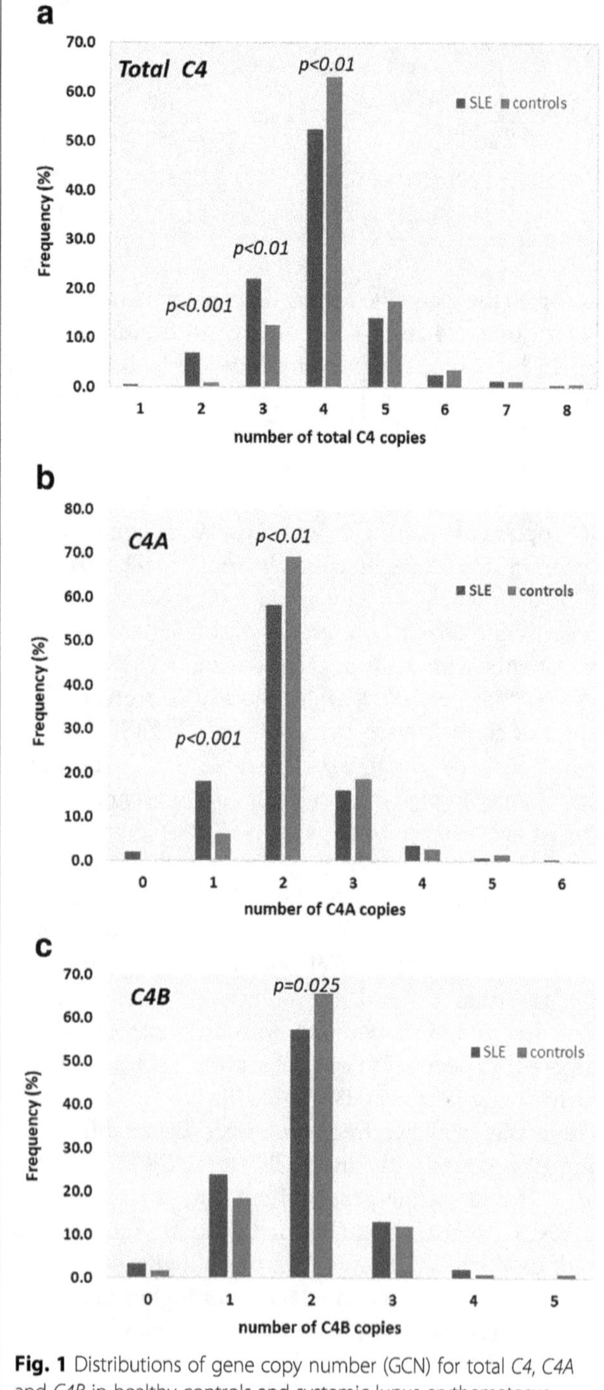

Fig. 1 Distributions of gene copy number (GCN) for total *C4, C4A* and *C4B* in healthy controls and systemic lupus erythematosus patients. GCN for total *C4* (**a**), *C4A* (**b**) and *C4B* (**c**) was determined in 427 patients with systemic lupus erythematosus (SLE) and 301 healthy controls by quantitative real time PCR

In addition, we investigated if the GCN for *C4, C4A* and *C4B* correlates with the progression of the disease in 335 SLE patients, using for that, the permanent damage index (DI) of the disease as measured by SLICC [23]. The Spearman correlation coefficient showed a mild but significant negative correlation between SLICC-DI and the GCN for total *C4* (rho = – 0.133, *p* = *0.015*) and *C4A* (rho = – 0.136, *p* = *0.012*), but not *C4B* (rho = 0.223, *p* = 0.675). Moreover, patients with low *C4A* GCN had higher permanent damage index (median = 1.5; 95% CI: 1.2–1.9) than patients with normal or high *C4A* GCN (median = 1.0; 95% CI: 0.8–1.1; *p* = *0.004*), regardless of age of onset and number of years of disease. This association was not observed for low total *C4* [1.3 (1.0–1.6) vs 1.0 (0.8–1.2); *p* = 0.087] or low *C4B* [1.0 (0.8–1.3) vs 1.0 (0.9–1.2); *p* = 0.916]. There was no correlation between the GCN for *C4, C4A* or *C4B* and age onset of SLE.

Discussion

The present study confirmed, also in the peculiar blended Brazilian ethnicity, the association between low total *C4* and *C4A* GCN and adult SLE previously reported in other ethnicities [7–9], and expanded this concept to low *C4B* GCN. This result corroborates a previous study with 90 patients with juvenile SLE and 170 patients with adult-onset SLE in Brazilian population, which showed a strong association with low number of copies of *C4, C4A* and *C4B* with SLE, remarkably in juvenile-onset lupus [26]. In addition, the present study originally demonstrated the impact of a lower *C4A* GCN on the progression of the disease. The distribution of total *C4, C4A* and *C4B* GCN in healthy controls was similar to that observed in other studies, with the majority of subjects presenting four copies of total *C4* (63.1%), two copies of *C4A* (69.4%) and two copies of *C4B* (65.8%). Interestingly, 20% of healthy subjects had less than two copies of *C4B,* whereas only 6% had less than two copies of C4A.

Although most SLE patients presented four copies of total *C4,* there was a higher percentage of subjects with less than four copies compared to controls, as well as less than two copies of *C4A*. Moreover, the risk of developing SLE was 2.6 and 3.6 times higher in subjects with lower total *C4* GCN and lower *C4A* GCN, respectively. These data are consistent with those previously observed in European, American and Asian samples, albeit with minor differences [7, 9, 27]. Only one study in the literature, performed with Japanese subjects, failed to demonstrate this association [28]. These genetic background differences had already been demonstrated, since *C4A* gene deletion has been more frequently reported in SLE patients in African American and Caucasian [11, 29, 30] than in Asian patients [12, 31, 32]. Moreover, the 2 bp insertion in exon 29, which leads to a *C4A*-null allele, was reported in Caucasian and African American SLE patients, but not in Asians [7, 28].

Although with a lower level of statistical significance, there was an association between low *C4B* GCN and SLE in our cohort. Previous studies have shown correlation between *C4B* deficiency and SLE in Spanish population [21, 27], in contrast to the UK cohort that

Table 3 Distribution of SLE and controls according to the gene copy number for total *C4, C4A* and *C4B*

GCN	*C4 n* (%)			*C4A n* (%)			*C4B n* (%)		
	Controls (n = 301)	SLE (n = 427)	*p*-value	Controls (n = 301)	SLE (n = 427)	*p*-value	Controls (n = 301)	SLE (n = 427)	*p*-value
0	0 (0)	0 (0)	1.00	1 (0.3)	9 (2.1)	0.053	5 (1.7)	14 (3.3)	0.239
1	0 (0)	1 (0.2)	1.00	19 (6.3)	78 (18.3)	< 0.001	56 (18.6)	102 (23.9)	0.100
2	3 (1.0)	30 (7.0)	< 0.001	209 (69.4)	249 (58.3)	< 0.01	198 (65.8)	245 (57.4)	0.025
3	38 (12.6)	94 (22.0)	< 0.01	57 (18.9)	69 (16.2)	0.371	36 (12.0)	56 (13.1)	0.734
4	190 (63.1)	224 (52.5)	< 0.01	9 (3.0)	16 (3.7)	0.682	3 (1.0)	9 (2.1)	0.377
5	53 (17.6)	60 (14.1)	0.213	5 (1.7)	4 (0.9)	0.500	3 (1.0)	1 (0.2)	0.312
6	11 (3.7)	11 (2.6)	0.510	1 (0.3)	2 (0.5)	1.00			
7	4 (1.3)	6 (1.4)	1.00						
8	2 (0.7)	1 (0.2)	0.573						

Fisher's exact test

revealed an association between high *C4B* GCN and SLE. Other studies failed to find association between *C4B* GCN and SLE [7, 9, 17]. Thus, the association between *C4B* GCN and SLE seems to be strongly influenced by ethnicity and further studies are needed to pinpoint the underlying genomic basis.

Despite the association of SLE with low GCN for *C4*, *C4*A and *C4*B, there were some SLE patients with normal or even high GCN for these genes. Conversely, some normal individuals had low GCN for these genes. This indicates that the SLE phenotype may be favored by low GCN of the *C4* gene system, but this is a relative factor that is integrated with a host of modulating genetic and environmental factors that ultimately define the fate of the phenotype.

While the association between low *C4* GCN and SLE has been consistently demonstrated, the impact of *C4* CNV on the disease phenotypes remains controversial. In our previous study in juvenile-onset SLE, the low GCN for total *C4* and *C4A* was associated with pericarditis [26]. A study in Chinese Han patients reported an association between low *C4A* deficiency and arthritis [7], while a more recent study reported serositis as the only clinical manifestation associated with low *C4A* GCN [17]. The current study adds some degree of complexity to this issue by showing a "protective" effect of low *C4B* GCN regarding the occurrence of arthritis, as well as between high *C4A* GCN and serositis. This apparent paradox of the "protective" effect of low *C4* GCN in the development of some SLE manifestations may reflect the dual role of the Complement system in autoimmune diseases. If C4 deficiency may favor autoimmune diseases onset, due to the impairment in the clearance of autoantigens and negative selection of auto-reactive B cells, on the other hand it may reduce inflammation, because the classical cascade of the Complement system will be also partially hampered in the context of low *C4A* GCN [33].

Recent studies have suggested that low *C4A* GCN may also be linked to increased susceptibility to infections [34]. However, this is also far from unanimous, since other authors found no association between low levels of *C4A* and *C4B* proteins or different haplotypes of *C4* with recurrent infections [35, 36]. In our series, there was no association between *C4* CNV and infectious diseases, and only 14% of SLE patients had recurrent infections. The differences in the results of the several studies may be secondary to the criteria used to define recurrent infections. In our study, we used the criteria suggested by Modell et al. for the definition of recurrent infections [24]. It is important to consider, however, that such information was collected by questionnaire or during the retrospective analysis of medical records. Although this bias could have affected equally the groups of lupus patients and healthy controls, it is reasonable to hypothesize that this could underestimate the prevalence of infections in the present study.

Table 4 Low gene copy number (GCN) for total *C4, C4A* and *C4B* genes is associated with systemic lupus erythematosus (SLE)

	Total C4 GCN category		*C4A* GCN category		*C4B* GCN category	
	< 4	≥4	< 2	≥2	< 2	≥2
Controls (n = 301)	41 (13.6)*	260 (86.3)	20 (6.6)	281 (93.3)	61 (20.2)	240 (79.7)
SLE (n = 427)	125 (29.2)	302 (70.7)	87 (20.3)	340 (79.6)	116 (27.1)	311 (72.8)
p-value**	< 0.001		< 0.001		0.033	
OR (95% CI)	2.62 (1.77–3.87)		3.59 (2.15–5.99)		1.46 (1.03–2.08)	

* Numbers within brackets are percentage; ** Fisher's exact test

Table 5 SLE clinical manifestations according to total *C4, C4A* and *C4B* gene copy number (GCN)

Clinical features		Total *C4* GCN n (%)			*C4A* GCN n (%)			*C4B* GCN n (%)		
		< 4 *n* = 125	≥4 *n* = 302	*p*-value	< 2 *n* = 87	≥2 *n* = 340	*p*-value	< 2 *n* = 116	≥2 *n* = 311	*p*-value
Cutaneous	+	116 (92.8)	278 (92.0)	1.000	82 (94.2)	312 (91.7)	0.509	106 (91.3)	288 (92.6)	0.686
	–	9 (7.2)	24 (8.0)		5 (5.8)	28 (8.2)		10 (8.7)	23 (7.4)	
Articular	+	104 (83.2)	269 (89.0)	0.110	76 (87.3)	297 (87.3)	1.000	94 (81.0)	279 (89.7)	0.022
	–	21 (16.8)	33 (11.0)		11 (12.7)	43 (12.7)		22 (19.0)	32 (10.3)	
Hematologic	+	90 (72.0)	204 (67.5)	0.422	65 (74.7)	229 (67.3)	0.197	82 (70.6)	212 (68.1)	0.640
	–	35 (28.0)	98 (32.4)		22 (25.3)	111 (42.7)		34 (29.4)	99 (31.9)	
Renal	+	72 (57.6)	174 (57.6)	1.000	53 (60.9)	193 (56.7)	0.544	63 (54.3)	183 (58.8)	0.441
	–	53 (42.4)	128 (42.4)		34 (39.1)	147 (43.3)		53 (45.7)	128 (41.2)	
Serositis	+	26 (20.8)	85 (28.1)	0.145	14 (16.0)	97 (28.5)	0.019	30 (25.8)	81 (26.0)	1.000
	–	99 (79.2)	217 (71.9)		73 (84.0)	243 (71.5)		86 (74.2)	230 (74.0)	
Neurologic	+	34 (27.2)	61 (20.1)	0.125	14 (16.0)	81 (23.8)	0.148	33 (28.4)	62 (19.9)	0.067
	–	91 (72.8)	241 (79.9)		73 (84)	259 (76.2)		83 (71.6)	249 (80.1)	
Infection	+	22 (17.6)	38 (12.5)	0.220	15 (17.2)	45 (13.2)	0.387	19 (16.3)	41 (13.1)	0.434
	–	103 (82.4)	264 (87.5)		72 (82.8)	295 (86.8)		97 (83.7)	270 (86.9)	
Oral ulcer[a]	+	9 (16.6)	55 (22.3)	0.463	9 (21.9)	55 (21.2)	1.000	17 (26.5)	47 (19.1)	0.301
	–	45 (83.3)	191 (77.6)		32 (78.1)	204 (78.8)		47 (73.5)	198 (80.9)	

[a]Information available only for 300 patients

An interesting and original finding of the present study was the association between low *C4A* GCN and permanent damage measured by SLICC-DI, suggesting that patients with low *C4A* GCN may have worse prognosis than those with normal or high GCN. The SLICC-DI measures permanent damage caused by SLE, by therapeutics and comorbidities. Actually, there are several studies associating *C4* CNV and obesity [4] diabetes mellitus [35] and cardiovascular disease [37]. It is, therefore, possible that non-SLE conditions related to low *C4* GCN may contribute to the observed increase in permanent damage in the present cohort.

Since C4 deficiency increases the activation of auto-reactive B cells and autoantibody production in animal models [38], we might expect an association between low GCN, especially of *C4A*, and the presence of events related to immune complex deposition, such as glomerulonephritis. However, such association was not observed either in the present study or in the one reported by Lv et al. [7], analyzing 924 Chinese SLE patients. It is possible that several genetic and adaptive factors interact, promoting or protecting against the disease and certain manifestations, what result in a wide and heterogeneous clinical spectrum.

Recently, several studies showed the association between lupus susceptibility or phenotypic features and polymorphism of different genes, such as PDCD1, BLK, TNIP1, TNFAIP3, SLC15A4, ETS1, and RasGRP3 IKZF1 [39–41]. The knowledge of the interplay between susceptibility genes and disease phenotypes can help us understand the clinical heterogeneity of this disease and its pathophysiology. Ultimately, this knowledge may contribute to the development of individualized approach for each patient.

In summary, the present study determined the distribution of *C4* GCN in a sample of the Brazilian SLE patients and healthy controls. We confirmed the association between low *C4A* and low total *C4* GCN and SLE, as previously described, and additionally showed similar findings for low *C4B* GCN. Furthermore, we originally documented a higher cumulative damage in patients with low *C4A* GCN as well as lower frequency of serositis in low *C4A* GCN patients. Finally, we observed an increased frequency of arthritis in patients with normal or high *C4B* GCN. Therefore, as demonstrated in this and in previous studies, low *C4* GCN may be a genetic risk factor for the development of SLE and may be related to other factors, culminating in a worse disease outcome.

Conclusions

Low gene copy number for *C4* genes, especially the *C4A* isoform, is a risk factor for development of systemic lupus erythematosus in the Brazilian population. In addition, low *C4A* gene copy number favors the occurrence of serositis and a more severe disease, while normal to high number of *C4B* genes favors the occurrence of arthritis in lupus patients. Therefore, the determination of *C4* gene copy number may be useful in sub-phenotyping and managing SLE patients.

Abbreviations

C4: Complement *C4* gene; *C4A*: Complement *C4A* gene; *C4B*: Complement *C4B* gene; CNV: Copy number variation; GCN: Gene copy number; SLE: Systemic lupus erythematosus; SLICC-DI: Systemic Lupus International Collaborating Clinics – Damage Index

Acknowledgements

We gratefully acknowledge Dr. Agnes Szilagyi, for all the support to develop the method for C4 quantification and for kindly providing the DNA samples with previously determined number of *C4A* and *C4B* genes.

Author's contributions

KMCP contributed with the conception, design of the work, collection of subject samples, acquisition, analysis and interpretation of data and have drafted the manuscript; SP contributed with the collection of subject samples and had a major contribution in writing the manuscript; AGAF contributed with the collection of subject samples and acquisition of the data; ESM contributed with the analysis and interpretation of data and revised the manuscript; VCS and MG contributed with the collection of subject samples; NPS contributed with the design of the work, analysis and interpretation of data; LECA contributed with the conception, design of the work, analysis and interpretation of data and substantively revised the manuscript.

Author details

[1]Disciplina de Reumatologia, Universidade Federal de São Paulo, Rua Botucatu 740, 3o andar, São Paulo, SP ZIP: 04023-062, Brazil. [2]Departamento de Genética e Biologia Evolutiva, Centro de Estudos do Genoma Humano, Instituto de Biociências, Universidade de São Paulo, São Paulo, SP, Brazil.

References

1. Law SK, Dodds AW, Porter RR. A comparison of the properties of two classes, C4A and C4B, of the human complement component C4. EMBO J. 1984;3:1819–23.
2. Yang Z, Mendoza AR, Welch TR, Zipf WB, Yu CY. Modular variations of the human major histocompatibility complex class III genes for serine/threonine kinase RP, complement component C4, steroid 21-hydroxylase CYP21, and tenascin TNX (the RCCX module). A mechanism for gene deletions and disease associations. J Biol Chem. 1999;274:12147–56.
3. Blanchong CA, Zhou B, Rupert KL, Chung EK, Jones KN, Sotos JF, et al. Deficiencies of human complement component C4A and C4B and heterozygosity in length variants of RP-C4-CYP21-TNX (RCCX) modules in caucasians. The load of RCCX genetic diversity on major histocompatibility complex-associated disease. J Exp Med. 2000;191:2183–96.
4. Yang Y, Chung EK, Zhou B, Blanchong CA, Yu CY, Füst G, et al. Diversity in intrinsic strengths of the human complement system: serum C4 protein concentrations correlate with C4 gene size and polygenic variations, hemolytic activities, and body mass index. J Immunol. 2003;171:2734–45.
5. Szilagyi A, Blasko B, Szilassy D, Fust G, Sasvari-Szekely M, Ronai Z. Real-time PCR quantification of human complement C4A and C4B genes. BMC Genet. 2006;7:1.
6. Fan Q, Uring-Lambert B, Weill B, Gautreau C, Menkes CJ, Delpech M. Complement component C4 deficiencies and gene alterations in patients with systemic lupus erythematosus. Eur J Immunogenet. 1993;20:11–21.
7. Lv Y, He S, Zhang Z, Li Y, Hu D, Zhu K, et al. Confirmation of C4 gene copy number variation and the association with systemic lupus erythematosus in Chinese Han population. Rheumatol Int. 2012;32:3047–53.
8. Wu YL, Yang Y, Chung EK, Zhou B, Kitzmiller KJ, Savelli SL, et al. Phenotypes, genotypes and disease susceptibility associated with gene copy number variations: complement C4 CNVs in European American healthy subjects and those with systemic lupus erythematosus. Cytogenet Genome Res. 2008;123:131–41.
9. Yang Y, Chung EK, Wu YL, Savelli SL, Nagaraja HN, Zhou B, et al. Gene copy-number variation and associated polymorphisms of complement component C4 in human systemic lupus erythematosus (SLE): low copy number is a risk factor for and high copy number is a protective factor against SLE susceptibility in European Americans. Am J Hum Genet. 2007;80:1037 54.
10. Man XY, Luo HR, Li XP, Yao YG, Mao CZ, Zhang YP. Polymerase chain reaction based C4AQ0 and C4BQ0 genotyping: association with systemic lupus erythematosus in Southwest Han Chinese. Ann Rheum Dis. 2003;62:71–3.
11. Olsen ML, Goldstein R, Arnett FC, Duvic M, Pollack M, Reveille JD. C4A gene deletion and HLA associations in black Americans with systemic lupus erythematosus. Immunogenetics. 1989;30:27–33.
12. Yamada H, Watanabe A, Mimori A, Nakano K, Takeuchi F, Matsuta K, et al. Lack of gene deletion for complement C4A deficiency in Japanese patients with systemic lupus erythematosus. J Rheumatol. 1990;17:1054–7.
13. Steinsson K, Jónsdóttir S, Arason GJ, Kristjánsdóttir H, Fossdal R, Skaftadóttir I, et al. A study of the association of HLA DR, DQ, and complement C4 alleles with systemic lupus erythematosus in Iceland. Ann Rheum Dis. 1998;57:503–5.
14. Yang Y, Lhotta K, Chung EK, Eder P, Neumair F, Yu CY. Complete complement components C4A and C4B deficiencies in human kidney diseases and systemic lupus erythematosus. J Immunol. 2004;173:2803–14.
15. Sturfelt G, Truedsson L, Johansen P, Jonsson H, Nived O, Sjöholm AG. Homozygous C4A deficiency in systemic lupus erythematosus: analysis of patients from a defined population. Clin Genet. 1990;38:427–33.
16. Petri M, Watson R, Winkelstein JA, McLean RH. Clinical expression of systemic lupus erythematosus in patients with C4A deficiency. Medicine (Baltimore). 1993;72:236–44.
17. Tsang-A-Sjoe MWP, Bultink IEM, Korswagen LA, et al. Comprehensive approach to study complement C4 in systemic lupus erythematosus: gene polymorphisms, protein levels and functional activity. Mol Immunol. 2017;92:125–31.
18. Fischer MB, Ma M, Goerg S, Zhou X, Xia J, Finco O, et al. Regulation of the B cell response to T-dependent antigens by classical pathway complement. J Immunol. 1996;157:549–56.
19. Davies KA, Erlendsson K, Beynon HL, Peters AM, Steinsson K, Valdimarsson H, et al. Splenic uptake of immune complexes in man is complement-dependent. J Immunol. 1993;151:3866–73.
20. Korb LC, Ahearn JM. C1q binds directly and specifically to surface blebs of apoptotic human keratinocytes: complement deficiency and systemic lupus erythematosus revisited. J Immunol. 1997;158:4525–8.
21. Naves M, Hajeer AH, Teh LS, Davies EJ, Ordi-Ros J, Perez-Pemen P, et al. Complement C4B null allele status confers risk for systemic lupus erythematosus in a Spanish population. Eur J Immunogenet. 1998;25:317–20.
22. Hochberg MC. Updating the American College of Rheumatology revised criteria for the classification of systemic lupus erythematosus. Arthritis Rheum. 1997;40:1725.
23. Gladman D, Ginzler E, Goldsmith C, Fortin P, Liang M, Urowitz M, et al. The development and initial validation of the systemic lupus international collaborating clinics/American College of Rheumatology damage index for systemic lupus erythematosus. Arthritis Rheum. 1996;39:363–9.
24. Modell V, Gee B, Lewis DB, Orange JS, Roifman CM, Routes JM, et al. Global study of primary immunodeficiency diseases (PI)--diagnosis, treatment, and economic impact: an updated report from the Jeffrey Modell Foundation. Immunol Res. 2011;51:61–70.
25. Livak KJ, Schmittgen TD. Analysis of relative gene expression data using real-time quantitative PCR and the 2(−Delta Delta C(T)) method. Methods. 2001;25:402–8.
26. Pereira KMC, Faria AGA, Liphaus BL, Jesus AA, Silva CA, Carneiro-Sampaio M, Andrade LEC. Low C4, C4A and C4B gene copy numbers are stronger risk factors for juvenile-onset than for adult-onset systemic lupus erythematosus. Rheumatology. 2016;55(5):869–73.
27. Boteva L, Morris DL, Cortés-Hernández J, Martin J, Vyse TJ, Fernando MM. Genetically determined partial complement C4 deficiency states are not independent risk factors for SLE in UK and Spanish populations. Am J Hum Genet. 2012;90:445–56.
28. Kamatani Y, Matsuda K, Ohishi T, Ohtsubo S, Yamazaki K, Iida A, et al. Identification of a significant association of a single nucleotide polymorphism in TNXB with systemic lupus erythematosus in a Japanese population. J Hum Genet. 2008;53:64–73.
29. Reveille JD, Anderson KL, Schrohenloher RE, Acton RT, Barger BO. Restriction fragment length polymorphism analysis of HLA-DR, DQ, DP and C4 alleles in Caucasians with systemic lupus erythematosus. J Rheumatol. 1991;18:14–8.
30. Hartung K, Baur MP, Coldewey R, Fricke M, Kalden JR, Lakomek HJ, et al. Major histocompatibility complex haplotypes and complement C4 alleles in systemic lupus erythematosus. Results of a multicenter study. J Clin Invest. 1992;90:1346–51.

31. Doherty DG, Ireland R, Demaine AG, Wang F, Veerapan K, Welsh KI, et al. Major histocompatibility complex genes and susceptibility to systemic lupus erythematosus in southern Chinese. Arthritis Rheum. 1992;35:641–6.
32. Hong GH, Kim HY, Takeuchi F, Nakano K, Yamada H, Matsuta K, et al. Association of complement C4 and HLA-DR alleles with systemic lupus erythematosus in Koreans. J Rheumatol. 1994;21:442–7.
33. Gilliam BE, Reed MR, Chauhan AK, Dehlendorf AB, Moore TL. Significance of complement components C1q and C4 bound to circulating immune complexes in juvenile idiopathic arthritis: support for classical complement pathway activation. Clin Exp Rheumatol. 2011;29:1049–56.
34. Kainulainen L, Peltola V, Seppänen M, Viander M, He Q, Lokki ML, et al. C4A deficiency in children and adolescents with recurrent respiratory infections. Hum Immunol. 2012;73:498–501.
35. Liberatore RR, Barbosa SF, Alkimin M, Bellinati-Pires R, Florido MP, Isaac L, et al. Is immunity in diabetic patients influencing the susceptibility to infections? Immunoglobulins, complement and phagocytic function in children and adolescents with type 1 diabetes mellitus. Pediatr Diabetes. 2005;6:206–12.
36. Guerra-Junior G, Grumach AS, de Lemos-Marini SH, Kirschfink M, Condino Neto A, de Araujo M, et al. Complement 4 phenotypes and genotypes in Brazilian patients with classical 21-hydroxylase deficiency. Clin Exp Immunol. 2009;155:182–8.
37. Arason GJ, Bödvarsson S, Sigurdarson ST, Sigurdsson G, Thorgeirsson G, Gudmundsson S, et al. An age-associated decrease in the frequency of C4B*Q0 indicates that null alleles of complement may affect health or survival. Ann N Y Acad Sci. 2003;1010:496–9.
38. Einav S, Pozdnyakova OO, Ma M, Carroll MC. Complement C4 is protective for lupus disease independent of C3. J Immunol. 2002;168:1036–41.
39. Thorburn CM, Prokunina-Olsson L, Sterba KA, Lum RF, Seldin MF, Alarcon-Riquelme ME, et al. Association of PDCD1 genetic variation with risk and clinical manifestations of systemic lupus erythematosus in a multiethnic cohort. Genes Immun. 2007;8:279–87.
40. Zhang Z, Zhu KJ, Xu Q, Zhang XJ, Sun LD, Zheng HF, et al. The association of the BLK gene with SLE was replicated in Chinese Han. Arch Dermatol Res. 2010;302:619–24.
41. He CF, Liu YS, Cheng YL, Gao JP, Pan TM, Han JW, et al. TNIP1, SLC15A4, ETS1, RasGRP3 and IKZF1 are associated with clinical features of systemic lupus erythematosus in a Chinese Han population. Lupus. 2010 Sep;19(10):1181–6.

11

Correlation of enthesitis indices with disease activity and function in axial and peripheral spondyloarthritis: A cross-sectional study comparing MASES, SPARCC and LEI

Penélope Esther Palominos[1*], Ana Paula Beckhauser de Campos[2], Sandra Lúcia Euzébio Ribeiro[3], Ricardo Machado Xavier[1,4], Jady Wroblewski Xavier[4], Felipe Borges de Oliveira[4], Bruno Guerra[4], Carla Saldanha[1], Aline Castello Branco Mancuso[5], Charles Lubianca Kohem[1,4], Andrese Aline Gasparin[1] and Percival Degrava Sampaio-Barros[6]

Abstract

Background: The presence of enthesitis is associated with higher disease activity, more disability and incapacity to work and a poorer quality of life in spondyloarthritis (SpA). There is currently no consensus on which clinical score should be used to assess enthesitis in SpA. The objective of the present work was to compare the correlation of three enthesitis indices (MASES, SPARCC and LEI) with measures of disease activity and function in a heterogeneous population of patients with axial and peripheral SpA.

Methods: A cross-sectional study was conducted in three Brazilian public university hospitals; patients fulfilling ASAS classification criteria for peripheral or axial SpA were recruited and measures of disease activity and function were collected and correlated to three enthesitis indices: MASES, SPARCC and LEI using Spearman's Correlation index. ROC curves were used to determine if the the enthesitis indices were useful to discriminate patients with active disease from those with inactive disease.

Results: Two hundred four patients were included, 71.1% ($N = 145$) fulfilled ASAS criteria for axial SpA and 28.9% ($N = 59$) for peripheral SpA. In axial SpA, MASES performed better than LEI ($p = 0.018$) and equal to SPARCC ($p = 0.212$) regarding correlation with disease activity (BASDAI) and function (BASFI). In peripheral SpA, only MASES had a weak but statistical significant correlation with DAS28-ESR (r_s 0.310 $p = 0.05$) and MASES had better correlation with functional measures (HAQ) than SPARCC ($p = 0.034$).

Conclusion: In this sample composed of SpA patients with high coexistence of axial and peripheral features, MASES showed statistical significant correlation with measures of disease activity and function in both axial and peripheral SpA.

Keywords: Spondyloarthritis, Enthesitis, Disease activity, Function

* Correspondence: penelopepalominos@gmail.com
[1]Serviço de Reumatologia, Hospital de Clínicas de Porto Alegre, Ramiro Barcelos 2350, sexto andar, Porto Alegre, Rio Grande do Sul CEP 90035-903, Brazil
Full list of author information is available at the end of the article

Background

A characteristic feature of the spondyloarthritis (SpA) is inflammation at tendon, fascia, capsule or ligament attachment sites, called enthesitis. Although enthesitis has traditionally been viewed as a focal abnormality, the inflammatory reaction intrinsic to enthesitis may be quite extensive [1]. In the clinical practice, the diagnosis of enthesitis is based on clinical examination, including interview (pain at the site of an enthesis that subsides following physical exercise) and observing pain in an enthesis upon compression [2]. Ultrasound and magnetic resonance image (RMI) are more direct ways to assess enthesitis although less feasible.

Recent publication comparing the clinical presentation of 2356 SpA patients from Europe (Spain and Belgium) and 1083 SpA patients from Latin America countries found a higher prevalence of peripheral arthritis and enthesitis in the Latin American patients [3].

The prevalence of enthesitis is high in Brazilian patients: among the 1505 patients included in the Brazilian Registry of Spondyloarthritis (Registro Brasileiro de Espondiloartrites - RBE), 54% had enthesitis; posterior iliac spine and Achilles tendon were the most common affected sites [4]. In this large cohort, enthesitis was found in 70.4% of the patients with undifferentiated SpA (USpA), 53.8% with psoriatic arthritis (PsA) and 53.5% with ankylosing spondylitis (AS) [4].

Patients with enthesitis present higher disease activity, disability and incapacity to work, frequently associated with a poorer quality of life [4–9]. In Brazilian patients, enthesitis was strongly associated with a more severe clinical picture, including axial as well as peripheral manifestations as well as higher Bath Ankylosing Disease Activity Index (BASDAI) [4, 7].

Although the Outcome Measures in Rheumatology (OMERACT) and the Assessment of Spondyloarthritis International Society (ASAS) recommend the assessment of enthesitis in SpA [10, 11] and besides the existence of several instruments proposed to entheseal evaluation there is no consensus on which tool should be used for subjects with axial and peripheral SpA [12–20].

There are 3 tools considered more feasible and usually employed in daily practice and clinical trials: the Maastricht Ankylosing Spondylitis Enthesitis Score (MASES), the Spondyloarthritis Research Consortium of Canada index (SPARCC), and the Leeds Enthesitis Index (LEI) [14–16]. Although there are several studies showing the correlation among one of these 3 indices with clinical variables, no single study compared the correlation among the three instruments and clinical variables in the same population [5, 8, 9, 21].

The present study aimed to compare the correlation of these three enthesitis indices (MASES, SPARCC and LEI) with measures of disease activity and function in a heterogeneous population of Brazilian patients with axial and peripheral SpA, as well as to establish if these enthesitis indices have good power at detecting active disease in this population.

Methods

An observational, cross-sectional study was conducted in three Brazilian public university hospitals: two of them located in the South of Brazil (Hospital de Clínicas de Porto Alegre, in Porto Alegre, Rio Grande do Sul and Hospital Universitário Evangélico, in Curitiba, Paraná) and one center located in the North of Brazil (Hospital Universitário Getúlio Vargas, in Manaus, Amazonas).

Inclusion criteria

Consecutive outpatients ≥ 18 years old attending Rheumatology Clinics in these three centers and fulfilling the ASAS classification criteria for axial or peripheral SpA were invited to participate [22, 23].

Exclusion criteria

Patients not willing and able to participate in a 1-h visit, illiterate patient that were not able to fulfill self-reported questionnaires. Patients with fibromyalgia (in whom tender points could be misdiagnosed as enthesitis) were not excluded from the study but additional analysis were conducted with exclusion of this subgroup.

Data collection

Data were collected from June to December 2015; the common data collection form included demographic data (gender, age and self-reported ethnicity), information about articular and extra-articular features, family history, measures of disease activity, functional status and quality of life, past and current treatment, laboratory tests and radiographic assessment.

Disease activity was assessed in subjects with axial SpA through the Bath Ankylosing Spondylitis Disease Activity Index (BASDAI), the inflammatory markers erythrocyte sedimentation rate (ESR) and C-reactive protein (CRP) and the Ankylosing Spondylitis Disease Activity Score (ASDAS) including CRP (ASDAS-CRP) and ESR (ASDAS-ESR) [24, 25]. In subjects with peripheral SpA and PsA, disease activity was assessed by the 28-Joints Disease Activity Score using ESR (DAS28-ESR) and by the inflammatory markers CRP and ESR [26]. Functional status was assessed through the Bath Ankylosing Spondylitis Functional Index (BASFI) in patients with axial SpA and the Health Assessment Questionnaire (HAQ) in patients with peripheral SpA and PsA [27, 28].

The enthesitis were assessed on each patient through three different tools recorded in the same visit: the Maastricht Ankylosing Spondylitis Enthesitis Score (MASES), the Spondyloarthritis Research Consortium of

Canada Index (SPARCC) and the Leeds Enthesitis Index (LEI) [14–16]. These three tools record tenderness on examination as either present (1) or absent (0) on each entheseal site after a firm palpation at a pressure of approximately 4 kg/cm^2 with the pulp of the thumb (the amount of pressure required to blanch a thumbnail).

It is relevant that MASES and SPARCC were developed in AS patients while LEI was a tool developed for PsA patients [14–16]. MASES analyses 13 sites: the bilateral first and seventh costochondral joints, the anterior and posterior superior iliac spines, the iliac crests, the fifth lumbar spinous process, and the proximal insertion of Achilles tendon (overall score range 0–13). SPARCC index evaluates 16 sites: the bilateral greater trochanter, quadriceps tendon insertion into the patella, patellar ligament insertion into the patella and tibial tuberosity, Achilles tendon insertion, plantar fascia insertion, medial and lateral epicondyles, and supraspinatus insertion (overall score range 0–16). LEI evaluates 6 sites: bilateral Achilles tendon insertions, medial femoral condyles, and lateral epicondyles of the humerus (overall score range 0–6).

Statistical analysis

In patients with axial SpA, the correlation between the three enthesitis indices (MASES, SPARCC and LEI) with measures of disease activity (BASDAI, ASDAS-CRP, ASDAS-ESR and inflammatory markers) and with function (BASFI) was calculated by the Spearman's Correlation index (r_s). The classification of Dancey was used to classify variables according to the intensity of correlation, with values from 0.10 to 0.39, 0.40 to 0.69, 0.70 to 0.99 representing, respectively, a weak, moderate and strong correlation [29]. ROC curves were used to determine if the three enthesitis indices were useful to discriminate patients with active disease using a cut off ≥4 for BASDAI and ≥ 1.3 for ASDAS-CRP. The usefulness of the enthesitis score to discriminate between active and inactive disease was interpreted according to the area under the curve as following: 0.50 to 0.75, 0.75 to 0.92, 0.92 to 0.97 and 0.97 to 1.00 representing, respectively, a fair, good, very good and excellent discrimination. The DeLong's test was used to compare ROC curves [30].

In subjects with peripheral SpA and in those patients fulfilling the CASPAR criteria for PsA [31], the correlation between the three enthesitis indices (MASES, SPARCC and LEI) and the disease activity measured by the DAS28-ESR and inflammatory markers was calculated using the Spearman's Correlation index. The correlation between the three enthesitis scores and function (HAQ) was also calculated.

In patients with peripheral SpA, the ROC curve analysis was conducted to investigate if the enthesitis indices could discriminate active disease using a DAS28-ESR ≥ 2.6 cut off.

Since the diagnosis of fibromyalgia could interfere in the assessment of entheseal sites (with tender points being misdiagnosed as enthesitis), all analysis conducted in the three groups (axial SpA, peripheral SpA and PsA) were repeated with the exclusion of patients who fulfilled the American College of Rheumatology 1990 criteria for the classification of fibromyalgia [32, 33].

Although the presence of peripheral involvement is quite common in Brazilian patients with axial SpA, it was considered as "axial SpA" all patients fulfilling ASAS classification criteria for axial SpA despite the peripheral involvement, and as "peripheral SpA" those fulfilling ASAS classification criteria for peripheral SpA (and not fulfilling criteria for "axial SpA"). Patients fulfilling both ASAS criteria for "axial SpA" and "peripheral SpA" were analyzed as "axial SpA".

The Win Pepi version 11.65 was used to calculate sample size; aiming to yield a 80% power to estimate the correlation of the enthesitis indices with disease activity scores and accepting a 5% margin of error, 109 subjects (55 with axial SpA and 54 with peripheral SpA) were deemed necessary [34]. The mean of the correlation coefficient (0,372) from previous work which studied correlation of MASES and SPARCC with BASDAI in AS was used to estimate the sample size of axial SpA since AS is the prototype of axial SpA [5, 8, 14, 15]. The mean of the correlation coefficients obtained by Healey et al. in their work which studied correlation of DAS 28 ESR with MASES and LEI (0.374) was used to estimate the number of subjects with peripheral SpA [16].

Ethics Committee approvals have been obtained by all participating centers prior to the start of the study and an informed consent form was obtained from all participants prior to enrollment.

Results

Characteristics of the population

The characteristics of patients included in the analysis are shown in Table 1.

Ankylosing Spondylitis was the most prevalent disease in this sample (N = 124, 60.8%), followed by psoriatic arthritis (N = 58, 28.4%), enteropathic arthritis (N = 9, 4.4%), undifferentiated SpA (N = 7, 3.4%), non-radiographic axial SpA (N = 5, 2.5%) and reactive arthritis (N = 1, 0.5%). The prevalence of subjects fulfilling ASAS criteria for axial SpA was 71.1% (N = 145) and for peripheral SpA was 28.9% (N = 59). Eighty-four patients (41.2% of the total sample) fulfilled criteria for both axial and peripheral criteria and these patients were analyzed in the group of "axial SpA".

About 54.4% of patients (N = 111/204) were treated with biological therapy. The 111 patients on biologic

Table 1 Characteristics of the 204 patients included in the analysis

	All Centers	Hospital de Clínicas de Porto Alegre, Porto Alegre (South Brazil)	Hospital Universitário Evangélico, Curitiba (South Brazil)	Hospital Universitário Getúlio Vargas, Manaus (North Brazil)	*P* value
Number of patients	204	54	84	66	
Male N (%)	131 (64.2)	28 (51.9)	55 (65.5)	48 (72.7)	0.057
Age in years (Mean ± SD, range)	48.6 ± 12.8 (18–87)	51.3 ± 12.2 (22–77)	47.8 ± 13.2 (18–87)	47.5 ± 12.7 (18–72)	0.213
Disease duration in years (Mean ± SD, range)	17.2 ± 10.6 (2–58)	17.4 ± 9.2 (4–44)	15.9 ± 10.9 (2–55)	18.5 ± 11.2 (2–58)	0.209
Self-reported ethnicity: white N (%)	126 (61.8)	41 (75.9)	67 (79.8)	18 (27.3)	< 0.001
Patients fulfilling ASAS classification criteria for Peripheral SpA N (%)	59 (28.9)	17 (31.5)	29 (34.5)	13 (19.7)	0.123
Patients fulfilling ASAS classification criteria for Axial SpA N (%)	145 (71.1)	37 (68.5)	55 (65.5)	53 (80.3)	0.123
Patients with at least one enthesitis N(%)	124 (60.8)	44 (81.5)	43 (51.2)	37 (56.1)	0.001
Composite activity index (mean ± SD)					
BASDAI*	3.5 (2.3)	4.7 (2.6)	3.1 (2.0)	3.0 (2.2)	0.002
ASDAS CRP*	2.3 (1.2)	2.8 (1.2)	2.4 (1.0)	1.8 (1.2)	0.001
ASDAS ESR*	2.6 (1.0)	2.8 (1.2)	2.6 (1.0)	2.5 (1.0)	0.610
DAS- 28 **	3.6 (1.4)	3.9 (1.4)	3.7 (1.5)	3.2 (1.2)	0.460
Enthesitis indices: Median (P25%, P75%), range / Mean ± SD					
MASES	1 (0, 5), 0–13/ 2.8 ± 3.9	3 (0, 7), 0–13/ 4.4 ± 4.3	0 (0, 3), 0–13/ 2.2 ± 3.5	0 (0, 3), 0–13/ 2.3 ± 3.6	< 0.001
SPARCC	0 (0, 3), 0–16/ 2.4 ± 3.9	2 (0, 6), 0–16/ 3.7 ± 4.6	0 (0, 3), 0–13/ 1.8 ± 3.0	0 (0, 2), 0–16/ 2.1 ± 4.0	0.005
LEI	0 (0, 2), 0–6/ 1.0 ± 1.6	0 (0, 2), 0–6/ 1.5 ± 2.0	0 (0, 1), 0–6/ 0.8 ± 1.5	0 (0, 1), 0–6/ 0.7 ± 1.4	0.016

SD: standard deviation; SpA: Spondyloarthritis; ASAS: Assessment of Spondyloarthritis International Society; MASES: Maastricht Ankylosing Spondylitis Enthesitis Score; SPARCC: Spondyloarthritis Research Consortium of Canada Index; LEI: Leeds Enthesitis Index * Reported only for the 145 patients fulfilling ASAS criteria for axial spondyloarthritis ** Reported only for the 59 patients fulfilling ASAS criteria for peripheral spondyloarthritis

therapy were receiving infliximab (21.6%, *N* = 24), adalimumab (36.9%, *N* = 41), etanercept (36.9%, N = 41), IL12/23 antagonists (1.8%, N = 2) and IL-17 antagonists (2.7%, *N* = 3). No patient was receiving golimumab or certolizumab. Furthermore, 54.4% (N = 111/204) were taking NSAIDs.

Among patients with axial SpA, that represented the majority of patients (N = 145), 57.2% (*N* = 83) had good disease control according to BASDAI score i.e., a BASDAI < 4. When the composite score ASDAS-CRP was considered to stablish the level of disease, 20% had inactive disease (*N* = 29), 21.3% had low disease activity (*N* = 31), 40.7% had high disease activity (*N* = 59) and 17.9% had very high disease activity (*N* = 26).

Enthesitis were common in all centers, 60.8% of Brazilian patients had at least one entheseal site with tenderness documented at physical exam, and the prevalence of enthesitis among the three centers ranged from 51.2 to 81.5%. The most prevalent site of tenderness on examination was the fifth lumbar spinous process, affected in 25% (*N* = 51) of the total sample, followed by the bilateral first and seventh costochondral joints, the right posterior superior iliac spine, and the left proximal insertion of Achilles tendon (each one affected in 24% / *N* = 49 of the total sample).

A comparison between patients < 60 years old and those ≥ 60 years old (who were expected to present lower disease activity) found no statistical difference in the distribution of MASES, SPARCC and LEI (*p*-value 0.222, 0.379 and 0.644 respectively). There was also no difference in the values of BASDAI, ASDAS CRP, ASDAS ESR and DAS28 between patients < 60 years old and those ≥ 60 years old (p-value 0.630, 0.851, 0.615, 0.820 respectively).

The involvement of bilateral enthesis was common: among the 109 patients with axial or peripheral SpA who reported tenderness in at least 2 enthesis in one of the three enthesitis scores (MASES, SPARCC or LEI), 88.0% (96/109) had bilateral enthesis involved; bilaterality was found in 86.1, 76.1 and 89.7% of patients reporting tenderness in at least two enthesis in MASES, SPARCC and LEI, respectively.

Correlation of enthesitis indices with disease activity and function in axial SpA

Among the 145 patients who fulfilled ASAS classification criteria for axial SpA the three enthesitis indices MASES, SPARCC and LEI were moderately correlated with disease activity measured by BASDAI (r_s 0.572 for MASES, r_s 0.508 for SPARCC and r_s 0.447 for LEI) (Table 2).

The comparison of the coefficients using the 95% confidence interval showed that MASES had a better correlation with BASDAI compared to LEI ($p = 0.018$). There was no statistical difference between MASES and SPARCC ($p = 0.212$) or between SPARCC and LEI ($p = 0.14$).

In the analysis of ROC curves, the three enthesitis scores could discriminate patients with suboptimal control of disease (BASDAI ≥4) from those with BASDAI< 4, but MASES and SPARCC performed better compared to LEI (Fig. 1). The DeLong's test for two correlated ROC curves showed statistically significant difference between MASES and LEI ($p = 0.02$) as well as between SPARCC and LEI (p = 0.02), but there was no statistically significant difference between MASES and SPARCC ($p = 0.60$). All the three enthesitis scores had only weak correlation with ASDAS-CRP and ASDAS-ESR (Table 2) and the three had only fair capability to discriminate subjects with inactive disease (ASDAS-CRP < 1.3) and active disease (ASDAS-CRP ≥1.3) (Area under the curve: MASES 0.647, SPARCC 0.638 and LEI 0.595). When the analysis was repeated using 2.1 as cut-off, the result was similar: the enthesitis indices had fair capability to discriminate between low (ASDAS-CRP < 2.1) and high disease activity (ASDAS-CRP ≥ 2.1) (Area under the curve: MASES 0.625, SPARCC 0.618 and LEI 0.579).

To evaluate if the three enthesitis scores had better correlation with BASDAI than ASDAS-CRP and ASDAS-ESR due to question 4 from BASDAI (which evaluates enthesitis), the correlation with every question from BASDAI was analyzed (data not shown). Question 4 had higher correlation with the three enthesitis scores than the remaining questions from BASDAI. However, when question 4 was excluded from BASDAI, this score continued to have better correlation with enthesitis indices compared to ASDAS-CRP and ASDAS-ESR (Table 2).

There was no statistical significant correlation between enthesitis indices and the inflammatory markers ESR and CRP (Table 2).

Functional status measured by BASFI had moderate correlation with MASES (r_s 0.465 $p \leq 0.01$) but only weak correlation with SPARCC (r_s 0.371 $p \leq 0.01$) and LEI (r_s 0.314 $p \leq 0.01$) (Table 2). Although the correlation coefficient of MASES was greater than SPARCC and LEI, the comparison of coefficients using the 95% confidence interval showed statistically significant difference only between MASES and LEI ($p = 0.008$). There was no statistically difference between the correlation coefficient of MASES and SPARCC ($p = 0.094$) or between SPARCC and LEI ($p = 0.2$).

The exclusion of patients with fibromyalgia ($N = 9$) did not change the correlation of enthesitis indices with scores of disease activity and function in patients with axial SpA.

Correlation of enthesitis indices with disease activity and function in peripheral SpA

Among the 59 patients fulfilling ASAS classification criteria for peripheral SpA, only MASES had a weak but statistically significant correlation with DAS28-ESR (r_s 0.310 $p = 0.05$) (Table 3).

The three enthesitis indices had only a fair capacity to discriminate active disease (DAS28-ESR ≥ 2.6) from inactive disease (DAS28-ESR < 2.6) (AUC 0.714 for MASES, 0.738 for SPARCC and 0.666 for LEI). The comparison of ROC curves using the DeLong's test showed no statistical significant difference among the three scores regarding their ability to discriminate active from inactive disease (comparison MASES/SPARCC $p = 0.733$; MASES/LEI $p = 0.466$; SPARCC/LEI $p = 0.06$).

There was no statistical significant correlation between enthesitis indices and the inflammatory markers ESR and CRP in patients with peripheral SpA (Table 3).

The correlation with function measured by HAQ was moderate for MASES (r_s 0.541) and LEI (r_s 0.497) and weak for SPARCC (r_s 0.347) (Table 3). The comparison of the 95% confidence interval of the three correlation coefficients showed that MASES had a better correlation with HAQ compared to SPARCC ($p = 0.034$) but it was not statistically different from LEI ($p = 0.628$). The exclusion of patients with fibromyalgia ($N = 2$) did not change the correlation between the enthesitis scores and clinical measures of disease activity and function in peripheral SpA.

Table 2 Correlation of the enthesitis indices with disease activity and function in 145 patients fulfilling ASAS criteria for axial SpA

	BASDAI	BASDAI without question 4	ASDAS- ESR	ASDAS-CRP	ESR	CRP	BASFI
MASES	,572[b]	,495[b]	,372[b]	,368[b]	-,085	-,091	,465[b]
SPARCC	,508[b]	,440[b]	,297[b]	,342[b]	-,066	-,065	,371[b]
LEI	,447[b]	,384[b]	,288[b]	,297[b]	-,074	-,064	,314[b]

[b]correlation is significant at the 0.01 level (2-tailed)

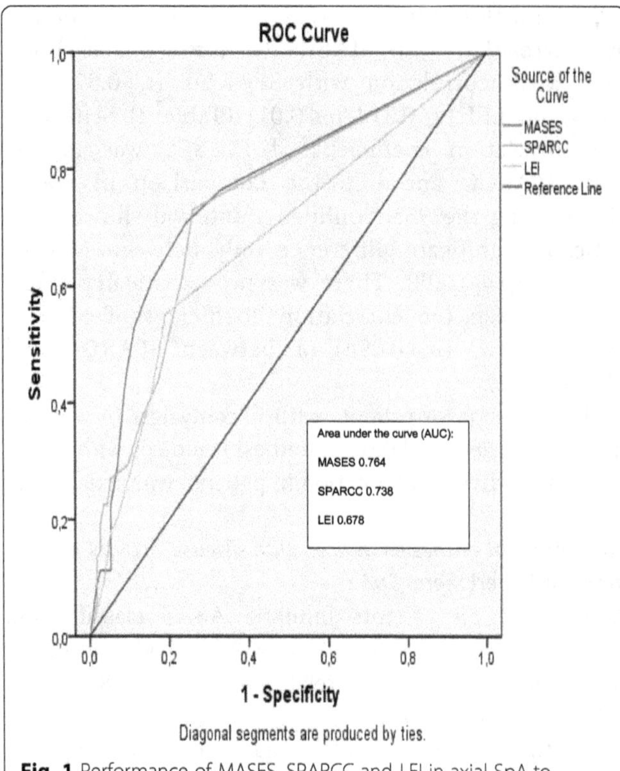

Fig. 1 Performance of MASES, SPARCC and LEI in axial SpA to discriminate between active disease (BASDAI ≥4) and inactive disease (BASDAI < 4)

Discussion

In this sample of Brazilian patients, MASES performed slightly better than SPARCC and LEI regarding correlation with disease activity and function in SpA patients. The three enthesitis scores had only fair capacity to discriminate active from inactive patients.

To the best of our knowledge, this is the first work to compare the correlation of the three indices MASES, SPARCC and LEI with disease activity and function in Brazilian patients studying their performance in categories of patients with SpA (axial x peripheral) regardless of the underlying individual disease. In the last years, the new ASAS criteria for axial and peripheral SpA emerged with the purpose to enhance design of clinical trials and allow an earlier and more effective diagnosis and treatment for patients. While previous work studied the correlation of enthesitis indices with clinical parameters in a specific entity, more frequently AS, our work incorporate the new tendency to group patients according to the pattern of manifestations and analyze the correlation of the instruments with disease activity and function among these groups rather than study their performance in a single, specific entity [5, 8, 14, 15].

Table 3 Correlation of the enthesitis indices with disease activity and function in 59 patients with peripheral SpA

	DAS28-ESR	ESR	CRP	HAQ
MASES	,318[a]	-,023	-,044	,541[b]
SPARCC	,250	-,006	-,093	,347[b]
LEI	,234	,008	-,002	,497[b]

[b]Correlation is significant at the 0.01 level (2-tailed)
[a]Correlation is significant at the 0.05 level (2-tailed)

In the present work, MASES, SPARCC and LEI were correlated to measures of disease activity in axial SpA and MASES was also correlated with DAS28-ESR in peripheral SpA. These findings are in accordance to previously published work which demonstrated that MASES index was correlated to BASDAI, patient global VAS and physician global VAS in AS patients [5, 8, 14].

Maksymowych et al. also found a correlation between SPARCC and the two measures of disease activity BASDAI and physician global VAS when studying 245 AS patients, while Healy et al.demonstrated a positive correlation between LEI and DAS28, tender joint count, swollen joint count, patient global VAS, physician global VAS and patient pain VAS in PsA patients [15, 16].

In this sample of Brazilian patients with axial SpA, the three enthesitis scores had better correlation with BASDAI than with ASDAS-CRP or ASDAS-ESR. The better correlation with BASDAI could be related to the item 4 of this questionnaire which evaluates entheseal pain although MASES has also been correlated with individual BASDAI items analyzed separately [5]. The absence of correlation between enthesitis and inflammatory markers contributes to decrease the correlation of the three enthesitis indices with ASDAS and has already been remarked in other studies [5, 8, 14] We can hypothesize that clinical entheseal scores are really a measurement of "pain" in the enthesis rather than true "inflammation" at entheseal sites and therefore correlate with item 4 of BASDAI. It would be interesting to obtain the correlation between inflammatory markers and the objective signs of inflammation detected through ultrasound or RMI.

There is a controversial result in literature regarding the correlation between the three enthesitis indices evaluated in this work and measures of function. Several trials are in line with our study and showed BASFI to be correlated with MASES and SPARCC in AS patients; a positive correlation was also found between HAQ and both MASES and LEI in PsA while other authors found no statistical significant correlation between enthesitis and function [5, 6, 8, 9, 15, 16].

Since the main difference among the three scores is the number and location of entheseal sites assessed, we could hypothesize that entheseal sites evaluated by MASES but not evaluated by SPARCC and LEI could be partially responsible for the better correlation of MASES with function and disease activity in the analyzed sample. MASES differs from the other two indices by evaluating enthesis with a more axial distribution as costochondral joints, antero and posterior iliac spines and the fifth lumbar spinous process. In the present work, the most prevalent site of entheseal tenderness was the fifth lumbar spinous process, affected in 25% ($N = 51$) of the total sample. Besides that, 24% of the 204 analyzed patients also had enthesitis in bilateral first and seventh costochondral joints and the right posterior superior iliac spine. The fact that there was a high prevalence of enthesitis in a more axial distribution could be partially responsible for the good performance of MASES in this sample.

Corroborating our findings, a high prevalence of enthesitis in a more axial location was also found when patients included in the Brazilian registry of SpA were analyzed, with posterior iliac spine and fifth lumbar spinous process being affected, respectively, in 22.8 and 19.2% of 1505 SpA patients [4]. Some sites evaluated exclusively by MASES as the iliac crests and posterior iliac spines were found to be associated with work incapacity in this large cohort of Brazilian patients, leading to the hypothesis that the enthesitis located in pelvis and lumbar spine, only evaluated by MASES, could play a significant role on functional disability [4].

Bilateral involvement of enthesis is a descriptive element suggested by the Group for Research and Assessment of Psoriasis and Psoriatic Arthritis (GRAPPA) which can aid physicians (mainly non-rheumatologists) to recognize enthesitis. In our sample, bilaterality was found in 86.1, 76.1 and 89.7% of patients reporting tenderness in at least two enthesis in MASES, SPARCC and LEI, respectively. This result reinforces the importance of "bilaterality" in the assessment of enthesitis [35].

This study has some weaknesses: the sample did not include patients from other states of Brazil outside the South and North region and the enthesitis were characterized only clinically, without imaging methods to confirm the diagnosis. More than 50% of patients were receiving biologic therapy and NSAIDs, therapies that could decrease the number of enthesitis. Despite the high prevalence of patients receiving biologic therapy in our sample (54.4%), the majority of axial SpA included in the study (58.6%) had high or very high disease activity. So, the probability to find enthesitis in the sample, in our opinion, was high.

We did not assess the University of California San Francisco (UCSF) Enthesitis Index which was specifically developed for AS and found to be slightly more sensitive than MASES in a previous study [18, 36]. Many clinical scores to assess enthesitis are currently available and MASES, SPARCC and LEI have been chosen because they were considered more feasible and usually employed in daily practice in the participating centers [12–20]. Furthermore, MASES and UCSF showed to be highly correlated [36].

There are many ways to classify the intensity of correlations and in this work we used the Dancey classification. The choice of other criteria could have changed the cut-offs to define weak, moderate and strong correlations, leading to a different interpretation of data [29].

Another important limitation is the utilization of the 28-joint count to evaluate peripheral arthritis. Although recent work showed that the DAS28 is not the most adequate tool to evaluate disease activity in PsA (since it can miss around 25% of active joint disease in oligoarticular patients), the 28-joint count was part of the routine care protocol in the three university hospitals at the time of data collection [37]. There is a lag of several years from study conception until data publication with continuous improvement in the SpA assessment along these years.

Another limitation is that the cross-sectional design of the study did not permit to assess the sensitive to change of the three enthesitis scores and whether they correlate to changes in other validated measures.

Conclusion

Regardless of its limitations, this study suggests that MASES performed statistically slightly better than SPARCC and LEI regarding correlation with disease activity and function in this Brazilian sample of SpA patients. However, in clinical practice it's difficult to stablish some superiority among the three scores since their performance was quite similar.

Acknowledgements

We would like to thanks Professor Eugenio de Miguel Mendieta for his suggestions to the manuscript.

Authors' contributions

PEP and PDS contributed to the conception and design of study. PEP, APBC, SLER, JWX, FBO, BG, CS, AAG contributed to acquisition of data. PEP, RMX, ACBM, CLK and PDS contributed to analysis and interpretations of data. PEP and PDS drafted the manuscript and all authors revised the manuscript critically for intellectual content. All authors read and approved the final manuscript.

Author details

[1]Serviço de Reumatologia, Hospital de Clínicas de Porto Alegre, Ramiro Barcelos 2350, sexto andar, Porto Alegre, Rio Grande do Sul CEP 90035-903, Brazil. [2]Serviço de Reumatologia, Hospital Universitário Evangélico, Alameda Augusto Stellfeld, 1908, Bigorrilho, Curitiba, Paraná CEP 80730-150, Brazil. [3]Serviço de Reumatologia, Hospital Universitário Getúlio Vargas, Universidade Federal do Amazonas, Avenida Apurinã 4, Manaus, Amazonas CEP 69020-170, Brazil. [4]Faculdade de Medicina, Universidade Federal do Rio Grande do Sul, Ramiro Barcelos 2400, Porto Alegre, Rio Grande do Sul CEP 90035-903, Brazil. [5]Departamento de Bioestatística, Hospital de Clínicas de Porto Alegre, Ramiro Barcelos 2350, Porto Alegre, Rio Grande do Sul CEP 90035-903, Brazil. [6]Serviço de Reumatologia, Faculdade de Medicina, Hospital das Clínicas HCFMUSP, Universidade de São Paulo, São Paulo, Brazil.

References

1. Benjamin M, McGonagle D. The enthesitis organ concept and its relevance to the spondyloarthropathies. AdvExp Med Biol. 2009;649:57–70.
2. Sudoł-Szopińska I, Kwiatkowska B, Prochorec-Sobieszek M, Maśliński WJ. Enthesopathies and *enthesitis*. Part 1. Etiopathogenesis. Ultrason. 2015;15(60):72–84.
3. Benegas M, Munoz-Gomariz E, Font P, Burgos-Vargas R, Chaves J, Palleiro D, et al. Comparison of the clinical expression. Of patients with ankylosing spondylitis from Europe and Latin America. J Rheumatol. 2012;39:2315–20.
4. Carneiro S, Bortoluzzo A, Gonçalves C, da Silva JAB, Ximenes AC, Bertolo M, et al. Effect of enthesitis on 1505 Brazilian patients with Spondyloarthritis. J Rheumatol. 2013;40:1719–25.
5. Rezvani A, Bodur H, Ataman S, Kaya T, Bugdayci DS, Demir SE, et al. Correlations among enthesitis, clinical, radiographic and quality of life parameters in patients with ankylosing spondylitis. Mod Rheumatol. 2014;24:651–6.
6. Kaya T, Bal S, Gunaydin R, et al. Relationship between the severity of enthesitis and clinical and laboratory parameters in patients with ankylosing spondylitis. Rheumatol Int. 2007;27:323–7.
7. Da Costa IP, Bortoluzzo AB, Gonçalves AR, da Silva JAB, Ximenes AC, Bértolo MB, et al. Evaluation of performance of BASDAI (Bath ankylosing spondylitis disease activity index) in a Brazilian cohort of 1492 patients with spondyloarthritis: data from the Brazilian registry of Spondyloarthritides (RBE). Rev Bras Reumatol. 2015;55:48–54.
8. Sivas F, Baskan BM, Ínal EE, Aktekin LA, Barça N. Ozoran, et al. the relationship between enthesitis índices and disease activity parameters in patients with ankylosing spondylitis. Clin Rheumatol. 2009;28:259–64.
9. Turan Y, Duruöz MT, Cerrahoglu L. Relationship between enthesitis, clinical parameters and quality of life in spondyloarthritis. Joint Bone Spine. 2009;76:642–7.
10. Gladman DD, Mease PJ, Strand V, Healy P, Helliwell PS, Fitzgerald O, et al. Consensus on a core set of domains for psoriatic arthritis. J Rheumatol. 2007;34:1167–70.
11. Van der Heidje D, Calin A, Dougados M, Khan MA, van der Linden S, Bellamy N. Selection of instruments in the core set for DC-ART, SMARD, physical therapy, and clinical record keeping in ankylosing spondylitis. Progress report of the ASAS working group. Assessment on ankylosing spondylitis. Ann Rheum Dis. 1999;26:951–4.
12. Mease PJ. Measures of psoriatic arthritis. Arthritis Care Res. 2011;63:S64–85.
13. Mander M, Simpson JM, McLellan A, Walker D, Goodacre JA, Dick WC. Studies with an enthesis index method of clinical assessment in ankylosing spondylitis. Ann Rheum Dis. 1987;46:197–202.
14. Heuft-Dorenbosch L, Spoorenberg A, van Tubergen R, Landewé R, van der Tempel H, Mielants H, et al. Assessment of enthesitis in ankylosing spondylitis. Ann Rheum Dis. 2003;62:127–32.
15. Maksymowych WP, Mallon C, Morrow S, Shojania K, Olszynski WP, Wong RL, et al. Development and validation of the Spondyloarthritis research consortium of Canada (SPARCC) Enthesitis index. Ann Rheum Dis. 2009;68: 948–53.
16. Healy PJ, Helliwell PS. Measuring clinical enthesitis in psoriatic arthritis: assessment of existing measures and development of an instrument specific to psoriatic arthritis. Arthritis Rheum. 2008;59:686–91.
17. Braun J, Brandt J, Listing J, et al. Treatment of active ankylosing spondylitis with infliximab: a randomized controlled multicenter trial. Lancet. 2002;359: 1187–93.
18. Gorman JD, Sack KE, Davis JC Jr. Treatment of ankylosing spondylitis by inhibition of tumor necrosis factor alpha. N Engl J Med. 2002;346:1349–56.
19. Gladman DD, Cook RJ, Schentag C, Feletar M, Inman RI, Hitchon C, et al. The clinical assessment of patients with psoriatic arthritis: results of a reliability study of the spondyloarthritis research consortium of Canada. J Rheumatol. 2004;31:1126–31.
20. Dawes PT, Sheeran TP, Beswick EJ, Hothersall TE. Enthesopathy index in ankylosing spondylitis. Ann Rheum Dis. 1987;46:717.
21. Laatiris A, Amine B, Yacoub YI, Hajjaj-Hassouni N. Enthesitis and its relationship with disease parameters in Moroccan patients with ankylosing spondylitis. Rheumatol Int. 2012;32:723–7.
22. Rudwaleit M, van der Heijde D, Landewé R, Listing J, Akkoc N, Brandt J, et al. The development of assessment of Spondyloarthritis international society classification criteria for axial spondyloarthritis (part II): validation and final selection. Ann Rheum Dis. 2009;68:777–83.
23. Rudwaleit M, van der Heijde D, Landewé R, Akkoc N, Brandt J, Chou CT, et al. The assessment of spondyloarthritis international society classification criteria for peripheral spondyloarthritis and for spondyloarthritis in general. Ann Rheum Dis. 2011;70:25–31.
24. Garrett S, Jenkinson T, Kennedy LG, Whitelock H, Gaisford P, Calin A, et al. A new approach to defining disease status in ankylosing spondylitis: the Bath ankylosing spondylitis disease activity index. J Rheumatol. 1994;21:2286–91.
25. Van der Heidje D, Lie E, Kvien TK, et al. ASDAS, a highly discriminatory ASAS-endorsed disease activity score in patients with ankylosing spondylitis. Ann Rheum Dis. 2009;68:181–8.
26. Prevoo MLL, Hof v't, MA KHH, van Leeuwen MA, van de Putte LBA, van Riel PLCM. Modified disease activity scores that include twenty eight-joint counts: development and validation in a prospective longitudinal study of patients with rheumatoid arthritis. Arthritis Rheum. 1995;38:44–8.
27. Calin A, Garret S, Whitelock H, Kennedy LG, O'Hea J, Malorie P, et al. A new approach to defining functional ability in ankylosing spondylitis: the development of the Bath ankylosing functional index. J Rheumatol. 1994;21:2281–5.
28. Bruce B, Fries JF. The Stanford health assessment questionnaire (HAQ): a review of its history, issues, progress, and documentation. J Rheumatol. 2003;30:167–78.
29. Dancey CP, Reidy J. Statistics without math for psychology: Prentice Hall; 2004.
30. DeLong ER, DeLong DM, Clarke-Pearson DL. Comparing the areas under two or more correlated receiver operating characteristic curves: a nonparametric approach. Biometrics. 1988;44:837–45.
31. Taylor W, Gladman D, Helliwell P, Marchesoni A, Mease P, Mielants H, et al. Classification criteria for psoriatic arthritis development of new criteria from a large international study. Arthritis Rheum. 2006;54: 2665–73.
32. Roussou E, Ciurtin C. Clinical overlap between fibromyalgia tender points and enthesitis sites in patients with spondyloarthritis who present with inflammatory back pain. Clin Exp Rheumatol. 2012;30:24–30.
33. Wolfe F, Smythe HA, Yunus MB, Bennett RM, Bombardier C, Goldenberg DL, et al. Arthritis Rheum. 1990;33:160–72.
34. Abramson JH. WINPEPI updated: computer programs for epidemiologists, and their teaching potential. Epidemiologic Perspectives & Innovations. 2011;8(1).
35. Mease PJ, Garg A, Helliwell PS, Park JJ, Gladman DD. Development of criteria to distinguish inflammatory from noninflammatory arthritis, Enthesitis, Dactylitis, and spondylitis: a report from the GRAPPA 2013 annual meeting. J Rheumatol. 2014;41:1249–51.
36. Van der Heijde D, Braun J, Deodhar A, Inman RD, Xu S, Mack ME, et al. Comparison of three enthesitis indices in a multicenter, randomizes, placebo-controlles trial of golimumab in ankylosing spondylitis (GO RAISE). Rheumatology (Oxford). 2013;52:321–5.
37. Coates LC, FitzGerald O, Gladman DD, McHugh N, Mease P, Strand V, et al. Reduced joint counts misclassify patients with oligoarticular psoriatic arthritis and miss significant numbers of patients with active disease. Arthritis Rheum. 2013;65:1504–9.

Human immunodeficiency virus in a cohort of systemic lupus erythematosus patients

Vanessa Hax[1*], Ana Laura Didonet Moro[1], Rafaella Romeiro Piovesan[2], Luciano Zubaran Goldani[3], Ricardo Machado Xavier[1] and Odirlei Andre Monticielo[1]

Abstract

Background: Systemic lupus erythematosus (SLE) and acquired immunodeficiency syndrome (AIDS) share many clinical manifestations and laboratory findings, therefore, concomitant diagnosis of SLE and human immunodeficiency virus (HIV) can be challenging.

Methods: Prospective cohort with 602 patients with SLE who attended the Rheumatology Clinic of the Hospital de Clínicas de Porto Alegre since 2000. All patients were followed until 01 May 2015 or until death, if earlier. Demographic, clinical and laboratory data were prospectively collected.

Results: Out of the 602 patients, 11 presented with the diagnosis of AIDS (1.59%). The following variables were significantly more prevalent in patients with concomitant HIV and SLE: neuropsychiatric lupus (10.9% vs. 36.4%; $p = 0.028$) and smoking (37.6% vs. 80%; $p = 0.0009$) while malar rash was significantly less prevalent in this population (56% vs. 18.2%; $p = 0.015$). Nephritis (40.5% vs. 63.6%; $p = 0.134$) and hemolytic anemia (28.6% vs. 54.5%; $p = 0.089$) were more prevalent in SLE patients with HIV, but with no statistical significance compared with SLE patients without HIV. The SLICC damage index median in the last medical consultation was significantly higher in SLE patients with HIV (1 vs. 2; p = 0,047).

Conclusions: Our patients with concomitant HIV and SLE have clinically more neuropsychiatric manifestations. For the first time, according to our knowledge, higher cumulative damage was described in lupus patients with concomitant HIV infection. Further studies are needed to elucidate this complex association, its outcomes, prognosis and which therapeutic approach it's best for each case.

Keywords: Systemic lupus erythematosus, Human immunodeficiency virus, Acquired immunodeficiency syndrome, Neuropsychiatric lupus, Opportunistic infections

Background

Concomitant diagnosis of systemic lupus erythematosus (SLE) and acquired immunodeficiency syndrome (AIDS) can be intriguing and challenging. SLE and human immunodeficiency virus (HIV) infection share many clinical manifestations, including musculoskeletal symptoms such as myalgia, arthralgia/arthritis, skin rashes, lymphadenopathy and organ involvement, such as kidneys, heart, lungs and central nervous system [1]. They also have several common laboratory findings such as anemia, leukopenia, lymphopenia, thrombocytopenia and hypergammaglobulinemia [1].

* Correspondence: vanessahax@gmail.com.br; vanessahax@gmail.com
[1]Division of Rheumatology, Hospital de Clínicas de Porto Alegre, Universidade Federal do Rio Grande do Sul, 2350 Ramiro Barcelos St, Room 645, Porto Alegre, RS 90035-903, Brazil
Full list of author information is available at the end of the article

There are few studies assessing the clinical and laboratory manifestations in SLE patients with HIV infection, as well as patient's profile and their evolution. Furthermore, there are no studies assessing the prognosis of this association until now. Therefore, the present study aimed to demonstrate the profile of these patients in our center, appointing their clinical and laboratory features, the significant differences between the patients with or without HIV, the treatment offered and their evolution considering infections, other diseases and mortality.

Methods

Study population

This prospective cohort consisted of 602 SLE patients who attended the Rheumatology Clinic of the Hospital de Clínicas de Porto Alegre since 2000. All patients fulfilled the American College of Rheumatology (ACR) revised criteria for the classification of SLE [2] and an informed consent form was obtained from all participants. The patients were followed until 01 May 2015 or until death, if earlier. The demographic, clinical and laboratory data were prospectively collected.

Clinical and laboratory variables

The following variables were recorded: age, gender, age at diagnosis of SLE and HIV (when the last was positive) , smoking status (current or previous), cardiovascular diseases, dyslipidemia, other autoimmune diseases and treatment performed. Clinical manifestations of SLE included the presence of photosensitivity, malar rash, discoid rash, oral or nasal ulcers, arthritis, serositis (pleuritis or pericarditis), nephritis and neurological disease, defined as seizures or psychosis. The assessment of the group of patients with concomitant HIV included infections, as well as CD4 and viral load at the diagnosis and the last count available. The laboratory evaluation included the presence of hematological disorders (hemolytic anemia, leukopenia, lymphopenia or thrombocytopenia), positive antinuclear antibody (ANA) (titer> 1:80) or other autoantibodies such as anti-dsDNA, anti-Sm, anti-RNP, anti-Ro, anti-La, anticardiolipin (aCL), lupus anticoagulant and false positive VDRL. The patients were also evaluated in regard to secondary antiphospholipid syndrome and secondary Sjogren's syndrome, according to the classification criteria for both diseases [3, 4]. The SLEDAI and the SLICC damage index of the last medical consultation were recorded too, as a measurement of disease activity and cumulative damage, respectively [5].

Statistical analyses

A descriptive analysis of data through calculation of mean and standard deviation (SD) for quantitative variables was performed while the frequency and percentage were calculated for categorical variables. The median and interquartile range were calculated to quantitative variables with asymmetrical distribution. We used the chi square test or Fisher's exact test to compare categorical variables, and continuous variable were analyzed with Mann-Whitney test. All statistical analyses were performed using SPSS 20.0. All tests were performed at the 0.05 level of significance and were two-sided.

Results

Our study consisted of 602 SLE patients, 75.2% European derived, 92% female and 11 (1.59%) of these patients presented with HIV. The patients mean age was 42.8±12.7 years and the mean SLE diagnostic age was 29.9±13.9 years. Demographic, clinical and laboratory profile were showed in Table 1. The following variables were significantly more prevalent in patients with concomitant HIV and SLE: neuropsychiatric lupus (10.9% vs. 36.4%; $p = 0.028$) and smoking (37.6% vs. 80%; $p = 0.0009$) while malar rash was significantly less prevalent in this population (56% vs. 18.2%; $p = 0.015$). The following features were more prevalent in SLE patients with HIV, but without to reach statistical significance compared with SLE patients without HIV: nephritis (40.5% vs. 63.6%; $p = 0.134$), hemolytic anemia (28.6% vs. 54.5%; $p = 0.089$), presence of anti-Ro (39.4% vs. 63.6%; $p = 0.125$) and anti-La (13.1% vs. 27.3%; $p = 0.172$), cardiovascular disease (18.1% vs. 36.4%; $p = 0.126$) and diabetes mellitus (7.7% vs. 18.2%; $p = 0.212$). Regarding the autoantibodies, in our cohort, amongst SLE patients with HIV, 72.7% had positive Coomb's test, 45.5% anti-dsDNA, 9.1% anti-Sm, 63.6% anti-Ro, 27.3% anti-La, 27.3% anti-RNP and 9.1% antiphospholipid antibodies. Hypergammaglobulinemia and hypocomplementenemia were observed in 81.8% of SLE patients with HIV.

The survival rate was 96.6% and 93.5% in 5 and 10 years, respectively, in SLE patients without HIV. Meanwhile, the survival rate was 90% in 5 and 10 years in SLE patients with HIV. There was no significant difference between the two groups. The SLICC damage index median in the last medical consultation was significantly higher in SLE patients with HIV (1 vs. 2; $p = 0.047$). The median of the last SLEDAI did not reach significant difference between groups (0 vs. 1; $p = 0.55$). In the HIV group, infections occurred in 54.5%, predominantly human papillomavirus infection, followed by tuberculosis and herpes zoster infection. Coinfection with C hepatitis virus occurred in two patients (18%).

Simultaneous diagnosis of SLE and HIV infection was done in one patient, while HIV following SLE was diagnosed in eight patients and HIV infection preceded SLE in two patients. All the patients were female and at diagnosis of HIV the mean CD4 count was 296 cells/μL and HIV-RNA 60.000 copies/ml. Antiretroviral therapy (ART) was taken by all the patients and, considering SLE, seven were treated with hydroxychloroquine (HCQ), two with azathioprine (AZA), two with cyclophosphamide (CYC), one with methotrexate (MTX) and one with mycophenolate mofetil (MMF), according to the severity of each case (Table 2).

Discussion

The coexistent infection of HIV and SLE is unusual and intriguing, because both diseases are characterized by multisystem involvement and immune dysfunction related to T lymphocytes, cytokine production alterations and polyclonal activation of B lymphocytes [6]. Despite these similarities, several theories have been formulated to explain the reason of the unexpectedly lower prevalence of concomitant diagnosis of HIV and SLE. SLE may prevent HIV infection as a result of polyclonal

Table 1 Demographic, clinical, and laboratory features of SLE patients with and without HIV infection

Patients features	All patients ($n = 602$)	SLE patients without HIV ($n = 591$)	SLE patients with HIV ($n = 11$)	P value[a]
Females	92% (602)	91.9% (591)	100% (11)	1.000
European derived	75.2% (584)	75.4% (573)	63.6% (11)	0.479
Smoking[b]	38.3% (582)	37.6% (215)	80% (11)	0.009
Obesity	25.3% (502)	25.9% (127)	0% (11)	0.074
Age (years)	48.2±14.9(597)	48.3±14.9 (586)	43.1±12.7 (11)	0.245
SLE age at diagnosis (years)	33.5±14.2 (591)	33.6±14.2 (580)	29.9±13.9 (11)	0.390
Malar rash	55.3% (597)	56% (586)	18.2% (11)	0.015
Photosensitivity	72.1% (598)	72.4% (587)	54.5% (11)	0.191
Oral ulcers	35.6% (598)	35.6% (587)	36.4% (11)	1.000
Arthritis	72.4% (597)	74.4% (586)	63.6% (11)	0.486
Serositis	25.2% (595)	25% (585)	36.4% (11)	0.482
Nephritis	40.9% (596)	40.5% (585)	63.6% (11)	0.134
Neurologic disorders	11.4% (596)	10.9% (585)	36.4% (11)	0.028
Psychosis	6.5% (597)	6.3% (586)	18.2% (11)	0.158
Seizures	6% (597)	6% (586)	9.1% (11)	0.498
Hematologic disorders	75.8% (598)	75.8% (587)	72.7% (11)	0.773
Hemolytic anemia	29.1% (598)	28,6% (587)	54,5% (11)	0.089
Leukopenia/Lymphopenia	55.9% (598)	56% (587)	45.5% (11)	0.549
Thrombocytopenia	21.4% (598)	21.5% (587)	18.2% (11)	1.000
Anti-dsDNA	46% (567)	46% (556)	45.5% (11)	1.000
Anti-Sm	20.8% (549)	21% (538)	9.1% (11)	0.474
Anticardiolipin	27.3% (550)	27.6% (539)	9.1% (11)	0.304
Lupus Anticoagulant	10% (548)	10.1% (537)	9.1% (11)	1.000
Anti-Ro	39.9% (516)	39.4% (505)	63.6% (11)	0.125
Anti-La	13.4% (515)	13.1% (504)	27.3% (11)	0.172
Anti-RNP	31.1% (515)	31.2% (504)	27.3% (11)	1.000
SLEDAI (median)[c]	1 (415)	1 (407)	0 (11)	0.550
SLICC damage index (median)[c]	1 (559)	1 (551)	2 (11)	0.047

Abbreviations: *SLE* systemic lupus erythematosus, *SLEDAI* systemic lupus erythematosus disease activity index, *SLICC* systemic lupus international collaborating clinics, *HIV* human immunodeficiency virus
[a]Chi square test for qualitative variables and Mann-Whitney test for quantitative variables
[b]Current or past smoker
[c]Median (interquartile interval)

antibody stimulation [7] and treatment with antimalarials [8]. Patients with SLE have higher levels of interleukin (IL)-16 and IL-16 inhibits HIV infection in vitro, representing a possible protective role against HIV in SLE patients [9]. Likewise, SLE cannot develop in the setting of CD4 cell depletion seen in HIV [10]. Zandman-Goddard and Shoenfeld proposed that autoimmune manifestations in patients with HIV occur after the restoration of immunological competence (CD4 count > 500 cells/μL and low viral load) using ART or during the first stage of HIV (the acute HIV infection), when the immune system is intact and, hence, autoimmune diseases may present [11].

Kopelman and Zolla-Pazner published in 1988 the first report of a patient with HIV infection and SLE [12]. Since then, there have been several case reports or small case series of patients with concomitant SLE and HIV. Literature review has identified a total of 58 patients reported until 2014, some of which did not fulfill the criteria for SLE [1]. Then, in 2014, Mody et al. published a relatively large case series of 13 patients with coexistent HIV infection and SLE evaluated in a hospital of Durban, South Africa [1].

Kopelman and Zolla-Pazner have tested 151 consecutive patients with HIV and found that 19 had positive ANA, most of it in low titers, which usually is not associated with clinical manifestations of SLE [12]. Medina-Rodriguez et al. also found a significant number of HIV-positive patients with positivity for aCL IgG (94%), and aCL IgM (44%) [13].

Table 2 Demographic, clinical and laboratory features, treatment and outcome of SLE patients with HIV

Case	Gender	First DX	Clinical features	Autoantibodies	SLE treatment	ART	CD4 at DX[a]	Last CD4	Outcome
1	F	SLE	Discoid lupus, photosensitivity, oral ulcers and arthritis	ANA and anti-Ro	CS	Yes	434	337	Good health condition, but loss of follow-up in the Rheumatology Clinic
2	F	SLE	Raynaud, arthritis and vasculitis	ANA, anti-dsDNA, anti-Ro and anti-La	CS	Yes	572	205	Disseminated TB at 2015, follow-up in the Infectious Diseases Clinic
3	F	SLE	Arthritis, leucopenia, lymphopenia, alopecia, Raynaud and photosensitivity	ANA	HCQ	Yes	424	1056	SLE in remission, HIV controlled
4	F	SLE	Discoid lupus, photosensitivity, nephritis, leucopenia and lymphopenia	ANA	HCQ	Yes	149	524	HCV coinfection SLE in remission and HIV controlled
5	F	SLE	Photosensitivity, oral ulcers, arthritis and nephritis	ANA, anti-Ro and anti-La	CS, AZA ➔ MMF and tacrolimus	Yes	273	991	Pulmonary TB in 2008, kidney transplantation in 2011
6	F	SLE	Photosensitivity, serositis and arthritis	ANA	None	Yes	172	391	HCV coinfection, SLE in remission and HIV controlled
7	F	SLE	Alopecia, arthritis, nephritis, hemolytic anemia and hypergammaglobulinemia	ANA, anti-dsDNA and anti-Ro	HCQ, CYC ➔ AZA	Yes	321	165	Good initial response, poor adherence to treatment with posterior reactivation of nephritis and CD4 count drop
8	F	HIV	Hemolytic anemia, serositis, oral ulcers and arthritis	ANA, anti-Sm and anti-RNP	HCQ, MTX	Yes	NA	477	CMV Retinitis in 2006, SLE in remission and HIV controlled
9	F	HIV	Hemolytic anemia and nephritis	ANA and anti-dsDNA	CS, HCQ CYC ➔ AZA	Yes	235	252	Complete response to CYC, posterior poor adherence and loss of follow-up due to drug addiction
10	F	SLE	Hemolytic anemia, serositis, leucopenia, lymphopenia, oral ulcers, arthritis and nephritis	ANA and anti-dsDNA	HCQ	Yes	203	323	SLE in remission and HIV controlled
11	F	Both	Alopecia, hemolytic anemia, nephritis, thrombocytopenia, leucopenia and lymphopenia	ANA	CS, HCQ ➔AZA	Yes	111	NA	Both diagnosed in hospital stay, progressing to death from sepsis

Abbreviations: *ACL IgG* anti-cardiolipin IgG, *ACL IgM* anti-cardiolipin IgM, *ANA* anti-nuclear antibody, *ART* active antiretroviral therapy, *AZA* azathioprine, *CMV* cytomegalovirus, *CS* corticosteroids, *CYC* cyclophosphamide, *dsDNA* anti-double-stranded DNA, *DX* diagnosis, *F* female, *HCQ* hydroxychloroquine, *HIV* human immunodeficiency virus, *M* male, *MMF* mycophenolate mofetil, *MTX* methotrexate, *NA* not available, *SLE* systemic lupus erythematosus, *TB* tuberculosis

[a]CD4 cell count at diagnosis of HIV-infection: cells/mm^3

However, Petrovas et al. in a case-control study that compared the prevalence of antiphospholipid antibodies in patients with HIV infection, SLE with or without antiphospholipid syndrome (APS) and in primary antiphospholipid syndrome (PAPS), also evaluating the reactivity of these antibodies with β2-glicoprotein (GPI). It was demonstrated that the prevalence of aCL antibodies in HIV-infection was 36%. However, anti-β2-GPI occurred in only 5% of HIV, which seems to reduce its thrombogenic potential [14]. Therefore, antiphospholipid antibodies occur in HIV-1 infection, but are not associated with thrombosis [14]. In our cohort, prevalence of antiphospholipid antibodies did not differ between patients with and without infection by HIV.

Additional studies evaluated the presence of other autoantibodies in HIV-positive patients and found multiple autoimmune phenomena HIV-associated, many of those seen in SLE, including besides the presence of ANAs, antiplatelet antibodies, antilymphocyte antibodies and antineutrophil cytoplasmic antibodies (ANCA), as well as Coomb's positivity, circulating immune complexes, rheumatoid factor and cryoglobulins [7, 13, 15, 16]. Furthermore, the presence of antibodies to extractable nuclear antigens (ENA) has also been described, although with controversial findings. Muller et al. have tested the presence of ENA by enzyme-linked immunosorbent assay (ELISA) in 100 HIV-positive patients, detecting anti-dsDNA, anti-histone, anti-Sm, anti-RNP and anti-Ro in 45% to 90% of these patients [17]. In its turn, Lafeuillade et al. in a study including 119 HIV-positive patients, found a lower frequency of those autoantibodies (4% had ANAs, 1% anti-dsDNA, 4% anti-Sm and 6% anti-histone) [18]. Thus, the presence of these autoantibodies in HIV patients is still controversial. Variations in the studied populations and in the analysis techniques employed explain, in part, these discrepancies [19]. In one study, the positivity for autoantibodies was significantly associated with lower CD4 lymphocyte counts and with increased mortality, which can indicate a prognostic implication of the autoimmunity in the context of HIV infection [15].

In patients with coexistence of HIV infection and diagnosis of SLE, three patterns of disease occurrence have been described: HIV following SLE diagnosis, SLE following the diagnosis of HIV infection and simultaneous diagnosis of HIV and SLE [20]. In our cohort, the most prevalent pattern was the one in which patients with established SLE were subsequently diagnosed with infection by HIV. Some studies suggest that HIV infection can attenuate the natural history of SLE [10, 21–23]. On the other hand, the impact of SLE in patients with pre-existing HIV infection is not well known. Some authors propose that SLE may contribute to a worst outcome of the HIV infection, keeping in mind that there are some reports describing a shorter time span until the development of AIDS in patients with concomitant SLE [23]. Nonetheless, this data is unavailable in many cases and there are some reports in which patients with coexistence of HIV infection and SLE did not developed AIDS even after long periods of observation [19]. Furthermore, some authors believe the immunologic effects of SLE and HIV may antagonize each other, contributing to the uncertainty regarding the clinical impact of this association [23].

Many of the clinical features of SLE overlap with either the primary features or secondary complications of HIV infection [24]: dermatologic findings such as alopecia, oral ulcers and facial rash; constitutional symptoms, including fever and malaise; musculoskeletal involvement such as arthralgias, arthritis and myalgias; renal abnormalities, including hematuria and proteinuria; central nervous system disorders, such as seizures and psychosis; hematologic alterations, including anemia, leucopenia, lymphopenia and thrombocytopenia; and immunologic features such as hypergammaglobulinemia and positive ANA [21, 25]. The term *pseudolupus* has been used to describe patients with HIV infection that present with rheumatic manifestations similar to SLE. In our cohort, nephritis, neuropsychiatric lupus, hemolytic anemia, hypergammaglobulinemia, presence of anti-Ro and anti-La were the most prevalent features amongst the SLE patients infected by HIV.

Besides, false positive HIV on ELISA tests have also been described in SLE patients, making the diagnosis even more difficult, and making it necessary to perform other confirmatory tests for HIV [26]. In these cases, viral RNA PCR assays were superior than the p24 antigen assay (less sensitive) to exclude the possibility of a false positive HIV on ELISA test [27]. Low complement due to HIV infection has not been reported. Therefore, hypocomplementenemia may be a helpful test to differentiate lupus activity from HIV-related manifestations [24]. In our cohort the majority of patients with AIDS presented with hypocomplementenemia and this finding contributed not only to assess the disease activity, but also to establish the diagnosis of SLE.

The treatment of patients with coexistent SLE and HIV infection is challenging and there aren't well established therapeutic guidelines thus far. Immunosuppressive medications may have a negative impact in patients with preexistent impaired immunity [25]. However, with the adequate suppression of the HIV viral load, it is postulated that the treatment of SLE would not anticipate the development of AIDS [19]. Associated to ART, HCQ seems to be a reasonable and safe approach, considering it also has antiviral properties in HIV patients [28] and that its anti-inflammatory effect doesn't appear to be associated with an increased risk of opportunistic infections [29]. Low-dose corticosteroids may be considered with caution for those with severe immunosuppression by AIDS [25]. Relative safety of using MMF in HIV-positive patients has been confirmed by its successful use in the solid organ transplantation in HIV patients on ART [30]. Therefore, the risks and benefits have to be considered carefully when deciding the therapeutic approach that is more adequate to each patient with concomitant HIV infection and SLE [20]. Patients of our cohort that used CYC for the induction treatment of nephritis, followed by maintenance with AZA, developed a complete response with no major infectious complications.

It is well known that there is an increased risk of opportunistic infection in SLE patients, as well as in patients infected by HIV and this is the leading cause of morbidity and mortality in both diseases [6]. In our cohort, survival in 5 and 10 years was similar in SLE patients with or without AIDS. Even though we emphasized a statistically significant difference in the SLICC, indicating a greater cumulative damage in patients with concomitant AIDS, the clinical and prognostic relevance of this finding is uncertain thus far, once there was no significant difference in the survival rate between the groups in our study population.

Special attention must also be paid to infections caused by Mycobacterium tuberculosis, due to its high prevalence in HIV patients [31] as well as SLE, especially in developing countries [32]. Patients with lupus and HIV seems to have a higher risk of developing tuberculosis as shown by the largest case series available on the subject, in which 7 out of 13 patients were diagnosed with tuberculosis [1]. In our cohort, only 2 patients infected by HIV developed tuberculosis, probably reflecting the demographic differences and the regional prevalences of this disease.

Conclusion

Patients with concomitant HIV and SLE presented with neuropsychiatric manifestations more often. Therefore, it is essential to pay attention to the early diagnosis of HIV, especially in the scenario of this severe manifestation and in light of the need to intensify the immunosuppression. Moreover, there was a higher prevalence of hypergammaglobulinemia and hypocomplementenemia, which in turn, can be an useful tool to identify disease activity. For the first time, higher cumulative damage was described in lupus patients with concomitant HIV infection, which can contribute to a worst life quality and reduction of the survival rates, although further studies are needed to elucidate this complex association, its outcomes and prognosis.

Abbreviations

aCL: Anticardiolipin; ACR: AMERICAN College of Rheumatology; AIDS: Acquired immunodeficiency syndrome; ANA: Antinuclear antibody; ANCA: Antineutrophil cytoplasmic antibodies; APS: Antiphospholipid syndrome; ART: Antiretroviral therapy; AZA: Azathioprine; CYC: Cyclophosphamide; ds-DNA: Anti-double-stranded DNA; ELISA: Enzyme-linked immunosorbent assay; ENA: Extractable nuclear antigens; GPI: Glicoprotein; HCQ: Hydroxychloroquine; IL: Interleukin; MMF: Mycophenolate mofetil; MTX: Methotrexate; PAPS: Primary antiphospholipid syndrome; SD: Standard deviation; SLE: Systemic lupus erythematosus; SLEDAI: Systemic Lupus Erythematosus Disease Activity Index; SLICC: Systemic Lupus International Collaborating Clinics

Authors' contributions

All the authors collaborated in the analysis and in writing the manuscript. All authors read and approved the final manuscript.

Author details

[1]Division of Rheumatology, Hospital de Clínicas de Porto Alegre, Universidade Federal do Rio Grande do Sul, 2350 Ramiro Barcelos St, Room 645, Porto Alegre, RS 90035-903, Brazil. [2]Medical School Student, Universidade Federal do Rio Grande do Sul, Porto Alegre, Brazil. [3]Division of Infectious Diseases, Hospital de Clínicas de Porto Alegre, Universidade Federal do Rio Grande do Sul, Porto Alegre, Brazil.

References

1. Mody GM, Patel N, Budhoo A, Dubula T. Concomitant systemic lupus erythematosus and HIV: case series and literature review. Semin Arthritis Rheum. 2014;44(2):186–94.
2. Hochberg MC. Updating the American College of Rheumatology revised criteria for the classification of systemic lupus erythematosus. Arthritis Rheum. 1997;40(9):1725.
3. Vitali C, Bombardieri S, Jonsson R, et al. Classification criteria for Sjögren's syndrome: a revised version of the European criteria proposed by the American-European consensus group. Ann Rheum Dis. 2002;61(6):554–8.
4. Miyakis S, Lockshin MD, Atsumi T, et al. International consensus statement on an update of the classification criteria for definite antiphospholipid syndrome (APS). J Thromb Haemost. 2006;4(2):295–306.
5. Griffiths B, Mosca M, Gordon C. Assessment of patients with systemic lupus erythematosus and the use of lupus disease activity indices. Best Pract Res Clin Rheumatol. 2005;19(5):685–708.
6. Sekigawa I, Okada M, Ogasawara H, et al. Lessons from similarities between SLE and HIV infection. J Inf Secur. 2002;44(2):67–72.
7. Kaye BR. Rheumatologic manifestations of HIV infections. Clin Rev Allergy Immunol. 1996;14:385–416.
8. Tsai WP, Nara PL, Kung HF, Oroszlan S. Inhibition of immunodeficiency virus infectivity by chloroquin. AIDS Res Hum Retrovir. 1990;6:481–9.
9. Sekigawa I, Lee S, Kaneko H, et al. The possible role of interleukin-16 in the low incidence of HIV infection in patients with systemic lupus erythematosus. Lupus. 2000;9:155–6.
10. Furie RA. Effects of human immunodeficiency virus infection on the expression of rheumatic illness. Rheum Dis Clin North Am. 1991;17:177–88.
11. Zandman-Goddard G, Shoenfeld Y. HIV and autoimmunity. Autoimmun Rev. 2002;1(6):329–37.
12. Kopelman RG, Zolla-Pazner S. Association of human immunodeficiency virus infection and autoimmune phenomena. Am J Med. 1988;84:82–8.
13. Medina-Rodriguez F, Guzman C, Jara LJ, et al. Rheumatic manifestations in human immunodeficiency virus positive and negative individuals: a study of 2 populations with similar risk factors. J Rheumatol. 1993;20:1880–4.
14. Petrovas C, Vlachouyiannopoulos PG, Kordossis T, Moutsopoulos M. Anti-phospholipid antibodies in HIV infection and SLE with or without anti-phospholipid syndrome: comparisons of phospholipid specificity, avidity and reactivity with B2-GPI. J Autoimmun. 1999;13:347–55.
15. Massabki PS, Accetturi C, Nishie IA, da Silva NP, Sato EI, Andrade LEC. Clinical implications of autoantibodies in HIV infection. AIDS. 1997;11:1845–50.
16. Stimmler MM, Quismorio FP Jr, McGehee WG, Boylen T, Sharma OP. Anticardiolipin antibodies in acquired immunodeficiency syndrome. Arch Intern Med. 1989;149:1833–5.
17. Muller S, Richalet P, Laurent-Crawford A, et al. Autoantibodies typical of non-organ-specific autoimmune disease in HIV-seropositive patients. AIDS. 1992;6:933–42.
18. Lafeuillade A, Ritter J, Pellegrino P, Qiulichini R, Monier JC. Lack of anti-nuclear antibodies during HIV infection (correspondence). AIDS. 1993;7:893.
19. Daikh BE, Holyst MM. Lupus-specific autoantibodies in concomitant human immunodeficiency virus and systemic lupus erythematosus: case report and literature review. Semin Arthritis Rheum. 2001;30:18–25.
20. Gindea S, Schwartzman J, Herlitz LC, et al. Proliferative glomerulonephritis in lupus patients with human immunodeficiency virus infection: a difficult clinical challenge. Semin Arthritis Rheum. 2010;40:201–9.
21. Molina JF, Citera G, Rosler D, et al. Coexistence of human immunodeficiency virus infection and systemic lupus erythematosus. J Rheumatol. 1995;22:347–50.
22. Byrd VM, Sergent JS. Suppression of systemic lupus erythematosus by the human immunodeficiency virus. J Rheumatol. 1996;23:1295–6.
23. Fox RA, Isenberg DA. Human immunodeficiency virus infection in systemic lupus erythematosus. Arthritis Rheum. 1997;40:1168–72.
24. Gould T, Tikly M. Systemic lupus erythematosus in a patient with human immunodeficiency virus infection – challenges in diagnosis and management. Clin Rheumatol. 2004;23:166–9.
25. López-López L, González A, Vilá LM. Long-term membranous glomerulonephritis as the presenting manifestation of systemic lupus erythematosus in a patient with human immunodeficiency virus infection. Lupus. 2012;21:900–4.
26. Gul A, Inanc M, Yilmaz G, et al. Antibodies reactive with HIV-1 antigens in systemic lupus erythematosus. Lupus. 1996;5:120–2.
27. UNAIDS/WHO Working Group on Global HIV/AIDS/STI Surveillance 2001 Guidelines for using HIV testing technologies in surveillance: selection, evaluation and implementation. Available at http://www.who.int/hiv/pub/epidemiology/pub4/en/.
28. Sperber K, Kalb TH, Stecher VJ, Banerjee R, Mayer L. Inhibition of human immunodeficiency virus type 1 replication by hydroxychloroquine in T cells and monocytes. AIDS Res Hum Retrovir. 1993;9:91–8.
29. Sperber K, Ornstein MH. The anti-inflammatory effect of hydroxychloroquine in two patients with acquired immunodeficiency syndrome and active inflammatory arthritis. Arthritis and Rheum. 1996;39:157–61.
30. Stock PG, Roland ME, Carlson L, et al. Kidney and liver transplantation in human immunodeficiency virus-infected patients: a pilot safety and efficacy study. Transplantation. 2003;76:370–5.

Autoimmune hepatitis in 847 childhood-onset systemic lupus erythematosus population

Verena A. Balbi[1†], Bárbara Montenegro[1†], Ana C. Pitta[1†], Ana R. Schmidt[1], Sylvia C. Farhat[1], Laila P. Coelho[1], Juliana C. O. Ferreira[1], Rosa M. R. Pereira[2], Maria T. Terreri[3], Claudia Saad-Magalhães[4], Nadia E. Aikawa[2], Ana P. Sakamoto[3], Kátia Kozu[1], Lucia M. Campos[1], Adriana M. Sallum[1], Virginia P. Ferriani[5], Daniela P. Piotto[3], Eloisa Bonfá[2†] and Clovis A. Silva[1,2*†]

Abstract

Objective: To evaluate autoimmune hepatitis (AIH) in a multicenter cohort of childhood-onset systemic lupus erythematosus (cSLE) patients.

Methods: This retrospective multicenter study included 847 patients with cSLE, performed in 10 Pediatric Rheumatology services of São Paulo state, Brazil. AIH was defined according to the International Autoimmune Hepatitis Group criteria (IAHGC). The statistical analysis was performed using the Bonferroni's correction ($p < 0.0033$).

Results: AIH in cSLE patients confirmed by biopsy was observed in 7/847 (0.8%) and all were diagnosed during adolescence. The majority occurred before or at cSLE diagnosis [5/7 (71%)]. Antinuclear antibodies were a universal finding, 43% had concomitantly anti-smooth muscle antibodies and all were seronegative for anti-liver kidney microsomal antibodies. All patients with follow-up ≥18 months (4/7) had complete response to therapy according to IAHGC. None had severe hepatic manifestations such as hepatic failure, portal hypertension and cirrhosis at presentation or follow-up. Further comparison of 7 cSLE patients with AIH and 28 without this complication with same disease duration [0 (0–8.5) vs. 0.12 (0–8.5) years, $p = 0.06$] revealed that the frequency of hepatomegaly was significantly higher in cSLE patients in the former group (71% vs. 11%, $p = 0.003$) with a similar median SLEDAI-2 K score [6 (0–26) vs. 7 (0–41), $p = 0.755$]. No differences were evidenced regarding constitutional involvement, splenomegaly, serositis, musculoskeletal, neuropsychiatric and renal involvements, and treatments in cSLE patients with and without AIH ($p > 0.0033$).

Conclusions: Overlap of AIH and cSLE was rarely observed in this large multicenter study and hepatomegaly was the distinctive clinical feature of these patients. AIH occurred during adolescence, mainly at the first years of lupus and it was associated with mild liver manifestations.

Keywords: Autoimmune hepatitis, Childhood systemic lupus erythematosus, Hepatomegaly, Multicenter study

* Correspondence: clovis.silva@hc.fm.usp.br
†Verena A. Balbi, Bárbara Montenegro, Ana C. Pitta, Eloisa Bonfá and Clovis A. Silva contributed equally to this work.
[1]Pediatric Rheumatology Unit, Children's Institute, Hospital das Clinicas HCFMUSP, Faculdade de Medicina, Universidade de Sao Paulo, Sao Paulo, SP, Brazil
[2]Division of Rheumatology, Hospital das Clinicas HCFMUSP, Faculdade de Medicina, Universidade de Sao Paulo, Sao Paulo, SP, Brazil
Full list of author information is available at the end of the article

Introduction

Childhood-onset systemic lupus erythematosus (cSLE) is an autoimmune and inflammatory disease that affects multiple organs and systems, including liver [1–3].

Of note, autoimmune hepatitis (AIH) is characterized by elevated hepatic enzymes, hypergammaglobulinemia, presence of autoantibodies and liver histology abnormalities, particularly interface hepatitis and lymphocytic infiltrates [4, 5]. To our knowledge the prevalence of overlap AIH and cSLE in a large population was not studied and analysis of this very rare association is restricted to few case reports or case series [1, 3, 6, 7].

Therefore, the objective of this multicenter cohort study was to evaluate cSLE and AIH and the possible association with demographic data, cumulative clinical manifestations, treatments and outcomes in a large cSLE population in Latin America.

Methods

This study was conducted in 10 Pediatric Rheumatology services in the state of São Paulo, Brazil including a population of 847 cSLE patients [8]. All patients fulfilled the American College of Rheumatology (ACR) criteria for SLE [9], with disease onset before the age of 18. The Ethical Committee of each University Hospital approved this study. An investigator meeting was held for this study in São Paulo city to define the protocol according to the clinical parameters and disease activity tool scoring. At least one investigator with Brazilian Board Pediatric Rheumatology Certifying Examination supervised data collection in each center, reviewed paper files and tried to solve discrepancies among investigators of these centers. Four rounds of queries were performed to check for accuracy and sort out discrepancies among groups.

Patients' medical charts were systematically reviewed according to demographic data, clinical features and AIH characteristics, laboratorial abnormalities, therapeutic data and outcomes. AIH was diagnosed according to International Autoimmune Hepatitis Group criteria (IAHGC) [4, 5]. Every medical visit from cSLE diagnosis to last visit or death was reviewed in each center. Percutaneous needle liver biopsy was performed in these centers in cSLE patients with elevation of liver enzymes (not related to hepatotoxic drugs, metabolic disease, alcohol or viral disease), associated with hypergammaglobulinemia and presence of at least one autoantibody [antinuclear antibodies (ANA), anti-type I liver-kidney microsomal (anti-LKM-1) antibody or liver and stomach tissue substrates and anti-smooth muscle antibody (anti-SMA)].

Descriptors of SLE Disease Activity Index 2000 (SLEDAI-2 K) were used to define clinical manifestations [10], and custom definitions as previously reported [8]. Cumulative clinical manifestations included constitutional involvement [defined as fever and lymphadenopathy (peripheral lymph node enlargement > 1.0 cm)], hepatomegaly [based on physical exam with liver edge ≥2 cm below the right costal margin or imaging (ultrasound or computer tomography when available)], splenomegaly [based on physical exam with palpable spleen or imaging (ultrasound or computer tomography when available)], musculoskeletal involvement, serositis, neuropsychiatric and renal involvement. Neuropsychiatric Lupus included 19 syndromes according to ACR classification criteria [11].

Antinuclear antibodies (ANA) were tested by indirect immunofluorescence. Anti-type I liver-kidney microsomal (anti-LKM-1) antibody on frozen sections of rodent kidney, liver and stomach tissue substrates and anti-smooth muscle antibody (anti-SMA) by indirect immunofluorescence on rat liver and kidney tissue sections on frozen sections of rodent kidney, liver and stomach tissue substrates. The cutoff values from the kit manufacturer were used to define abnormal.

Drug treatment data (prednisone, intravenous methylprednisolone, chloroquine diphosphate, hydroxychloroquine sulfate, methotrexate, azathioprine, cyclosporine, mycophenolate mofetil, intravenous cyclophosphamide, intravenous immunoglobulin and rituximab) were also recorded.

Patients were divided in two groups with similar disease duration: cSLE patients with AIH (evaluated at AIH diagnosis) and cSLE patients without AIH (evaluated at last visit).

Statistical analysis

Results were presented as absolute number (frequency) for categorical variables and median (range) or mean ± standard deviation for continuous variables. Categorical variables comparisons were assessed by Pearson χ-Square or Fisher's exact test. Continuous variables from cSLE patients with and without AIH were compared by Mann-Whitney test or t test as appropriate. Statistical analysis was performed using Bonferroni correction ($p < 0.0033$).

Results

Demographic data, clinical and laboratorial features, outcomes and treatments in cSLE patients with AIH are described in Table 1. AIH in cSLE patients confirmed by biopsy was observed in 7/847 (0.8%) and all were diagnosed during adolescence. The majority occurred before or at cSLE diagnosis [5/7 (71%)]. Antinuclear antibodies were a universal finding, 43% had concomitantly anti-SMA and all were seronegative for anti-LKM-1 antibodies. All 7 patients with follow-up ≥18 months (4/7) had complete response to therapy according to IAHGC. None of cSLE patients with AIH had severe hepatic manifestations such as hepatic failure, portal hypertension, cirrhosis or deceased at presentation or at follow-up (Table 1).

Liver biopsy was performed in only 7/847 (0.8%) cSLE that fulfilled the AIH criteria (IAHGC) [4, 5]. Regarding

Table 1 Demographic data, clinical and laboratorial features, outcomes and treatments in childhood-onset systemic lupus erythematosus (cSLE) patients with autoimmune hepatitis (AIH)

	Cases						
	1	2	3	4	5	6	7
Demographic data							
Age, years	12.5	12.3	10.3	15	10.3	15.6	11.7
Female gender	+	+	+	+	+	+	–
Time between AIH and cSLE, years	−1.5	0	−4.75	0	2.3	8.5	0
cSLE duration, years	0	0	0	0	2.3	8.5	0
Clinical/laboratorial features							
Constitutional symptoms	–	+	+	+	+	+	+
Jaundice/ascites	+/–	–/–	+/–	+/–	–/–	+/–	+/–
Hepatomegaly/Splenomegaly	–/–	+/+	–/–	+/+	+/–	+/–	+/+
AST, IU/L	93	652	35	345.7	245	4466	1260
ALT, IU/L	113	268	122	244.6	552	1411	949
GGT, IU/L	258	604	91	51.2	613	69	606
Hypergammaglobulinemia	+	+	+	+	+	+	+
ANA > 1:80	+	+	+	+	+	+	+
Anti-SMA > 1:80	+	+	+	–	–	–	–
Anti-LKM1 > 1:80	–	–	–	–	–	–	–
Viral hepatitis markers	–	–	–	–	–	–	–
Alcohol intake	–	–	–	–	–	–	–
Liver histology with interface hepatitis and lymphocytic infiltrates	+	+	+	+	+	+	+
Outcomes							
Liver failure/portal hypertension/cirrhosis	- /–/–	- /–/–	- /–/–	- /–/–	- /–/–	- /–/–	- /–/–
Death	–	–	–	–	–	–	–
Therapy							
AIH complete response therapy (> 18 months)	+	NP	+	NP	+	+	NP
cSLE treatments	PD, AZA	PD, AZA, AM	PD, AZA, AM	PD, AZA	PD, AZA, AM	PD, AZA	PD

AST aspartate aminotransferase (normal value 15–40 IU/L), *ALT* alanine aminotransferase (normal value 10–40 IU/L), *GGT* gamma glutamyl transferase (normal value 3–25 IU/L), *ANA* antinuclear antibodies, anti-SMA - anti-smooth muscle antibody, anti-LKM1 - anti-liver kidney microsomal antibody type1, *NP* not possible, *PD* prednisone, *AZA* azathioprine, *AM* antimalarial

the remaining 840 cSLE patients without AIH, 86% patients were females. The median of age was 12 years (0.25–18) and the median of disease duration was 5 years (0–23). Leukopenia (45%), thrombocytopenia (21%), ANA (99%), anti-dsDNA antibodies (71%) and anti-Sm antibodies (32%) were observed in these cSLE patients.

Deaths occurred in 69/840 (8%) cSLE patients that were not affected by AIH. Infections accounted for 54/69 (78%) of overall deaths and 70% of these had concomitant disease activity. Other causes of death were: nephritis (acute kidney injury or chronic renal disease) (9%), alveolar hemorrhage (4%), massive intracranial bleeding (1.4%), multiple thrombosis due to catastrophic antiphospholipid syndrome (1.4%), B-cell lymphoma (1.4%) and unknown etiologies (4%).

Further analysis of 7 cSLE patients with AIH compared to 28 cSLE patients without AIH and with the same disease duration [0 (0–8.5) vs. 0.12 (0–8.5) years, $p = 0.06$] revealed that the frequency of hepatomegaly was significantly higher in cSLE patients with AIH compared to those without AIH (71% vs. 11%, $p = 0.003$). The median of age at diagnosis [12.25 (10.3–15.6) vs. 12.9 (3.3–19.7) years, $p = 0.650$] and SLEDAI-2 K score [6 (0–26) vs. 7 (0–41) years, $p = 0.755$] were similar in both groups. No differences were evidenced between constitutional involvement, splenomegaly, serositis, musculoskeletal, neuropsychiatric and renal manifestations, and treatments in cSLE patients with and without AIH ($p > 0.0033$) (Table 2).

The comparisons of last visit of cSLE patients with AIH ($n = 7$) versus last visit of cSLE without AIH ($n = 840$) revealed similar age [12.25 (7.1–15) vs. 11.83 (0.25–17.8) years, $p = 0.94$] and disease duration [4.3 (0.58–11.8) vs. 4.58 (0–23.4) years, $p = 0.56$] in both groups. The frequency

Table 2 Demographic data, disease activity, cumulative clinical manifestations and treatments in childhood-onset systemic lupus erythematosus (cSLE) patients with autoimmune hepatitis (AIH) at diagnosis compared to those without AIH evaluated at last visit

Variables	cSLE with AIH (at AIH diagnosis) ($n = 7$)	cSLE without AIH (at last visit) ($n = 28$)	*P*
Demographic data			
Age at diagnosis, years	12.25 (10.3–15.6)	12.9 (3.3–19.7)	0.650
Disease duration, years	0 (0–8.5)	0.12 (0–8.5)	0.060
Disease activity parameter			
SLEDAI-2 K	6 (0–26)	7 (0–41)	0.755
Cumulative clinical manifestations			
Constitutional involvement	6 (86)	7 (25)	0.006
Hepatomegaly	5 (71)	3 (11)	**0.003***
Splenomegaly	3 (43)	1 (4)	0.019
Musculoskeletal involvement	4 (57)	3 (11)	0.018
Serositis	0 (0)	4 (7)	1.000
Neuropsychiatric involvement	0 (0)	5 (18)	0.559
Renal involvement	2 (29)	11 (39)	0.689
Treatment			
Prednisone dose, mg/kg/day	1.07 (0.5–2.4)	0.9 (0.1–2.8)	0.365
Antimalarial use	3 (43)	14 (50)	1.000
Immunosuppressive use	6 (86)	8 (29)	0.009

Results are presented in n (%) and median (range), *P - value according to Bonferroni correction for multiple comparisons ($p < 0.0033$), SLEDAI-2 K - SLE Disease Activity Index 2000

of female gender (85.7% vs. 85.9%, $p = 1.0$) and median of SLEDAI-2 K [4 (2–10) vs. 2 (0–45), $p = 0.45$] and SLICC-ACR/damage index [0 (0–1) vs. 0 (0–9), $p = 0.77$] were also similar in both groups. The frequencies of chronic renal failure (0% vs. 6.1%, p = 1.0), prednisone (100% vs. 97%, $p = 1.0$), azathioprine (86% vs. 61%, $p = 0.26$), methotrexate (29% vs. 23%, $p = 0.66$), mycophenolate mofetil (14% vs. 21%, $p = 1.0$) and intravenous cyclophosphamide (0% vs. 42%, $p = 0.05$) were alike in both group. The lower frequency of death in AIH patients did not reach statistical significance (0% vs. 8%, $p = 1.0$).

The Kaplan-Meier overall survival curve was significantly higher in cSLE patients with AIH compared to those without this complication ($p = 0.001$). After 11.6 years of disease onset the survival percentage of cSLE patients with AIH was 100% and for those without AIH was 83% (Fig. 1).

Discussion

This multicenter study demonstrated that overlap of AIH and cSLE is a very rare association. This liver autoimmune disease occurred mainly at the first years of cSLE diagnosis, without liver complication and associated with mild disease manifestations.

The strength of this study was the large cohort including 10 different Pediatric Rheumatology and tertiary centers of cSLE. All AIH patients fulfilled the IAHGC definite criteria (score > 15) with typical histological features in liver biopsy [4, 5]. We also used a standardized cSLE protocol with definitions for clinical and disease activity parameters [10]. The limitations were the possible missing data due to retrospective design, the collinearity of the variables and the limited indication for liver biopsy.

We have confirmed and extended previous observation that liver involvement is rarely observed in cSLE and adult SLE patients, with a variety of clinical and laboratorial manifestations [1, 12–16]. The rigorous selection criteria of AIH and cSLE patients excluding viral infections, malignancies and alcohol intake was relevant to avoid other confounding etiologies of hepatitis [1, 7, 12, 14].

AIH was solely observed in adolescents and the majority occurred before or at cSLE diagnosis. Hepatomegaly was a distinctive feature of AIH in this age group contrasting with our previous observation that liver enlargement was usually not common in adolescent at lupus diagnosis [17]. Hepatomegaly was not associated with liver congestion, fatty infiltration, viral hepatitis, metabolic disorders, thrombosis or hepatotoxic drugs usage, since histological findings excluded these issues. The concomitant presences of jaundice, splenomegaly and hypergammaglobulinemia reinforced the AIH diagnosis [1], as observed in more than 50% of cases.

AIH occurred in cSLE patients with mild lupus manifestations. Of note, the majority of our patients had a

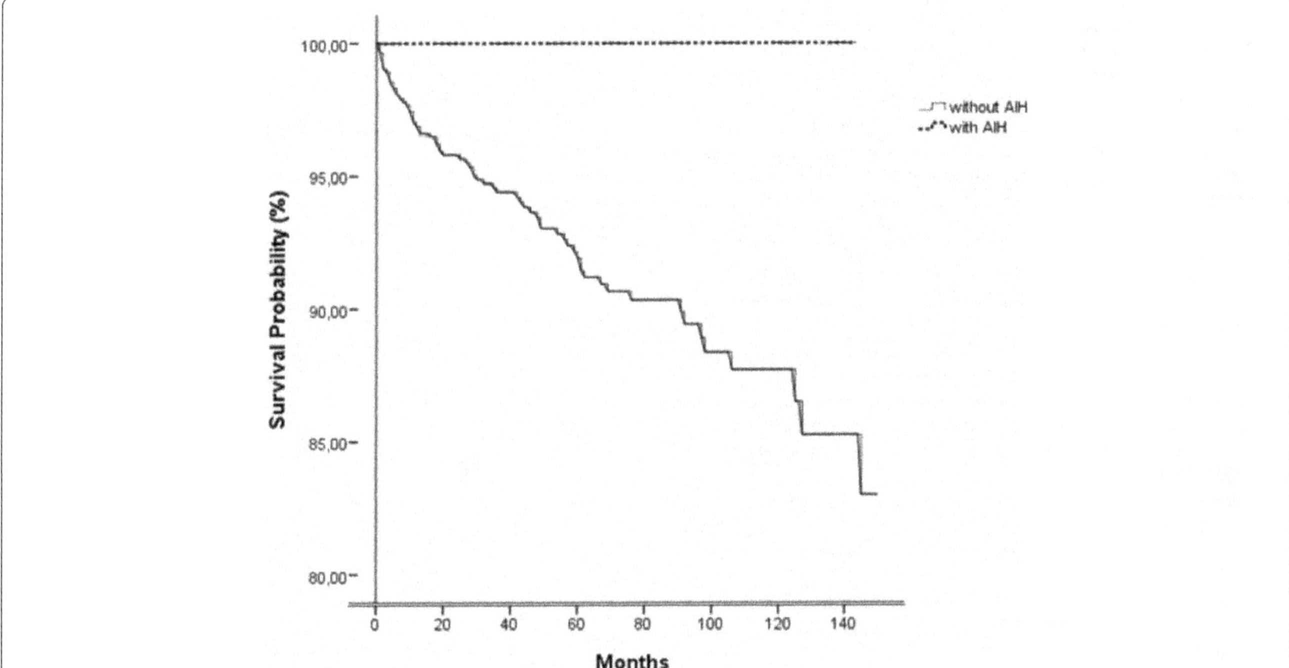

Fig. 1 Kaplan-Meier overall survival curve in childhood-onset systematic lupus erythematosus patients with autoimmune hepatitis (AIH) compared to those without this complication

complete response to the classical AIH prednisone and azathioprine combination therapy. Reinforcing this finding none of our patients had hepatic failure, portal hypertension and cirrhosis suggesting that AIH phenotype in lupus was a non-severe pattern [1, 3]. Additionally, none of our cSLE patients had anti-LKM1 antibodies.

Conclusion

Overlap AIH and cSLE was rarely observed in this large multicenter study and hepatomegaly was the distinctive clinical feature of these patients. AIH occurred during adolescence, mainly at the first years of lupus and it was associated with mild liver manifestations.

Acknowledgements

Our gratitude to Ulysses Doria-Filho for the statistical analysis. The authors thank the following Pediatric Rheumatology Divisions and colleagues for including their patients: Pediatric Rheumatology Unit, Children's Institute, FMUSP (Adriana Maluf Elias Sallum, Cristina Miuki Abe Jacob, Gabriela Blay, Gabriela Nunes Leal, Heloisa Helena de Souza Marques, João Domingos Montoni da Silva, Joaquim Carlos Rodrigues, Juliana Caíres de Oliveira Achili Ferreira, Kátia Kozu, Laila Pinto Coelho, Luciana dos Santos Henriques, Magda Carneiro-Sampaio, Maria Helena Vaisbich, Roberta Cunha Gomes, Victor Leonardo Saraiva Marques, Werther Brunow de Carvalho); Pediatric Rheumatology Unit, UNIFESP (Anandreia Simões Lopes, Claudio Len, Daniela Petry Piotto, Giampaolo Faquin, Gleice Clemente, Maria Odete Esteves Hilário, Melissa Fraga, Octavio Augusto Bedin Peracchi, Vanessa Bugni); Division of Rheumatology, FMUSP (Juliane A Paupitz, Glauce L Lima); UNESP (Priscila R. Aoki, Juliana de Oliveira Sato, Silvana Paula Cardin, Taciana Albuquerque Pedrosa Fernandes), Irmandade da Santa Casa de Misericórdia de São Paulo (Andressa Guariento, Eunice Mitiko Okuda, Silvana Brasília Sacchetti), State University of Campinas (Simone Appenzeller, Renata Barbosa, Roberto Marini), Ribeirão Preto Medical School – University of São Paulo (Francisco Hugo Gomes, Gecilmara Salviatto Pileggi, Luciana Martins de Carvalho, Paola Pontes Pinheiro), Hospital Infantil Darcy Vargas (Cássia Maria Passarelli Lupoli Barbosa, Luciana Tudech Pedro Paulo), Pontifical Catholic University of Sorocaba (Valeria Cristina Santucci Ramos); Hospital Municipal Infantil Menino Jesus (Simone Lotufo and Tânia Caroline Monteiro Castro).

Authors' contributions

VAB, BM, ACP, ARS, LPC, JCOF, RMRP, MTT, CSM, NEA, APS, KK, LMC, AMS, VPF, DPP, EB and CAS analyzed and interpreted the patient data regarding autoimmune hepatitis in childhood onset systemic lupus erythematosus. VAB, BM, ACP, EB and CAS were the major contributor in writing the manuscript. All authors read and approved the final manuscript.

Author details

[1]Pediatric Rheumatology Unit, Children's Institute, Hospital das Clinicas HCFMUSP, Faculdade de Medicina, Universidade de Sao Paulo, Sao Paulo, SP, Brazil. [2]Division of Rheumatology, Hospital das Clinicas HCFMUSP, Faculdade de Medicina, Universidade de Sao Paulo, Sao Paulo, SP, Brazil. [3]Pediatric Rheumatology Unit, Universidade Federal de São Paulo, São Paulo, Brazil. [4]Pediatric Rheumatology Unit, São Paulo State University (UNESP) – Faculdade de Medicina de Botucatu, São Paulo, Brazil. [5]Pediatric Rheumatology Unit, Ribeirão Preto Medical School, University of São Paulo, São Paulo, Brazil.

References

1. Deen ME, Porta G, Fiorot FJ, Campos LM, Sallum AM, Silva CA. Autoimmune hepatitis and juvenile systemic lupus erythematosus. Lupus. 2009;18:747–51.
2. Aikawa NE, Jesus AA, Liphaus BL, Silva CA, Carneiro-Sampaio M, Viana VS, et al. Organ-specific autoantibodies and autoimmune diseases in juvenile systemic lupus erythematosus and juvenile dermatomyositis patients. Clin Exp Rheumatol. 2012;30:126–31.
3. Sönmez HE, Karhan AN, Batu ED, Bilginer Y, Gümüş E, Demir H, et al. Gastrointestinal system manifestations in juvenile systemic lupus erythematosus. Clin Rheumatol. 2017;36:1521–6.
4. Alvarez F, Berg PA, Bianchi FB, Bianchi L, Burroughs AK, Cancado EL, et al. International autoimmune hepatitis group report: review of criteria for diagnosis of autoimmune hepatitis. J Hepatol. 1999;31:929–38.

5. European Association for the Study of the Liver. EASL clinical practice guidelines: autoimmune hepatitis. J Hepatol. 2015;63:971–1004.
6. Battagliotti C, Rispolo Klubek D, Karakachoff M, Costaguta A. An overlap syndrome involving lupus erythematosus and autoimmune hepatitis in an adolescent girl. Arch Argent Pediatr. 2016;114:155–8.
7. Alves SC, Fasano S, Isenberg DA. Autoimmune gastrointestinal complications in patients with systemic lupus erythematosus: case series and literature review. Lupus. 2016;25:1509–19.
8. Lopes SRM, Gormezano NWS, Gomes RC, Aikawa NE, Pereira RMR, Terreri MT, et al. Outcomes of 847 childhood-onset systemic lupus erythematosus patients in three age groups. Lupus. 2017;26:996–1001.
9. American College of Rheumatology. 1997 update of the 1982 American College of Rheumatology revised criteria for classification of systemic lupus erythematosus. Arthritis Rheum. 1997;40:1725.
10. Gladman DD, Ibañez D, Urowitz MB. Systemic lupus erythematosus disease activity index 2000. J Rheumatol. 2002;29:288–91.
11. American College of Rheumatology Ad Hoc committee on neuropsychiatric Lupus Syndromes. The American College of Rheumatology nomenclature and case definitions for neuropsychiatric lupus syndromes. Arthritis Rheum. 1999;42:599–8.
12. Irving KS, Sen D, Tahir H, Pilkington C, Isenberg DA. A comparison of autoimmune liver disease in juvenile and adult populations with systemic lupus erythematosus-a retrospective review of cases. Rheumatology. 2007;46:1171–3.
13. Silva CA. Childhood-onset systemic lupus erythematosus: early disease manifestations that the paediatrician must know. Expert Rev Clin Immunol. 2016;12:907–10.
14. Guariento A, Silva MF, Tassetano PS, Rocha SM, Campos LM, Valente M, et al. Liver and spleen biometrics in childhood-onset systemic lupus erythematosus patients. Rev Bras Reumatol. 2015;55:346–51.
15. Lim DH, Kim YG, Lee D, Min Ahn S, Hong S, Lee CK, et al. Immunoglobolin G levels as a prognostic factor for autoimmune hepatitis combined with systemic lupus erythematosus. Arthritis Care & Res (Hoboken). 2016;68:995–1002.
16. Teufel A, Weinmann A, Kahaly GJ, Centner C, Piendl A, Wörns M, et al. Concurrent autoimmune diseases in patients with autoimmune hepatitis. J Clin Gastroenterol. 2010;44:208–13.
17. Gomes RC, Silva MF, Kozu K, Bonfá E, Pereira RM, Terreri MT, et al. Features of 847 Childhood-Onset Systemic Lupus Erythematosus Patients in Three Age Groups at Diagnosis: A Brazilian Multicenter Study. Arthritis Care Res (Hoboken). 2016;68:1736–41.

Diffuse alveolar hemorrhage in childhood-onset systemic lupus erythematosus: A severe disease flare with serious outcome

Gabriela Blay[1,2], Joaquim C. Rodrigues[2], Juliana C. O. Ferreira[1], Gabriela N. Leal[1], Natali W. Gormezano[3], Glaucia V. Novak[1], Rosa M. R. Pereira[3], Maria T. Terreri[4], Claudia S. Magalhães[5], Beatriz C. Molinari[1], Ana P. Sakamoto[4], Nadia E. Aikawa[1,3], Lucia M. A. Campos[1], Taciana A. P. Fernandes[5], Gleice Clemente[4], Octavio A. B. Peracchi[4], Vanessa Bugni[4], Roberto Marini[6], Silvana B. Sacchetti[7], Luciana M. Carvalho[8], Melissa M. Fraga[9], Tânia C. M. Castro[10], Valéria C. Ramos[11], Eloisa Bonfá[1], Clovis A. Silva[1,2*] and Brazilian Childhood-onset Systemic Lupus Erythematosus Group

Abstract

Objective: To evaluate prevalence, clinical manifestations, laboratory abnormalities and treatment in a multicenter cohort study including 847 childhood-onset systemic lupus erythematosus (cSLE) patients with and without diffuse alveolar hemorrhage (DAH), as well as concomitant parameters of severity.

Methods: DAH was defined as the presence of at least three respiratory symptoms/signs associated with diffuse interstitial/alveolar infiltrates on chest x-ray or high-resolution computer tomography and sudden drop in hemoglobin levels. Statistical analysis was performed using Bonferroni correction ($p < 0.0022$).

Results: DAH was observed in 19/847 (2.2%) cSLE patients. Cough/dyspnea/tachycardia/hypoxemia occurred in all cSLE patients with DAH. Concomitant parameters of severity observed were: mechanical ventilation in 14/19 (74%), hemoptysis 12/19 (63%), macrophage activation syndrome 2/19 (10%) and death 9/19 (47%). Further analysis of cSLE patients at DAH diagnosis compared to 76 cSLE control patients without DAH with same disease duration [3 (1–151) vs. 4 (1–151) months, $p = 0.335$], showed higher frequencies of constitutional involvement (74% vs. 10%, $p < 0.0001$), serositis (63% vs. 6%, $p < 0.0001$) and sepsis (53% vs. 9%, $p < 0.0001$) in the DAH group. The median of disease activity score(SLEDAI-2 K) was significantly higher in cSLE patients with DAH [18 (5–40) vs. 6 (0–44), $p < 0.0001$]. The frequencies of thrombocytopenia (53% vs. 12%, $p < 0.0001$), intravenous methylprednisolone (95% vs. 16%, $p < 0.0001$) and intravenous cyclophosphamide (47% vs. 8%, $p < 0.0001$) were also significantly higher in DAH patients.

Conclusions: This was the first study to demonstrate that DAH, although not a disease activity score descriptor, occurred in the context of significant moderate/severe cSLE flare. Importantly, we identified that this condition was associated with serious disease flare complicated by sepsis with high mortality rate.

Keywords: Diffuse alveolar hemorrhage, Childhood, Systemic lupus erythematosus, Multicenter study

* Correspondence: clovisaasilva@gmail.com
[1]Pediatric Rheumatology Unit, Children's Institute, Faculdade de Medicina da Universidade de São Paulo (FMUSP), Av. Dr. Eneas Carvalho Aguiar, 647 - Cerqueira César, São Paulo, SP 05403-000, Brazil
[2]Pediatric Pulmonology Unit, Children's Institute, FMUSP, Av. Dr. Eneas Carvalho Aguiar, 647 - Cerqueira César, São Paulo, SP 05403-000, Brazil
Full list of author information is available at the end of the article

Introduction

Systemic lupus erythematosus (SLE) is a multisystemic autoimmune disease characterized by the involvement of several organs and systems [1–3]. Pleuropulmonary manifestations were described as initial feature from 17 to 42% childhood-onset SLE (cSLE) patients, particularly mild to moderate pleuritis [1, 3–5]. These respiratory complications may be classified as acute or chronic [6].

Of note, diffuse alveolar hemorrhage (DAH) is an acute, rare and life-threatening pulmonary manifestation characterized by sudden onset of respiratory symptoms, such as dyspnea; hypoxemia; hemoptysis; tachycardia and/or cough; associated with new lung infiltrates on chest x-ray (CXR) or high-resolution computer tomography (HRCT); and sudden drop in serum hemoglobin levels [7, 8].

Data of DAH in cSLE patients are limited due to the small representation of this complication in previous case series or the focus on the comparison to adult SLE, precluding an accurate analysis of associated factors and outcomes in patients with and without this severe complication [4, 7–15].

Therefore, the objective of the present multicenter cohort study was to assess the prevalence and the possible DAH association with demographic, clinical manifestations, laboratory abnormalities, disease activity score, treatments and outcomes in a large cSLE population.

Methods

This was a retrospective multicenter cohort study including 1017 patients followed in 10 Pediatric Rheumatology tertiary referral services in São Paulo state, Brazil. One hundred and sixty five patients were excluded due to: incomplete medical charts ($n = 96$), undifferentiated connective tissue disorder with 3 or fewer American College of Rheumatology (ACR) criteria ($n = 43$), isolated cutaneous lupus erythematosus ($n = 11$), neonatal lupus erythematosus ($n = 8$), drug-induced lupus ($n = 5$) and mixed connective tissue disease ($n = 2$). Therefore, this study group comprised 852 cSLE patients. All of them fulfilled the ACR criteria for SLE [16], with disease onset before the age of 18 [17].

An investigator meeting was held for protocol training according to the clinical parameters definitions and disease activity tool scoring, as previously reported [3, 18]. Patient's medical charts were systematically reviewed according to demographic data, clinical characteristics, DAH features, laboratorial abnormalities, therapies and outcomes.

DAH was defined as the presence of at least three respiratory symptoms and signs (dyspnea, hypoxemia, hemoptysis, tachycardia and/or cough) associated with diffuse interstitial and/or alveolar infiltrates on CXR or HRCT, and sudden drop in hemoglobin level at least of 1.5 g/dL [7, 10, 11]. Bronchoalveolar lavage with hemosiderin-laden macrophages evidence was also recorded [14]. Patients were divided in two groups with similar disease duration: cSLE patients with DAH (assessed at DAH diagnosis) and cSLE patients without DAH (assessed at last visit).

Descriptors and definitions of SLE Disease Activity Index 2000 (SLEDAI-2 K) score were used to characterize disease parameters and to calculate disease activity score [19]. Custom definitions were defined as previously reported [3, 18]. Neuropsychiatric lupus included 19 syndromes according to ACR classification criteria [20]. Antiphospholipid syndrome was diagnosed taking into account the presence of arterial and/or venous thrombosis concomitant to high titers of antiphospholipid antibodies [21]. Macrophage activation syndrome was diagnosed considering the preliminary cSLE diagnostic guidelines, requiring the presence of at least one clinical plus two laboratorial criteria [22].

Laboratorial assessment included complete blood cell count and urine test. Anti-double-stranded DNA (anti-dsDNA), IgG and IgM anticardiolipin antibodies (aCL) were carried out at each center and the cutoff values were considered valid. Lupus anticoagulant was detected according to the guidelines of the International Society on Thrombosis and Hemostasis [23].

Drug treatment data (prednisone, intravenous methylprednisolone, chloroquine diphosphate, hydroxychloroquine sulfate, methotrexate, azathioprine, cyclosporine, mycophenolate mofetil, intravenous cyclophosphamide and intravenous gammaglobulin) were also recorded.

Statistical analysis

Results were presented as an absolute number (frequency) for categorical variables and median (range) or mean ± standard deviation (SD) for continuous variables. Categorical variables comparisons were assessed by Pearson χ-Square or Fisher's exact test. Continuous variables from cSLE patients with and without DAH were compared by Mann-Whitney test or t test as appropriate. Statistical analysis was performed using Bonferroni correction ($p < 0.0022$).

Results

DAH was observed in 19/847 (2.2%) cSLE patients. Cough, dyspnea, tachycardia and hypoxemia occurred in all 19 cSLE patients with DAH; hemoptysis in 12/19 and endotracheal tube bleeding in 14/19. New infiltrates on CXR or HRCT and hemoglobin drop at least of 1.5 g/dL were evidenced in all cSLE patients with DAH (Table 1). Bronchoalveolar lavage was performed in two cSLE patients and hemosiderin-laden macrophage was observed in both of them.

Table 1 Demographic, clinical manifestations and imaging in 19 childhood-onset systemic lupus erythematosus (cSLE) patients with diffuse alveolar hemorrhage

Patient	Disease duration, Months	Cough	Dyspnoea	Tachycardia	Hypoxemia	Hemoptysis/bleeding in endotracheal tube	New Infiltrates CXR or HRCT	Drop Hbg/dL
1	60	+	+	+	+	+ / +	+	1.8
2	151	+	+	+	+	+ / +	+	1.5
3	5	+	+	+	+	+ / +	+	2.0
4	0	+	+	+	+	+ / +	+	1.6
5	33	+	+	+	+	+ / +	+	1.9
6	0	+	+	+	+	+ / +	+	2.7
7	3	+	+	+	+	+ / +	+	1.7
8	90	+	+	+	+	+ / -	+	2.5
9	42	+	+	+	+	+ / +	+	4.5
10	4	+	+	+	+	+ / +	+	3.0
11	0	+	+	+	+	- / -	+	3.2
12	47	+	+	+	+	- / +	+	1.5
13	5	+	+	+	+	- / +	+	1.5
14	0	+	+	+	+	+ / -	+	2.0
15	0	+	+	+	+	- / +	+	7.0
16	0	+	+	+	+	- / -	+	2.0
17	3	+	+	+	+	- / +	+	2.0
18	1	+	+	+	+	- / -	+	1.7
19	0	+	+	+	+	+ / +	+	8.0

CXR Chest x-ray, *HRCT* High resolution computer tomography, *Hb* Hemoglobulin, *ND* Not done

Regarding outcomes, hospitalization in pediatric intensive care unit occurred in 17/19 cSLE patients with DAH and mechanical ventilation in 14/19. DAH associated with sepsis was observed in 10/19 cSLE patients. Concomitant macrophage activation syndrome was evidenced in 2/19 patients. Death was observed in 9/19 cSLE patients. The median duration between DAH onset and death was 2 days (0.5–25). Blood erythrocyte transfusion and broad-spectrum antibiotics were administered in all cSLE patients with DAH. Intravenous methylprednisolone pulse therapy was used in 18/19 cSLE and intravenous cyclophosphamide in 9/19 (Table 2). None of them had recurrence of DAH.

Further comparison between cSLE patients with DAH compared to 76 cSLE control patients without DAH with same disease duration [3 (1–151) vs. 4 (1–151) months, $p = 0.335$], showed significantly higher frequencies of constitutional involvement (74% vs. 10%, $p < 0.0001$), serositis (63% vs. 6%, $p < 0.0001$) and sepsis (53% vs. 9%, $p < 0.0001$) in the former group. The median of SLEDAI-2 K was significantly higher in cSLE patients with DAH compared to cSLE patients without this complication [18 (5–40) vs. 6 (0–44), $p < 0.0001$]. Frequencies of nephritis and neuropsychiatric involvements were similar in both groups ($p > 0.0022$) (Table 3).

The frequencies of thrombocytopenia (53% vs. 12%, $p < 0.0001$), intravenous methylprednisolone (95% vs. 16%, $p < 0.0001$) and intravenous cyclophosphamide (47% vs. 8%, $p < 0.0001$) were also significantly higher in the former group. The median of prednisone dose was higher in cSLE patients with DAH compared to those without DAH [1.4 (0.3–2) vs. 0.5 (0.03–3) mg/Kg, $p < 0.0001$] (Table 4).

Discussion

This is the largest study to evaluate DAH, a rare and acute life-threatening pulmonary manifestation, in cSLE population.

The multicenter study design with a large cohort of children and adolescents patients allowed a more precise assessment of this rare and severe cSLE respiratory complication. An investigator meeting was also taken in place to standardize the protocol study in all centers. However, the limitation was the retrospective design with potential missing data.

The prevalence of DAH in cSLE patients in the present study was similar to other reports, varying from 2 to 5% [6, 7, 24]. Diagnosis of this condition included the typical respiratory symptoms and signs, drop in hemoglobin levels and the radiographic evidence of pulmonary infiltrates, as well as the assessment of

Table 2 Outcomes and immunosuppressive treatment in 19 childhood-onset systemic lupus erythematosus (cSLE) patients with diffuse alveolar hemorrhage

Patient	ICU	Mechanical ventilation	Sepsis	MAS	Death	IV methylprednisolone pulse therapy	IV cyclophosphamide
1	+	+	+	–	+	+	–
2	+	+	+	–	–	+	+
3	+	+	+	–	+	+	–
4	+	+	+	–	–	+	+
5	+	+	–	–	+	+	–
6	+	+	–	–	–	+	+
7	+	+	+	–	+	+	+
8	+	–	+	–	+	+	+
9	+	+	–	–	+	+	–
10	+	+	–	–	–	+	+
11	+	–	–	–	–	+	–
12	+	+	–	+	+	+	–
13	+	+	–	–	+	–	–
14	+	–	+	–	–	+	+
15	+	+	+	+	–	+	+
16	–	–	+	–	–	+	–
17	+	+	+	–	–	+	+
18	–	–	–	–	–	+	–
19	+	+	–	–	+	+	–

ICU Intensive care unit, *MAS* Macrophage activation syndrome, *IV* Intravenous

Table 3 Demographic data, clinical manifestations and disease activity score in childhood-onset systemic lupus erythematosus (cSLE) patients according to the presence of diffuse alveolar hemorrhage (DAH)

Variables	With DAH (at diagnosis) ($n = 19$)	Without DAH (at last visit) ($n = 76$)	*P*
Demographic data			
Female gender	14 (74)	66 (87)	0.172
Disease duration, months	3 (1–151)	4 (1–151)	0.335
Current age, years	13 (9–18)	13 (3–23)	0.889
Current clinical manifestations			
Constitutional	14 (74)	8 (10)	< 0.0001*
Mucocutaneous	9 (47)	31 (41)	0.614
Musculoskeletal	5 (26)	8 (10)	0.127
Serositis	12 (63)	5 (6)	< 0.0001*
Neuropsychiatric	4 (21)	11 (14)	0.491
Nephritis	16 (84)	42 (55)	0.033
Current autoimmune thrombosis (APS), $n = 90$	0/16 (0)	1/74 (1)	1.000
Sepsis	10 (53)	7 (9)	< 0.0001*
Macrophage activation syndrome	2 (10)	2 (3)	0.113
Death, $n = 94$	9 (47)	15/75 (20)	0.020
Current disease activity			
SLEDAI-2 K, $n = 82$	18 (5–40)	6 (0–44)	< 0.0001*

**P*-value according to Bonferroni correction for multiple comparisons ($p < 0.0022$). Results are presented in *n* (%) and median (range), *APS* Antiphospholipid syndrome, *SLEDAI-2 K* Systemic Lupus Erythematosus Disease Activity Index 2000

Table 4 Current laboratory tests and drug therapy of childhood-onset systemic lupus erythematosus (cSLE) according to the presence of diffuse alveolar hemorrhage (DAH)

Variables	With DAH (at diagnosis) (*n* = 19)	Without DAH (at last visit) (*n* = 76)	*P*
Current laboratory exams			
Autoimmune hemolytic anemia	5 (26)	8 (10)	0.127
Thrombocytopenia, < 150,000/mm^3, *n* = 93	10 (52)	9/74 (12)	< 0.0001*
Anti-ds-DNA, *n* = 75	8/13 (61)	30/62 (48)	0.544
Drug therapy			
Prednisone current dose, mg/Kg, *n* = 82	1.4 (0.3–2)	0.5 (0.03–3)	< 0.0001*
Intravenous methylprednisolone	18 (95)	12 (15)	< 0.0001*
Antimalarial drugs	14 (74)	41 (54)	0.193
Azathioprine	2 (10)	16 (21)	0.513
Mycophenolate mofetil	1 (5)	5 (6)	1.000
Intravenous cyclophosphamide	9 (47)	6 (8)	< 0.0001*

**P*-value according to Bonferroni correction for multiple comparisons ($p < 0.0022$). Results are presented in n (%) and median (range), anti-ds-DNA – anti-double-stranded DNA antibodies

hypoxemia due to acute respiratory distress [7]. In addition, in two of our cSLE patients the presence of haemosiderin-laden macrophages in the absence of bloody fluid suggested recent bleeding [6], analyzed by the bronchoalveolar lavage.

We demonstrated that DAH, although not a disease activity score descriptor of SLEDAI-2 K [19], was associated with high moderate or severe disease activity scores, particularly thrombocytopenia, serositis and constitutional involvement. In contrast to previous reports DAH was not associated with lupus nephritis [13].

Of note, we identified that DAH was a severe manifestation requiring pediatric intensive care unit hospitalization and mechanical ventilation for the vast majority of our patients. We extended previous observation of high frequency of severe infection in adults/cSLE patients with DAH [7], thus demonstrating the catastrophic nature of DAH, since more than half of cSLE patients developed concomitant sepsis.

Reinforcing this finding of poor outcome, 10% of the cSLE patients were diagnosed with concomitant macrophage activation syndrome. In fact, this is a rare condition characterized by an excessive activation and proliferation of T lymphocytes and macrophages with massive hypersecretion of proinflammatory cytokines, and may induce severe hemorraghae [25, 26].

We observed a high mortality rate in cSLE patients with DAH, as also observed in other studies [6, 10, 11]. This unfavorable outcome revealed that sepsis and macrophage activation syndrome may have contributed to the death of more than half of the patients.

Early detection of this severe pulmonary complication, prompt immunosuppressive agents treatment [9, 15, 27], empirical antibiotics and mechanical ventilation are therefore essential to improve cSLE outcome [6, 7].

Conclusion

This was the first study to demonstrate that DAH, although not a disease activity score descriptor, occurs in the context of significant moderate/severe cSLE flare. Importantly, we identified that this condition is associated with serious disease flare complicated by sepsis and high mortality rate.

Acknowledgements
Our gratitude to Ulysses Doria-Filho for the statistical analysis. The authors thank the following Pediatric Rheumatology Divisions and colleagues for including their patients: Children's Institute, FMUSP (Marco F. Silva, Mariana Ferriani, Roberta C. Gomes, Victor L. Marques, Gabriella E. Lube, Sandra R. M. Lopes, Glaucia V. Novak, Beatriz C. Molinari, Clarissa C. Valões, Verena Balbi, João D. Montoni, Laila P. Coelho, Luciana S. Henriques, Pedro Anuardo, Monica Verdier, Juliana B. Brunelli, Adriana A. Jesus, Antonio C. Pastorino, Heloisa H. Marques, Andrea Watanabe, Benita G. Schvartsman, Maria H. Vaisbich, Werther B. Carvalho, Magda Carneiro-Sampaio, Vicente Odone-Filho); Division of Rheumatology, FMUSP (Juliane A. Paupitz, Glauce L. Lima, Ana Paula L. Assad); UNIFESP (Maria O. E. Hilário, Andreia S. Lopes, Aline Alencar, Daniela P. Piotto, Giampaolo Faquin); UNESP (Priscila R. Aoki, Juliana O. Sato, Silvana P. Cardin); Irmandade da Santa Casa de Misericórdia de São Paulo (Andressa Guariento, Eunice Okuda, Maria Carolina dos Santos); UNICAMP (Maraísa Centeville, Renata Barbosa, Simone Appenzeller); Ribeirão Preto Medical School, FMUSP (Paola P. Kahwage, Gecilmara Pileggi, Francisco Hugo Gomes, Virginia Ferriani), Hospital Infantil Darcy Vargas (Jonatas Libório, Cássia Barbosa, Luciana T. P. Paulo); Hospital Municipal Infantil Menino Jesus (Simone Lotufo).

Authors' contributions
All authors analyzed and interpreted the patient data regarding autoimmune hepatitis in childhood onset systemic lupus erythematosus. GB, EB and CAS were the major contributor in writing the manuscript. All authors read and approved the final manuscript.

Author details
[1]Pediatric Rheumatology Unit, Children's Institute, Faculdade de Medicina da Universidade de São Paulo (FMUSP), Av. Dr. Eneas Carvalho Aguiar, 647 - Cerqueira César, São Paulo, SP 05403-000, Brazil. [2]Pediatric Pulmonology Unit,

Children's Institute, FMUSP, Av. Dr. Eneas Carvalho Aguiar, 647 - Cerqueira César, São Paulo, SP 05403-000, Brazil. [3]Division of Rheumatology, FMUSP, Sao Paulo, Brazil. [4]Pediatric Rheumatology Unit, Universidade Federal de São Paulo, Sao Paulo, Brazil. [5]São Paulo State University (UNESP), Faculdade de Medicina de Botucatu, Sao Paulo, Brazil. [6]São Paulo State University of Campinas (UNICAMP), Sao Paulo, Brazil. [7]Irmandade da Santa Casa de Misericórdia de São Paulo, Sao Paulo, Brazil. [8]Ribeirão Preto Medical School – University of São Paulo, Sao Paulo, Brazil. [9]Hospital Darcy Vargas, Sao Paulo, Brazil. [10]Hospital Menino Jesus, Sao Paulo, Brazil. [11]Pontifical Catholic University of Sorocaba, Sao Paulo, Brazil.

References

1. Silva CA. Childhood-onset systemic lupus erythematosus: early disease manifestations that the paediatrician must know. Expert Rev Clin Immunol. 2016;12:907–10.
2. Silva CA, Aikawa NE, Pereira RM, Campos LM. Management considerations for childhood-onset systemic lupus erythematosus patients and implications on therapy. Expert Rev Clin Immunol. 2016;12:301–13.
3. Gomes RC, Silva MF, Kozu K, Bonfá E, Pereira RM, Terreri MT, et al. Features of 847 childhood-onset systemic lupus Erythematousus patients in three age groups at diagnosis: a Brazilian multicenter study. Arthritis Care Res (Hoboken). 2016;68:1736–41.
4. Veiga CS, Coutinho DS, Nakaie CM, Campos LM, Suzuki L, Cunha MT, et al. Subclinical pulmonary abnormalities in childhood-onset systemic lupus erythematosus patients. Lupus. 2016;25:645–51.
5. Bader-Meunier B, Armengaud JB, Haddad E, Salomon R, Deschênes G, Koné-Paut I, et al. Initial presentation of childhood-onset systemic lupus erythematosus: a French multicenter study. J Pediatr. 2005;146:648–53.
6. Richardson AE, Warrier K, Vyas H. Respiratory complications of the rheumatological diseases in childhood. Arch Dis Child. 2016;101:752–8.
7. Araujo DB, Borba EF, Silva CA, Campos LM, Pereira RM, Bonfa E, et al. Alveolar hemorrhage: distinct features of juvenile and adult onset systemic lupus erythematosus. Lupus. 2012;21:872–7.
8. Singla S, Canter DL, Vece TJ, Muscal E, DeGuzman M. Diffuse Alveolar Hemorrhage as a Manifestation of Childhood-Onset Systemic Lupus Erythematosus. Hosp Pediatr. 2016;6:496–500.
9. Godfrey S. Pulmonary hemorrhage/hemoptysis in children. Pediatr Pulmonol. 2004;37:476–84.
10. Liu MF, Lee JH, Weng TH, Lee YY. Clinical experience of 13 cases with severe pulmonary hemorrhage in systemic lupus erythematosus with active nephritis. Scand J Rheumatol. 1998;27:291–5.
11. Chang MY, Fang JT, Chen YC, Huang CC. Diffuse alveolar hemorrhage in systemic lupus erythematosus: a single center retrospective study in Taiwan. Ren Fail. 2002;24:791–802.
12. Koh WH, Thumboo J, Boey ML. Pulmonary haemorrhage in oriental patients with systemic lupus erythematosus. Lupus. 1997;6:713–6.
13. Shen M, Zeng X, Tian X, Zhang F, Zeng X, Zhang X, et al. Diffuse alveolar hemorrhage in systemic lupus erythematosus: a retrospective study in China. Lupus. 2010;19:1326–30.
14. Martinez-Martinez MU, Sturbaum AK, Alcocer-Varela J, Merayo-Chalico J, Gómez-Martin D, Gómez-Bañuelos Jde J, et al. Factors associated with mortality and infections in patients with systemic lupus erythematosus with diffuse alveolar hemorrhage. J Rheumatol. 2014;41:1656–61.
15. Kimura D, Shah S, Briceno-Medina M, Sathanandam S, Haberman B, Zhang J, et al. Management of massive diffuse alveolar hemorrhage in a child with systemic lupus erythematosus. J Intensive Care. 2015;7(3):10.
16. Hochberg MC. Updating the American College of Rheumatology revised criteria for the classification of systemic lupus erhytematosus. Arthrits Rheum. 1997;40:1725.
17. Silva CA, Avcin T, Brunner HI. Taxonomy for systemic lupus erythematosus with onset before adulthood. Arthritis Care Res (Hoboken). 2012;64:1787–93.
18. Marques VL, Gormezano NW, Bonfá E, Aikawa NE, Terreri MT, Pereira RM, et al. Pancreatitis subtypes survey in 852 childhood-onset systemic lupus erythematosus patients. J Pediatr Gastroenterol Nutr. 2016;62:328–34.
19. Gladman DD, Ibañez D, Urowitz MB. Systemic lupus erythematosus disease activity index 2000. J Rheumatol. 2002;29:288–91.
20. American College of Rheumatology Ad Hoc committee on neuropsychiatric Lupus Syndromes. The American College of Rheumatology nomenclature and case definitions for neuropsychiatric lupus syndromes. Arthritis Rheum. 1999;42:599 608.
21. Avcin T, Cimaz R, Rozman B. The Ped-APS Registry: the antiphospholipid syndrome in childhood. Lupus. 2009;18:894–9.
22. Parodi A, Davì S, Pringe AB, Pistorio A, Ruperto N, Magni-Manzoni S, et al. Lupus Working Group of the Paediatric Rheumatology European Society. A macrophage activation syndrome in juvenile systemic lupus erythematosus: a multinational multicenter study of thirty-eight patients. Arthritis Rheum. 2009;60:3388–99.
23. Brandt JT, Triplett DA, Alving B, Scharrer I. Criteria for the diagnosis of lupus anticoagulants: an update. On behalf of the subcommittee on lupus anticoagulant/antiphospholipid antibody of the scientific and standardisation committee of the ISTH. Thromb Haemost. 1995;74:1185–90.
24. Fatemi A, Matinfar M, Saber M, Smiley A. The association between initial manifestations of childhood-onset systemic lupus erythematosus and the survival. Int J Rheum Dis. 2016;19:974–80. in press.
25. Gormezano NW, Otsuzi CI, Barros DL, da Silva MA, Pereira RM, Campos LM, et al. Macrophage activation syndrome: A severe and frequent manifestation of acute pancreatitis in 362 childhood-onset compared to 1830 adult-onset systemic lupus erythematosus patients. Semin Arthritis Rheum. 2016;45:706–10.
26. Aikawa NE, Carvalho JF, Bonfá E, Lotito AP, Silva CA. Macrophage activation syndrome associated with etanercept in a child with systemic onset juvenile idiopathic arthritis. Isr Med Assoc J. 2009;11:635–6.
27. Klumb EM, Silva CA, Lanna CC, Sato EI, Borba EF, Brenol JC, et al. Consensus of the Brazilian Society of Rheumatology for the diagnosis, management and treatment of lupus nephritis. Rev Bras Reumatol. 2015;55:1–21.

15

Panniculitis in childhood-onset systemic lupus erythematosus

Mônica Verdier[1], Pedro Anuardo[1], Natali Weniger Spelling Gormezano[1,2], Ricardo Romiti[3], Lucia Maria Arruda Campos[1], Nadia Emi Aikawa[2], Rosa Maria Rodrigues Pereira[2], Maria Teresa Terreri[4], Claudia Saad Magalhães[5], Juliana C. O. A. Ferreira[1], Marco Felipe Castro Silva[1], Mariana Ferriani[1], Ana Paula Sakamoto[4], Virginia Paes Leme Ferriani[6], Maraísa Centeville[7], Juliana Sato[5], Maria Carolina Santos[8], Eloisa Bonfá[2†] and Clovis Artur Silva[1,2*†]

Abstract

Objective: To evaluate prevalence, clinical manifestations, laboratory abnormalities, treatment and outcome in a multicenter cohort of childhood-onset systemic lupus erythematosus (cSLE) patients with and without panniculitis.

Methods: Panniculitis was diagnosed due to painful subcutaneous nodules and/or plaques in deep dermis/subcutaneous tissues and lobular/mixed panniculitis with lymphocytic lobular inflammatory infiltrate in skin biopsy. Statistical analysis was performed using Bonferroni correction($p < 0.004$).

Results: Panniculitis was observed in 6/847(0.7%) cSLE. Painful subcutaneous erythematosus and indurated nodules were observed in 6/6 panniculitis patients and painful subcutaneous plaques in 4/6. Generalized distribution was evidenced in 3/6 and localized in upper limbs in 2/6 and face in 1/6. Cutaneous hyperpigmentation and/or cutaneous atrophy occurred in 5/6. Histopathology features showed lobular panniculitis without vasculitis in 5/6(one of them had concomitant obliterative vasculopathy due to antiphospholipid syndrome) and panniculitis with vasculitis in 1/6. Comparison between cSLE with panniculitis and 60 cSLE without panniculitis with same disease duration [2.75(0–11.4) vs. 2.83(0–11.8) years,$p = 0.297$], showed higher frequencies of constitutional involvement (67% vs. 10%,$p = 0.003$) and leukopenia (67% vs. 7%,$p = 0.002$). Cutaneous atrophy and hyperpigmentation occurred in 83% of patients.

Conclusions: Panniculitis is a rare skin manifestation of cSLE occurring in the first three years of disease with considerable sequelae. The majority of patients have concomitant mild lupus manifestations.

Keywords: Lupus erythematosus panniculits, Childhood, Systemic lupus erythematosus and multicenter study

Introduction

Systemic lupus erythematosus (SLE) is an autoimmune disease that affects multiple organs and systems. Mucocutaneous involvement was described as initial manifestation in up to 81% childhood-onset SLE (cSLE) patients and in up to 100% of them during the disease course [1–3]. Chronic cutaneous lupus erythematosus was reported as first manifestation in up to 4% cSLE patients and in up to 10% during the course of disease [1, 3].

Lupus erythematosus panniculitis (LEP) is a rare form of chronic cutaneous lupus erythematosus described from 2 to 5% of adult SLE [4–6]. In cSLE, LEP data are limited to few case reports [7–10].

Therefore, the objective of the present multicenter cohort study was to evaluate the prevalence of LEP and its possible association with demographic data, clinical manifestations, laboratory abnormalities,

* Correspondence: clovis.silva@hc.fm.usp.br
†Eloisa Bonfá and Clovis Artur Silva contributed equally to this work.
[1]Pediatric Rheumatology Unit, Children's Institute, Hospital das Clinicas HCFMUSP, Faculdade de Medicina, Universidade de Sao Paulo, Sao Paulo, SP, BR, Brazil
[2]Division of Rheumatology, Hospital das Clinicas HCFMUSP, Faculdade de Medicina, Universidade de Sao Paulo, Av. Dr. Eneas Carvalho Aguiar, 647 - Cerqueira César, São Paulo, SP 05403-000, Brazil
Full list of author information is available at the end of the article

disease activity score, treatment and outcome in a large cSLE population.

Methods

This study was conducted in 10 pediatric rheumatology services in the state of São Paulo, Brazil including a population of 847 cSLE patients [3]. All patients fulfilled the American College of Rheumatology (ACR) criteria for SLE [11], with disease onset before the age of 18 [12]. This study was approved by the Ethical Committee of University of São Paulo (CAPPESq number 09231912.2.1001.0068) and the consent from the patient for publication of these images was also obtained. The study was also approved by the others University Hospital participating in the present study. An investigator meeting was held for this study in São Paulo city to delineate the protocol according to the clinical parameters definitions and disease activity tool scoring. Investigators in each one of the centers, using the same specific database, conducted data collection locally. One or more rounds of queries were performed to check for accuracy and sort out discrepancies [3, 13].

Patient's medical charts were systematically reviewed according to demographic data, clinical features and LEP characteristics, laboratorial abnormalities, therapeutic data and outcome. LEP was diagnosed by the presence of painful subcutaneous nodules or plaques in deep dermis and subcutaneous tissues. Skin biopsy confirmed lobular or mixed panniculitis with lymphocytic lobular inflammatory infiltrate in all patients [8]. Patients were divided in two groups with similar disease duration: cSLE patients with LEP (evaluated at LEP diagnosis) and cSLE patients without LEP (evaluated at last visit).

Descriptors of SLE Disease Activity Index 2000 (SLEDAI-2 K) were used to define clinical manifestations [14], and custom definitions as previously reported [3, 13]. Constitutional involvement included fever, lymphadenopathy (peripheral lymph node enlargement > 1.0 cm), hepatomegaly [based on physical exam with liver edge ≥2 cm below the right costal margin or imaging (ultrasound or computer tomography when available)] and/or splenomegaly [based on physical exam with palpable spleen or imaging (ultrasound or computer tomography when available)] [3]. Neuropsychiatric lupus included 19 syndromes according to ACR classification criteria [15]. Antiphospholipid syndrome (APS) was diagnosed according to the presence of arterial and/or venous thrombosis and antiphospholipid antibodies [16].

Laboratorial assessment included complete blood cell count and urine examination. Anti-double-stranded DNA (anti-dsDNA), anticardiolipin antibodies (aCL) IgG and IgM were carried out at each center and the cutoff values were considered to be valid. Lupus anticoagulant was detected according to the guidelines of the International Society on Thrombosis and Hemostasis [17].

Drug treatment data [prednisone, intravenous methylprednisolone, chloroquine diphosphate, hydroxychloroquine sulfate, methotrexate, azathioprine, cyclosporine, mycophenolate mofetil, intravenous cyclophosphamide (IVCYC), intravenous immunoglobulin (IVIG) and rituximab] were also recorded.

Statistical analysis

Results were presented as an absolute number (frequency) for categorical variables and median (range) or mean ± standard deviation for continuous variables. Categorical variables comparisons were assessed by Pearson χ-Square or Fisher's exact test. Continuous variables from cSLE patients with and without LEP were compared by Mann-Whitney test or t test as appropriate. Statistical analysis was performed using Bonferroni correction ($p < 0.004$).

Results

LEP was observed in 6/847 (0.7%) cSLE patients. LEP was the first disease manifestation in 1/6 cSLE patient (2.5 years before cSLE diagnosis), occurred at diagnosis in 2/6 patients and after diagnosis in 3/6 patients (with 5.5, 9.91 and 11.4 years after cSLE diagnosis) (Table 1). Painful subcutaneous erythematous and indurated nodules were observed in 6/6 LEP patients, and concomitant painful subcutaneous erythematous plaques in 4/6. Generalized distribution (including face, trunk and limbs) was evidenced in 3/6 LEP patients and it was localized in upper limbs in 2/6 and face in 1/6. Cutaneous hyperpigmentation and/or cutaneous atrophy occurred in 5/6. Histopathology findings showed lobular panniculitis without vasculitis in 5/6 and panniculitis with vasculitis in 1/6 (Table 1). One female patient (Case 4) had sepsis and LEP as initial cSLE manifestation and she deceased before lupus diagnosis and prior to immunosuppressive treatment. Her biopsy revealed LEP associated with skin obliterative vasculopathy with positive serology for antiphospholipid antibodies.

Figure 1 shows LEP with cutaneous atrophy affecting the back and limbs. Figure 2 shows details of LEP patient with subcutaneous nodules, cutaneous atrophic and hyperpigmentated skin. Figure 3 shows histopathology of a skin biopsy of a LEP cSLE patient.

Treatment for LEP included: prednisone in 5/6 (83%), antimalarial drugs in 4/6 (67%), methotrexate in 3/6 (50%), azathioprine in 2/6 (33%) and one patient used cyclosporine. Regarding response for LEP treatment, 3/6 had refractory LEP to glucocorticoid, anti-malarial drugs and immunosuppressive agents (cases 2, 5 and 6). These cSLE patients improved the recurrent painful subcutaneous erythematous nodules and plaques after IVIG (case 2), rituximab (case 5)

Table 1 Cutaneous manifestations, demographic data, disease activity, outcome, skin biopsy and treatment in six childhood-onset systemic lupus erythematosus (cSLE) patients with lupus erythematosus panniculitis (LEP)

Patient	Interval between LEP and cSLE diagnosis, years	SLEDAI-2 K	Painful Plaques / painful subcutaneous nodules	Cutaneous hyperpigmentation / hypopigmentation / atrophy	Skin biopsy findings; direct immunofluorescence staining (DIF)	Treatments
1	−2.5	3	- / +	+ / - / +	LP; mild GCD of IgM at DEJ)	PD, AM, NSAID, AZA
2	11.4	13	+ / +	+ / - / +	LP with vasculitis; moderate GCD of IgM at DEJ)	PD, MP, AM, AZA, MTX, IVIG
3	5.5	13	+ / +	+ / + / +	LP; intense GCD of IgG, IgG, IgA and C3 at DEJ	PD, MP, CY, MTX
4	0	25	- / +	- / - / -	LP, vasculopathy obliterans; absence of IgG, IgM, IgA, C3 and C4 at DEJ	No treatment[a]
5	0	0	+ / +	+ / + / +	LP; absence of IgG, IgM, IgA, C3 and C4 at DEJ	PD, AM, NSAID, MMF, rituximab
6	9.91	5	+ / +	+ / - / +	LP; ND	PD, MP, AM, MTX, MMF, IVCYC

[a]deceased before starting any treatment, + presence, – absence, *LP* lobular panniculitis, *APS* antiphospholipid syndrome *PD* prednisone, *MP* methylprednisolone, *NSAID* nonsteroidal anti-inflammatory, *AM* antimalarial, *AZA* azathioprine, *IVCYC* intravenous cyclophosphamide, *CY* cyclosporine, *MTX* methotrexate, *MMF* mycopheneolate mofetil, *IVIG* intravenous immunoglobulin, *GCD* granular and continuous deposits, *DEJ* dermo-epidermal junction, *ND* not done, *SLEDAI-2 K* Systemic Lupus Erythematosus Disease Activity Index 2000

and IVCYC (case 6). Regarding outcomes, skin hyperpigmentation was observed in 5/6 LEP patients, skin hypopigmentation in 2/6 and cutaneous atrophy in 5/6.

LEP patients ($n = 6$) were compared with 60 patients without LEP (ratio of 1:10). These 60 patients without LEP were randomly selected of 841 cSLE patients without LEP and that presented same disease duration of LEP patients. Further comparison between 6 cSLE patients with LEP compared to 60 cSLE patients without LEP with the same disease duration [2.75 (0–11.4) vs. 2.83 (0–11.8) years, $p = 0.297$], showed higher frequencies of constitutional involvement (67% vs. 10%, $p = 0.003$) and leukopenia (67% vs. 7%, $p = 0.002$) in the former group. The median of serum CRP values was significantly higher in cSLE patients with LEP compared to cSLE control patients without LEP (10.5 vs. 0.5 mg/L, $p = 0.001$). Frequencies of major organ involvements such as renal and neuropsychiatric were similar in both groups ($p > 0.004$). The median of SLEDAI-2 K was similar in the two groups [9 (0–25) vs. 4 (0–41), $p = 0.352$] (Table 2).

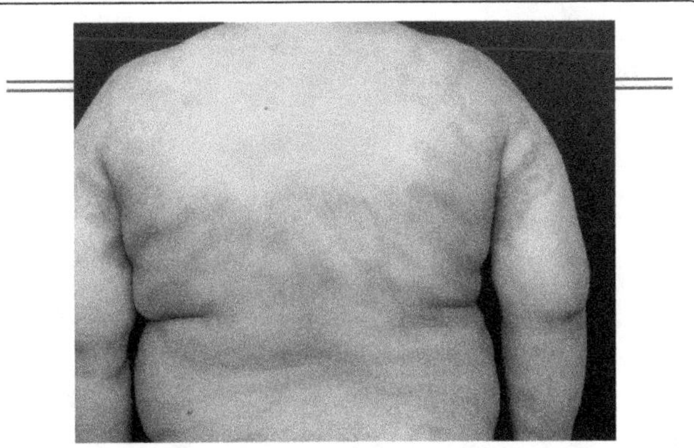

Fig. 1 Lupus erythematosus panniculitis showing extense areas of cutaneous atrophy affecting the back and limbs.

Discussion

This was the first study to assess panniculitis in a large cSLE population. LEP was a rare skin manifestation of cSLE occurring mainly in the first three years of disease.

The multicentric design with a large cohort of pediatric patients allowed a more precise evaluation of this rare lupus manifestation. All cSLE patients with suspect of LESP were included in the present study and the diagnoses were confirmed according to the histopathology

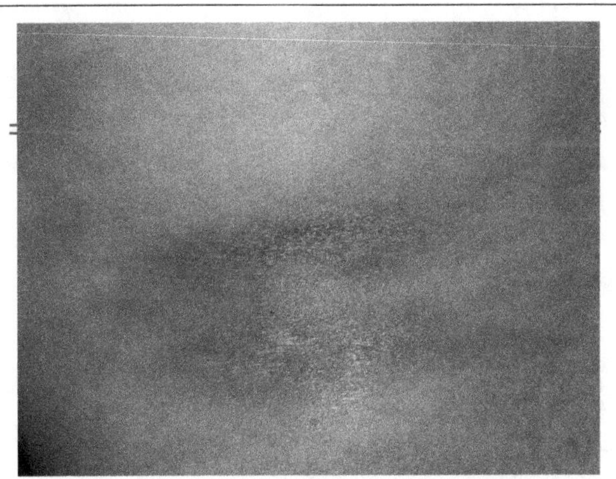

Fig. 2 Detail of lupus panniculitis presenting subcutaneous nodules with cutaneous atrophic and hyperpigmentated skin.

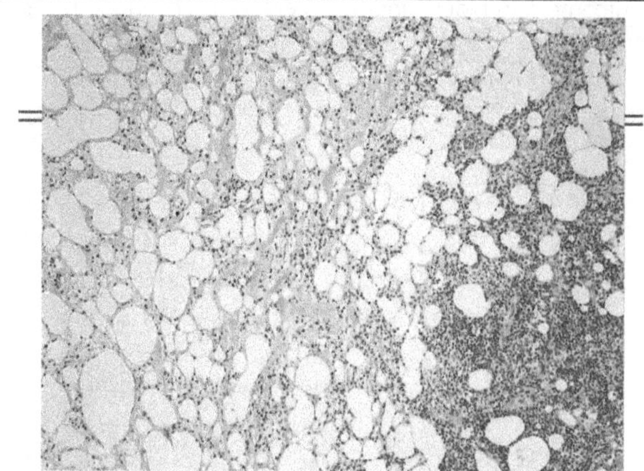

Fig. 3 Histopathology of a skin biopsy of the arm presenting septal and lobular panniculitis, with inflammatory infiltrate predominantly composed of lymphocytes in fat lobules and hyaline fat necrosis

findings. The limitation was the retrospective analysis with potential missing data and for this reason an investigator meeting was performed to standardize the protocol study in all centers involved. The low number of cSLE patients with LEP observed herein was also the limitation of the present study. However to minimize bias, the comparisons of clinical manifestations, laboratorial abnormalities and treatments were performed in both groups assessing same disease duration, with a ratio of 1:10 (1 cSLE with LEP, 10 cSLE without LEP patients).

Importantly, the diagnosis of panniculitis in all patients was based not only on the typical clinical manifestations with nodules and/or plaques in deep dermis and subcutaneous adipose tissues, but it was also confirmed through histopathological features [18]. In fact, skin biopsy is essential to exclude other causes of inflammation of the fatty tissue, such as lymphoma, deep morphea, erythema nodosum and sarcoidosis [18]. Lymphocytic vasculitis may also be an additional and typical cutaneous histopathology abnormality in LEP patients [4, 5, 19]. Interestingly one of our cSLE patients had LEP associated with vasculopathy obliterans probably due to APS, as also described in two adult SLE [20].

We confirmed previous observation that LEP in cSLE patients has a predilection for face [4] and we described that in half of our cases the distribution of skin lesions were generalized, a condition reported to be extremely rare [21].

In our study children and adolescents with lupus panniculitis had a mild systemic disease, characterized by constitutional involvement and leukopenia. Indeed other studies observed that this cutaneous chronic manifestation might be an indicator of a less severe systemic lupus [4, 9, 22–24].

Treatment for cSLE includes corticosteroids, antimalarial and immunosuppressive drugs [25, 26], as also prescribed for LEP patients evaluated in this study. Depressed lipoatrophic areas were very frequent

Table 2 Demographic data, cumulative clinical manifestations and laboratory parameters, and SLEDAI-2 K in childhood-onset systemic lupus erythematosous (cSLE) patients with lupus erythematosus panniculitis (LEP)

Variables	cSLE with LEP (at diagnosis) (n = 6)	cSLE without LEP (at last visit) (*n* = 60)	*P*
Demographic data			
Age at diagnosis, years	15 (10–21)	15 (2–25)	0.624
Female gender	4 (67)	52 (87)	0.222
Disease duration, years	2.75 (0–11.4)	2.83 (0–11.8)	0.297
Cumulative clinical manifestations			
Constitutional involvement	4 (67)	6 (10)	0.003
Cutaneous vasculitis	3 (50)	6 (10)	0.029
Musculoskeletal involvement	3 (50)	4 (7)	0.013
Serositis	0 (0)	4 (7)	1.000
Neuropsychiatric involvement	0 (0)	8 (13)	1.000
Nephritis	1 (17)	19/59 (32)	0.657
Cumulative laboratory parameters			
Leukopenia, < 4000/mm^3	4 (67)	4/55 (7)	0.002
Anti-ds-DNA	4 (67)	17/47 (36)	0.200
Disease activity at diagnosis			
SLEDAI-2 K	9 (0–25)	4 (0–41)	0.352

* *P* - value according to Bonferroni correction for multiple comparisons ($p < 0.004$). Results are presented in n (%) and median (range), SLEDAI-2 K - Systemic Lupus Erythematosus Disease Activity Index 2000

sequelae at cSLE diagnosis, reinforcing the concept that this residual scarring induces great morbidity associated with cosmetic abnormalities [4]. Hyperpigmentation and hypopigmentation are described in these patients and the former was more often observed in our patients [4, 5, 8, 9, 27].

Conclusion

Panniculitis is a rare skin manifestation of cSLE occurring in the first three years of disease with a high frequency of sequelae. The majority of patients presented concomitant mild lupus manifestations.

Authors' contributions

All authors analyzed and interpreted the patient data regarding autoimmune hepatitis in childhood onset systemic lupus erythematosus. MV, PA, NWSG, EB and CAS were the major contributor in writing the manuscript. All authors read and approved the final manuscript.

Author details

[1]Pediatric Rheumatology Unit, Children's Institute, Hospital das Clinicas HCFMUSP, Faculdade de Medicina, Universidade de Sao Paulo, Sao Paulo, SP, BR, Brazil. [2]Division of Rheumatology, Hospital das Clinicas HCFMUSP, Faculdade de Medicina, Universidade de Sao Paulo, Av. Dr. Eneas Carvalho Aguiar, 647 - Cerqueira César, São Paulo, SP 05403-000, Brazil. [3]Division of Dermatology, Hospital das Clinicas HCFMUSP, Faculdade de Medicina, Universidade de Sao Paulo, Sao Paulo, SP, BR, Brazil. [4]Pediatric Rheumatology Unit, Universidade Federal de São Paulo, São Paulo, Brazil. [5]São Paulo State University (UNESP) – Faculdade de Medicina de Botucatu, Botucatu, Brazil. [6]Pediatric Rheumatology Unit, Ribeirão Preto Medical School – University of São Paulo, Ribeirão Preto, Brazil. [7]São Paulo State University of Campinas (UNICAMP), Campinas, Brazil. [8]Irmandade da Santa Casa de Misericórdia de São Paulo, São Paulo, Brazil.

References

1. Silva CA. Childhood-onset systemic lupus erythematosus: early disease manifestations that the paediatrician must know. Expert Rev Clin Immunol. 2016;12:907–10.
2. Chiewchengchol D, Murphy R, Edwards SW, Beresford MW. Mucocutaneous manifestations in juvenile-onset systemic lupus erythematosus: a review of literature. Pediatr Rheumatol Online J. 2015;13:1.
3. Gomes RC, Silva MF, Kozu K, Bonfá E, Pereira RM, Terreri MT, et al. Features of 847 childhood-onset systemic lupus Erythematousus patients in three age groups at diagnosis: a Brazilian multicenter study. Arthritis Care Res. 2016;68:1736–41.
4. Fraga J, García-Díez A. Lupus erythematosus panniculitis. Dermatol Clin. 2008;26:453–63.
5. Park HS, Choi JW, Kim BK, Cho KH. Lupus erythematosus panniculitis: clinicopathological, immunophenotypic, and molecular studies. Am J Dermatopathol. 2010;32:24–30.
6. Bednarek A, Bartoszak L, Samborski W. Case report on a patient with lupus panniculitis. Postepy Dermatol Alergol. 2015;32:59–62.
7. Fernandes S, Santos S, Freitas I, Salgado M, Afonso A, Cardoso J. Linear lupus erythematosus profundus as an initial manifestation of systemic lupus erythematosus in a child. Pediatr Dermatol. 2014;31:378–80.
8. Guissa VR, Trudes G, Jesus AA, Aikawa NE, Romiti R, Silva CA. Lupus erythematosus panniculitis in children and adolescents. Acta Reumatol Port. 2012;37:82–5.
9. Weingartner JS, Zedek DC, Burkhart CN, Morrell DS. Lupus erythematosus panniculitis in children: report of three cases and review of previously reported cases. Pediatr Dermatol. 2012;29:169–76.
10. Wimmershoff MB, Hohenleutner U, Landthaler M. Discoid lupus erythematosus and lupus profundus in childhood: a report of two cases. Pediatr Dermatol. 2003;20:140–5.
11. Hochberg MC. Updating the American College of Rheumatology revised criteria for the classification of systemic lupus erhytematosus. Arthritis Rheum. 1997;40:1725.
12. Mina R, Brunner HI. Update on differences between childhood-onset and adult-onset systemic lupus erythematosus. Arthritis Res Ther. 2013;15:218.
13. Marques VL, Gormezano NW, Bonfá E, Aikawa NE, Terreri MT, Pereira RM, et al. Pancreatitis subtypes survey in 852 childhood-onset systemic lupus erythematosus patients. J Pediatr Gastroenterol Nutr. 2016;62:328–34.
14. Gladman DD, Ibañez D, Urowitz MB. Systemic lupus erythematosus disease activity index 2000. J Rheumatol. 2002;29:288–91.
15. American College of Rheumatology Ad Hoc committee on neuropsychiatric Lupus Syndromes. The American College of Rheumatology nomenclature and case definitions for neuropsychiatric lupus syndromes. Arthritis Rheum. 1999;42:599–608.
16. Avcin T, Cimaz R, Rozman B. The Ped-APS Registry: the antiphospholipid syndrome in childhood. Lupus. 2009;18:894–9.
17. Brandt JT, Triplett DA, Alving B, Scharrer I. Criteria for the diagnosis of lupus anticoagulants: an update. On behalf of the subcommittee on lupus anticoagulant/antiphospholipid antibody of the scientific and standardisation committee of the ISTH. Thromb Haemost. 1995;74:1185–90.
18. Moraes AJ, Soares PM, Zapata AL, Lotito AP, Sallum AM, Silva CA. Panniculitis in childhood and adolescence. Pediatr Int. 2006;48:48–53.
19. Chopra R, Chhabra S, Thami GP, Punia RP. Panniculitis: clinical overlap and the significance of biopsy findings. J Cutan Pathol. 2010;37:49–58.
20. Arai S, Katsuoka K, Eto H. An unusual form of lupus erythematosus profundus associated with antiphospholipid syndrome: report of two cases. Acta Derm Venereol. 2013;93:581–2.
21. Nousari HC, Kimyai-Asadi A, Provost TT. Generalized lupus erythematosus profundus in a patient with genetic partial deficiency of C4. J Am Acad Dermatol. 1999;41:362–4.
22. Martens PB, Moder KG, Ahmed I. Lupus panniculitis: clinical perspectives from a case series. J Rheumatol. 1999;26:68–72.
23. Koransky JS, Esterly NB. Lupus panniculitis (profundus). J Pediatr. 1981;98:241–4.
24. Taïeb A, Hehunstre JP, Goetz J, Surlève Bazeille JE, Fizet D, Hauptmann G, et al. Lupus erythematosus panniculitis with partial genetic deficiency of C2 and C4 in a child. Arch Dermatol. 1986;122:576–82.
25. Silva CA, Aikawa NE, Pereira RM, Campos LM. Management considerations for childhood-onset systemic lupus erythematosus patients and implications on therapy. Expert Rev Clin Immunol. 2016;12:301–13.
26. Klumb EM, Silva CA, Lanna CC, Sato EI, Borba EF, Brenol JC, et al. Consensus of the Brazilian Society of Rheumatology for the diagnosis, management and treatment of lupus nephritis. Rev Bras Reumatol. 2015;55:1–21.
27. Vera-Recabarren MA, García-Carrasco M, Ramos-Casals M, Herrero C. Comparative analysis of subacute cutaneous lupus erythematosus and chronic cutaneous lupus erythematosus: clinical and immunological study of 270 patients. Br J Dermatol. 2010;162:91–101.

16

Nailfold capillaroscopy as a risk factor for pulmonary arterial hypertension in systemic lupus erythematosus patients

Juliana Fernandes Sarmento Donnarumma[1], Eloara Vieira Machado Ferreira[2], Jaquelina Ota-Arakaki[2] and Cristiane Kayser[1,3*]

Abstract

Background: Pulmonary arterial hypertension (PAH) is a rare and severe complication of systemic lupus erythematosus (SLE). This study aimed to evaluate clinical and laboratory risk factors associated with PAH in SLE patients.

Methods: This was a retrospective case-control study in which patients with SLE with PAH (SLE-PAH) confirmed by right heart catheterization (RHC) were compared with SLE patients without PAH. Clinical and demographic variables related to SLE and PAH and nailfold capillaroscopy were evaluated by reviewing the medical records of the patients.

Results: Twenty-one patients with SLE-PAH and 44 patients with SLE without PAH matched for sex and disease duration were included. The scleroderma (SD) pattern on nailfold capillaroscopy was more frequently found in patients with SLE-PAH than in those without PAH (56.3% versus 15.9%, respectively, $p = 0.002$). By univariate analysis, Raynaud's phenomenon, history of abortion, and SD pattern on capillaroscopy were associated with PAH. Arthritis was a protective factor for PAH development. Multivariate analysis showed that the SD pattern on capillaroscopy was the only variable associated with a significantly higher risk of PAH, with an odds ratio of 6.393 (95% confidence interval, 1.530–26.716; $p = 0.011$).

Conclusion: In this study, SD pattern was associated with a 6.3-fold increased risk for PAH development in SLE patients, suggesting that nailfold capillaroscopy might be useful as a screening method to identify SLE patients with a high risk of developing this severe complication.

Keywords: Systemic lupus erythematosus, Pulmonary arterial hypertension, Risk factors, Nailfold capillaroscopy

Background

Systemic lupus erythematosus (SLE) is a rare chronic autoimmune disease of multifactorial etiology. Symptoms are heterogeneous and vary from mild to severe and potentially fatal systemic manifestations [1].

Pulmonary hypertension (PH) is a complex condition defined as an elevation of the mean pulmonary artery pressure (MPAP) (≥ 25 mmHg) at rest on right heart catheterization (RHC). The term pulmonary arterial hypertension (PAH) is used to designate a group of patients with pulmonary hypertension hemodynamically defined by precapillary PH, with pulmonary capillary wedge pressure (PCWP) ≤ 15 mmHg and an increase in the pulmonary vascular resistance (PVR) [2, 3].

PAH associated with autoimmune rheumatic diseases represent 30% of all adult PAH cases [4–6]. Among the rheumatic diseases associated with PAH, systemic sclerosis (SSc) and SLE are the most common [7, 8]. The prevalence of PAH among SLE patients varies from 0.5 to 14% according to the analyzed population [9–13]. Such wide variation is mainly attributed to the diagnostic methods used. Indeed, many studies were based on estimates of the right ventricular systolic pressure

* Correspondence: criskayser@terra.com.br
[1]Rheumatology Division, Medicine Department, Escola Paulista de Medicina, Universidade Federal de São Paulo (UNIFESP), São Paulo, SP, Brazil
[3]Disciplina de Reumatologia da Universidade Federal de São Paulo, Rua Botucatu 740, 3 ° andar, São Paulo, SP 04023-062, Brazil
Full list of author information is available at the end of the article

measured on transthoracic echocardiogram, using a variety of cutoff points (> 30 to 45 mmHg) to define PAH. Moreover, although PAH is the most frequent etiology of PH, it can be associated with other aetiologies, including pulmonary veno-occlusive disease, and pulmonary fibrosis and the differential diagnosis is not always simple [7].

Among patients with SLE, PAH is associated with high morbidity and mortality [14, 15]. Despite advances in the treatment of PAH in recent decades, patients with associated autoimmune rheumatic diseases exhibit a more severe form of disease and a poorer prognosis than do patients with other forms of PAH [8, 16]. According to reports in the literature, the 1- and 3-year survival rates for patients with SLE and PAH are 78 and 74%, respectively [17]. However, in a recent cohort study of 2967 patients with PAH at various American centers, the 1-year survival rate for patients with SLE was 94% [8].

Several risk factors have been associated with the development of PAH among SLE patients, including the presence of Raynaud's phenomenon (RP), anti-ribonucleoprotein (anti-RNP) and anti-cardiolipin antibodies, digital vasculitis, livedo reticularis, serositis, and high serum endothelin-1 levels [14, 16, 18–20]. However, most studies employed echocardiography for the diagnosis of PAH, which is a substantial limitation given its low accuracy.

Nailfold capillaroscopy (NC) is a noninvasive method that is widely used in the investigation of patients with RP. Patients with RP secondary to SSc and SSc spectrum disorders exhibit a classic microangiopathy pattern known as the scleroderma (SD) pattern, which is characterized by loss of capillary loops, capillary dilatation, and disorganization of the capillary structure [21]. Some studies of patients with SSc have found an association between NC abnormalities and the presence and severity of PAH, which suggests that changes in the microcirculation might play a role in the development or pathogenesis of PAH [22–25].

The aim of the present study was to identify risk factors for the development of PAH among SLE patients by analyzing clinical aspects and complementary tests, with an emphasis on NC as a possible method for the identification of patients with SLE and PAH.

Materials and methods

Patients and study design

In the present single-center, retrospective, case-control study conducted from 2013 to 2015, risk factors for PAH were investigated among SLE patients who developed PAH (SLE-PAH) or who did not (SLE-nPAH). Both groups were matched for sex and duration of disease (up to the outcome in group SLE-PAH) at a 2:1 ratio.

For the SLE-PAH group, the diagnosis of PAH met established criteria, especially confirmation on RHC [2]. Patients were identified through a review of medical records and via the database of PH patients of the Pulmonary Circulation Service, of the Pneumology Department of the Federal University of São Paulo.

Patients with SLE and without known diagnosed PAH (SLE-nPAH) were randomly selected from the SLE outpatient clinic, and those with SLE-PAH were also followed-up at the pulmonary outpatient clinic at the Federal University of São Paulo Medical School Hospital. The inclusion criteria were as follows: age of 18 years old or older; fulfilling the American College of Rheumatology (ACR) 1997 revised criteria for the classification of SLE [26]; and availability of clinical and laboratory data in the medical records at the time of inclusion. Patients with SSc overlap syndrome, rheumatoid arthritis, or polymyositis/dermatomyositis were excluded. The study was approved by the local research ethics committee (no. 503,630).

Thirty patients with PAH were identified. Five of them had not performed RHC for diagnosis and thus did not meet the inclusion criteria. Four patients had missing data in their medical records and had been subjected to one single outpatient evaluation; therefore, they could not be included in the study. As a result, the study sample comprised 21 SLE-PAH and 44 SLE-nPAH patients.

Right heart catheterization

RHC was indicated for patients with clinical suspicion of PAH and pulmonary artery pressure (PAP) ≥ 35 mmHg on Doppler echocardiogram. PAH was defined as MPAP ≥25 mmHg at rest, PCWP ≤15 mmHg, and an elevated PVR (> 3 Wood units-WU). The following parameters were analyzed on RHC at the time of PAH diagnosis: MPAP, cardiac index (CI), PCWP, and PVR index (PVRI). All exams were performed at the hemodynamics service of São Paulo Medical School Hospital. Interstitial lung disease, chronic thromboembolic pulmonary hypertension, congenital heart disease, significant valvular heart disease, chronic obstructive pulmonary disease, portal hypertension, schistosomiasis, immunodeficiency virus, and thyroid disorders had been previously ruled out.

Clinical and laboratory data

All the analyzed data were extracted from the patients' medical records. Attention was paid to the following variables: age, sex, ACR classification criteria for SLE, time since diagnosis of SLE and PAH, smoking, obstetric history, presence of RP and livedo reticularis, laboratory data, NC data, thrombotic events, and deaths in the SLE-PAH group. SLE activity was analyzed for all patients based on their score on the Systemic Lupus Erythematosus Disease Activity Index (SLEDAI) [27].

Laboratory tests included the detection of antinuclear (ANA) and anti-dsDNA antibodies by indirect immunofluorescence using HEp-2 cells and *Crithidia luciliae* as the substrate, respectively. Anti-Sm, anti-RNP, anti-Ro, and anti-La were investigated based on double immunodiffusion. Complement fractions (C2 and C100) were measured with radial immune hemolysis. Anti-cardiolipin antibodies (anti-aCL IgG and IgM) were detected using an enzyme-linked immunosorbent assay (ELISA). Serum creatinine levels, complete blood counts, C-reactive protein (CRP) levels, and 24-h urine protein levels, were also evaluated in all subjects.

NC was performed with a stereomicroscope (SZ40, Olympus) at 10-25x magnification. The NC parameters considered in the analysis were as follows: SD, normal or unspecific pattern, number of loops per mm, avascular score, number of giant and enlarged capillaries, and microhemorrhages [28]. The avascular score was determined semiquantitatively on a scale from 0 to 3 as previously described [29]. The mean score for each parameter was calculated from the analysis of all fingers except the thumbs.

Patients with PAH were also evaluated based on the New York Heart Association (NYHA) functional classification [30], distance walked in the 6-min walk test (6MWT), forced vital capacity (FVC) and carbon monoxide diffusing capacity (Dco) on pulmonary function tests, and echocardiogram at the time of PAH diagnosis. The echocardiogram parameters considered were as follows: PAP, right ventricular size, tricuspid regurgitation velocity (TRV), and presence of pericardial effusion.

Clinical and demographic data were collected at the time of diagnosis. The data on SLEDAI and current or previous SLE treatment were obtained at the time of inclusion in the study. For the SLE-PAH group, clinical and laboratory data on PAH were collected at the time of PAH diagnosis.

Statistical analysis

The data are presented as the mean and standard deviation and as absolute and relative frequencies in the case of categorical variables. The Shapiro-Wilk test was used to investigate the normality of the variable distribution. Continuous variables were compared between groups using Student's t-test or the Mann-Whitney test. Categorical data were analyzed using the chi-square or Fisher's exact test. The significance level was set at $p < 0.05$. To identify risk factors in the SLEP-PAH group, uni- and multivariate logistic regression analyses were performed, and the odds ratio (OR) for each factor was calculated with the corresponding 95% confidence interval (95% CI) relative to the SLE-nPAH group. All variables with $p < 0.10$ in the univariate analysis were included in the multivariate analysis. Statistical analyses were performed using *SPSS* software for Windows version 19.0 (Chicago, IL).

Results

The clinical, demographic, and laboratory characteristics of the 21 patients with SLE-PAH and the 44 SLE-nPAH patients are described in Table 1. The mean age at the time of SLE onset was 28.8 and 31.2 years in the SLE-PAH and SLE-nPAH groups, respectively. Female patients predominated in both groups. The mean duration of SLE at the time of PAH diagnosis was 6.7 ± 6.4 years in the SLE-PAH group. Regarding the ACR criteria, arthritis and photosensitivity were more frequent in the SLE-nPAH group (93.2 and 79.5%, respectively) than in the SLE-PAH group (70 and 55%, respectively). The SLEDAI score was not significant different between the groups; 29% of the patients in the SLE-nPAH group and 19% of those in the SLE-PAH group exhibited active disease (SLEDAI ≥4). Forty-two patients (64.6%) exhibited RP, with a trend toward a higher frequency in the SLE-PAH group than in the SLE-nPAH group (81% versus 56.8%, respectively; $p = 0.057$).

Forty patients (61.5%) had been pregnant at least once, without a significant difference between the groups. Only one patient in the SLE-PAH group had become pregnant after the diagnosis of PAH, and the outcome was a preterm birth. Ten patients (15.4%) had at least one miscarriage, with a significantly higher frequency in the SLE-PAH group than in the SLE-nPAH group (28.6% versus 9.1%, respectively; $p = 0.042$) (Table 1). Secondary antiphospholipid syndrome was diagnosed in two patients in the SLE-PAH group and in five patients in the SLE-nPAH group.

Nailfold capillaroscopy was performed in 16 patients in the SLE-PAH group and 44 patients in the SLE-nPAH group. The SD pattern was detected in 56.3% of the SLE-PAH patients. Most patients (84.1%) in the SLE-nPAH group exhibited a normal or unspecific pattern on capillaroscopy, and only 15.9% exhibited the SD pattern ($p = 0.002$). The number of dilated capillaries and the avascular score were significantly higher in the SLE-PAH group ($p = 0.027$ and $p = 0.010$, respectively) (Table 2).

The mean RHC findings for the SLE-PAH group were as follows: MPAP 48.9 ± 11.7 mmHg, CI 2.47 ± 0.7 L/min/m^2, and PVRI 10.9 ± 8.8 WU/m^2 (Table 3). The most frequent functional class (NYHA) at the time of diagnosis was functional class III (47.6%), followed by class II (33.3%); two patients (9.5%) were categorized as class I and another two (9.5%) as class IV. The mean distance walked in the 6MWT was 416.6 ± 80.6 m. The mean FVC was 79.6 ± 15.2%, and the mean Dco was 47.4 ± 18.9%. Regarding the echocardiography parameters, the mean PAP was 63.1 ± 14.1 mmHg, the mean TRV was 3.71 ± 0.41 m/s, and the mean right ventricular

Table 1 Clinical and demographic characteristics of patients with SLE associated with PAH (SLE-PAH) or not associated with PAH (SLE-nPAH)

	SLE-nPAH $n = 44$	SLE-PAH $n = 21$	P-value
Age at SLE diagnosis (years)	31.2 ± 12.3	28.8 ± 10.2	0.411
Age at PAH diagnosis (years)	–	35.5 ± 11.8	–
Duration of disease at recruitment (years)	5.6 ± 3.2	6.7 ± 6.4	0.437
Female sex, n (%)	42 (95.5)	20 (95.2)	0.969
Smoker, n (%)	0 (0)	1 (4.8)	0.145
Ex-smoker, n (%)	4 (9.1)	1 (4.8)	0.295
ACR SLE criteria, n (%)			
Malar rash	34 (77.3)	13 (65)	0.303
Photosensitivity	35 (79.5)	11 (55)	0.043
Discoid rash	3 (6.8)	0 (0)	0.232
Oral ulcers	7 (15.9)	4 (20)	0. 688
Arthritis	41 (93.2)	14 (70)	0.013
Serositis	2 (40%)	12 (60)	0.112
Hematologic involvement	27 (61.4)	14 (70)	0.504
Renal involvement	18 (40.9)	7 (35)	0.635
Neuropsychiatric involvement	8 (18.2)	4 (20)	0.863
ANA	44(100)	19 (90.4)	0.189
Anti-dsDNA, anti-Sm, or antiphospholipid	25 (56.8)	11 (57.9)	0.937
Raynaud's phenomenon, n (%)	25 (56.8)	17 (81)	0.057
Livedo reticularis, n (%)	0 (0)	1 (4.8)	0.145
Arterial thrombosis, n (%)	0 (0)	1 (4.8)	0.145
Venous thrombosis, n (%)	7 (15.9)	5 (23.8)	0.443
SLEDAI	1.91 ± 3.16	2.56 ± 3.79	0.559
Pregnancy, n (%)	26 (59.1)	14 (66.7)	0.557
Miscarriage, n (%)	4 (9.1)	6 (28.6)	0.042
Anti-SM, n (%)	10 (22.7)	4 (23.5)	0.947
Anti-RNP, n (%)	19 (43.2)	11 (64.7)	0.132
Anti-Ro, n (%)	11 (25)	5 (29.4)	0.725
Anti-La, n (%)	5 (11.4)	2 (11.8)	0.965
Positive anti- aCL IgM, n (%)	3 (7)	2 (11.1)	0.591
Positive anti- aCL IgG, n (%)	7 (16.3)	3 (16.7)	0.970
Positive anti-dsDNA, n (%)	15 (34.1)	3 (17.6)	0.207
C2 (mg/dL)	91.4 ± 25.7	86.9 ± 29.8	0.690
CH100 (mg/dL)	91.5 ± 24.8	89.4 ± 30.2	0.957
Hemoglobin (g/dL)	12.5 ± 1.3	13.2 ± 1.5	0.138
Leukocytes (/mm^3)	6.317 ± 3.120	6.149 ± 3.766	0.977
Lymphocytes (/mm^3)	1.643 ± 899	1.477 ± 675	0.617
Platelets (/mm^3)	251.295 ± 101.691	197.500 ± 68.534	0.028
Creatinine (mg/dL)	0.73 ± 0.23	0.86 ± 0.36	0.077
CRP (mg/dL)	9.02 ± 14.3	12.10 ± 37.32	0.314
24-h urine protein (mg/kg/24 h)	0.36 ± 0.52	0.26 ± 0.25	0.785

Data are expressed as the mean ± standard deviation or n (%). *ACR* American College of Rheumatology, *ANA* antinuclear antibodies, *anti-aCL* anticardiolipin, *CRP* C-reactive protein, *nPAH* no PAH, *PAH* pulmonary arterial hypertension, *SLE* systemic lupus erythematosus, *SLEDAI* Systemic Lupus Erythematosus Disease Activity Index

Table 2 Abnormalities on nailfold capillaroscopy among patients with SLE associated with PAH (SLE-PAH) or not associated with PAH (SLE-nPAH)

	SLE-PAH *n* = 16	SLE-nPAH *n* = 44	*P*-value
Capillaroscopy pattern			
SD, n (%)	9 (56.3)	7 (15.9)	0.002
Normal or unspecific, n (%)	7 (43.7)	37 (84.1)	
Number of loops/mm	8.63 ± 1.28	9.18 ± 1.77	0.081
Microhemorrhages	1.03 ± 1.67	0.3 ± 0.52	0.134
Dilated capillaries	1.39 ± 1.46	0.85 ± 1.72	0.027
Giant capillaries	0.04 ± 0.11	0.03 ± 0.44	0.468
Avascular score	0.45 ± 0.63	0.12 ± 0.28	0.010

Data are expressed as the mean ± standard deviation or n (%). *NC* nailfold capillaroscopy, *nPAH* no PAH, *PAH* pulmonary arterial hypertension, *SD* scleroderma pattern, *SLE* systemic lupus erythematosus

area was 26.2 ± 5.5 cm^2. Pericardial effusion was detected in 9.5% of the patients.

Among the medications for the treatment of SLE, current or previous use of corticosteroids and antimalarial agents was significantly more frequent in the SLE-nPAH group than in the SLE-PAH group (100% versus 85%, respectively, for both medications; $p = 0.009$). Mycophenolate and cyclophosphamide was also significantly more frequently used in the SLE-nPAH group than in the SLE-PAH group (29.5% versus 5%, respectively, $p = 0.028$; 56.8% versus 15%, respectively, $p = 0.002$) (Table 4). A higher proportion of patients used contraceptives in the SLE-PAH group than in the SLE-nPAH group (52.6% versus 22.7%, respectively; $p = 0.019$). Regarding the medications used for the treatment of PAH, 57.1% of the participants used sildenafil and 47.6% bosentan; five patients (23.8%) received combined therapy. Ten patients (47.6%) had received intravenous cyclophosphamide pulse therapy and eight (38.1%) intravenous corticosteroids at the time of diagnosis of PAH (Table 4). Thirteen patients (61.9%) had received oral anticoagulants. Six patients (28.6%) in the SLE-PAH group died during follow-up.

As shown in Table 5, there were no significant differences in demographic, clinical, or laboratory variables between NYHA class I/II and NYHA class III/IV SLE-PAH patients. Although MPAP, CI, and PVRI were worse in class III/IV patients than in class I/II patients, these differences were not significant. There were 5 deaths in the NYHA class III and IV group and only one death in the NYHA class I and II group. No association was found between MPAP or CI values on RHC and clinical or laboratory variables (data not shown).

Table 3 Results of right heart catheterization for patients with PAH

	SLE-PAH *n* = 21
MPAP (mm Hg)	48.9 ± 11.7
CI (L/min/m^2)	2.47 ± 0.7
PCWP (mm Hg)	10.7 ± 2.5
PVRI (WU/m^2)	10.9 ± 8.8

Data are expressed as the mean ± standard deviation. *MPAP* mean pulmonary artery pressure, *CI* cardiac index, *PAH* pulmonary arterial hypertension, *PCWP* pulmonary capillary wedge pressure, *PVRI* pulmonary vascular resistance index, *SLE* systemic lupus erythematosus

In the univariate analysis, miscarriage, RP, and SD pattern on capillaroscopy were significant risk factors for PAH ($p = 0.05$; $p = 0.06$; $p = 0.003$, respectively). In turn, arthritis was a protective factor against the development of PAH (p = 0.05) (Table 6). In the multivariate analysis, SD pattern on NC was the single variable associated with an increased risk of PAH, with an OR of 6.393 (95% CI: 1.530–26.716; $p = 0.011$).

Discussion

PAH is a devastating disorder that might lead to right ventricular dysfunction and, consequently, death. Recent studies have suggested that PAH associated with SLE involves heterogeneous conditions with a variable response to treatment. The identification of risk factors might contribute to improved screening and treatment management. To the best of our knowledge, this is the first study to analyze NC among patients with SLE associated with PAH. Thus, in the present study there was a 6.3-fold higher risk of PAH development in patients with the SD pattern on capillaroscopy.

NC is useful for analyses of microvascular abnormalities in the peripheral circulation and for the early diagnosis of SSc [28]. The SD pattern occurs in up to 98% of patients with SSc, and it may be found in 2 to 15% of patients with SLE [28, 31]. In a study of SLE patients, the SD pattern was associated with the presence of RP and anti-RNP antibodies, which were associated with PAH in other studies [31].

NC abnormalities in SSc are associated with more severe visceral involvement and digital ulcers [21, 32]. Studies evaluating NC in patients with scleroderma and PAH found a reduced capillary density among patients

Table 4 Treatment for SLE and PAH

	SLE-PAH *n* = 21	SLE-nPAH *n* = 44	*P*-value
Corticosteroids, n (%)	17 (85)	44(100)	0.009
Antimalarial agents, n (%)	17 (85)	44(100)	0.009
Immunosuppressants, n (%)			
Azathioprine	8 (40)	25 (56.8)	0.212
Mycophenolate	1 (5)	13 (29.5)	0.028
Cyclophosphamide	3 (15)	25 (56.8)	0.002
Methotrexate	11 (55)	19 (43.2)	0.380
PAH treatment			
Sildenafil, n (%)	12 (57.1)	–	
Bosentan, n (%)	10 (47.6)	–	
Cyclophosphamide IV, n (%)	10 (47.6)	–	
Methylprednisolone IV, n (%)	8 (38.1)	–	
Oral anticoagulants, n (%)	13 (65)	–	

nPAH no PAH, *PAH* pulmonary arterial hypertension, *SLE* systemic lupus erythematosus

with PAH compared with those without PH [22, 24]. In a study of 24 patients with SSc, 12 with and 12 without PAH, Riccieri et al., observed greater devascularization and a higher frequency of the active and late NC pattern compared with the early pattern among patients with PAH [23]. In addition, more severe NC abnormalities, such as a higher avascular score and lower capillary density, have been associated with a higher MPAP, suggesting an association between pulmonary arterial disease and the degree of abnormalities on NC [22, 23]. Interestingly, Hofstee et al., observed an inverse correlation between pulmonary arterial pressure and capillary density among patients with PAH, either idiopathic or secondary to SSc [22].

In our study, in addition to the higher frequency of the SD pattern among patients with PAH, we also found a higher degree of devascularization and larger number of dilated capillaries among patients with PAH compared with those without PAH. Although not fully elucidated, the pathogenesis of PAH involves an imbalance between vasodilation and vasoconstrictor mediators, and excessive vasoconstriction and increased PVR have been associated with endothelial and smooth muscle proliferation and pulmonary vascular remodeling [16, 18]. The findings of the present study suggest that the peripheral microangiopathy might have a similar pathogenesis to pulmonary vascular bed microangiopathy. Our findings further suggest that patients with SSc and SLE share similar pathogenic mechanisms involved in the development of PAH.

The multivariate analysis did not reveal an association with variables previously reported as correlating with a higher risk of PAH, such as the presence of RP, serositis, and anti-RNP and anticardiolipin antibodies. This discrepancy might derive from the sample characteristics or the small number of patients with PAH analyzed.

Several studies have described an association of RP and digital vasculitis with PAH [19, 33–36]. In the present study, 81% of the patients with SLE and PAH and 56% of the patients without PAH exhibited RP. By univariate analysis, the presence of RP was associated with a 3.2-fold higher risk of PAH, which suggests that this variable might be relevant for the identification of this subpopulation of patients.

Anti-RNP and antiphospholipid antibodies have also been associated with an elevated risk of PAH among patients with SLE [19, 37–39]. Several autoantibodies might cause endothelial damage, vasoconstriction, and immunocomplex formation, and might be deposited on the pulmonary arterial wall [37]. In a study of Chinese individuals, anti-RNP and anticardiolipin antibodies were independent predictors of PAH among SLE patients, with ORs of 5.3 and 3.7, respectively [19]. A systematic review also of Chinese patients reported a higher frequency of anti-RNP (51.5%) and anticardiolipin (46.6%) antibodies among patients with SLE and PAH [38]. While some studies found a higher prevalence of anti-RNP antibodies among patients with SLE and PAH, other did not find a significant difference between SLE patients with or without PAH [11, 36]. In the present study, 65% of the patients with PAH had positive anti-RNP compared with 43% of the patients without PAH.

Antiphospholipid antibodies are classically associated with antiphospholipid syndrome and a higher risk of arterial or venous thrombosis and recurrent pregnancy loss. Cefle et al. (2011), found a higher frequency of antiphospholipid antibodies among SLE patients diagnosed with PAH on echocardiogram compared with patients without PAH [37]. However, other studies have failed to find such association [11, 33, 36, 40]. In the present

Table 5 Demographic and clinical characteristics of patients with SLE and PAH by NYHA functional classes I/II and III/IV

	NYHA class I/II *n* = 9	NYHA class III/IV *n* = 12	*P*-value
Female sex, n (%)	9 (100)	11 (91.7)	0.375
Age at SLE diagnosis	26.7 ± 10.9	30.3 ± 9.9	0.219
Age at PAH diagnosis	35.8 ± 11.7	35.3 ± 12.3	0.922
SLE length at PAH diagnosis	9.1 ± 7.5	4.9 ± 4.9	0.138
Smoking, n (%)	1 (11)	0 (0)	0.352
Miscarriage, n (%)	3 (33)	3 (25)	0.676
Pregnancy, n (%)	6 (66.7)	8 (66.7)	1.000
Raynaud's phenomenon, n (%)	7 (77.8)	10 (81)	0.748
Livedo reticularis, n (%)	1 (11.1)	0 (0)	0.237
Arterial thrombosis, n (%)	0 (0)	1 (8.3)	0.375
Venous thrombosis, n (%)	4 (44.4)	1 (8.3)	0.055
Anti-SM, n (%)	2 (25)	2 (22.2)	0.893
Anti-RNP, n (%)	4 (50)	7 (77.8)	0.232
Anti-Ro, n (%)	2 (25)	3 (33.3)	0.707
Anti-La, n (%)	0 (0)	2 (22.2)	0.156
Positive anti- aCL IgM, n (%)	1 (12.5)	1 (10)	0.867
Positive anti- aCL IgG, n (%)	1 (12.5)	2 (20)	0.671
Positive anti-dsDNA, n (%)	2 (25)	1 (11.1)	0.453
C2 (mg/dL)	85.2 ± 34.3	88.1 ± 28.6	0.859
CH100 (mg/dL)	83.8 ± 30.2	93.1 ± 31.4	0.579
CRP (mg/dL)	3.43 ± 2.01	19.20 ± 50.20	1.000
SLEDAI	2 ± 4.5	3.0 ± 3.4	0.299
6-min walk test	413 ± 14.8	417.7 ± 92.9	0.934
FVC (%)	84.1 ± 17.5	75.7 ± 13.2	0.143
Dco (%)	52.2 ± 8.3	44.5 ± 23.2	0.548
Death, n (%)	1 (11.1)	5 (41.7)	0.125
Nailfold capillaroscopy			
SD pattern, n (%)	4 (66.7)	5 (50)	0.515
Normal or unspecific	2 (33.3)	5 (50)	
RHC			
MPAP	47.6 ± 7.7	50.0 ± 14.6	0.654
CI	2.61 ± 0.66	2.36 ± 0.75	0.441
PVRI	8.86 ± 3.0	12.62 ± 11.47	0.824
Treatment			
Sildenafil, n (%)	4 (44.4)	8 (67)	0.309
Bosentan, n (%)	5 (55.6)	5 (41.7)	0.528
Cyclophosphamide IV, n (%)	4 (44.4)	6 (50)	0.801
Methylprednisolone IV, n (%)	3 (33.3)	5 (41.7)	0.697
Oral anticoagulants, n (%)	6 (66.7)	7 (63.6)	0.642

Data are expressed as the mean ± standard deviation or n (%). *SLE* systemic lupus erythematosus, *PAH* pulmonary arterial hypertension, *anti-aCL* anticardiolipin, *CI* cardiac index, *CRP* C-reactive protein, *Dco* carbon monoxide diffusing capacity, *FVC* forced vital capacity, *IV* intravenous, *MPAP* mean pulmonary artery pressure, *NYHA* New York Heart Association, *PVRI* pulmonary vascular resistance index, *SLE* systemic lupus erythematosus, *SLEDAI* Systemic Lupus Erythematosus Disease Activity Index

Table 6 Variables associated with PAH among SLE patients in the univariate logistic regression analysis

Variables	Odds ratio	95% CI	*P*-value
Sex	0.952	0.081–11.134	0.969
Age at SLE diagnosis	1.019	0.972–1.069	0.437
Pregnancy	1.385	0.466–4.111	0.558
Miscarriage	4.000	0.989–16.179	0.052
Smoking	0.526	0.055–5.035	0.577
Raynaud's phenomenon	3.230	0.933–11.182	0.064
Venous thrombosis	1.652	0.455–5.993	0.445
SLEDAI (total)	0.945	0.802–1.113	0.501
Malar rash	0.812	0.141–4.640	0.809
Photosensitivity	0.313	0.057–1.703	0.179
Arthritis	0.136	0.018–1.003	0.050
Serositis	3.172	0.708–14.213	0.131
Renal involvement	0.881	0.191–4.068	0.871
Neuropsychiatric involvement	0.560	0.105–2.989	0.498
Anti-Sm	1.046	0.278–3.932	0.947
Anti-RNP	2.412	0.756–7.694	0.137
Anti-La	1.040	0.182–5.953	0.965
Anti-Ro	1.250	0. 359–4.348	0.726
Anticardiolipin IgM	1.667	0.254–10.931	0.594
Anticardiolipin IgG	1.029	0.234–4.521	0.970
Anti-DNA	0.414	0.103–1.670	0.215
C2	1.006	0.984–1.029	0.574
CH 100	1.003	0.981–1.026	0.787
CRP	1.005	0.984–1.027	0.634
SD pattern on capillaroscopy	6.796	1.897–24.345	0.003

95% CI 95% confidence interval, *CRP* C-reactive protein, *PAH* pulmonary arterial hypertension, *SD* scleroderma pattern, *SLE* systemic lupus erythematosus

study, we did not observe a significant difference in the proportion of aCL IgM and IgG between the groups. One should note that the measurement of lupus anticoagulants and anti-beta-2 glycoprotein I is not available at our service, and thus the levels of antiphospholipid antibodies might have been underestimated.

In agreement with previous studies, we did not find an association between disease activity as assessed by SLEDAI and the development of PAH [34, 39, 41].

Miscarriage occurred in a significantly higher proportion of patients in the SLE-PAH group, all of which occurred prior to the diagnosis of PAH. It is noteworthy that termination of pregnancy should be considered for patients with PAH due to the high risk of maternal death [42].

NYHA functional class, 6MWT, and hemodynamic parameters have considerable clinical relevance, as they are the main final outcomes in PAH and have strong association with mortality [3]. Upon investigating possible correlations between the severity of PAH and clinical and laboratory markers, we did not find a difference between patients with a higher (NYHA class III/IV) or lower (NYHA class I/II) functional class severity. In addition, we did not identify an association between CI and MPAP in the RHC with the analyzed variables. However, five deaths occurred among the NYHA class III/IV patients versus only one among the NYHA class I/II patients, indicating more severe disease among patients with higher functional class.

The treatment for PAH has undergone substantial changes over the past decades. Pulmonary vasodilators, such as prostacyclin analogs, endothelin receptor antagonists, and phosphodiesterase-5 inhibitors, have significantly improved symptoms and reduced the rate of clinical deterioration [3]. In the present study, 57% of the patients had received sildenafil, 47% bosentan, and 23.8% combined treatment; none of the patients had received prostacyclin analogs, which remain scarcely available in our country. Because the immune system and/or inflammatory response abnormalities seem to be involved in the pathogenesis of PAH, especially among patients with SLE, immunosuppressant therapy is suggested for patients with SLE and PAH [42–45]. In our study, 47% of the patients had received cyclophosphamide pulse therapy for PAH.

The present study has some limitations, such as the small number of patients with PAH and prior exposure of some patients in the control group to NC, which might have resulted in selection bias, i.e., the inclusion of a larger number of patients with RP. A further limitation derives from the retrospective design of the study, which was based on a review of medical records, hindering the analysis of relevant aspects such as the response to PAH treatment. In addition, only a portion of the patients with SLE but without PAH (43%) underwent an echocardiogram for PAH screening, and thus, we could not rule out the possible inclusion of some asymptomatic PAH patients in the normal control group. Although we excluded patients with SSc overlap syndrome, we could not rule out the possible inclusion of patients with subclinical SSc in the study.

It is worth noting that this study included only patients with PAH confirmed on RHC, which is considered the gold standard for both the diagnosis and analysis of factors related to a poorer prognosis, such as elevated right atrial pressure and reduced CI [2, 3]. Due to its low prevalence, there is no recommendation for screening patients with SLE for PAH, in contrast to patients with SSc. Nevertheless, Khanna et al. (2013) [45], recently suggested that screening with Doppler echocardiography, pulmonary function tests with Dco, and serum markers, such as N-terminal pro-B-type natriuretic peptide (NT-proBNP), should be performed for patients with mixed connective tissue disease or SLE with SSc-related manifestations and symptoms suggestive of PAH.

Conclusions

In conclusion, the frequency of the SD pattern on NC was significantly increased among SLE patients with PAH compared with those without PAH. The presence of the SD pattern was associated with a 6.7 times higher risk of PAH. Thus, the present results lead us to consider the relevance of capillaroscopy evaluation for SLE patients, who are also at high risk of developing this serious and potentially fatal complication. We suggest the utilization of NC, a non-invasive method, as a screening method for patients with SLE and further annual PH screening for patients who present the SD pattern, as currently conducted for patients with SSc. Prospective and multicenter studies are needed to better elucidate the role of NC in the determination of the risk of PAH development among patients with SLE, as well as to confirm the present results.

Acknowledgements
Not applicable.

Authors' contributions
JFSD, EVMF, JOA, and CK contributed to the conception and design of the study, and to the acquisition of the data. JFSD and CK contributed to analysis and interpretations of data, and were the major contributor in writing the manuscript. All authors read and approved the final manuscript.

Author details
[1]Rheumatology Division, Medicine Department, Escola Paulista de Medicina, Universidade Federal de São Paulo (UNIFESP), São Paulo, SP, Brazil. [2]Division of Pneumology, Medicine Department, Escola Paulista de Medicina, Universidade Federal de São Paulo (UNIFESP), São Paulo, SP, Brazil. [3]Disciplina de Reumatologia da Universidade Federal de São Paulo, Rua Botucatu 740, 3 ° andar, São Paulo, SP 04023-062, Brazil.

References

1. Tsokos GC. Sytemic lupus erythematosus. N Engl J Med. 2011;365:2110–21.
2. Hoeper MM, Bogaard HJ, Condliffe R, Frantz R, KhannaD KM, et al. Definitions and diagnosis of pulmonary hypertension. J Am Coll Cardiol. 2013;(62 Suppl):D42–50.
3. Galiè N, Humbert M, Vachiery JL, Gibbs S, Lang I, Torbicki A, et al. 2015 ESC/ERS Guidelines for the diagnosis and treatment of pulmonary hypertension. Eur Heart J. 2016;37:67–119.
4. Galiè N, Manes A, Farahani KV, Pelino F, Palazzini M, Negro L, et al. Pulmonary arterial hypertension associated to connective tissue diseases. Lupus. 2005;14:713–7.
5. McGoon MD, Miller DP. REVEAL: a contemporary US pulmonary arterial hypertension registry. Eur Respir Rev. 2012;21(123):8–18.
6. Peacock AJ, Murphy NF, McMurray JJV, Caballero L, Stewart S. An epidemiological study of pulmonary arterial hypertension. Eur Respir J. 2007;30:104–9.
7. Johnson SR, Granton JT. Pulmonary hypertension in systemic sclerosis and systemic lupus erythematosus. Eur Respir Rev. 2011;20:277–86.
8. Chung L, Liu J, Parsons L, Hassoun PM, McGoon M, Badesch DB, et al. Characterization of connective tissue disease-associated pulmonary arterial hypertension from REVEAL: identifying systemic sclerosis as a unique phenotype. Chest. 2010;138:1383–94.
9. Haas C. Pulmonary hypertension associated with systemic lupus erythematosus. Bull Acad Natl Med. 2004;188:985–97.
10. Pope J. An update in pulmonary hypertension in systemic lupus erythematosus – do we need to know about it? Lupus. 2008;17:274–7.
11. Prabu A, Patel K, Yee CS, Nightingale P, Situnayake RD, Thickett DR, et al. Prevalence and risk factors of pulmonary arterial hypertension in patients with lupus. Rheumatology. 2009;48:1506–11.
12. Simonson JS, Schiller NB, Petri M, Hellman DB. Pulmonary hypertension in systemic lupus erythematosus. J Rheumatol. 1989;16:918–25.
13. Foïs E, Le Guern V, Dupuy A, Humbert M, Mouthon L, Guillevin L. Noninvasive assessment of systolic pulmonary artery pressure in systemic lupus erythematosus: retrospective analysis of 93 patients. Clin Exp Rheumatol. 2010;28:836–41.
14. Chow SL, Chandran V, Fazelzad R, Johnson SR. Prognostic factors for survival in systemic lupus erythematosus associated pulmonary hypertension. Lupus. 2012;21:353–64.
15. Qian J, Wang Y, Huang C, Yang X, Zhao J, Wang Q, et al. Survival and prognostic factors of systemic lupus erythematosus-associated pulmonary arterial hypertension: a PRISMA-compliant systematic review and meta-analysis. Autoimmun Rev. 2016;15:250–7.
16. Tselios K, Gladman DD, Urowitz MB. Systemic lupus erythematosus and pulmonary arterial hypertension: links, risks, and management strategies. Open Access Rheumatol. 2016;9:1–9.
17. Condliffe R, Kiely DG, Peacock AJ, Corris PA, Gibbs JS, Vrapi F, et al. Connective tissue disease-associated pulmonary arterial hypertension in the modern treatment era. Am J Respir Crit Care Med. 2009;179:151–7.
18. Dhala A. Pulmonary arterial hypertension in systemic lupus erythematosus: current status and future direction. Clin Dev Immunol 2012;2012:854–941.
19. Lian F, Chen D, Wang Y, Ye Y, Wang X, Zhan Z, et al. Clinical features and independent predictors of pulmonary arterial hypertension in systemic lupus erythematosus. Rheumatol Int. 2012;32:1727–31.
20. Huang C, Li M, Liu Y, Wang Q, Guo X, Zhao J, et al. Baseline characteristics and risk factors of pulmonary arterial hypertension in systemic lupus erythematosus patients. Medicine (Baltimore). 2016;95:e2761.
21. Souza EJ, Kayser C. Nailfold capillaroscopy: relevance to the practice of rheumatology. Rev Bras Reumatol. 2015;55:264–71.
22. Hofstee HM, Vonk Noordegraaf A, Voskuyl AE, Dijkmans BA, Postmus PE, Smulders YM, et al. Nailfold capillary density is associated with the presence and severity of pulmonary arterial hypertension in systemic sclerosis. Ann Rheum Dis. 2009;68:191–5.
23. Riccieri V, Vasile M, Iannace N, Stefanantoni K, Sciarra I, Vizza CD, et al. Systemic sclerosis patients with and without pulmonary arterial hypertension: a nailfold capillaroscopy study. Rheumatology. 2013;52:1525–8.
24. Ong YY, Nikoloutsopoulos T, Bond CP, Smith MD, Ahern MJ, Roberts-Thomson PJ. Decreased nailfold capillary density in limited scleroderma with pulmonary hypertension. Asian Pac J Allergy Immunol. 1998;16:81–6.
25. Ohtsuka T, Hasegawa A, Nakano A, Yamakage A, Yamaguchi M, Miyachi Y. Nailfold capillary abnormality and pulmonary hypertension in systemic sclerosis. Int J Dermatol. 1997;36:116–22.
26. Hochberg MC. Updating the American College of Rheumatology revised criteria for the classification of systemic lupus erythematosus. Arthritis Rheum. 1997;40:1725.
27. Bombardier C, Gladman DD, Urowitz MB, Caron D, Chang CH. Derivation of the SLEDAI. A disease activity index for lupus patients. The committee on prognosis studies in SLE. Arthritis Rheum. 1992;35:630–40.
28. Maricq HR, LeRoy EC, D'Angelo WA, Medsger TA Jr, Rodnan GP, Sharp GC, et al. Diagnostic potential of in vivo capillary microscopy in scleroderma and related disorders. Arthritis Rheum. 1980;23:183–8.
29. Sekiyama JY, Camargo CZ, Andrade LE, Kayser C. Reliability of Widefield Nailfold Capillaroscopy and Videocapillaroscopy in the assessment of patients with Raynaud's Phenomenon. Arthritis Care Res. 2013;65:1853–61.
30. The Criteria Committee of the New York Heart Association. Nomenclature and criteria for diagnosis of diseases of the heart and great vessels. 9th ed. Boston: Lippincott Williams and Wilkins; 1994.
31. Furtado RN, Pucinelli ML, Cristo VV, Andrade LE, Sato EI. Scleroderma-like nailfold capillaroscopic abnormalities are associated with anti-U1-RNP antibodies and Raynaud's phenomenon in SLE patients. Lupus. 2002;11:35–41.
32. Herrick AL, Moore TL, Murray AK, Whidby N, Manning JB, Bhushan M, et al. Nail-fold capillary abnormalities are associated with anti-centromere antibody and severity of digital ischemia. Rheumatology. 2010;49:1776–82.
33. Li EK, Tam LS. Pulmonary hypertension in systemic lupus erythematosus: clinical association and survival in 18 patients. J Rheumatol. 1999;26:1923–9.
34. Asherson RA, Higenbottam TW, Dinh Xuan AT, Khamashta MA, Hughes GR. Pulmonary hypertension in a lupus clinic: experience with twenty-four patients. J Rheumatol. 1990;17:1292–8.

35. Kasparian A, Floros A, Gialafos E, Kanakis M, Tassiopoulos S, Kafasi N, et al. Raynaud's phenomenon is correlated with elevated systolic pulmonary arterial pressure in patients with systemic lupus erythematosus. Lupus. 2007; 16:505–8.
36. Min HK, Lee JH, Jung SM, Lee J, Kang KY, Kwok SK, et al. Pulmonary hypertension in systemic lupus erythematosus: an independent predictor of patient survival. Korean J Intern Med. 2015;30:232–41.
37. Cefle A, Inanc M, Sayarlioglu M, Kamali S, Gul A, Ocal L, et al. Pulmonary hypertension in systemic lupus erythematosus: relationship with antiphospholipid antibodies and severe disease outcome. Rheumatol Int. 2011;31:183–9.
38. Xia YK, Tu SH, Hu YH, Wang Y, Chen Z, Day HT, et al. Pulmonary hypertension in systemic lupus erythematosus: a systematic review and analysis of 642 cases in Chinese population. Rheumatol Int. 2013;33:1211–7.
39. Kamel SR, Omar GM, Darwish AF, Asklany HT, Ellabban AS. Asymptomatic pulmonary hypertension in systemic lupus erythematosus. Clin Med Insights Arthritis Musculoskelet Disord. 2011;4:77–86.
40. Petri M, Rheinschmidt M, Whiting-O'Keefe Q, Hellmann D, Corash L. The frequency of lupus anticoagulant in systemic lupus erythematosus. A study of sixty consecutive patients by activated partial thromboplastin time, Russell viper venom time, and anticardiolipin antibody level. Ann Intern Med. 1987;106:524–31.
41. Chung SM, Lee CK, Lee EY, Yoo B, Lee SD, Moon HB. Clinical aspects of pulmonary hypertension in patients with systemic lupus erythematosus and in patients with idiopathic pulmonary arterial hypertension. Clin Rheumatol. 2006;25:866–72.
42. Galiè N, Hoeper MM, Humbert M, Torbicki A, Vachiery JL, Barbera JA, et al. Guidelines for the diagnosis and treatment of pulmonary hypertension: the Task Force for the Diagnosis and Treatment of Pulmonary Hypertension of the European Society of Cardiology (ESC) and the European Respiratory Society (ERS), endorsed by the International Society of Heart and Lung Transplantation (ISHLT). Eur Heart J. 2009;30:2493–537.
43. Tanaka E, Harigai M, Tanaka M, Kawaguchi Y, Hara M, Kamatani N. Pulmonary hypertension in systemic lupus erythematosus: evaluation of clinical characteristics and response to immunosuppressive treatment. J Rheumatol. 2002;29:282–7.
44. Sanchez O, Sitbon O, Jaïs X, Simonneau G, Humbert M. Immunosuppressive therapy in connective tissue diseases-associated pulmonary arterial hypertension. Chest. 2006;130:182–9.
45. Khanna D, Gladue H, Channick R, Chung L, Distler O, Furst DE, et al. Recommendations for screening and detection of connective tissue disease-associated pulmonary arterial hypertension. Arthritis Rheum. 2013;65:3194–201.

17

Effect of food intake and ambient air pollution exposure on ankylosing spondylitis disease activity

Narjes Soleimanifar[1,2,3], Mohammad Hossein Nicknam[1,3], Katayoon Bidad[4], Ahmad Reza Jamshidi[5], Mahdi Mahmoudi[5], Shayan Mostafaei[6], Zahra Hosseini-khah[2] and Behrouz Nikbin[1,2,3*]

Abstract

Background: Ankylosing spondylitis (AS) is a chronic inflammatory disease characterized by axial arthritis. The genetic–environmental factors seem to be involved in the pathogenesis of the disease and the disease debilitates patients during the most productive stages of their lives. The aim of this study was to examine the relationships between two environmental factors, diet and air pollution with disease activity and functional impairment in AS.

Methods: A case-control study was carried out. Thirty patients with AS and 30 age and sex-matched healthy controls were included. Disease scores including BASMI, BASDAI, BASFI, and BASG were calculated by means of the international Ankylosing Spondylitis Assessment working group consensus recommendations. The food intake was evaluated by semi-quantitative food frequency questionnaire (147 items FFQ). Level of air pollution indices, PM10 and PM2.5 information was obtained from the Tehran air quality control network.

Results: Total energy and fat intake, some vitamins (A, B1, B2, C) and mineral intake (potassium, calcium, iron, phosphorus, magnesium, zinc, copper and selenium) were significantly higher in patients with AS compared to controls. Fat component consumption especially Saturated Fat of Food was moderately correlated with BASFI score. PM2.5 long term exposure was strongly correlated with BASMI, BASFI and BASDAI scores of patients.

Conclusion: High-fat diet and long term exposure to air pollution are associated with worse disease outcomes reported in patients with AS. This is an interesting area of investigation in AS pathogenesis and management.

Keywords: Diet, Food intake, PM10, PM2.5, Air pollution, Ankylosing spondylitis

Introduction

Ankylosing spondylitis (AS) is a chronic progressive inflammatory disease among adults and is classified as an immune-mediated inflammatory rheumatic disease grouped under the term spondyloarthritis. It mainly Involves the axial skeleton including back, neck, or the sacroiliac joints [1, 2]. AS is often associated with physical impairments due to decreased spinal mobility and can lead to early mortality.

The Globally mean prevalence of AS per 10,000 is reported to be 16.7 in Asia, 10.2 in Latin America, 31.9 in North America, 23.8 in Europe, and 7.4 in Africa [3]. Disease activity in AS patients differs extensively, i.e., some patients have only minimal symptoms whilst others suffer from an aggressive and widespread disease which can rapidly lead to severe disability. It has been suggested that this heterogeneity can be explained by genetic factors as well as environmental factors [4–6]. Air pollution and nutrition are amongst the two crucial environmental issues that can affect this disease.

Recently, the World Health Organization (WHO) cited exposure to outdoor urban air pollution (14th) among the top 15 risk factors for the Global Burden of Disease (WHO 2009) [7]; There is a growing interest on the role of air pollution, especially particulate matter (PM), on inflammation and diseases. Sources of PM are mostly from human activities and include industrial emissions and road vehicles. Particles come in a wide range of

* Correspondence: bnik33@hotmail.com; dnik@ams.ac.ir
[1]Molecular immunology research center, Tehran University of Medical Sciences, Tehran, Iran
[2]Department of Molecular Medicine, School of Advanced Technologies in Medicine, Tehran University of Medical Sciences, Tehran, Iran
Full list of author information is available at the end of the article

sizes. Particles less than or equal to 10 μm in diameter (PM 10) are so small that they can get into the lungs, potentially causing serious health problems. Especially when fine PM with a median diameter < 2.5 μm (PM 2.5) enter the body through airways, it can trigger a systemic inflammatory response [8, 9].

Nutritional habits and food intakes can also be involved in both promoting and combating inflammatory processes. Some evidence shows correlations between nutrients and induction of chronic inflammatory diseases. Excessive energy intake stimulates adipose cell growth and proliferation, hence promotes abdominal obesity, increasing the risk of diabetes, metabolic syndrome and other chronic diseases [10, 11].We conducted the present study to evaluate relations between these two environmental risk factors, urban air pollution exposures and food intakes with disease activity of AS patients.

Methods

Patients and controls

Thirty patients with AS, diagnosed based on modified New York criteria [12], and 30 healthy age- and sex-matched controls were included. Patients with AS were recruited from the Iranian Ankylosing Spondylitis Association and healthy controls were employees of Tehran University of Medical Sciences. A questionnaire on disease information, medications, and demographic data was completed. [13, 14]. BASDAI and BASFI are recommended by the international Ankylosing Spondylitis Assessment working group consensus [15], in the clinical evaluation of patients with AS and have been shown to be specific to the disease and sensitive to change [16]. We examined possible confounders by age and race, and to control for smoking, we calculated pack-years for the whole life of each participant (number of packs/day multiplied by number of years of cigarette smoking) and current smoking status (current/former/never). The patients which had used biological drugs like TNF blockers were excluded because it as a confounding factor could mask clinical score of disease.

The study protocol was approved by the ethics board of Tehran University of Medical Sciences and written informed consent was obtained from all participants after explaining the research protocol to them.

Food intake

Food intake was evaluated by semi-quantitative food frequency questionnaire (147 items FFQ). Energy (kcal), carbohydrates (g), lipids (g), proteins (g), cholesterol mg/dl, fiber (g) and micronutrients were measured through the software N4. All anthropometric and food intake assessments were conducted by one expert in order to minimize the possible errors.

Measures of ambient PM2.5 and PM10 levels

Hourly measurements at fixed-site monitoring stations in Tehran were obtained from the Tehran air quality control network (http://air.tehran.ir/). We assigned a concentration from the operational monitor closest to the area of residence of each participant within 10 km each day. Hourly PM2.5 and PM10 concentrations were recorded across all Tehran stations; these mean hourly levels, averaged for the day of all subjects' clinical evaluations, the previous week, the previous month and the previous 3 months. In the case of an incomplete series, each missing value was imputed by using an algorithm that integrates the annual average of the incomplete series and the PM concentrations of the nearest and more correlated monitors.

Statistical analysis

All analyses were performed by SPSS 20.0 software. All variables were examined by 1-sample Kolmogorov-Smirnov test to test their normal distribution. Parametric variables were described by mean ± SD and nonparametric variables by median (range). Independent-sample t-test was used to compare means between parametric variables and the Mann-Whitney U test used to determine relationships between smoking with BASDAI and BASFI scores. Correlation analysis was performed using the Pearson and Spearman correlation coefficient for parametric and non-parametric variables, respectively. A value of $p < 0.05$ was considered statistically significant.

Results

Patients and controls

Thirty patients with AS (24 men, 6 women) with a mean age of 35 ± 10 years and 30 age-matched and sex-matched healthy controls with a mean age of 33 ± 8 years were included in the study. 13 (43%) patients and 9 (30%) healthy controls were smokers and in the patient's group, there were no significant differences between smokers and non-smokers regarding BASMI, BASFI and BASDAI score. The mean body mass index (BMI) was 21.73 (± 3.14) kg/m^2 and 21.61 (± 3.23) kg/m^2 in the AS group and healthy group, respectively without significant differences ($p > 0.05$). Mean disease duration was 10 (± 7) years and BMI was weakly correlated to disease duration in patients group ($r = 0.36$; $p = 0.049$). Of the patients studied, 22 (73.3%) were using non-steroidal anti-inflammatory drugs (NSAIDs)or disease-modifying anti-rheumatic drugs (DMARDs) or both, none were using corticosteroids or biological DMARDs and 8 (26.7%) patients were not using any drugs. The characteristics of patients are shown in Table 1.

The mean caloric consumption was 2061.66 (± 751) Kcal in AS group vs. 1652.18(± 551) Kcal in healthy group ($p = 0.028$) and the mean of total fat intake was

Table 1 Demographic characteristics of AS patients and controls

	Cases	Controls
Numbers	30	30
Age (yrs) (SD)	35.4 (10.1)	33.4 (8.1)
BMI (kg/cm^2) (SD)	21.7 (3.1)	21.6 (3.2)
Smoking status N (%)		
smoker	13 (43%)	9 (30%)
Non-smoker	17 (57%)	21 (70%)
Cigarette (pack/year) (SD)	2.6 (3.5)	2.2 (5.2)
Disease duration (yrs) (SD)	10.7 (6.7)	–
BASDAI score (SD)	4.02 (2.3)	–
BASFI Score(SD)	3.33 (2.6)	–
BASMI Score (SD)	3.38 (2.0)	–
BASG Score (SD)	4.06 (2.6)	–
Treatment N (%)		
NSAID	10 (33.3%)	
DMARD	2 (6.7%)	
NSAID+DMARD	10 (33.3%)	
No Treatment	8 (26.7%)	

BMI Body mass index, *BASDAI* Bath Ankylosing Spondylitis Disease Activity Index, *BASFI* Bath Ankylosing Spondylitis Functional Index, *BASMI* the Bath Ankylosing Spondylitis Metrology Index, *BAS-G* Bath Ankylosing Spondylitis Global Score, *NSAID* Non-steroidal anti-inflammatory drugs, *DMARD* Disease-modifying anti-rheumatic drugs

74.58 g/d in AS group and 60.57 g/d in healthy group (p = 0.02). Total energy and fat intake in patients group were significantly higher than the controls and total fat intake was weakly correlated with BASFI score of disease activity (r = 0.37; p = 0.04) in the patient group.

Analysis of the lipid intake quality showed us that the consumption of Saturated fat (SF), mono unsaturated fatty acids (MUFA) and poly unsaturated fatty acids (PUFA) was significantly higher in AS patients compared to healthy controls and the intake of all the three components was moderately correlated with BASFI score and MUFA was also moderately correlated with BASMI score of patients (Table 6).

Interestingly the diet of studied AS patients contained satisfactory levels of vitamins and minerals as compared with recommended daily allowance [17, 18]. Patients' diets contained significantly more vitamins (A, B1, B2, C) and minerals (potassium, calcium, iron, phosphorus, magnesium, zinc, copper and selenium) compared to the diet of the control group (Tables 2,3,4). Vitamin E intake was moderately correlated to BASMI score in the patient group (Table 6).

The distribution of air pollution exposure in time intervals is shown in Table 5. There was no significant difference between cases and controls air pollution exposure in the time intervals studied.

Table 2 Dietary intake of food components in AS and healthy groups

	AS patients N = 30 mean (SD)	Controls N = 30 mean (SD)	*P*-value t Test
Energy (kj/d)	2061.66 (751)	1652.18 (551)	0.02*
Carbohydrate (g/d)	71.05 (22.8)	63.35 (22.6)	0.02*
Protein (g/d)	280.09 (105)	217.75 (89)	0.21
Fat (g/d)	74.58 (29.7)	60.547 (16.1)	0.03*
Cholesterol (mg/d)	211.59 (130.7)	206.75 (90.6)	0.87
SF	21.36 (7.1)	18.96 (6.7)	0.02*
MUFA	26.04 (12.5)	19.55 (6.5)	0.018**
PUFA	18.82 (8.7)	13.83 (3.8)	0.007**
Fiber (gr/d)	29.53 (23.4)	19.56 (16.5)	0.07

SF Saturated fat of food, *MUFA* Mono unsaturated fatty acids, *PUFA* Poly unsaturated fatty acid
*: *P*-value 0.01 to 0.05, **: *P*-value 0.001 to 0.01

Mean concentration of PM 2.5 in the previous month before sampling was strongly correlated with BASFI, BASDI and BASMI score with r = 0.63, r = 0.62, and r = 0.66 respectively and p-value was less than 0.05 Table 6.

Discussion

The main purpose of our study was to find the relationship between environmental factors like diet and air pollution exposure with disease activity in a group of Iranian AS patients. There was a mild correlation between diet and disease activity, as assessed by BASFI and BASMI. This wasreflected by the results of the FFQ and nutritional calculations. Among all the essential components that were measured like proteins, the amount of carbohydrates, energy intake and fat intake in the patient group was significantly higher than the control group. In statistical analysis, only total fat intake, saturated fatty acids (SFA), mono unsaturated fatty acids (MUFA) and poly unsaturated fatty acids (PUFA) consumption was correlated with patient indices of disease, namely BASMI and BASFI.

Table 3 Dietary intake of vitamins in AS and healthy groups

Vitamins	AS patients N = 30 mean (SD)	Controls N = 30 mean (SD)	*P*-value t Test
Vitamin A (μg/d)	506.62 (250.1)	376.93 (153.8)	0.028*
Vitamin C (mg/d)	77.19 (34.5)	43.85 (29.7)	0.001**
Vitamin E (mg/d)	11.22 (6.05)	7.01 (2.5)	0.001**
Vitamin B1 (mg/d)	1.75 (0.8)	1.28 (0.7)	0.04*
Vitamin B2 (mg/d)	1.77 (0.6)	1.20 (0.3)	0.000**
Vitamin B3 (mg/d)	20.23 (8.5)	16.09 (8.8)	0.84
Vitamin B6 (mg/d)	1.53 (0.6)	1.18 (0.5)	0.03*
Vitamin B12 (mg/d)	2.72 (1.1)	2.29 (1.1)	0.17

*: *P*-value 0.01 to 0.05, **: *P*-value 0.001 to 0.01

Table 4 Dietary intake of minerals in AS and healthy groups

Minerals	AS patients N = 30 mean (SD)	Controls N = 30 mean (SD)	P-value t Test
Sodium (g/d)	2.497 (1.6)	2.00 (1.4)	0.25
Potassium (g/d)	2.80 (1.2)	1.86 (0.7)	0.002**
Calcium (mg/d)	962.34 (529.1)	608.12 (286.6)	0.003**
Iron (mg/d)	22.72 (18.1)	11.76 (6.0)	0.004**
Phosphorus (mg/d)	1237.63 (547.3)	937.08 (421.5)	0.029*
Magnesium (mg/d)	329.3 (186.6)	223.80 (114.7)	0.017*
Zinc (μg/d)	10.0 (4.1)	7.97 (3.2)	0.041*
Copper (mg)	1.42 (0.5)	1.10 (0.5)	0.029*
Selenium (ug)	135.87 (62.2)	103.26 (40.7)	0.029*

*: *P*-value 0.01 to 0.05, **: *P*-value 0.001 to 0.01

Lipid components can directly or indirectly modify immune responses [19, 20], some toward pro-inflammatory and others immunosuppressive effects. Studies have shown that saturated fatty acids (SFA) play a key role in the inflammatory process by stimulating macrophage induction and the secretion of the pro-inflammatory cytokines TNF-alpha, IL-6, and IL-8 [21, 22]. Moreover, SFA intake can trigger IL-1β secretion and also is known to cause lipemia that is more noticeable than the lipemia due to mono unsaturated fatty acids (MUFA) and PUFA and can lead to a higher pro-inflammatory state [23].

However, monounsaturated fatty acid (MUFA) and polyunsaturated fatty acid (PUFA) consumption exhibit an anti-inflammatory profile and a less pronounced pro-inflammatory response particularly in comparison with SFAs, dietary polyunsaturated fatty acids (PUFA) like linoleic acid (LA; 18:2n6) can convert into arachidonic acid (AA; 20:4n6) by a series of enzymatic reactions which is a source of more proinflammatory eicosanoids, such as prostaglandin E2 (PGE2). Recently, SUNDSTRÖM et al. have shown the correlation between plasma phospholipid levels of AA and the BASDAI score in AS patients which can explain the results of our study more [24]. In concordance, we observed that higher consumptions of SFA were more strongly correlated with BASFI score than MUFA and PUFA. Recently, serum free fatty acids have been shown as a biomarker of AS and some evidence of fat metaplasia in the pathogenesis of this disease has been revealed [25, 26]. Moreover, diet strongly influences the composition of the gut microbiota in this regards diet rich in fat and carbohydrates might impact the gut microbiota of AS patients thus subclinical gut inflammation in AS might restrict the absorption and despite high energy intake in AS, BMI is not higher than controls [27, 28].

Regarding FFQ results, most of vitamins and minerals that we measured had elevated intake levels in AS patients compared to control group, although we did not measure them in blood, this satisfactory level of vitamins and mineral consumption might be due to the willingness of the patients to improve their diseases. There is some evidence that AS patients have less vitamin A level in serum, despite higher intakes there might be some genetic polymorphisms or other reasons for poor absorption [29]. Therefore, it is highly recommended to measure dietary food components in blood to help a firm conclusion.

Our findings have shown that long term exposure (at least 1 month) to fine PM can exacerbate AS manifestations measured by BASDAI, BASFI and BASMI score. Air pollutants, especially particulate matters, can enter the body through the respiratory tract and deal with the immune system. PM10 includes a mixture of soil and road dust along with industrial emissions that makes coarse particles suspensions that is not small enough to penetrate to blood circulation and usually face with first responders immune cell types like dendritic cells and alveolar macrophages and could make local respiratory inflammations [30]. Whereas PM2.5 are mainly derived from combustion processes of diesel fuel, gasoline, and industrial processes and due to their tiny size they can pass the respiratory barriers and spread to the whole body through the bloodstream, therefore, are more associated with triggering systemic inflammations [31, 32]. Also the sustainability of pollutants and prolonged exposure to them could result in a chronic inflammation which provides a proper opportunity for unbalancing the T cell subsets toward Th1 and Th17 in a macrophage dependent fashion that can produce more elevated level of FN-γ, IL-10, IL-17 and IL-21 cytokines [33]. These activated T cells have shown to exacerbate the autoimmune disease conditions particularly in the AS [34]. However, many previous studies have shown that chronic inflammation plays

Table 5 Mean daily concentration of particulate matters exposure in time intervals in studied subjects

Day of sampling	Case		Control	
	PM 2.5 μg/m3- mean (SD)	Pm10 μg/m3-mean (SD)	PM2.5 μg/m3-mean (SD)	Pm10 μg/m3-mean (SD)
	28.2 (13.2)	85.4 (49.2)	25.9 (20.5)	60.0 (31.4)
1 month before sampling	28.7 (10.5)	76.6 (39.3)	30.0 (13.4)	73.33 (27.8)
3 months before sampling	26.4 (6.8)	76.7 (36.6)	27.6 (9.2)	67.44 (11.38)

PM Particulate Matter

Table 6 Correlations between disease activity and environmental factors in AS patients

$n = 30$	BASDAI Score correlation coefficient (*P* value)	BASFI Score correlation coefficient (*P*-value)	BASMI Score correlation coefficient (*P*-value)
Total fat of food	NS	0.37 (0.04)	NS
SF	NS	0.43 (0.01)	NS
MUFA	NS	0.36 (0.04)	0.39 (0.03)
PUFA	NS	0.37 (0.04)	NS
Vitamin E	NS	NS	0.42 (0.02)
PM2.5 in the 1 month before sampling	0.63 (0.03)	0.62 (0.04)	0.66 (0.02)

SF Saturated fat of food, *MUFA* Mono unsaturated fatty acids, *PUFA* Poly unsaturated fatty acids, *NS* Not significant

an important role in the pathogenesis of AS, there is no evidence of air born particulate matters effect on AS disease activity. Therefore our findings in the strong correlation results between long term exposure to PM2.5 and clinical manifestations of AS patients reveal a new perspective to air pollution effects on AS.

Conclusion

We found a higher consumption of total energy and fat, higher intake of some vitamins (A, B1, B2, C) and minerals (potassium calcium iron phosphorus magnesium zinc copper and selenium) in AS patients compared to controls. This can be due to the fact that patients are more aware of the effect of nutrition and they try to have a better diet. Fat component intake, especially Saturated Fat of Food was moderately correlated with BASFI score. This might be a field for further research and intervention in patients. Although air pollution exposure were not different among patients and controls, PM2.5 long term exposure was strongly correlated with BASMI, BASFI and BASDAI score of disease in the patient group. Living in areas with lower air pollution might be a solution for AS patients.

Acknowledgements
We thank Maryam Chamari for excellent FFQ analysis.

Authors' contributions
NS performed the experimental work, data analysis and wrote the manuscript, MN conceived the idea and co-supervised the project, KB designed the study and reviewed and corrected the manuscript, AJ evaluated patients and confirmed their disease, MM acquisition of patients' clinical data and revised the manuscript, SHM and NS analyzed and interpreted the data, ZH and NS contributed to the air quality control data collection, BN supervised the project, obtained funds. All authors were involved in the final approval of the manuscript.

Author details
[1]Molecular immunology research center, Tehran University of Medical Sciences, Tehran, Iran. [2]Department of Molecular Medicine, School of Advanced Technologies in Medicine, Tehran University of Medical Sciences, Tehran, Iran. [3]Department of Immunology, Tehran University of Medical Sciences, Tehran, Iran. [4]Immunology, Asthma and Allergy Research Institute, Tehran University of Medical Sciences, Tehran, Iran. [5]Rheumatology Research Center, Tehran University of Medical Sciences, Tehran, Iran. [6]Department of Community Medicine, Faculty of Medicine, Kermanshah University of Medical Sciences, Kermanshah, Iran.

References

1. Dakwar E, et al., A review of the pathogenesis of ankylosing spondylitis. 2008.
2. Raychaudhuri SP, Deodhar A. The classification and diagnostic criteria of ankylosing spondylitis. J Autoimmun. 2014;48:128–33.
3. Dean LE, et al. Global prevalence of ankylosing spondylitis. Rheumatology. 2014;53(4):650–7.
4. Shiue I. Relationship of environmental exposures and ankylosing spondylitis and spinal mobility: US NHAENS, 2009–2010. Int J Environ Health Res. 2015; 25(3):322–9.
5. Fallahi S, et al. The correlation between pack-years of smoking and disease activity, quality of life, spinal mobility, and sacroiliitis grading in patients with ankylosing spondylitis. Turk J Rheumatol. 2013;28(3):181–8.
6. Soleimanifar N, et al. Study of programmed cell death 1 (PDCD1) gene polymorphims in Iranian patients with ankylosing spondylitis. Inflammation. 2011;34(6):707–12.
7. Organization, W.H, Global health risks: mortality and burden of disease attributable to selected major risks. 2009: World Health Organization.
8. Bernatsky S, et al. Fine particulate air pollution and systemic autoimmune rheumatic disease in two Canadian provinces. Environ Res. 2016;146:85–91.
9. Hamra, G.B., et al., Outdoor particulate matter exposure and lung cancer: a systematic review and meta-analysis. 2014.
10. Hajer GR, van Haeften TW, Visseren FL. Adipose tissue dysfunction in obesity, diabetes, and vascular diseases. Eur Heart J. 2008;29(24):2959–71.
11. Rayssiguier Y, et al. High fructose consumption combined with low dietary magnesium intake may increase the incidence of the metabolic syndrome by inducing inflammation. Magnes Res. 2006;19(4):237–43.
12. Linden SVD, Valkenburg HA, Cats A. Evaluation of diagnostic criteria for ankylosing spondylitis. Arthritis Rheumatol. 1984;27(4):361–8.
13. Garrett S, et al. A new approach to defining disease status in ankylosing spondylitis: the Bath ankylosing spondylitis disease activity index. J Rheumatol. 1994;21(12):2286–91.
14. Bidad K, et al. Evaluation of the Iranian versions of the bath ankylosing spondylitis disease activity index (BASDAI), the bath ankylosing spondylitis functional index (BASFI) and the patient acceptable symptom state (PASS) in patients with ankylosing spondylitis. Rheumatol Int. 2012;32(11):3613–8.
15. Zochling J, Braun J. Quality indicators, guidelines and outcome measures in ankylosing spondylitis. Clin Exp Rheumatol. 2007;25(6):S147.
16. Yanık B, et al. Adaptation of the Bath ankylosing spondylitis functional index to the Turkish population, its reliability and validity: functional assessment in AS. Clin Rheumatol. 2005;24(1):41–7.
17. Intakes, I.o.M.S.C.o.t.S.E.o.D.R., Dietary reference intakes for thiamin, riboflavin, niacin, vitamin B6, folate, vitamin B12, pantothenic acid, biotin, and choline. 1998: National Academies Press (US).
18. Alaimo, K., et al., Dietary intake of vitamins, minerals, and fiber of persons ages 2 months and over in the United States: third National Health and nutrition examination survey, phase 1, 1988-91. Adv Data, 1994(258): p. 1–28.
19. Calder PC. Dietary fatty acids and lymphocyte functions. Proc Nutr Soc. 1998;57(04):487–502.

20. Harbige LS, Fisher BA. Dietary fatty acid modulation of mucosally-induced tolerogenic immune responses. Proc Nutr Soc. 2001;60(04):449–56.
21. Rocha D, et al. Saturated fatty acids trigger TLR4-mediated inflammatory response. Atherosclerosis. 2016;244:211–5.
22. Chait A, Kim F. Saturated fatty acids and inflammation: who pays the toll? Am Heart Assoc. 2010.
23. L'homme L, et al. Unsaturated fatty acids prevent activation of NLRP3 inflammasome in human monocytes/macrophages. J Lipid Res. 2013;54(11): 2998–3008.
24. Sundström B, et al. Plasma phospholipid fatty acid content is related to disease activity in ankylosing spondylitis. J Rheumatol. 2012;39(2):327–33.
25. Chen R, et al. Serum fatty acid profiles and potential biomarkers of ankylosing spondylitis determined by gas chromatography–mass spectrometry and multivariate statistical analysis. Biomed Chromatogr. 2015; 29(4):604–11.
26. Maksymowych WP, et al. Fat metaplasia and backfill are key intermediaries in the development of sacroiliac joint ankylosis in patients with ankylosing spondylitis. Arthritis Rheumatol. 2014;66(11):2958–67.
27. Xiao L, et al. High-fat feeding rather than obesity drives taxonomical and functional changes in the gut microbiota in mice. Microbiome. 2017;5(1):43.
28. Sundström B, Wållberg-Jonsson S, Johansson G. Diet, disease activity, and gastrointestinal symptoms in patients with ankylosing spondylitis. Clin Rheumatol. 2011;30(1):71–6.
29. O'Shea FD, et al. Retinol (vitamin a) and retinol-binding protein levels are decreased in ankylosing spondylitis: clinical and genetic analysis. J Rheumatol. 2007;34(12):2457–9.
30. Fujii T, et al. Interaction of alveolar macrophages and airway epithelial cells following exposure to particulate matter produces mediators that stimulate the bone marrow. Am J Respir Cell Mol Biol. 2002;27(1):34–41.
31. Ristovski ZD, et al. Respiratory health effects of diesel particulate matter. Respirology. 2012;17(2):201–12.
32. Zhang Y, et al. Effect of atmospheric PM2. 5 on expression levels of NF-κB genes and inflammatory cytokines regulated by NF-κB in human macrophage. Inflammation. 2018;41(3):784–94.
33. Ma Q-Y, et al. Exposure to particulate matter 2.5 (PM2. 5) induced macrophage-dependent inflammation, characterized by increased Th1/Th17 cytokine secretion and cytotoxicity. Int Immunopharmacol. 2017;50:139–45.
34. Rezaiemanesh A, et al. Immune cells involved in the pathogenesis of ankylosing spondylitis. Biomed Pharmacother. 2018;100:198–204.

Clinical and epidemiologic characterization of patients with systemic lupus erythematosus admitted to an intensive care unit in Colombia

Maria Fernanda Alvarez Barreneche[1,5*], William Dario Mcewen Tamayo[2], Daniel Montoya Roldan[3], Libia Maria Rodriguez Padilla[2], Carlos Jaime Velasquez Franco[2,4] and Miguel Antonio Mesa Navas[2,4]

Abstract

Objective: Describe the clinical and epidemiologic characteristics of patients with systemic lupus erythematosus (SLE) admitted to the intensive care unit (ICU).

Methods: a retrospective study with medical records review of patients with systemic lupus erythematosus (SLE) admitted to the ICU between 2004 and 2015 were included. Qualitative variables were described using absolute and relative frequencies. For quantitative variables mean value and standard deviation (SD) or median value with the interquartile range (IQR) depending on data distribution. To compare groups, it was used the Student t-test or Mann Whitney U test as appropriate and Fisher's exact test.

Results: 33 patients were included, with a total of 45 ICU admissions, 29 (87.9%) were females with a median age of 26 years. The median time of diagnosis of SLE was two years, (IQR 1.5–5). The most common SLE manifestation and comorbidity were renal disease and hypertension with 27 (81.8%) and 14 (42.4%) respectively. The main reason for admittance was lupus flare with 25 events (55.5%). Infection was the second cause of admission with 19 events (42.2%). The median stay time in the ICU was four days (IQR 2–7). LODS score was 6 (RIQ 5–8), and APACHE II score was 13 (RIQ 11–17.7). There were 29 infections (64.5%) of which 20 (69%) were hospital-acquired. Four (12.1%) patients died.

Conclusion: Unlike most of the previously reported series, in this study SLE activity was the most common cause of admission in the ICU. A more aggressive disease and difficulties in the ambulatory setting could explain this behavior. Despite the higher percentage of lupus flares, there was lower mortality.

Keywords: Lupus erythematosus, Systemic, Intensive care unit, Symptom flare up, Infection, Mortality

Introduction

Rheumatological diseases (RD) are a heterogeneous group of entities with a chronic course and multisystemic involvement associated with significant morbidity and mortality. The complexity of the management of these diseases in the intensive care unit (ICU) lies in the fact that their complications do not derive only from the activity of RD, but from other associated factors such as the side effects of treatment and the lower functional reserve derived from cumulative damage to this type of diseases [1, 2].

Historically, patients with rheumatoid arthritis (RA) have occupied the first place of RD admitted to the ICU [3]. However, this has changed in recent decades secondary to therapeutic advances that have allowed better control of the disease and less dependence on steroidal therapy and non-steroidal anti-inflammatory drugs (NSAIDs). This has led to less prevalent diseases such as systemic lupus erythematosus (SLE) occupy their place as a cause of admission to ICU within the RD [3–5], generating a knowledge gap, which is particularly important given that the behavior of SLE differs significantly from other ERs.

* Correspondence: mariafernandaalvarezbarrenech@gmail.com
[1]Clínica Cardiovid, Calle 78 # 75-21, Medellín, Antioquia, Colombia
[5]Medellin, Colombia
Full list of author information is available at the end of the article

At the local level, few studies provide information on patients with SLE and admission to the ICU, and those that do exist to RD in general [2, 6–9]. It is therefore essential to have data of SLE in Latin America since certain factors vary with a geographic location such as race and access to health services that can significantly affect the prognosis of this disease [10, 11]. Additionally, the therapeutic advances in the different rheumatological diseases have not been the same, which accentuates the differences between them.

The objective of this study is to define the epidemiological and clinical characteristics of patients with SLE who enter to ICU in a reference hospital, with experience in the management of autoimmune diseases in the city of Medellin, Colombia. This study will serve to determine the characteristics of patients that enter to ICU and plan management strategies.

Patients and methods

Study design and patient selection

A retrospective descriptive study of medical records from adult patients with SLE admitted to ICU at Clinica Universitaria Bolivariana (CUB) (Medellin, Colombia) between the years 2004 and 2015. The inclusion criteria were: patients over 18 years of age, diagnosed with SLE according to the classification criteria of ACR [12]. admitted to the ICU during the study period. We excluded patients with concomitant oncological diseases, transplanted with active graft and immunosuppressive therapy and those whose records of clinical history were incomplete for the variables of interest.

Data collection

The information was obtained through the review of the physical and electronic histories of patients who met the eligibility criteria of the study and was recorded in an electronic format (Magpi) designed considering the study variables (at admission, hospital stay and discharge from the ICU). A pilot test was carried out with ten clinical histories to assess the quality of the form and the need to adjust. The data was collected by two researchers if there were missing information in the selected ICU records; the data was searched in the laboratory results, nurse registry, and the patient's treatment specialties notes.

The variables that were investigated in the registries to fulfill the objectives of the study were demographic, clinical, treatment and outcomes (conditions of discharge, overall mortality, days of ICU stay, nosocomial infections, surgical interventions required). For the sepsis criteria, the Surviving Sepsis 2012 guidelines were considered [13], the renal failure was diagnosed according to the diagnostic criteria of acute kidney injury of KDIGO 2012 [14].

Statistical analysis

To describe the qualitative variables, absolute and relative frequencies were used and for the quantitative variables mean and standard deviation (SD) or the median with interquartile range (RIQ) were used depending on the distribution of the data. To compare groups it was used the Student t-test or Mann Whitney U test as appropriate and Fisher's exact test. P values < 0.05 were considered statistically significant. All the analyses were carried out in the statistical package IBM SPSS version 24.

Results

Demographic characteristics and comorbidities

A total of 959 records were reviewed, of which 33 patients met the eligibility criteria, presenting 45 episodes of admission to the ICU. Of the 33 patients, 29 (87.9%) were female, with an median age of 26 years. Regarding comorbidities, 21 (63.6%) had at least one comorbidity at the time of admission to the ICU, the most frequent being arterial hypertension 14 (42.4%), followed by chronic kidney disease (18.1%) (Table 1).

Baseline characteristics

The median time of SLE diagnosis was two years (RIQ 1–5.5 years), the most frequent clinical manifestation was renal involvement, in 27 patients (81.8%), followed by joint in 19 (57.6%). Regarding the place from which the patients were transferred to the ICU, most of them entered from the emergency department, 19 (57.6%) patients. Eleven patients (33.3%) were referred from other institutions, and four patients (12.1%) had had a previous hospitalization, mainly due to disease activity. The most frequent

Table 1 Demographic characteristics of SLE patients admitted to the ICU

Characteristic	$N = 33$ n (%)
Female sex	29 (87,9)
Age[a]	26 (23–35)
Comorbidities	21 (63,6)
• Arterial hypertension	14 (42,4)
• Chronic renal failure	6 (18,1)
o Dyalisis	3
• Hypothyroidism	5 (15,1)
• Cerebrovascular disease	5 (15,1)
• Tuberculosis	3 (9,0)
• Diabetes	2 (6,0)
• Cardiac failure	1 (3,0)
• Asthma	1 (3,0)
• Peripheral artery disease	1 (3,0)

[a]Median/Interquartile range (IQR)

ambulatory therapeutic strategy was steroids 28 (84.8%), followed by antimalarials 22 (66.6%). (Table 2).

Clinical and paraclinical characteristics upon admission to the ICU

During the evaluated period there were 45 ICU admissions, corresponding to 33 patients, from this moment onward we will refer to the 45 admission events. The leading cause of admission was disease activity with 25 events (55.5%), followed by infection with 19 events (42.2%). The most frequent organic involvement was renal with 24 events (53.3%) explained mainly by lupus nephritis (Table 3). Table 4 shows the vital signs and the paraclinical signs on admission. The calculation of the SELENA SLEDAI was possible only in 23 events, with an average score of 20 (SD 11).

When comparing at baseline the patients who presented infection (Table 5) versus those who did not, it was found that the APACHE was higher, as well as the CRP, other variables such as the time of diagnosis of the disease, type of baseline commitment or the previous use of steroids were not more at the time of admission due to infection. When comparing at baseline patients who were admitted for disease activity with those who did not (Table 5), more renal involvement, hemolytic anemia, and thrombocytopenia were found.

Table 2 Baseline clinical characteristics

Baseline clinic characteristics	*N* = 33 *n* (%)
Disease diagnosis time in years[a]	2 (1–5,5)
SLE manifestation	
• Renal	27 (81,8)
• Articular	19 (57,6)
• Hematological	19 (57,6)
• Mucocutaneous	18 (54,5)
• Serositis	8 (24,2)
• Central Nervous System	8 (24,2)
• Pulmonary	4 (12,1)
Previous hospitalization	28 (84,8)
Previous hospitalization days[a]	5 (1–15)
Previous ICU admission	4 (12,1)
Outpatient treatment	
• Steroids	28 (84,8)
• Chloroquine	22 (66,6)
• Rituximab	4 (12,1)
• Azathioprine	4 (12,1)
• Mycophenolate	4 (12,1)
• Cyclophosphamide	2 (6,0)
• Methotrexate	1 (3,0)
• Leflunomide	1 (3,0)
• Calcineurin inhibitors	1 (3,0)

[a]Median/Interquartile range (IQR)

Table 3 Clinical characteristics upon admission to ICU in 45 events

Clinical characteristics upon admission to ICU	*N* = 45 n (%)
Reasons for UCI admission	
• Disease activity	25 (55,5)
• Infection	19 (42,2)
• Ventilatory failure	18 (40,0)
• Cardiovascular emergency	12 (26,7)
• Hemorrhage	7 (15,5)
• Dialytic urgency	6 (13,3)
• Postsurgery care	5 (11,1)
Organic commitment	
• Renal involvement	24 (53,3)
• Haematological commitment	19 (42,2)
o Hemolytic anemia	13 (28,9)
o Thrombocytopenia	13 (28,9)
o Lymphopenia	10 (22,2)
o Neutropenia	6 (13,3)
• Lung commitment	18 (40,0)
o Acute Pulmonary Edema	8 (17,8)
o ARDS[a]	5 (11,1)
o Pleural effusion	4 (8,9)
o Alveolar hemorrhage	4 (8,9)
o Pneumonitis	3 (6,7)
o Pulmonary embolism	1 (2,2)
• Commitment of CNS[b]	9 (20,0)
o Vasculitis	4 (8,8)
o Hemorrhage	2 (4,4)
o Optic neuritis	1 (2,2)
o Myelopathy	1 (2,2)
o Autoimmune encephalitis	1 (2,2)
• Cardiac commitment	5 (11,1)
o Myocarditis	1 (2,2)
o Pericarditis	4 (8,9)
• Gastrointestinal commitment	5 (11,1)
o Hepatitis	4 (8,9)
o Digestive tract hemorrhage	1 (2,2)
o Pancreatitis	1 (2,2)

[a]Acute Respiratory Distress Syndrome, [b]CNS central nervous system

Management during the stay in ICU

Antibiotics were used in 31 (68.9%) of the 45 admissions with carbapenems and piperacillin/tazobactam as the most

Table 4 Vital signs and laboratory upon admission to the ICU

Vital signs and laboratory	$N = 45$ Media (SD)
Heart rate (bpm)	101 (22,1)
Systolic pressure (mmHg)	126 (39,0)
Diastolic pressure (mmHg)	77 (23,6)
PaFi	313 (158,8)
Hemoglobin (g / dL)	9,2 (2,3)
INR	1,14 (0,2)
Apache II[a]	13 (11–17,7)
SLEDAI[b]	20 (11,0)
LODS Score [a]	6 (5–8)
Creatinine (mg / dL)[a]	1,3 (0,8-3,55)
Platelets (cel / mm3)	204593 (116.000)
CRP[a]	5,0 (2,4-11,0)
Glasgow	
• < 15	9 (20,0)
• 15	36 (80,0)

[a]Median (RIQ), [b]It could only be taken in 23 patients, CRP c reactive protein

frequently used in 15 (33.1%) and 12 (26.7%) respectively. Treatment for tuberculosis was used in three cases (6.7%) and seven (15.5%) received antifungal treatment. Immunosuppression was mainly used in the form of pulses of methylprednisolone in 22 admissions (48.9%). Concerning additional supports, mechanical ventilation was used in 14 cases (31.1%), hemodialysis in 16 events (35.5%) and the latter could be removed while in the ICU in two cases (Table 6).

The most frequent diagnostic procedures were renal biopsies 5/17 (29.4%), in addition, five abdominal procedures were performed, two emergent cesarean deliveries, one embolization of an arteriovenous fistula, two bronchoalveolar lavages, one pleural decortication, and one femoropopliteal arterial bypass.

Complications and outcomes

Infections occurred in 29 events (64.4%), 20 (69.0%) corresponding to nosocomial infections, of these, pneumonia was the most frequent 12/20 (60.0%). Seven events were community-acquired infections consisting mainly in urinary tract infections which occurred in three patients (42.9%) (Table 7). Of the 29 infectious events in 21 (72.2%), microbiological isolation was obtained with a total of 43 germs, of them there were 24 g negative bacilli (BGN) (55.8%), being the most frequent *E.coli* with five (11.6%) isolates. Twelve of the isolates were gram positive cocci (CGP) (27.9%), with *S.aureus* as the most frequent one with five isolates (11.6%). There were five fungal isolations (11.6%) and two (4.7%) of *Mycobacterium tuberculosis.*

Table 5 Comparison of principals reasons for admission and main variables

	Infection	NO Infection	*P* value	Disease activity	NO disease activity	*P* value
Age	30	24.5	0.345	25	32	0.146
Disease diagnosis time in years	2	2	0.972	2	2	0.470
Comorbidities	11	21	0.091	17	15	0.429
Organic basal commitment						
• Renal	16	22	0.641	23	15	0.126
• CNS	4	9	0.257	8	5	0.429
• Pulmonary	4	4	0.456	5	3	0.498
• Hematologic	12	11	0.140	14	9	0.333
APACHE score	16	12	**0.007**	14	12	0.457
LODS score	7	6	0.199	6	6	0.806
CRP	8.3	3.6	**0.011**	5.1	4.3	0.585
Previously steroid use	16	21	0.544	21	16	0.513
Organic commitment during hospitalization						
• Renal	9	11	0.486	16	4	**0.004**
• Pulmonary	7	11	0.477	13	5	0.062
• Hemolytic anemia	7	6	0.250	13	0	**0.001**
• Thrombocytopenia	7	6	0.250	12	1	**0.001**
Dyalisis support	6	19	0.438	10	6	0.352
Immunoglobulin use	5	2	0.1	6	1	0.089
Time at ICU	5	4	0.224	3	4.5	0.818

Boldface is the values with stadistic signficance $p < 0.05$

Table 6 Therapeutic management during the stay in the ICU

Therapeutic treatment	N = 45 n(%)
Required antibiotic	31 (68,9)
• Carbapenem	15 (33,1)
• Piperacillin / tazobactam	12 (26,7)
• Vancomycin	10 (22,2)
• Ceftriaxone	7 (15,5)
• Ampicillin sulbactam	5 (11,1)
• Anti MRSA does not vancomycin *	5 (11,1)
• Ciprofloxacin	4 (8,9)
• Tuberculosis treatment	3 (6,7)
• Cefazolin	3 (6,7)
• Clarithromycin	2 (4,4)
• Polymyxin B	1 (2,2)
• Penicillin	1 (2,2)
Required Antifungal	7 (15,5)
• Fluconazole	4 (8,9)
• Voriconazole	2 (4,4)
• Caspofungin	1 (2,2)
• Anidulafungin	1 (2,2)
Immunosuppression	
• Pulses Methylprednisolone	22 (48,9)
• Cyclophosphamide	18 (40,0)
• Immunoglobulin	7 (15,5)
• Rituximab	3 (6,7)
Supports	
• Mechanical ventilation	14 (31,1)
• Days, Medium (RIQ)	5,5 (3–17,75)
• Dialytic support	16 (35,5)
• Vasopressor support	9 (20,0)
Procedures	17 (37,7)
Red blood cells transfusion	31 (68,9)
Platelet aferesis	7 (15,5)
Fresh frozen plasma	8 (17,7)
Plasmaferesis	1 (2,2)

* Anti MRSA not vancomycin (Daptomycin, clindamycin and linezolid)

Acute kidney injury was observed in 24 events (53.3%), of these 12/24 (50.0%) KDIGO 3. The LODS score on admission (was available in 38 events) was 6 (RIQ 5–8). The median number of days of mechanical ventilation was 5.5 (RIQ 3–17), the median time of stay in the ICU was four days (RIQ 2–7).

Finally, in terms of mortality, four patients died (12.1%), two of them were men. Three deaths were due to septic shock and subsequent multiple organ failure and the remaining one due to accidental decannulation after tracheostomy with secondary ventilatory failure, all had an infection at the time of death, and three were receiving dialysis support.

Table 7 Complications and outcomes

Complications	n/N (%)
Infections	**29/45 (64,4)**
• Nosocomial	20/29 (69,0)
o Pneumonia	12/20 (60,0)
o Urinary tract infection	7/20 (35,0)
o Bacteriemia	7/20 (35,0)
o Soft tissue	2/20 (10,0)
o Intrabdominal	1/20 (5,0)
• Acquired in the community	7/29 (24,1)
o Urinary tract infection	3/7 (42,9)
o Pneumonia	2/7 (28,6)
o Bacteriemia	2/7 (28,6)
o Soft tissue	1/7 (14,3)
o Intrabdominal	1/7 (14,3)
• Nosocomial and acquiered in community	2/29 (6,9)
Acute kidney injury	24/45 (53,3)
Re-admissions to ICU	7/45 (21,2)
Death	4/33 (12,1)

Boldface is the values with stadistic signficance $p < 0.05$

Discussion

The present study describes the characteristics of all the admissions to the ICU of patients in a reference center for RD. As expected, there is a predominance of women of reproductive age typical of the behavior of the disease [1, 12, 15]. Compared with different series, both the age and the predominance of the female sex are similar; this is important because although the SLE tends to be thought of as a single entity, its behavior varies significantly according to sex, race, and age [16]. This is evidenced, for example, in Abramovich's study [17] that evaluated the mortality of patients with SLE who were admitted to the ICU due to sepsis. In this study, the average age of admission was 55 years with an accumulated damage scale in SLICC lupus [18, 19] between 5 and 7, which is a high value and with cardiovascular comorbidity in 27%. The mortality found was 31%, with the main risk factor being cardiovascular dysfunction due to sepsis, a finding that is not found in other series and was expected considering their baseline characteristics.

Despite the young age of the patients, it was found a high rate of comorbidities, especially high blood pressure, which was present in 42% and renal failure with 18%, these being unusual in such a high proportion in this age group and making more difficult the management of these patients [3, 8]. Interestingly, patients entered with high levels of disease activity (SLEDAI 20) but with an APACHE median score of 13, which is low compared to other series of both rheumatologic diseases in general [2, 8, 20] as well as those that consider SLE only [1, 4, 16, 21–24]. This aspect is important given that mortality in this study is one of the lowest reported even though the SLEDAI score was elevated whether it is compared with the oldest series (40%) [1, 16, 24] or with the most recent ones, where mortality is around 20% [23, 25]. A possible explanation for this finding is the low APACHE score of these patients reflecting an early admission strategy to the ICU.

The leading cause of admission was activity; this differs from several series, where infection plays a preponderant role [1, 21, 23]. Only a few cohorts report disease activity as a cause of hospitalization [25, 26] and in some, as in the study by Whitelaw et al. [27] more than half of the patients had less than six months of diagnosis of SLE, which would explain the predominance of activity. In the present cohort, the average time of diagnosis was two years; the high activity was possibly a reflection of difficulties in outpatient management. This should be highlighted given that reduced access to health services has been associated with a worse prognosis in SLE [28] and is usually associated with the requirement of greater immunosuppressive therapy for more extended periods and consequently greater cumulative damage. When comparisons were made between patients with infections as a reason for admission to ICU, It was found that APACHE was higher, as well as the CRP. Also, in patients with activity of disease at baseline was more common renal involvement, hemolytic anemia, and thrombocytopenia. However, it should be noted that this analysis is merely exploratory and should be verified with other types of studies. In addition, the cause of infection with disease activity was sometimes overlapped, given the difficulties that often exist in differentiating one from the other and that the same infection can lead to disease activity.

Infections were nosocomial in 69%, which explains the broad antimicrobial spectrum used. There was a large amount of gram-negative bacillus being *E.coli* the leading isolation, nonetheless, there were other germs that are not common in the non-immunosuppressed population as previously reported [1, 28]. This high percentage of infection can be explained by the high number of patients in whom a high dose of methylprednisolone treatment was required to control the activity of the disease. Previous studies have shown that the use of steroids is an independent risk factor for infection [4, 28].

Mechanical ventilation was used in 31% of the patients for a median of 5 days, which is lower than that reported in other cohorts, where it was used between 68 and 77% of patients for an average of 10 days [7, 9, 20, 29]. This may be due to the cause of admission in our patients in which renal involvement predominated. This could be one of the reasons for the overall low mortality, and possibly reflects the transfer of less ill patients to the ICU as evidenced by its APACHE score as has been mentioned previously.

The median of LODS score was 6 and of APACHE II score was 13, which predicts mortality of 18.6%, higher than the observed. Concerning the APACHE II score, some series have shown their correlation with mortality, although in most of them with confidence intervals close to unity [9, 22, 30]. The mean value of APACHE II in this study was low if the series mentioned above are considered, even more, when the predictive value found in several studies is between 18 and 20 [9, 22, 30].

One aspect that is worth mentioning is that all cases of mortality were related to infectious processes; which emphasizes the need to perform subsequent analyzes in order to detect factors that may be modifiable. Finally, it is striking that half of the patients who died were men, which is in agreement with the prognosis that has been established, where sex has a significant weight in manifestations and mortality [31–33].

This study has several limitations, due to its retrospective nature it was frequent that the medical records lacked some data. On the other hand, having been performed in a single center of the third level of complexity may limit the applicability of these findings.

Conclusions

In this cohort, it was the activity of the disease and not infectious complications the main reason for admittance to the ICU. This may be due to difficulties in monitoring and continuity of treatments, which makes relapse more frequent and immunosuppression more aggressive. Mortality was low, but it occurred more frequently in patients with infections, especially of nosocomial origin. Given these characteristics of the population, it is necessary to improve the conditions of access to health and generate more strict protocols in the ICU to avoid infections.

Acknowledgments

Clínica Universitaria Bolivariana.

Authors' contributions

All authors contributed equally in the design of the study, collection, analysis of the data and in the writing of the manuscript. All authors read and approved the final manuscript.

Author details

[1]Clínica Cardiovid, Calle 78 # 75-21, Medellín, Antioquia, Colombia. [2]Universidad Pontificia Bolivariana, Calle 78B # 72a-109, Medellín, Antioquia, Colombia. [3]Hospital la Maria, Calle 92 EE #67-61, Medellín, Antioquia, Colombia. [4]Cínica Universitaria Bolivariana, Cra 72A #78b -50, Medellín, Antioquia, Colombia. [5]Medellin, Colombia.

References

1. Siripaitoon B, Lertwises S, Uea-Areewongsa P, Khwannimit B. A study of Thai patients with systemic lupus erythematosus in the medical intensive care unit: epidemiology and predictors of mortality. Lupus. 2015;24(1):98–106.

2. Camargo JF, Tobón GJ, Fonseca N, Diaz JL, Uribe M, Molina F, et al. Autoimmune rheumatic diseases in the intensive care unit: experience from a tertiary referral hospital and review of the literature. Lupus. 2005;14(4):315–20.
3. Quintero OL, Rojas-Villarraga A, Mantilla RD, Anaya J-M. Autoimmune diseases in the intensive care unit. An update. Autoimmun Rev. 2013 Jan;12(3):380–95.
4. Han BK, Bhatia R, Traisak P, Hunter K, Milcarek B, Schorr C, et al. Clinical presentations and outcomes of systemic lupus erythematosus patients with infection admitted to the intensive care unit. Lupus. 2013 Jun;22(7):690–6.
5. Alzeer AH, Al-Arfaj A, Basha SJ, Alballa S, Al-Wakeel J, Al-Arfaj H, et al. Systemic lupus erythematosus in the intensive care unit.Pdf. Lupus. 2004:537–42.
6. Hancevic M, Gobbi C, Babini A, Albiero E. Evolución y factores pronósticos en pacientes lúpicos con admisión en unidad de terapia intensiva. Rev Argent Reum. 26(1):23–8.
7. Carrizosa JA, Aponte J, Cartagena D, Cervera R, Ospina MT, Sanchez A. Factors associated with mortality in patients with autoimmune diseases admitted to the intensive care unit in Bogota, Colombia. Front Immunol. 2017;8:337.
8. Bernal-Macías S, Reyes-Beltrán B, Molano-González N, Augusto Vega D, Bichernall C, Díaz LA, et al. Outcome of patients with autoimmune diseases in the intensive care unit: a mixed cluster analysis. Lupus Sci Med. 2015;2(1):e000122.
9. Cavallasca JA, Del Rosario Maliandi M, Sarquis S, Nishishinya MB, Schvartz A, Capdevila A, et al. Outcome of patients with systemic rheumatic diseases admitted to a medical intensive care unit. J Clin Rheumatol Pract Rep Rheum Musculoskelet Dis. 2010;16(8):400–2.
10. McAlindon T, Giannotta L, Taub N, D'Cruz D, Hughes G. Environmental factors predicting nephritis in systemic lupus erythematosus. Ann Rheum Dis. 1993 Oct;52(10):720–4.
11. Barbhaiya M, Costenbader KH. Environmental exposures and the development of systemic lupus erythematosus. Curr Opin Rheumatol. 2016 Sep;28(5):497–505.
12. Hochberg MC. Updating the American college of rheumatology revised criteria for the classification of systemic lupus erythematosus. Arthritis Rheum. 1997 Sep;40(9):1725.
13. The Surviving Sepsis Campaign Guidelines Committee including The Pediatric Subgroup*, Dellinger RP, Levy MM, Rhodes A, Annane D, Gerlach H, et al. Surviving Sepsis Campaign: International Guidelines for Management of Severe Sepsis and Septic Shock, 2012. Intensive Care Med. 2013;39(2):165–228.
14. Khwaja A. KDIGO clinical practice guidelines for acute kidney injury. Nephron Clin Pract. 2012;120(4):c179–84.
15. Kaul A, Gordon C, Crow MK, Touma Z, Urowitz MB, van Vollenhoven R, et al. Systemic lupus erythematosus. Nat Rev Dis Primer. 2016;2:16039.
16. Gladman DD, Urowitz MB, Goldsmith CH, Fortin P, Ginzler E, Gordon C, et al. The reliability of the systemic lupus international collaborating clinics/ American College of Rheumatology Damage Index in patients with systemic lupus erythematosus. Arthritis Rheum. 1997 May;40(5):809–13.
17. Abramovich E, Barrett O, Dreiher J, Novack V, Abu-Shakra M. Incidence and variables associated with short and long-term mortality in patients with systemic lupus erythematosus and sepsis admitted in intensive care units. Lupus. 2018 Oct 5;27(12):1936–43.
18. Gladman D, Ginzler E, Goldsmith C, Fortin P, Liang M, Urowitz M, et al. The development and initial validation of the systemic lupus international collaborating clinics/American College of Rheumatology damage index for systemic lupus erythematosus. Arthritis Rheum. 1996;39(3):363–9.
19. Griffiths B, Mosca M, Gordon C. Assessment of patients with systemic lupus erythematosus and the use of lupus disease activity indices. Best Pract Res Clin Rheumatol. 2005 Oct;19(5):685–708.
20. Antón JM, Castro P, Espinosa G, Marcos M, Gandía M, Merchán R, et al. Mortality and long term survival prognostic factors of patients with systemic autoimmune diseases admitted to an intensive care unit: a retrospective study. Clin Exp Rheumatol. 30(3):338–44.
21. Hsu C-L, Chen K-Y, Yeh P-S, Hsu Y-L, Chang H-T, Shau W-Y, et al. Outcome and prognostic factors in critically ill patients with systemic lupus erythematosus: a retrospective study. Crit Care Lond Engl. 2005;9(3):R177–83.
22. Ranzani OT, Battaini LC, Moraes CE, Prada LFL, Pinaffi JV, Giannini FP, et al. Outcomes and organ dysfunctions of critically ill patients with systemic lupus erythematosus and other systemic rheumatic diseases. Braz J Med Biol Res Rev Bras Pesqui Medicas E Biol. 2011;44(11):1184 93.
23. Namendys-Silva SA, Baltazar-Torres JA, Rivero-Sigarroa E, Fonseca-Lazcano JA, Montiel-López L, Domínguez-Cherit G. Prognostic factors in patients with systemic lupus erythematosus admitted to the intensive care unit. Lupus. 2009 Dec;18(14):1252–8.
24. Fatemi A, Shamsaee S, Raeisi A, Sayedbonakdar Z, Smiley A. Prognostic factors of mortality in Iranian patients with systemic lupus erythematosus admitted to intensive care unit. Clin Rheumatol. 2017 Nov;36(11):2471–7.
25. Ñamendys-Silva S, Reyes-Ruiz M, Rivero-Sigarroa E, Domínguez Cherit G. Pronóstico de pacientes con lupus eritematoso generalizado en una unidad de cuidados intensivos. Gac México. 2018;154(4):468–72.
26. Lee J, Dhillon N, Pope J. All-cause hospitalizations in systemic lupus erythematosus from a large Canadian referral Centre. Rheumatol Oxf Engl. 2013;52(5):905–9.
27. Whitelaw DA, Gopal R, Freeman V. Survival of patients with SLE admitted to an intensive care unit-a retrospective study. Clin Rheumatol. 2005 Jun 25;24(3):223–7.
28. Alarcón GS, McGwin G, Uribe A, Friedman AW, Roseman JM, Fessler BJ, Bastian HM, Baethge BA, Vilá LM, Reveille JD. Systemic lupus erythematosus in a multiethnic lupus cohort (LUMINA). XVII. Predictors of self-reported health-related quality of life early in the disease course. Arthritis & Rheumatism. 2004;51:465–74. doi: https://doi.org/10.1002/art.20409.
29. Mohamed DF, Habeeb RA, Hosny SM, Ebrahim SE. Incidence and risk of infection in Egyptian patients with systemic lupus erythematosus. Clin Med Insights Arthritis Musculoskelet Disord. 2014;7:41–8.
30. Faguer S, Ciroldi M, Mariotte E, Galicier L, Rybojad M, Canet E, et al. Prognostic contributions of the underlying inflammatory disease and acute organ dysfunction in critically ill patients with systemic rheumatic diseases. Eur J Intern Med. 2013 Apr;24(3):e40–4.
31. Campbell R, Cooper GS, Gilkeson GS. Two aspects of the clinical and humanistic burden of systemic lupus erythematosus: mortality risk and quality of life early in the course of disease. Arthritis Rheum. 2008 Apr 15;59(4):458–64.
32. Ward MM, Pyun E, Studenski S. Long-term survival in systemic lupus erythematosus. Patient characteristics associated with poorer outcomes. Arthritis Rheum. 1995 Feb;38(2):274–83.
33. Tan TC, Fang H, Magder LS, Petri MA. Differences between male and female systemic lupus erythematosus in a multiethnic population. J Rheumatol. 2012 Apr;39(4):759–69.

Axial Spondyloarthritis after bariatric surgery: A 7-year retrospective analysis

Thauana Luiza de Oliveira[1*], Hilton Telles Libanori[2] and Marcelo M. Pinheiro[1]

Abstract

Background: In recent decades, obesity has become a public health problem in many countries. The objective of this study was to evaluate the main joint and extra-articular manifestations related to spondyloarthritis (SpA) after bariatric surgery (BS) in a retrospective cohort.

Methods: Demographic, clinical, laboratory and imaging data from nine patients whose SpA symptoms started after a BS have been described. Modified New York (mNY) criteria for ankylosing spondylitis (AS) and the Assessment of Spondyloarthritis International Society (ASAS) criteria for axial (ax-SpA) and peripheral (p-SpA) spondyloarthritis were applied.

Results: The mean weight reduction after BS was 49.3 ± 21.9 kg. The BS techniques were Roux-en-Y gastric bypass (n = 8; 88.9%) and biliopancreatic diversion with duodenal switch (n = 1; 11.1%). Four (44.4%) patients had no axial or peripheral pain complaints before BS, while the other four (44.4%) had sporadic non-inflammatory back pain that had been attributed to obesity. One patient (11.1%) had persistent chronic back pain. In all nine cases, patients reported back pain onset or pattern (intensity or night pain) change after BS (mean time 14.7 ± 18 months). In addition, 8 of them (88.9%) were human leukocyte antigen (HLA)-B27 positive. All nine patients could be classified according to ASAS criteria as ax-SpA and five (55.6%) patients were classified as AS, according to the mNY criteria.

Conclusion: Our data highlight a temporal link between SpA onset symptoms and the BS, suggesting a possible causal plausibility between the two events.

Keywords: Spondyloarthritis, Bariatric surgery, HLA-B27

Key message

1- Spondyloarthritis could arise after surgical interventions for the treatment of obesity.
2- Microbiota changes may play a key role as trigger in this setting and Human leukocyte antigen (HLA)-B27 could be considered as screening tool before BS.

Background

In recent decades, obesity has become a public health problem in many Western countries related to lifestyle changes, including higher low-nutritional value and high-calorie foods intake, as well as no regular physical activity. These aspects partly explain the increase of bariatric surgeries (BS) rate for treating of morbid obese patients and overweight individuals with comorbidities, because it has provided global benefits, especially for quality of life, self-esteem, control of peripheral insulin resistance and metabolic syndrome. Moreover, it is considered the most effective treatment for obesity, since the non-pharmacological approach, based on lifestyle changes and psychotherapeutic support, as well as drug therapy, has a high recurrence rate of weight gain [1, 2].

BS may cause several neuroendocrine changes, especially those related to the leptin axis, ghrelin, glucagon-like peptide-1 (GLP-1) and other incretins, promoting an early satiety state, weight loss, and better glucose control. However, many complications can occur. In the short-term, these include infections, bleeding, and pulmonary thromboembolism; and in the long-term, they include nutritional deficiencies, anastomotic stenosis, osteoporosis, gallstones and kidney stones [2].

* Correspondence: thauanareumato@gmail.com
[1]Rheumatology Division, Spondyloarthritis Section, Universidade Federal de São Paulo, Rua Leandro Dupré, 204, Conjunto 74, Vila Clementino, São Paulo, SP CEP 04025-010, Brazil
Full list of author information is available at the end of the article

From an immunological perspective, some immune-mediated manifestations related to intestinal bypass (BP) surgeries have been described. These are mainly associated with jejunoileal BP, including arthritis, immune complex glomerulonephritis, cutaneous vasculitis, pericarditis, Raynaud's phenomenon, psoriasis and pyoderma gangrenosum [3–5]. The Bowel-associated Dermatosis-Arthritis Syndrome (BADAS), described in 1979 by Dicken and Seehafer, is one of the manifestations better associated with intestinal BP [6, 7]. It is characterized by recurrent episodes of fever, polyarthralgia or polyarthritis associated with skin lesions. It has also been described after other types of surgery and intestinal anastomoses, such as Billroth II gastrectomy, biliopancreatic diversion, ileocolic BP, appendectomy, and bariatric surgery with more recent surgical techniques [8, 9].

The main rheumatic manifestation associated with the jejunoileal BP is arthritis, commonly episodic, migratory, and polyarticular, with a predominantly self-limited course, but sometimes with a chronic evolution similar to rheumatoid arthritis [10, 11]. The axial involvement is less frequent and may be associated with the HLA-B27 positivity [12, 13]. Conversely, obese patients with rheumatoid arthritis or systemic lupus erythematosus may benefit from BS since it contributes to better disease control and dose reduction of immunosuppressants [14, 15].

The pathophysiology of these immune-mediated manifestations is unknown, although both innate and adaptive immunity are involved. Among the most accepted theories, the intestinal microbiome changes after surgery stand out, such as bacterial overgrowth due to the increase of pH, and the blind loop syndrome. Altogether they could cause alterations of intestinal permeability and bacterial translocation, which would work as a trigger for the intestinal and systemic immune activation through molecular mimicry between peptides from gram-negative bacteria and structures of the synovial membrane and synovio-entheseal complex [16]. Some histopathological studies of the intestinal blind loop from patients with BADAS demonstrated a non-specific chronic inflammatory response [3].

The objective of this study was to describe patients who underwent BS before onset of spondyloarthritis (SpA) symptoms.

Methods

Among 429 patients from the Spondyloarthritis database from the Rheumatology Division at the Federal University of São Paulo, nine (2.1%) had SpA-onset symptoms after BS from 2010 to 2016. These patients denied any inflammatory back pain (IBP), enthesitis, dactilitis, arthritis or extra-articular manifestations such as uveitis, colitis or psoriasis before being submitted to BS.

Demographic, clinical, laboratory and imaging data from these patients, including plain pelvic radiograph and sacroiliac joint (SIJ) and spine magnetic resonance imaging (MRI), when applicable, are shown. Furthermore, the modified New York (mNY) criteria for ankylosing spondylitis (AS) and the Assessment of Spondyloarthritis International Society (ASAS) criteria for axial (ax-SpA) and peripheral (p-SpA) spondyloarthritis were applied [17]. The first clinical evaluation data were considered to measure disease activity, functional impairment and structural damage measurements, including BASDAI (Bath Ankylosing Spondylitis Disease Activity Index) and ASDAS (Ankylosing Spondylitis Disease Activity Score), BASFI (Bath Ankylosing Spondylitis Functional Index), BASMI (Bath Ankylosing Spondylitis Metrology Index) and mSASSS (modified Stoke Ankylosing Spondylitis Spinal Score) [17].

Patients signed an Informed Consent Form, and the study was approved by the Ethics Committee of the Federal University of São Paulo (1478/09).

Numerical data were presented as the mean ± standard deviation and categorical variables as percentages. P below 0.05 was set as significant. The Statistical Package for Social Science software (SPSS version 20.0) was used for descriptive analysis.

Results

The demographic and clinical manifestations of these nine patients are described in Table 1. The mean weight loss after BP surgery was 49.3 ± 21.9 kg. The BS techniques were Roux-en-Y gastric bypass (n = 8; 88.9%) and biliopancreatic diversion with duodenal switch (n = 1; 11.1%).

Four (44.4%) patients had no axial or peripheral pain complaints before BS, while the other four (44.4%) had sporadic non-inflammatory back pain that had been attributed to obesity. One patient (11.1%) had persistent chronic back pain and had been submitted to surgery for spinal stenosis correction (L5-S1 segment). In all nine cases, patients reported back pain onset or pattern (from unspecified or non-inflammatory to IBP, according to the ASAS criteria) or intensity (from mild to moderate or severe) change after BS (mean time of 14.7 ± 18.0 months). In addition to axial manifestation, all of them had calcaneal enthesitis, and more than half had arthritis at the onset of symptoms. In addition, 8 of them (88.9%) were human leukocyte antigen (HLA)-B27 positive.

Regarding extra-articular manifestations, one patient had recurrent anterior uveitis and IBP after 12 months of BS. Another patient had chronic non-specific colitis. One patient had psoriasis, and no cutaneous manifestation suggestive of BADAS was observed in any of them.

Five (55.6%) patients were classified as AS, according to the mNY criteria. The plain pelvic radiograph demonstrated grade II bilateral sacroiliitis in four patients and grade III unilateral in one. The other four patients (44.4%) were classified as non-radiographic axial SpA, according to the ASAS criteria (Table 1).

At the time of the first clinical evaluation, they had high disease activity according to BASDAI, ASDAS-CRP, with significant function and mobility impairment. After two years, the mSASSS data showed structural spine damage progression, defined as a new syndesmophyte, in 5 patients (Table 2).

Concerning treatment, all nine patients were taking nonsteroidal anti-inflammatory drugs on demand. Two (22.2%) patients were taking methotrexate and two (22.2%) were on sulfasalazine and other four (44.4%) were taking anti-tumor necrosis factor agents. It was necessary to reverse the BS of one patient due to intensity and refractoriness of axial and peripheral SpA complaints. After that, he had significant clinical improvement but did not reach complete remission.

Table 2 Assessment of disease activity and structural damage

Assessment of disease activity and structural damage (n = 9)	
BASDAI	5.0 ± 1.4
ASDAS-ESR	3.9 ± 0.6
ASDAS-CRP	3.2 ± 1.2
BASFI	3.7 ± 2.4
BASMI	3.6 ± 1.7
ESR (mm/h)	52.4 ± 27.5
CRP(mg/L)	11.7 ± 16.8
mSASSS Cervical (0–36) $^{\Delta}$	13 ± 12.4 (10)
mSASSS Lumbar (0–36) $^{\Delta}$	9 ± 8.6 (7)
mSASSS Total (0–72) $^{\Delta}$	22.7 ± 20.7 (17)

Numeric variables expressed as mean ± standard deviation. $^{\Delta}$Data presented as mean ± standard deviation (median). *BASDAI* (Bath Ankylosing Spondylitis Disease Activity Index); *BASFI* (Bath Ankylosing Spondylitis Functional Index); *BASMI* (Bath Ankylosing Spondylitis Metrology Index); *ASDAS* (Ankylosing Spondylitis Disease Activity Score); *ESR* (erythrocyte sedimentation rate); *CRP* (C-reactive protein), *mSASSS* (modified Stoke Ankylosing Spondylitis Spinal Score)

Discussion

This series of cases highlights the possible temporal link between the onset of symptoms related to SpA and the BS, suggesting a possible causal plausibility between them. Although with a variable time interval, there was a clear temporal relationship between BS and the onset of axial and/or peripheral joint symptoms, as well as extra-articular manifestations in previously asymptomatic patients or patients with vague complaints, such as occasional non-inflammatory non-chronic back pain and that were attributed to overweight and physical inactivity. To the best of our best knowledge, this is the more consistent case series, including sampling and clinical characterization, showing axial SpA after BS with current surgical techniques. Previously, most of the case reports were from patients with arthritis or BADAS, especially after BS using an obsolete and disabsorptive techniques.

Table 1 Clinical, demographic and imaging characteristics of patients with new onset axial Spondyloarthritis after bariatric surgery

Patient characteristics (n = 9)	
Sex (M:F)	4:5
Current age (years)	49.5 ± 10.1
Age at the onset of symptoms (years)	42.0 ± 9.1
Disease duration (years)	5.7 ± 3.0
Time between surgery and symptoms (months)	14.7 ± 18.0
White color	7 (77.8%)
HLA-B27 positive	8 (88.9%)
Chronic low back pain (> 3 months)	9 (100%)
Inflammatory low back pain	7 (77.8%)
Arthritis	5 (55.6%)
Calcaneal enthesitis	9 (100%)
Dactylitis	0 (0%)
Recurrent anterior uveitis	3 (33.3%)
Colitis	1 (11.1%)
Balanitis circinata/ urethritis	0 (0%)
Psoriasis	1 (11.1%)
Radiographic evidence of sacroiliitis (n = 9) Grade II bilateral Grade III unilateral or higher	5 (55.6%) 4 (80%) 1 (20%)
Sacroiliac Joint MRI* (n = 4)	4 (100%)

Mean ± standard deviation, frequency (%). MRI: magnetic resonance imaging. *MRI was performed only in patients without radiographic sacroiliitis and was classified according to Assessment of Spondyloarthritis International Society (ASAS) criteria

Our data suggest that there may be a link between the intestinal microbiome changes (dysbiosis), after BS, and the clinical manifestations related to SpA. Likely, these mechanisms could be associated with HLA-B27 regarding antigen presentation and other innate immunity ways. Recently, it was demonstrated that AS patients had qualitative differences in their intestinal microbiome, including a higher frequency of five families of bacteria (*Lachnospiraceae, Ruminococcaceae, Rikenellaceae, Porphyromonadaceae, Bacteroidaceae*) and reduction in the abundance of two others (*Veilonellaceae and Prevotellaceae*) [18]. Although some evidence has demonstrated the role of genetic factors on gut microbiome composition, it is believed that the interaction with the HLA-B27 plays a relevant role, especially by the mis-folding theory or formation of homodimers on the surface of antigen-presenting cells, leading to the induction of immunological pathways, such as IL-23/IL-17 axis. Furthermore, it was shown that there is a relationship between the presence of chronic ileocolic inflammation and increased inflammatory activity on SIJ MRI in patients with AS, emphasizing the close link between gut inflammation and the axial involvement [19].

Bacterial overgrowth induced by changes in peristalsis, drainage pathways and chemical composition of digestive juices, as well as pH elevation, could be an additional pathophysiological mechanism, but none of the patients showed any clinical evidence of these symptoms, including malaise, fever, hypoglycemia and stool bulk modifications. On the other hand, the dumping phenomenon was common to all.

Additionally, this setting could be the clinical translation of the HLA-B27 transgenic mice models that do not develop the symptoms of joint disease in a germ-free microenvironment [20]. The partial clinical and laboratory improvement of a patient following reversal of BS, as observed by other authors, reinforces this hypothesis [11].

All nine patients had heel pain at the time of first clinical evaluation. We did not perform any ultrasound or magnetic resonance imaging of this specific entheseal site, because calcaneal enthesopathy is common in obese individuals, and we cannot guarantee that it was associated with inflammatory SpA background or just related to overweight mechanical stress itself.

Considering the HLA-B27 has a crucial role in four theoretical models to explain the pathophysiological aspects related to articular and extra-articular manifestations in SpA experimental models, we could explore that SpA features after BS, where huge microbiota changes can occur, could be more frequent in HLA-B27 positive patients [21, 22]. Interestingly, none of the patients reported any family history of diseases related to the SpA concept. Thus, the HLA-B27 status definition could be to take account by surgeons and patients before making decision for BS choosing. Nonetheless, it is worthy emphasizing that more prospective studies with larger sampling are needed to establish the cause and effect relationship between both conditions.

Our study has some limitations, such as the retrospective design and problems inherent to remembering medical complaints, including dates and characteristics of pain and articular and extra-articular manifestations. Secondly, the intestinal microbiome was not evaluated. In contrast, it has other relevant aspects, such as the description of a case series and assessment and detailed characterization of patients over time, demonstrating the possible temporal link between BS and onset of SpA symptoms.

Conclusion

Our data showed SpA could arise after surgical interventions for obesity treatment, especially Roux-en-Y, in patients with genetic susceptibility conferred by the presence of HLA-B27.

Acknowledgements
To our study group of Spondyloarthritis.

Authors' contributions
TLO did the clinical evaluations of patients and wrote the article; HTL revised the article and MMP idealized the project and did revision of the manuscript. All authors read and approved the final manuscript.

Author details
Rheumatology Division, Spondyloarthritis Section, Universidade Federal de São Paulo, Rua Leandro Dupré, 204, Conjunto 74, Vila Clementino, São Paulo, SP CEP 04025-010, Brazil. [2]Hospital Israelita Albert Einstein, São Paulo, Brazil.

References

1. Fruhbeck G. Bariatric and metabolic surgery: a shift in eligibility and success criteria. Nat Rev Endocrinol. 2015;11(8):465–77. https://doi.org/10.1038/nrendo.2015.84.
2. Pories WJ. Bariatric surgery: risks and rewards. J Clin Endocrinol Metab. 2008; 93(11 Suppl 1):S89–96. https://doi.org/10.1210/jc.2008-1641.
3. Drenick EJ, Ament ME, Finegold SM, Corrodi P, Passaro E. Bypass enteropathy. Intestinal and systemic manifestations following small-bowel bypass. JAMA. 1976;236(3):269–72. https://doi.org/10.1001/jama.1976.03270030023022.
4. Gamble CN, Kimchi A, Depner TA, Christensen D. Immune complex glomerulonephritis and dermal vasculitis following intestinal bypass for morbid obesity. Am J Clin Pathol. 1982;77(3):347–52. https://doi.org/10.1093/ajcp/77.3.347.
5. Zapanta M, Aldo-Benson M, Biegel A, Madura J. Arthritis associated with jejunoileal bypass. clinical and immunologic evaluation Arthritis Rheum. 1979;22(7):711–7. https://doi.org/10.1002/art.1780220704.
6. Dicken CH, Seehafer JR. Bowel bypass syndrome. Arch Dermatol. 1979; 115(7):837–9. https://doi.org/10.1001/archderm.1979.04010070013012.
7. Stein HB, Schlappner OL, Boyko W, Gourlay RH, Reeve CE. The intestinal bypass: arthritis-dermatitis syndrome. Arthritis Rheum. 1981;24(5):684–90. https://doi.org/10.1002/art.1780240509.
8. Tu J, Chan JJ, Yu LL. Bowel bypass syndrome/bowel-associated dermatosis arthritis syndrome post laparoscopic gastric bypass surgery. Australas J Dermatol. 2011;52(1):e5–7. https://doi.org/10.1111/j.1440-0960.2009.00614.x.
9. Slater GH, Kerlin P, Georghiou PR, Fielding GA. Bowel-associated dermatosis-arthritis syndrome after biliopancreatic diversion. Obes Surg. 2004;14(1):133–5. https://doi.org/10.1381/096089204772787446.
10. Le Quintrec JL, Puechal X, Marin A, Lamy P, Gendre JP, Menkes CJ. Chronic erosive arthritis associated with an unusual intestinal bypass. Clin Exp Rheumatol. 1991;9(5):529–32.
11. Kudo H. A case of chronic erosive polyarthirits which developed 14 years after an intestinal bypass operation with subsequent remission by intestinal revision. Ryumachi. 2001;41(5):880–7.
12. Ribeiro DS, Fernandes JL, Rangel L, de Araújo Neto C, D'Almeida F, Moura CG, et al. Spondyloarthritis after bariatric surgery: is there a link? Clin Rheumatol. 2010;29(4):435–7. https://doi.org/10.1007/s10067-009-1351-4.
13. Rose E, Espinoza LR, Osterland CK. Intestinal bypass arthritis: association with circulating immune complexes and HLA B27. J Rheumatol. 1977;4(2):129–34.
14. Corcelles R, Daigle CR, Talamas HR, Batayyah E, Brethauer SA, Schauer PR. Bariatric surgery outcomes in patients with systemic lupus erythematosus. Surg Obes Relat Dis. 2015;11(3):684–8. https://doi.org/10.1016/j.soard.2014.10.006.
15. Sparks JA, Halperin F, Karlson JC, Karlson EW, Bermas BL. Impact of bariatric surgery on patients with rheumatoid arthritis. Arthritis Care Res (Hoboken). 2015;67(12):1619–26. https://doi.org/10.1002/acr.22629.
16. Carubbi F, Ruscitti P, Pantano I, Alvaro S, Benedetto PD, Liakouli V, et al. Jejunoileal bypass as the main procedure in the onset of immune-related conditions: the model of BADAS. Expert Rev Clin Immunol. 2013;9(5):441–52.
17. Sieper J, Rudwaleit M, Baraliakos X, Brandt J, Burgos-Vargas R, Dougados M, et al. The assessment of Spondyloarthritis international society (ASAS) handbook: a guide to assess spondyloarthritis. Ann Rheum Dis. 2009;68:1–44.

18. Costello M-E, Ciccia F, Willner D, Warrington N, Robinson PC, Gardiner B, et al. Brief report: intestinal dysbiosis in ankylosing spondylitis. Arthritis Rheumatol. 2015;67(3):686–91. https://doi.org/10.1002/art.38967.
19. Van Praet L, Jans L, Carron P, Jacques P, Glorieus E, Colman R, et al. Degree of bone marrow oedema in sacroiliac joints of patients with axial spondyloarthritis is linked to gut inflammation and male sex: results from the GIANT cohort. Ann Rheum Dis. 2014;73:1186–9. https://doi.org/10.1136/annrheumdis-2013-203854.
20. Rath H, Herfarth H, Ikeda J, Grenther WB, Hamm TE Jr, Balish E, et al. Normal luminal bacteria, especially bacteroides species, mediate chronic colitis, gastritis, and arthritis in HLA-B27/human beta2 microglobulin transgenic rats. J Clin Invest. 1996;98:945–53. https://doi.org/10.1172/JCI118878.
21. Lin P, Bach M, Asquith M, Lee AY, Akileswaran L, Stauffer P, et al. HLA-B27 and human β2-microglobulin affect the gut microbiota of transgenic rats. PLoS One. 2014;9(8):e105684. https://doi.org/10.1371/journal.pone.0105684.
22. Asquith M, Brooks SR, Rosenbaum JT, Colbert RA. Effects of HLA-B27 on gut microbiota in experimental Spondyloarthritis implicate an ecological model of Dysbiosis. Arthritis Rheumatol. 2018;70(4):555–65.

20

The effect of therapies on the quality of life of patients with systemic lupus erythematosus

Tassia Catiuscia da Hora[1], Kelly Lima[2] and Roberto Rodrigues Bandeira Tosta Maciel[3*]

Abstract

Introduction: Systemic lupus erythematosus (SLE) is a multi-systemic, chronic inflammatory disease of autoimmune nature, which can impair performance in daily life activities, causing to a compromised quality of life. Thus, the aim of this study was to evaluate the effect of therapies, such as physical activity, cognitive behavioral therapy, pharmacological treatment and phytotherapy in the quality of life of patients with systemic lupus erythematosus.

Materials and methods: A systematic review with a meta-analysis of randomized clinical trials was conducted by searching the PubMed database, including studies comparing patients who participated in cognitive therapy, physical activity, pharmacological treatment or phytotherapeutic treatment.

Results: Of the seven studies included in this meta-analysis, a significant difference was observed in the quality of life of patients with lupus who participated in the intervention groups compared to the control groups (− 10.27 95% CI: − 15, 77 at − 4.77, $p = 0.0003$, I2 = 0%).

Conclusion: Interventions improve the Quality of life of patients with SLE. However, the methodological quality of the included articles and the sizes of the samples for being small propose that new randomized clinical trials be performed.

Keywords: Systemic lupus erythematosus, Quality of life, Meta-analysis

Introduction

Systemic lupus erythematosus (SLE) is a chronic, autoimmune, multisystemic inflammatory disease that can cause skin lesions, inflammation of the joints and membranes that cover the lungs and heart, nephritis, cardiovascular, hematological, gastrointestinal and neuropsychiatric disorders. In this way, the symptoms can appear slowly and progressively or quickly and vary with phases of activity and remission [1], which may impair performance in daily activities, leading to impairment of quality of life (QoL).

Since the World Health Organization advocates that QoL reflects on individuals' perceptions that their needs are being met, or that they are being denied opportunities to achieve happiness and self-realization, regardless of their physical state of health or social and economic conditions [2], therapies and/or treatments are used for these patients, in order to minimize the implications imposed by the disease and improve the quality of life. Randomized clinical trials (RCTs) that demonstrated the effects of these therapies and/or treatments on the health aspect in general, reported an improvement in quality of life [3, 4]. However, the studies have relatively small samples.

Because of the greater statistical power, a systematic review with meta-analysis of randomized clinical trials may provide more accurate estimates of the efficacy of the intervention than individual trials. A RCT meta-analysis was performed comparing patients who were part of the intervention group (cognitive therapy, physical activity, pharmacological and phytotherapeutic treatment) with control groups, in order to identify if the

* Correspondence: rmaciel@uneb.br
[3]Universidade do Estado da Bahia- Silveira Martins, 2555 - Cabula, Salvador, BA 41150-000, Brazil
Full list of author information is available at the end of the article

interventions provided statistically significant improvements in QoL. Thus, the objective of this study was to evaluate the effect of therapies, such as physical activity, cognitive behavioral therapy, pharmacological treatment and phytotherapy, and identify whether interventions provide statistically significant improvements on the quality of life of patients with systemic lupus erythematosus.

Methodology

A systematic review with a meta-analysis of randomized clinical trials was performed, observing the criteria defined by the Preferred Reporting Items for Systematic Reviews and Meta-Analyses (PRISMA) guideline.

Eligibility criteria

Randomized clinical trials evaluating the quality of life of patients with SLE were included. We included studies comparing patients who participated in cognitive therapy, physical activity, pharmacological treatment or phytotherapeutic treatment. To carry out such a study, the PubMed database was consulted. The search was not restricted by language. The publications were selected if they reported on quality of life in patients with SLE and specified the use of a quality of life scale.

The exclusion criteria were studies that included children, those who did not specify the general health domain of the patient, the studies that reported only baseline measurements, those who did not clearly identify the presence of a control group and those who did not provide standard deviation nor confidence interval.

Search

In the PubMed search strategy, keywords were used according to their description in MeSH, the complete search strategy was: ((((((((Systemic Lupus Erythematosus) OR Lupus Erythematosus) OR Libman-Sacks Disseminatus) OR Disease, Libman-Sacks) OR Libman Sacks Disease) OR "lupus erythematosus, systemic"[MeSH Terms])) AND (((((Life Quality) OR Health-Related Quality Of Life) OR Health-Related Quality Of Life) OR HRQOL) OR ("quality of life"[MeSH Terms] OR quality of life [Text Word])))) AND ((((clinical [Title/Abstract] AND trial [Title/Abstract]) OR clinical trials as topic [MeSH Terms] OR clinical trial [Publication Type] OR random*[Title/Abstract] OR random allocation [MeSH Terms] OR therapeutic use [MeSH Subheading]))).

Data collect

The relevant articles published in the period between 2010 and 2017 were initially selected by the screening of titles and abstracts, going to the stage of reading the articles in full, collected through database searches.

A previous exploratory reading of all the selected material was carried out, followed by a more selective and analytical reading of the parts that really mattered. Subsequently, the information extracted from the articles (authors, title, journal, year, abstract and conclusions) was recorded in order to order and summarize the material, so as to enable the obtaining of information relevant to the research.

The process of identifying the methodological aspects and extracting the data of the articles was carried out by two independent reviewers. In the event of any disagreement between them, the article was read again in full for re-evaluation based on pre-determined eligibility criteria.

Subsequently, a meta-analysis was performed using Review Manager Analysis software (RevMan 5.3), from Cochrane Collaboration. The effects were summarized using differences between means with 95% confidence intervals, using a fixed effects model. Heterogeneity was assessed using the statistics I^2.

Risk of Bias

To assess the risk of bias, we used the Cochrane Collaboration criterion, which evaluated the following domains: 1) sequence generation (randomization): We identified the method used to generate the random sequence, in order to evaluate if it was possible to produce comparable groups; 2) allocation concealment: We identified the method used to conceal the random sequence, in order to know if the allocation of the interventions could be predicted before or during the recruitment of the participants; 3) blindness of participants and blindness of professional: We analyzed whether there was an adequate description of the measures used to blind participants of the studies and professionals involved 4) Results Evaluator Blindness: We evaluated if the studies described the measures used to blind the evaluators of the outcome, in relation to the knowledge of the intervention provided to each participant; 5) incomplete follow-up data: We evaluated whether the studies reported loss of outcome data, whether losses were balanced between groups, as well as whether data were allocated in an appropriate way; 6) Report of selective outcome: We evaluated the possibility that the studies included in this review reported incomplete outcomese and 7) Other sources of bias: We judged this item considering the quality and extent of the information reported in the included studies.

Results

The search strategy resulted in 292 articles, of which 28 studies were selected for a detailed reading. Of these, 07 studies met the eligibility criteria and were included in the present study. Figure 1 shows the flowchart of the studies included in this analysis and Table 1 summarizes the characteristics of these studies.

Two trials compared physical activity with usual care (total $n = 73$, of which 38 were in the physical activity

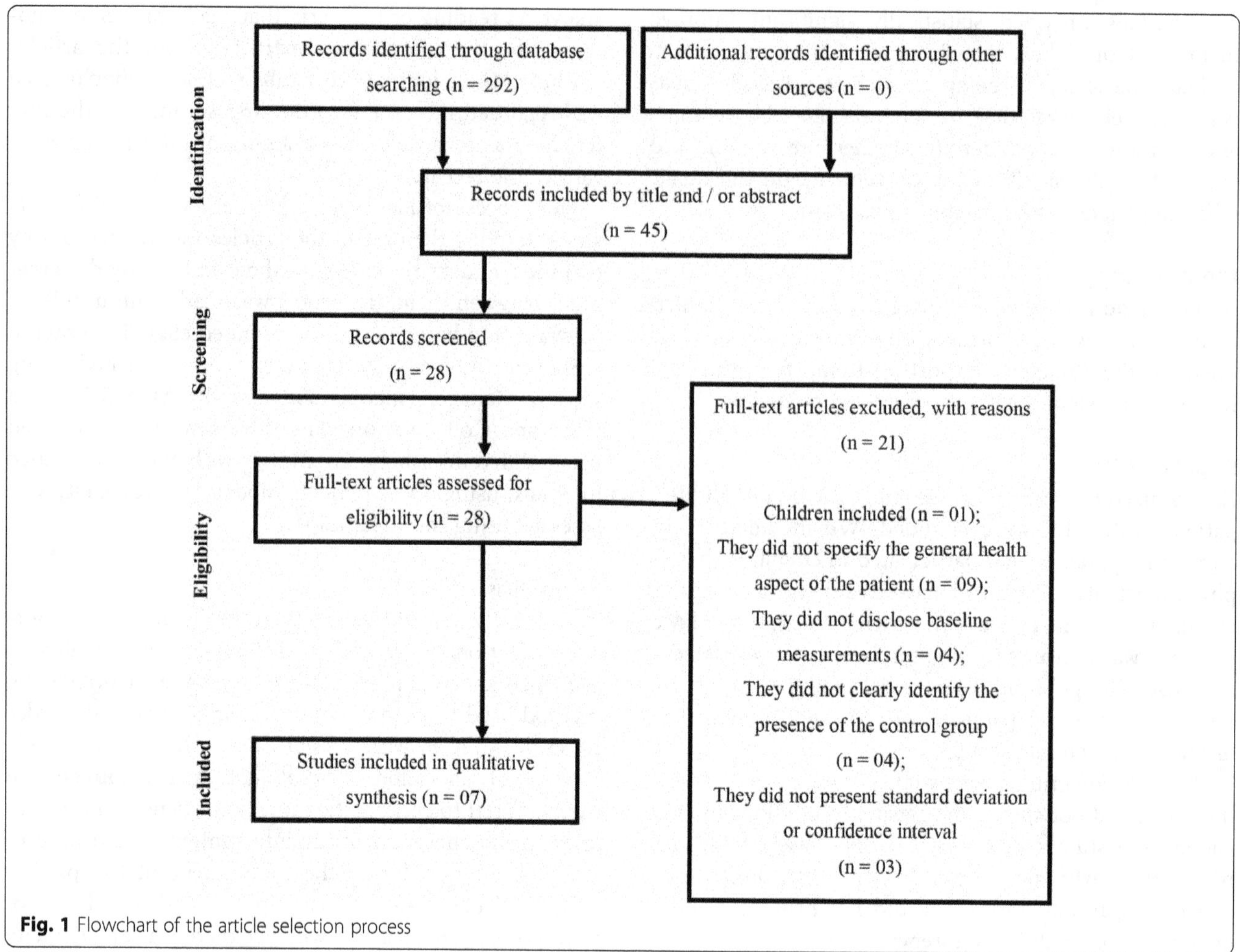

Fig. 1 Flowchart of the article selection process

group); two trials compared cognitive behavioral therapy with conventional care (total n = 79, of which 39 were in the cognitive therapy group); two trials compared phytotherapeutic treatment with placebo (total 100, of which 50 were in the phytotherapeutic group); and one study compared pharmacological treatment with placebo (total n = 48, of which 11 were in the epratuzumab group).

Risk of bias

Of the studies that were included in the review, in the field of random sequence generation (randomization), 03 studies presented low risk of bias, 3 were not clear and 01 was not randomized. Only 01 study presented low risk of bias in the concealment domain of the allocation and 06 were not clear. Only 03 studies had low risk of bias of blind participants, 02 were not clear and 02 presented high risk of bias. Regarding the blindness of the evaluators, only 01 study presented low risk of bias, while 03 were uncertain and 03 had high risk of bias. In the 07 studies, losses in follow-up and exclusions were described. Regarding the selective reporting of outcome, 03 studies presented low risk of bias and 04 presented high risk of bias. Only 01 study presented low risk of bias in the intention to treat domain, 03 were not clear and 03 presented high risk of bias (Fig. 2).

Effects of interventions

Of the seven studies included in this meta-analysis (n = 300), a significant difference in quality of life was observed in SLE patients who participated in the intervention groups compared to the control groups (-10.27 95% CI: -15.77 to -4.77, p = 0.0003, I2 = 0%) (Fig. 3).

Physical activity

Two studies, Abrahão et al [5] and Boström et al [6] evaluated QOL (n = 73). It was verified that the physical activity program provided a non-significant improvement in the QoL compared to the control groups (-6.46 95% CI: -19.85 to 6.93, p = 0.34, I^2 = 0) (Fig 4).

In this meta-analysis, Abrahão et al [5] and Boström et al [6], performed a physical activity program during 03 and 12 months, respectively, including patients who have SLE in a physical activity program, and had control groups that received only usual care, was observed that there was a significant difference in relation to physical

Table 1 Characteristics of the studies included in the review

Author year	Population	Intervention	Follow-up	Outcome	Result
Abrahão, 2015 [6]	42	Intervention ($n = 21$) cardiovascular training Control group ($n = 21$) (usual care and information about the disease)	03 months	Quality of life	The intervention group presented a significant improvement in the physical health and vitality aspect, in the general health aspect no significant differences were found (SF36 health survey questionnaire)
Arriens, 2015 [9]	32	Intervention ($n = 18$) (supplementation with fish oil) Control group ($n = 14$) (placebo)	06 months	Quality of life	The intervention group presented a significant improvement in the mental health and vitality aspect (SF36 health survey questionnaire)
Boström, 2016 [7]	31	Intervention ($n = 17$) (physical activity) Control group ($n = 14$) (usual care)	12 months	Quality of life	The intervention group had improved mental health, there was no significant improvement in the general health aspect (SF36 health survey questionnaire).
Navarrete, 2010 [4]	45	Intervention ($n = 21$) (cognitive behavioral therapy) Control group ($n = 24$) (health care, moderate exercise, balanced diet and plenty of rest)	15 months	Quality of life	The intervention group had a significant reduction in the level of depression, anxiety and daily stress and a significant improvement in QoL and somatic symptoms (SF36 health survey questionnaire).
Navarrete et al, 2010 [8]	34	Intervention (n = 18) cognitive behavioral therapy Control group ($n = 16$) (usual care)	15 months	Quality of life	The intervention group presented improvement in the level of physical function, vitality, general health perception andmental health (SF36 health survey questionnaire).
Shamehki, 2017 [5]	68	Intervention ($n = 32$) (supplementation of green tea extract) Control group ($n = 36$) (placebo)	03 months	Quality of life	The intervention group presented a significant increase in hrvitality and general health (SF36 health survey questionnaire).
Strand, 2013 [10]	48	Intervention ($n = 11$) (epratuzumab 720 mg/m2) Control group ($n = 37$) (placebo)	12 months	Quality of life	The intervention group showed evident improvements in the mean SF-36 scores (SF36 health survey questionnaire).

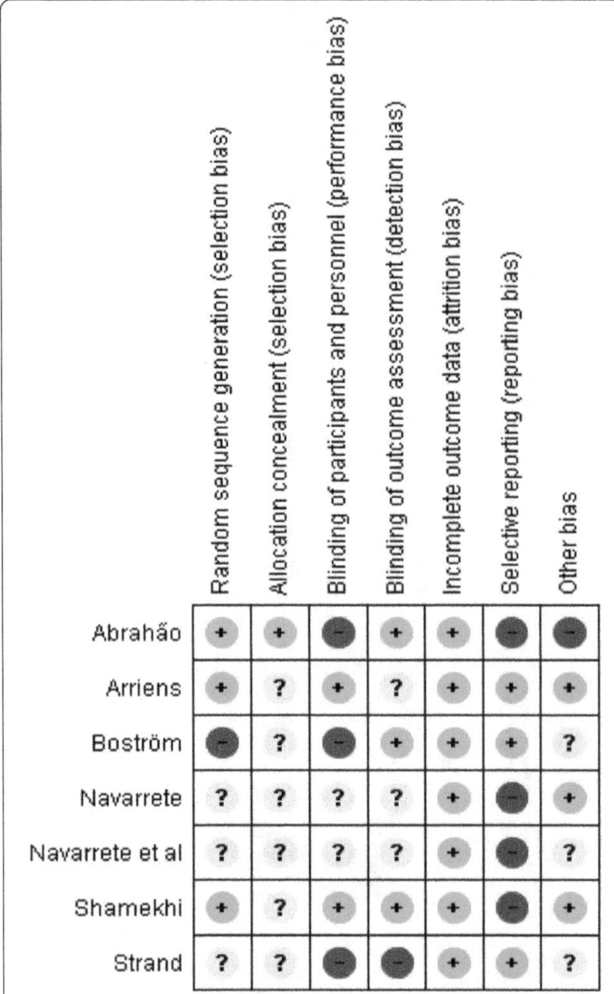

Fig. 2 Review author judgments about the risk for each bias item in all included trials

function (Fig. 4), but not to vitality (Fig. 5), but in general health the results were not statistically significant.

Cognitive behavioral therapy (CBT)

Navarrete et al [3, 7], assessed in two studies the QoL of patients with SLE who participated in cognitive behavioral therapy (n = 79). It was observed that the CBT group provided a significant improvement in the QoL of these patients when compared to the control groups (-17.66 95% CI: -26.69 to -8.63, p = 0.0001, I^2 = 7%) (Additional file 1).

During 15 months, Navarrete et al [3, 7] performed a CBT program with SLE patients and the control groups received conventional care. It was shown that the group that performed CBT presented a reduction in the level of depression and anxiety, improvement in the level of physical function and vitality, as well as an improvement in the general perception of health and a statistically significant improvement in the QoL.

Phytotherapeutic treatment

Two studies, Arriens et al [8] and Shamehki et al [4], evaluated QoL after treatment with herbal medicines (n = 100). It was observed that the phytotherapeutic treatment for QoL was not statistically significant when purchased from the placebo groups (-4.94 95% CI: -16.31 to 6.43), p = 0.39, I^2 = 0%) (Additional file 1).

In this meta-analysis, Arriens et al [8] and Shamehki et al [4] carried out a program with herbal medicines for a period of 06 and 03 months, respectively. It was observed that supplementation resulted in improvement in vitality and in the general health aspect of QoL.

Pharmacological treatment

Strand et al [9] carried out a 12-month study (n = 48) comparing QOL in SLE patients who used epratuzumab compared to the placebo group. It was not possible to conduct a meta-analysis due to the fact that only one study met the eligibility criteria of this review. However, mean SF-36 scores showed evident improvements in the intervention group.

Discussion

In this systematic review, it was found that the treatments/therapies were associated with a statistically significant improvement in the QoL of patients with SLE. However, if observed separately, physical activity and phytotherapy programs did not achieve significant improvements. It is worth

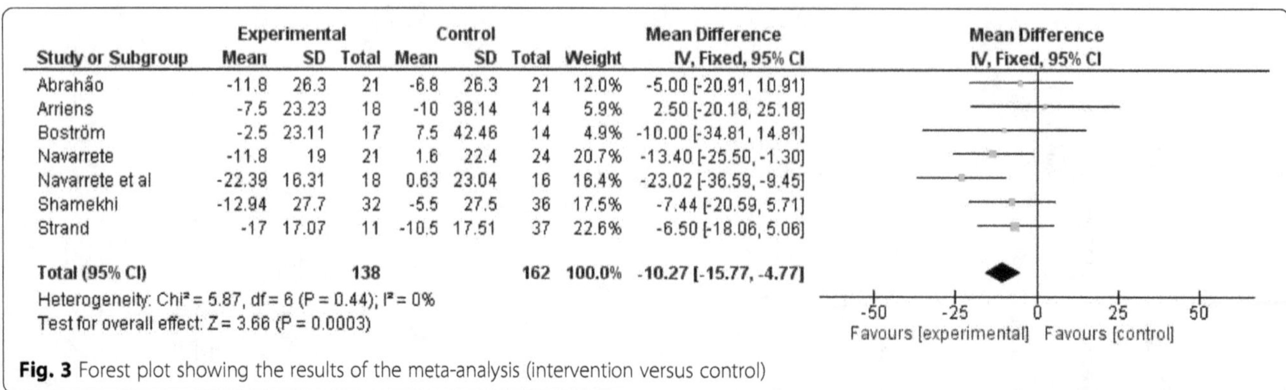

Study or Subgroup	Experimental Mean	SD	Total	Control Mean	SD	Total	Weight	Mean Difference IV, Fixed, 95% CI
Abrahão	-11.8	26.3	21	-6.8	26.3	21	12.0%	-5.00 [-20.91, 10.91]
Arriens	-7.5	23.23	18	-10	38.14	14	5.9%	2.50 [-20.18, 25.18]
Boström	-2.5	23.11	17	7.5	42.46	14	4.9%	-10.00 [-34.81, 14.81]
Navarrete	-11.8	19	21	1.6	22.4	24	20.7%	-13.40 [-25.50, -1.30]
Navarrete et al	-22.39	16.31	18	0.63	23.04	16	16.4%	-23.02 [-36.59, -9.45]
Shamekhi	-12.94	27.7	32	-5.5	27.5	36	17.5%	-7.44 [-20.59, 5.71]
Strand	-17	17.07	11	-10.5	17.51	37	22.6%	-6.50 [-18.06, 5.06]
Total (95% CI)			**138**			**162**	**100.0%**	**-10.27 [-15.77, -4.77]**

Heterogeneity: Chi² = 5.87, df = 6 (P = 0.44); I² = 0%
Test for overall effect: Z = 3.66 (P = 0.0003)

Fig. 3 Forest plot showing the results of the meta-analysis (intervention versus control)

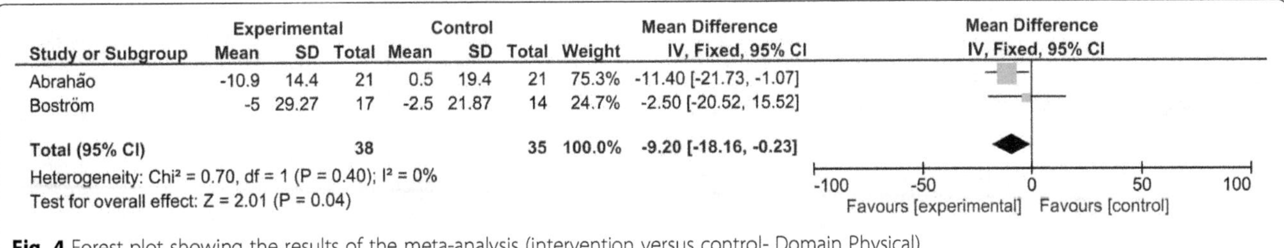

Fig. 4 Forest plot showing the results of the meta-analysis (intervention versus control- Domain Physical)

mentioning that it was not possible to perform the meta-analysis with the pharmacological treatment.

Patients with SLE may develop with limitations in exercise capacity and reduction in QoL [10], due to the great amount of pathophysiological and psychosocial symptoms imposed by the disease [11]. Regular physical exercise has as main objectives for SLE patients, increase the perception of physical function and reduce fatigue, besides providing numerous benefits for mental health, which directly interfere in the perception of QoL [12].

Abrahão et al [5] found higher SF-36 scores in physical aspects and vitality, however, no significant differences were found in the score referring to the general health aspect. The same was reported by Boström et al [6], who after 12 months, concluded an improvement in the mental health field and considered it a positive effect, since there were lower feelings of nervousness and depression. However, regarding the general health aspect of QoL, no significant results were obtained.

Behavioral cognitive therapies focus on the psychological aspect as a positive effect in the therapeutic approach in anxiety and mood disorders, depression and chronic pain. The purpose of CBTs is to minimize the interference of the disease in patients' daily lives, improving the social aspect and the independence levels and, consequently, the well-being of these individuals [13]. This was demonstrated by Navarrete et al [3, 7] in their studies, where they found a significant reduction in levels of depression, anxiety and daily stress, and at the same time, obtained improvements in levels of physical function, vitality, mental health and general health perception.

The results found by Navarrete et al [3, 7], suggest that CBT relieves somatic symptoms, facilitating coping with the disease and improving the implications of long-term health behaviors.

The phytotherapeutic treatment is used as a way to intervene in the health-disease process, aiming to establish a balance between innumerable dimensions that establish the human being, contributing to better well-being and QoL.

The changes in the perception of QoL refer to the greater capacity to perform activities and the achievement of satisfactory levels of health [14].

Arriens et al [8] presented in their study with fish oil an improvement in disease activity, inflammatory biomarkers and QoL. However, this improvement in QOL was not statistically significant, since most of the SF-36 scores remained unchanged. There has been an improvement in vitality and emotional well-being. This can be complemented by Shamekhi et al [4], who obtained results favorable to general health, physical appearance and vitality.

Pharmacological treatment for SLE has been shown to be essential, since patient survival has increased in the last two decades. However, QoL has decreased due to the fact that currently available treatments are often associated with adverse factors [15], leading to a reduction in physical well-being and a negative impact on daily living activities [16]. This is not consistent with the study by Strand et al [9].

The study lasted for 12 months and it was observed that the patients who were part of the intervention group (epratuzumab 720 mg/m2) exceeded the normative values in pain scores, social, emotional, mental health and vitality scores, and no improvement was identified in the general aspect of health.

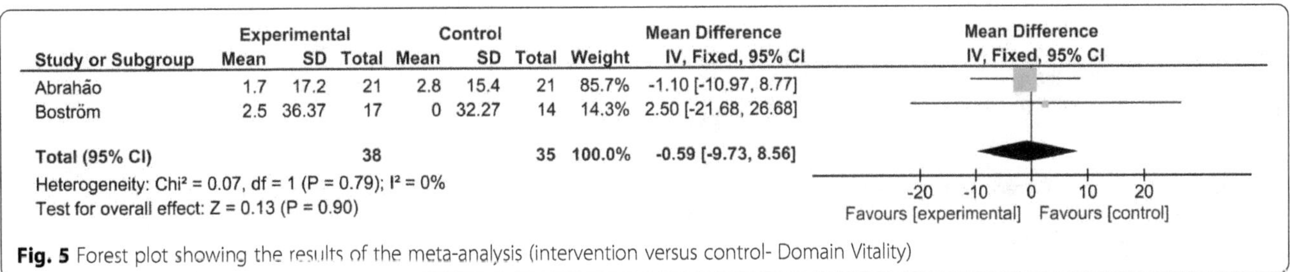

Fig. 5 Forest plot showing the results of the meta-analysis (intervention versus control- Domain Vitality)

This systematic review with meta-analysis has some limitations. First, this review was limited to only a single database. In addition, few studies were included and the studies included in this review consisted of small samples (between 31 and 68 participants), which may suggest the possibility of type II errors. We also believe that there may have been multiple publication bias for the subgroup of cognitive behavioral therapy, since part of the population may have been computed in two studies, which may compromise the results of the analysis for this subgroup. However, in order to avoid compromising the outcome of the meta-analysis in which we included all studies (fig. 06), we performed a new analysis in which we included only one study from Navarrete, and we identified that there was no statistically significant change (see Additional file 1).

The presence of bias in these studies leads to conclusions that systematically tend not to be completely reliable [17]. Only two studies clearly described the blinding of participants and practitioners and the confidentiality of concealment of allocation, and only three trials reported blinding of outcome assessors. However, as previously described, the analysis was hampered by the small number of studies and participants.

Conclusion

This systematic review with meta-analysis suggests that interventions such as physical activity, cognitive behavioral therapy, phytotherapy, and pharmacological treatment improve QOL in patients with SLE, being more evident in cognitive behavioral therapy. However, the methodological quality of the included articles and the small sample sizes propose that new randomized clinical trials be performed. The studies should be elaborated with greater methodological rigor and a greater number of patients.

Additional file

Additional file 1: Figure S1. Forest plot showing the results of the meta-analysis (One study was excluded)

Acknowledgments
Not applicable.

Authors' contributions
RRBTM; KL and TCH drafted the manuscript. RRBTM and TCH carried out the analysis. All authors read and approved the final manuscript.

Author details
[1]Faculdade Metropolitana de Camaçari- Jorge Amado, Ponto Certo, Camaçari, BA 42.801-120, Brazil. [2]Centro Universitário Estácio da Bahia, Xingu Street, 179 - Stiep, Salvador, BA, Brazil. [3]Universidade do Estado da Bahia-Silveira Martins, 2555 - Cabula, Salvador, BA 41150-000, Brazil.

References

1. Piga M, Congia M, Gabba A, Figus F, Floris A, Mathieu A, et al. Musculoskeletal manifestations as determinants of quality of life impairment in patients with systemic lupus erythematosus. Sage J. 2017.
2. Pereira EF, Teixeira CS, Santos A. Qualidade de vida: abordagens, conceitos e avaliação. Rev. Bras. Educ. Fís. Esporte. 2012;26:241–50.
3. Navarrete-Navarrete N, Peralta-Ramírez MI, Sabio-Sánchez JM, Coín MA, Robles-Ortega H, Hidalgo-Tenorio C, et al. Efficacy of cognitive Behavioural therapy for the treatment of chronic stress in patients with lupus erythematosus: a randomized controlled trial. Psychother Psychosom. 2010; 79:107–15.
4. Shamekhi Z, Amani R, Habibagahi Z, Namjoyan F, Ghadiri A, Malehi AS. A Randomized, Double-blind, Placebo-controlled Clinical Trial Examining the Effects of Green Tea Extract on Systemic Lupus Erythematosus Disease Activity and Quality of Life. Phytother Res. 2017;31(7):1063–71.
5. Abrahão MI, Gomiero AB, Peccin MS, Grande AJ, Trevisani VFM. Cardiovascular training vs. resistance training for improving quality of life and physical function in patients with systemic lupus erythematosus: a randomized controlled trial. Scand J Rheumatol. 2015:1–5.
6. Boström C, Elfving B, Dupré B, Opava CH, Lundberg IE, Jansson E. Effects of a one-year physical activity programme for women with systemic lupus erythematosus – a randomized controlled study. Sage Journals. 2016;25: 602–16.
7. Navarrete-Navarrete N, Peralta-Ramírez MI, Sabio JM, Martínez-Egea I, Santos-Ruiz A, Jiménez-Alonso J. Quality-of-life predictor factors in patients with SLE and their modification after cognitive behavioural therapy. Sage Journals. 2010;19:1632–9.
8. Arriens C, Hynan LS, Lerman RH, Karp DR, Mohan C. Placebo-controlled randomized clinical trial of fish oil's impact on fatigue, quality of life, and disease activity in systemic lupus erythematosus. Nutr J. 2015;14:82.
9. Strand V, Petri M, Kalunian K, Gordon C, Wallace DJ, Hobbs K, et al. Epratuzumab for patients with moderate to severe flaring SLE: health-related quality of life outcomes and corticosteroid use in the randomized controlled ALLEVIATE trials and extension study SL0006. Rheumatology. 2014;53:502–11.
10. Carvalho MR, Sato EI, Tebexreni AS, Heidecher RT, Schenkman S, Neto TL. Effects of supervised cardiovascular training program on exercise tolerance, aerobic capacity, and quality of life in patients with systemic lupus erythematosus. Rev Arthritis & Rheumatism. 2005;53:838–44.
11. Yuen HK, Cunningham MA. Optimal management of fatigue in patients with systemic lupus erythematosus. Rev. Ther Clin Risk Manag. 2014;10: 775–86.
12. Mancuso CA, Perna M, Sargent AB, Salmon JE. Perceptions and measurements of physical activity in patients with systemic lupus erythematosus. Sage Journals. 2010;20:231–42.
13. Solati K, Mousavi M, Kheiri S, Hasanpour-Dehkordi A. The effectiveness of mindfulness-based cognitive therapy on psychological symptoms and quality of life in systemic lupus erythematosus patients: a randomized controlled trial. Oman Med J. 2017;32:378–85.
14. Loures MC, Porto CC, Siqueira KM, Barbosa MA, Medeiros M, Brasil W, et al. Contribuições da fitoterapia para a qualidade de vida: percepções de seus usuários. Rev. Enfermagem - UERJ. 2010;18:278–83.
15. Tian J, Luo Y, Wu H, et al. Risk of adverse events from different drugs for SLE: a systematic review and network meta-analysis. Lupus Sci Med. 2018;5: e000253. https://doi.org/10.1136/lupus-2017-000253.
16. Medeiros MM, Menezes AP, Silveira VA, Ferreira FN, Lima GR, Ciconelli RM. Health-related quality of life in patients with systemic lupus erythematosus and its relationship with cyclophosphamide pulse therapy. Eur J Intern Med. 2008;19:122–8.
17. Carvalho AP, Silva V, Grande AJ. Avaliação do risco de viés de ensaios clínicos randomizados pela ferramenta da colaboração Cochrane. Diagn Tratamento. 2013;18:38–44.

21

The use of ultrasonography in the diagnosis of nail disease among patients with psoriasis and psoriatic arthritis

José Alexandre Mendonça[1*], Sibel Zehra Aydin[2] and Maria-Antonietta D'Agostino[3,4]

Abstract

Background: Nail involvement has been described as a key clinical feature for both psoriasis (PsO) and psoriatic arthritis (PsA) and is an important risk factor in PsA. Thus, early diagnosis of nail involvement may be essential for better management of PsO and PsA. Ultrasonography is considered a highly promising method to visualize nail disease. The main aim of this review was to evaluate the use of ultrasonography for the diagnosis of nail disease in patients with PsO and PsA by reviewing ultrasound parameters with the best diagnostic accuracy.
Main body of the abstract: A systematic search was performed in MEDLINE via the PubMed and LILACS databases. Conference proceedings of relevant rheumatology scientific meetings were also screened.

Results: After applying eligibility criteria, only 13 articles and 5 abstracts were included in this review. The selected studies showed a huge variability in evaluation methods (and therefore in the results) and were mainly focused on the assessment of nails ultrasound parameters that may differ among patients and healthy controls, especially the morphological aspects in B-mode ultrasonography and vascularization of the nail bed by Doppler ultrasonography. Our research indicated that the evaluation of nail disease in PsO and PsA is still underrepresented in the literature, probably reflecting a restricted use in clinical practice, despite the widespread use of ultrasonography in the management of chronic arthritis.

Short conclusions: Despite the potential relevance of ultrasonography for the diagnosis of nail disease, additional studies are needed to determine which features are more reliable and clinically pertinent to ensure accuracy in the evaluation of nail involvement in PsO and PsA.

Keywords: Psoriasis, Psoriatic arthritis, Ultrasonography, Spectral Doppler, Power Doppler, Ungueal disease

Background

Psoriasis (PsO) is defined as a chronic, immune-mediated, gene-based disease with an inflammatory background that affects the skin, semi-mucosa, and joints. When joints and surrounding structures are involved, patients are classified as having psoriatic arthritis (PsA) [1–4]. The prevalence of PsO may range from 0.5 to 11.8% around the world [5–9], while the prevalence of PsA amongst patients with PsO varies from 5.9 to 48%, according to the patient characteristics and classification criteria used [1, 3, 4, 8]. PsO manifestations may vary; however, plaque PsO (or psoriasis vulgaris) is the most frequent skin phenotype, affecting approximately 90% of patients with PsO [9]. The disease may also affect the scalp, joints, creases, or nails, even in patients without skin lesions [10].

Fifty to 80 % of patients with PsO have concurrent nail lesions [11–13], which can lead to functional impairment, pain and discomfort, and decreased quality of life and general well-being [14, 15]. Despite its significant prevalence (around 50% of patients), nail manifestations are often neglected in daily clinical practice, probably

* Correspondence: mendoncaja.us@gmail.com
[1]Department of Rheumatology and Postgraduate Program of the Pontifical Catholic, University of Campinas, Rua da Fazenda, 125, Condomínio Dálias, casa 10, Residencial Vila Flora, Sumaré, São Paulo 13175665, Brazil
Full list of author information is available at the end of the article

due to a lack of recognition of its impact on patients or its relevance as an indicator of disease extension [15].

Psoriatic arthritis leads to impairments in a patient's life, decreasing functional capacity and quality of life, which also increases the burden of disease to society. This burden highlights the need for early diagnosis and timely treatment for all comorbidities. In this sense, nail disease has been reported as a relevant risk factor for PsA [16] and may be employed as an early diagnostic parameter among patients with PsO.

Imaging techniques such as ultrasonography (US) have been increasingly used to diagnose and to monitor clinical features of PsO and PsA [17–20]. US findings usually include measures of thickness of the nail bed and the ventral and dorsal plates, as well as loss of definition, morphologic changes, and blood flow disturbances [21, 22]. Power Doppler (PD) and spectral Doppler (SD) are US techniques that are used to visualize nail inflammation. PD semiquantitatively shows nail inflammation through the detection of increased flow in blood vessels, whereas SD calculates the resistive index (RI) using systolic and diastolic peak flows of small vessels, which expresses the resistance to blood flow in the nail bed [22, 23]. Despite the relevance of US, discordant data are available on the usefulness of Doppler techniques for the evaluation of nail disease in PsO and PsA. Thus, the aims of this review are (i) to investigate the usefulness of nail US for the diagnosis of nail disease in patients with PsO and PsA; (ii) to gather data about parameters obtained through Doppler techniques (PD and SD) indicating inflammation of the nail bed, including but not limited to RI and vascularization of the nail unit; and (iii) to observe the differences between PsO, PsA, and healthy controls in RI and morphologic changes.

Main text

Methods

A systematic search was performed using MEDLINE via PubMed and LILACS (Latin American and Caribbean Health Sciences Literature) in order to identify studies addressing the use of US in nail assessment in terms of variables relevant in the context of PsO and PsA, to meet the previously mentioned goals. Two search strategies using a combination of controlled vocabulary (MeSH and DeCs keywords, for Pubmed and LILACS, respectively) and text words were adopted, as shown in Table 1. Searches were performed until March 20, 2018.

Conference proceedings of relevant scientific meetings in rheumatology (European League Against Rheumatism and American College of Rheumatology, as selected by the authors) were also screened. Only studies published during the past 10 years were considered eligible. Language selection was made manually by the reviewers.

After applying the predefined search strategies, the records were screened by two different reviewers using the following inclusion criteria: i) observational or non-therapy interventional studies; ii) patients with PsO and/or PsA; iii) studies assessing the use of US for nail assessment; and iii) papers reported in English, French, Portuguese, and Spanish only. Studies were deemed non-eligible if they consisted of any of the following exclusion criteria: i) clinical trials of any phase or study design or ii) case reports.

Initially, it was planned that in cases of discordance, a third reviewer would be the responsible for the final decision to include a selected article or not. No disagreements were identified in the review process; therefore, this strategy was unnecessary. Data extraction was performed by the reviewers, using a data collection tool specifically designed for this review. Variables abstracted from individual studies were: author, year, study design, sample size, baseline disease (if applicable), primary and secondary aims (if applicable), US assessments performed, nail parameters described, results. Assessment of bias was based on the Joanna Briggs Institute Critical Appraisal Instrument for Studies Reporting Prevalence Data [24, 25]. The risk assessment tool is descriptive and does not provide scores.

Results

A total of 48 records were initially identified. After application of the eligibility criteria, 13 were selected and included in this review. In addition, five abstracts were manually identified in the conference proceedings searched (Fig. 1), which provided the final number of 18 studies analyzed.

The main characteristics of the 18 studies included in this review are summarized in Table 2.

Assessment of bias

The Joanna Briggs Institute Critical Appraisal Instrument for Studies Reporting Prevalence Data was applied to all of the included studies. In terms of sample frame and sampling, most studies used a clinic-based approach

Table 1 Search strategy

Database	Search Strategy
PubMed	("Arthritis, Psoriatic"[Mesh] OR "Psoriasis"[Mesh] OR "psoriatic arthritis" OR "psoriasis") AND ("Ultrasonography"[Mesh] OR "ultrasound" OR "Ultrasonography, Doppler"[Mesh] OR "Doppler" OR "Power doppler" OR "spectral") AND ("nail" OR "ungueal")
LILACS	("Psoríase" or "Psoriasis" or "Arthritis, Psoriatic" or "Artrite Psoriásica") and ("ultrasonography" or "ultrasound" or "ultrassonografia" or "doppler") and ("unha" or "nail" or "ungueal")

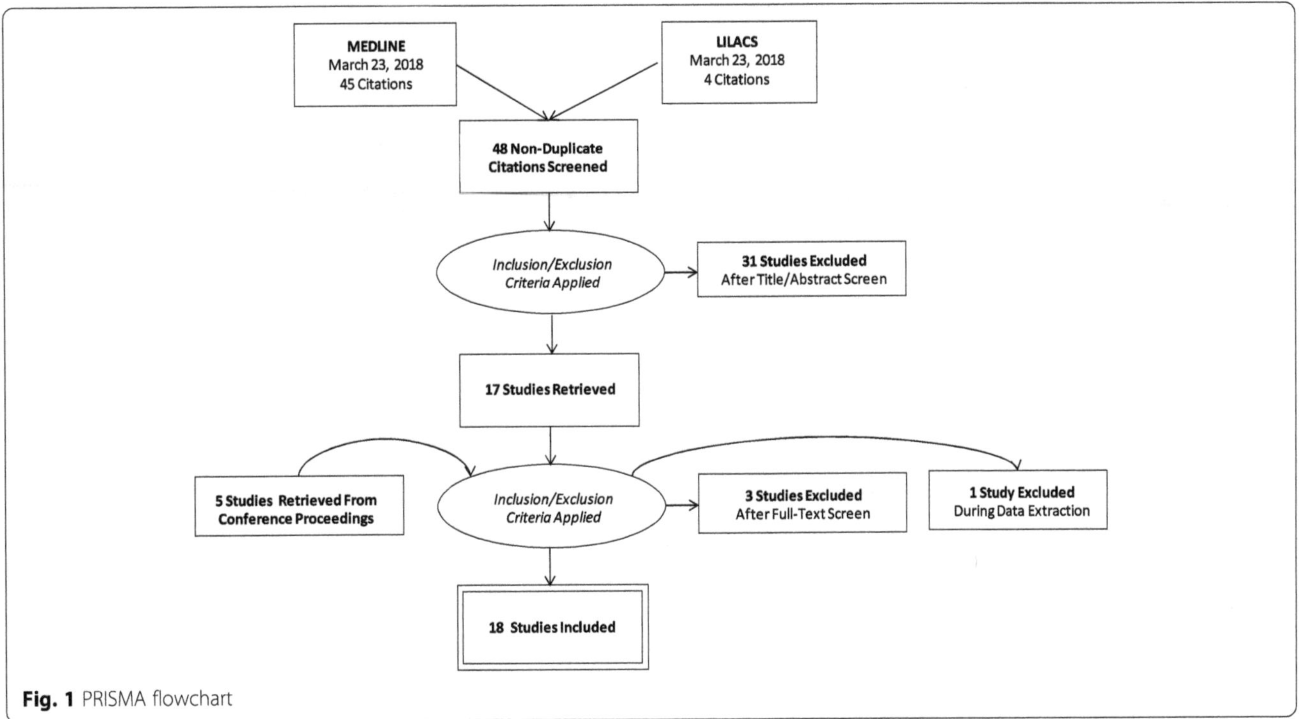

Fig. 1 PRISMA flowchart

and described how the potential participants were recruited. Sample sizes varied from 10 to 238 patients, and all of them relied upon convenience, without clearly stating a sample size calculation rationale. Study subjects were appropriately described in all included studies, and valid methods to determine the presence of the pathological condition were used and extensively described. The statistical analysis plan was deemed appropriate for the 15 studies [26–40]. Overall, the risk of bias was assessed as moderate to high due to the small sample size of the studies.

Main findings of included studies

After full text analysis of the 18 records included in the review, a wide range of variables and methodologic approaches was identified. Tables 3, 4, and 5 summarize the key features that are relevant to this systematic literature review. Due to the methodologic variability of the included studies (as shown in Table 2), comparability or further data pooling was deemed not feasible. The descriptive data regarding grey-scale features, presence of Doppler vascularity, and RI measurement of nails' vascularization are presented below.

Gray-scale features of the nail by ultrasonography

Twelve studies reviewed gray-scale findings [26, 28–31, 33–39]. Three of these studies were only pictorial essays, which were purely descriptive [41–43]. The terminology that was used by different investigators to describe gray-scale findings widely varied across studies, such as "loss of definition," "hyperechoic definition," "fusion," or "hyperechoic focal involvement of the ventral plate," all of which are likely to correspond to the loss of trilaminar appearance. The normal nail plate was usually described as "two hyperechoic white bands surrounding an anechoic well defined layer in between" and the lack of visibility of the latter anechoic layer may technically be named using one of these definitions. Although it was impossible to compare studies in the absence of a uniform definition, there were consistently more nail lesions as measured using US in patients with PsA (46–54%) [29, 35] and PsO (48.8–77.8%) [33, 35–37] compared with healthy controls (10%) [37]. In addition, patients with clinical nail disease were consistently found to have more lesions on US (57/101 [56.4%] vs 6/68 [8.8%]; $p < 0.0001$) [37] and had more frequent ventral nail plate deposits (median, 17.72 [Q1–Q3 = 10.14–27.83] vs 4.65 [Q1–Q3 = 0.05–16.23]; $p = 0.0410$) [31]. US results have a good agreement with clinical assessment for nail disease (kappa value = 0.79 for PsA patients and controls; $p < 0.001$) [33] and also a strong correlation (chi-square test, 10.769 for PsA and osteoarthritis patients; $p = 0.001$) [29]. However, it was not possible to confirm that US was more sensitive to detect nail disease versus clinical assessment. While there was higher number of nails with US features in the absence of clinical findings, there were also patients with positive clinical nail disease and no US features [36]. Nails with a false negative US test had mainly mild lesions, such as onycholysis or pitting with lower modified nail psoriasis severity index (mNAPSI, a psoriatic nail grading instrument used to

Table 2 Studies included in the review

Author	Year	Study Design	Sample characteristics[a]	Aim	Ultrasonography assessment	Ultrasonography variables reported for the nail	Risk of bias
Arbault et al [26]	2017	Cross-sectional	27 patients with PsA Severity level: NR Duration (mean): 13.4 ± 9.4 years Age (mean): age 55 ± 16.2 years Female:40.74 %	To determine the feasibility, reliability, and validity of nail US in PsA as an outcome measure.	• ESAOTE MyLab 70 XVG fitted with a high frequency transducer of 22 mHz. (PRF: 500 Hz, Doppler frequency: 6.3 MHz, Gain: 30%)	• Nail bed thickness • Nail plate thickness	High
Aydin et al [27]	2017	Cross-sectional	86 patients with PsO and 19 healthy controls Severity level: NR Duration (mean): NR Age (mean): NR Female: NR	To find the frequency and severity of PD signals in psoriatic nail disease compared with healthy controls to understand whether PD signals are associated with disease.	• Logiq E9 machine (General Electric, Wauwatosa, WI, USA) • Linear probe at 10–18 MHz • PD settings: pulse repetition frequency of 800 Hz, a Doppler frequency of 9.1, and low wall filters	• PD changes on the nail bed	Moderate
Fassio et al [28]	2017	Case-control	82 cases (31 PsO, 51 PsA, and 50 controls) Severity level: NR Duration (mean): NR Age (mean): NR Female: NR	To evaluate the presence of the nail involvement and subclinical alterations using US in PsO and PsA.	• Not informed	• Nail bed thickness • Nail plate thickness	Moderate
Paramalingam et al [29]	2017	Cross-sectional	10 patients with PsA Severity level: NR Duration (mean): NR Age (mean): 55.0 (48.0–63.2) years Female: NR	To investigate the nail bed changes seen in patients with PsA and OA using US and MRI, and to determine the impact of nail bed changes on quality of life.	• Not informed	• Pitting • Nail structural abnormalities • Trilaminar appearance	High
Acquitter et al [30]	2016	Cross-sectional	37 patients with PsO (18 with nail disease and19 with scalp PsO and/or inverse PsO) Severity level: NR Duration (mean): (years/SD) 13.28/10.34 Nail psoriasis 17.11/13.14; Inverse and scalp psoriasis Age (mean): 47.61 (15.88) years Nail psoriasis; 47.11 (12.65) years Inverse and scalp psoriasis Female: 44.44% Nail psoriasis; 63.15% Inverse and scalp psoriasis	To detect subclinical entheses and nail abnormalities using gray-scale and PD US between patients with nail PsO and those with inverse and scalp PsO.	• IU 22 machine (Philips) and a linear probe at 12.5 MHz (PRF = 500 Hz)	• Nail matrix thickness • PD signal in nail bed • Trilaminar appearance	High

Table 2 Studies included in the review *(Continued)*

Author	Year	Study Design	Sample characteristics[a]	Aim	Ultrasonography assessment	Ultrasonography variables reported for the nail	Risk of bias
Marina et al [31]	2016	Case-control	23 cases with PsO and 11 controls Severity level: moderate-to-severe chronic plaque psoriasis Duration (mean): lasting at least 6 months Age (mean): 52.43±14.28SD years Female: 21%	To evaluate both the morphologic appearance and blood flow changes in the nail apparatus of patients with PsO compared with disease-free controls using gray-scale and color and PD HRUS.	• Transducer ranging from 8–40 MHz (focal range 0.2–3 cm, image field 16 mm) – nail anatomy • Hitachi EUB 8500 System with a variable-frequency transducer ranging from 6.5–13 MHz – blood flow • Doppler (color Doppler: PRF 500–1000 Hz, wall filter 25–50 Hz, PD: PRF 350–700 Hz, wall filter 22–50 Hz; color and PD) • Esaote US machine with 18 MHz – morphostructural changes	• Ventral nail plate deposits • Nail plate aspect • Color Doppler spots • PD spots • Nail bed thickness • Nail plates thickness • Nailfold vessel RI	High
Mendonça et al [32]	2015	Case-control	44 cases (PsA and 16 controls (10 healthy controls, 6 OA) Severity level: NR Duration (mean): NR Age (mean): NR Female: NR	To compare PD and SD US indexes (semiquantitative gray-scale and PD scores) and RI in the nails of patients with PsA and their controls.	• PD and SD techniques with frequency ranging from 6–8 MHz	• RI	High
El Miedany et al [33]	2014	Case-control	126 cases (PsO) and 112 controls Severity level: PASI 12.4± 10.4 Duration (mean): 4.8±3.1 mo Age (mean): 35.9±8.7 years Female: 43.4%	To identify the clinical predictors of arthritis in patients with PsO and to evaluate the use of musculoskeletal US as a predictor for inflammatory structural progression consistent with early PsA in psoriatic patients, using rheumatologic evaluation as the gold standard for diagnosis.	• Multi-frequency linear array 14–21 MHz transducer; • Gray-scale and PD techniques.	• Trilaminar appearance	Moderate
Mendonça et al [34]	2014	Case-control	28 cases (PsA) and 7 controls Severity level: PASI 6.03± 12.27 Duration (mean): 10.05± 10.49 mo Age (mean): 45.3±14.61 years Female: 54.5% women	To assess the RI in the nail bed in longitudinal and transverse planes and correlate with the presence of PD in the nail bed, change in standard trilaminar appearance of the nail, measure of the nail bed, and clinical measurements.	• Esaote US machine , with 6–18 MHz broadband multifrequency linear transducer • Doppler frequency ranging from 7.1–14.3 MHz	• RI in the nail bed in longitudinal plane • RI in the nail bed in transverse plane • PD in the nail bed • Trilaminar appearance • Nail bed thickness	High
Sandobal et al [35]	2014	Case-control	35 cases with PsA, 20 with PsO, 28 healthy subjects, and 27 with RA Severity level: PASI 3 Duration (mean): 9±1.6 mo Age (mean): 51±13 years Female: NR	To show findings at finger nails level revealed by high-frequency gray-scale US and PD in patients with PsA, and cutaneous PsO compared with RA and control subjects.	• MyLab 25 XVG system with a variable-frequency transducer ranging from 10–18 MHz • Doppler frequency ranging from 6–8 MHz	• Wortsman typology • PD signal in nail beds • Nail thickness	High

Table 2 Studies included in the review *(Continued)*

Author	Year	Study Design	Sample characteristics[a]	Aim	Ultrasonography assessment	Ultrasonography variables reported for the nail	Risk of bias
Aydin et al [36]	2013	Case-control	5 cases with PsO, 13 with PsA and 12 controls Severity level: NR Duration (mean): NR Age (mean): NR Female: NR	To compare optical coherence tomography US for nail disease assessment in psoriatic disease.	• Logiq E9 machine with a linear probe at 9–14 MHz • Multiplanar technique • Gray-scale technique	• Trilaminar appearance • Pitting	High
Aydin et al [37]	2012	Case-control	86 cases (PsO) and 20 controls Severity level: mNAPSI 15 Duration (mean): 16 mo Age (mean): NR Female: 38.4%	To compare US with the modified NAPSI, to investigate the nail plate, nail matrix, and adjacent tendons in subjects with psoriatic nail disease and to test the hypothesis that nail involvement was specifically linked to extensor tendon enthesopathy.	• Logiq E9 machine with a linear probe at 18–10 MHz • Gray-scale technique - frequency at 14 MHz, gain at 18 dB, and a dynamic range at 36 dB	• Pitting • Nail thickness • Nail matrix	Moderate
Gisondi et al [38]	2012	Case-control	138 cases (PsO) and 83 controls Severity level: NAPSI 18.4 ± 17.5 Duration (mean): 20 ± 12 mo Age (mean): |NR Female: 15%	To estimate nail involvement in patients with chronic plaque PsO using US.	• Voluson I portable US machine (General Electrics, United States) with linear 10–18 MHz probe equipped with a variable-frequency transducer of 18 MHz • Gray-scale technique	• Thickening of the nail plate • Sub-nail hyperkeratosis • Pitting	Moderate
Haddad et al [39]	2012	Case-control	10 PsA cases, 10 PsO cases, and 20 controls Severity level: NR Duration (mean): 21.1 ± 11.7 mo Age (mean): 54.7 ± 12.6 years Female: 22.2%	To investigate the association between clinical and ultrasonographic features of psoriatic nail disease and to identify specific nail features associated with PsA.	• 10-MHz linear array transducer • Doppler signal standardized with a pulse repetition frequency of 400 Hz, a gain of 20 dB, and a low wall	• Loss of definition of the ventral plate • Hyperechoioc focal involvement of the ventral plate • Thickening of both the and dorsal and ventral plates • Nail bed thickness • Nail matrix thickness • Nail bed vascularity • Nail matrix vascularity	High
El-Ahmed et al [40]	2011	Case-control	23 PsO cases (16 with nail disease and 7 without) and 23 controls Severity level: NR Duration (mean): NR Age (mean): 42 years Female: 34.78%	To evaluate the vascularity in the nails of patients with PsO treated with classic and biologic therapies for comparison with disease-free controls, and to evaluate whether there are differences in nail vascularity among patients with and without nail involvement.	• Echo Doppler examination	• Nailfold vessel RI	High

Table 2 Studies included in the review *(Continued)*

Author	Year	Study Design	Sample characteristics[a]	Aim	Ultrasonography assessment	Ultrasonography variables reported for the nail	Risk of bias
Gutierrez et al [41]	2010	Pictorial essay	30 cases (PsA) Severity level: PASI 12.4 Duration (mean): NR Age (mean): NR Female: NR	To show the main high-frequency gray-scale US and PD findings in patients with PsA at joint, tendon, enthesis, skin, and nail level.	• MyLab 70 XVG with 6–18 MHz broadband multifrequency linear transducer and Doppler frequency ranging from 7.1 to 14.3 MHz • Technos "Partner" System with 8–14 MHz multifrequency linear band transducer and Doppler frequency ranging from 8.3–12.5 MHz • Logiq with 8–15 MHz multifrequency linear transducer	• Hyperechoic definition of the nail plate • Fusion of nail plate • Thickening of nail plate • Nail bed • Blood flow	High
Gutierrez et al [42]	2009	Case-control	20 cases (PsO) and 10 controls Severity level: NR Duration (mean): NR Age (mean): 32-52 years Female: 65%	To show the main sonographic findings obtainable with "last-generation" high-frequency transducers and PD technique in patients with PsO.	• MyLab 70 XVG with a variable-frequency transducer ranging from 6–18 MHz	• Only descriptive approach of morphologic characteristics of nail; • Nail homogeneity • Trilaminar aspect • Nail bed • Blood flow	High
Gutierrez et al [43]	2009	Case-control	30 cases (PsO) and 15 controls Severity level: PASI 12.3 Duration (mean): 20 mo Age (mean): 46 years Female: 40%	To show the potential of the latest sonographic equipment using high-frequency probes and a very sensitive PD technique in depicting both skin and nail changes in patients affected by PsO.	• MyLab 70 XVG system with a variable-frequency transducer ranging from 6–18 MHz and a Doppler frequency ranging from 7–14 MHz • Gray-scale – to detect mosphostructural changes • PD to detect abnormal blood flow • SD to confirm PD signal	• Nail plate • Nail bed • Thickening measurement • Blood flow	High

Studies reported as abstracts: Fassio et al (2017) [28], Paramalingam et al (2017) [29], Mendonça et al (2015) [32], Mendonça et al (2014) [34], and Haddad et al (2012) [39]

[a]Cases indicate the number of patients with an actual diagnosis, as compared to healthy controls, and only data for patients is presented; HRUS=high-resolution ultrasonography; *MRI* Magnetic resonance imaging, *NAPSI* Nail Psoriasis Severity Index, *NR* Not Reported, *OA* Osteoarthritis, *OCR* Optical coherence tomography, *PD* Power Doppler, *PASI* Psoriasis Area Severity Index, *PsA* Psoriatic arthritis, *PsO* Psoriasis, *RA* Rheumatoid arthritis, *RI* Resistive Index, *SD* Spectral Doppler, *US* Ultrasonography

Table 3 Studies comprising measurements on gray-scale[a]

Studies	Population	Gray-scale	Result
Arbault et al. (2017) [26]	PsA	Nail bed thickness Mean (SD): 0.5 mm (0.04) Nail plate thickness Mean (SD): 2.0 mm (0.42)	–
Fassio et al. (2017) [28]	PsO	Nail bed thickness Mean (SD): 0.25 mm (0.05) Nail plate thickness Mean (SD): 0.063 mm (0.011)	Healthy controls had lower nail plate and nail bed thickness.
	PsA	Nail bed thickness Mean (SD): 0.25 mm (0.04) Nail plate thickness Mean (SD): 0.065 mm (0.014)	
	Controls	Nail bed thickness Mean (SD): 0.22 mm (0.02) Nail plate thickness Mean (SD): 0.051 mm (0.006)	
Acquitter et al. (2016) [30]	Patients with PsO with nail disease	Nail matrix thickness Median (SD): 1.94 mm (0.69)	Patients with PsO with nail disease presented with significantly higher nail matrix thickness than patients with scalp PsO and/or inverse PsO ($p < 0.01$).
	Patients with scalp PsO and/or inverse PsO	Nail matrix thickness Median (SD): 1.77 mm (0.54)	
Marina et al. (2016) [31]	PsO	Nail bed thickness Median (IQR): 1.88 mm (1.71–2.03) Nail plate thickness Median (IQR): 0.86 mm (0.60–1.14)	Healthy controls had a statistically significant lower nail plate thickness than patients with PsO ($p < 0.0001$). No significant differences were observed in nail bed thickness variability among groups ($p = 0.4621$).
	Controls	Nail bed thickness Median (IQR): 1.89 mm (1.78–2.00) Nail plate thickness Median (IQR): 0.63 mm (0.59–0.67)	
Mendonça et al. (2014) [34]	PsA	NGS Mean (SD): 0.48 mm (0.50)	Healthy controls had lower NGS than patients with PsA.
	Controls	NGS Mean (SD): 0.00 mm (0.00)	
Aydin et al. (2012) [37]	PsO	Nail thickness Median (range): 0.56 mm (0.3–1.9)	Healthy controls had slightly lower NGS than patients with PsO.
	Controls	Nail thickness Median (range): 0.5 mm (0.3–0.6)	
Gisondi et al. (2012) [38]	PsO	Nail plate thickness 70 patients (50%)	–
Haddad et al. (2012) [39]	PsO	Nail bed thickness Mean (SD): 16.0 mm (2.9) Nail matrix thickness Mean (SD): 17.5 mm (2.9)	Comparing the three groups, patients with PsO and PsA presented with statistically significant higher values of nail bed thickness and nail matrix thickness than controls ($p < 0.0001$). Comparing patients with PsO and PsA, patients with PsO presented with a significantly lower nail matrix thickness than patients with PsA ($p = 0.002$). No statistically significant differences were observed in nail bed thickness among those groups ($p = 0.81$).
	PsA	Nail bed thickness Mean (SD): 15.9 mm (3.0) Nail matrix thickness Mean (SD): 18.8 mm (3.0)	
	Controls	Nail bed thickness Mean (SD): 14.1 mm (1.2) Nail matrix thickness Mean (SD): 15.8 mm (0.92)	

IQR interquartile range, *NGS* standard trilaminar appearance of the nail, *PD* power Doppler, *PsA* psoriatic arthritis, *PsO* psoriasis, *SD* standard deviation
[a]Only studies with quantitative results regarding nail thickness, trilaminar appearance, presence of PD signal, and nail resistive index were included in this table

Table 4 Studies comprising quantitative results on PD[a]

Studies	Population	PD	Results
Aydin et al. (2017) [27]	PsO	NPD: 84.6%	Presence of nail bed with PD signal was similar among patients with PsO and healthy controls.
	Controls	NPD: 81.6%	
Paramalingam et al. (2017) [29]	PsA	NPD: 96.0%	Patients with PsA presented with a slightly higher percentage of nails with PD signal than patients with OA.
	OA	NPD: 95.0%	
Acquitter et al. (2016) [30]	Patients with PsO with nail disease	NPD: 44.5%	NPD was higher in patients with PsO with nail disease; however, differences among groups were not significant.
	Patients with scalp PsO and/or inverse PsO	NPD: 39.0%	
Mendonça et al. (2014) [34]	PsA	NPD mean (SD): 0.88 (0.31)	NPD was slightly lower in patients with PsA than controls.
	Controls	NPD mean (SD): 1.0 (0.00)	
Sandobal et al. (2014) [35]	PsO	Increase PD signal in nail beds: 20.5%	Patients with psoriatic arthropathy showed increased PD signal in nail bed ($p = 0.0001$).
	PsA	Increase PD signal in nail beds: 23.4%	
	RA	Increase PD signal in nail beds: 2.2%	
	Controls	Increase PD signal in nail beds: 19.6%	
Haddad et al. (2012) [39]	PsO	Nail bed vascularity: 14%	Comparing the three groups, patients with PsO and PsA presented with statistically significantly lower values of nail bed vascularity than controls ($p < 0.001$). Comparing patients with PsO and PsA, patients with PsO presented with lower nail bed vascularity than patients with PsA; however, no statistically significant differences were observed ($p = 0.44$).
	PsA	Nail bed vascularity: 18%	
	Controls	Nail bed vascularity: 20%	

NPD presence of power Doppler in the nail bed, *OA* osteoarthritis, *PD* power Doppler, *PsA* psoriatic arthritis, *PsO* psoriasis, *RI* Resistive Index, *SD* standard deviation
[a]Only studies with quantitative results regarding nail thickness, trilaminar appearance, presence of PD signal, and nail RI were included in this table

Table 5 Studies comprising quantitative results on spectral Doppler[a]

Studies	Population	Spectral Doppler	Results
Marina et al. (2016) [31]	PsO	NVRI Median (IQR): 0.62 (0.55–0.69)	Patients with PsO presented with significantly higher median NVRI measurements than controls ($p < 0.0001$)
	Controls	NVRI Median (IQR): 0.57 (0.55–0.58)	
Mendonça et al. (2014) [34]	PsA	LRI Mean (SD): 0.50 (0.13) TRI Mean (SD): 0.48 (0.09)	RI measurements in both the transverse and longitudinal planes were lower for patients with PsA than controls.
	Controls	LRI Mean (SD): 0.86 (0.41) TRI Mean (SD): 0.70 (0.16)	
El-Ahmed et al. (2011) [40]	PsO	NVRI Mean (SD): 0.56 (0.09)	The mean NVRI was significantly higher in PsO than controls ($p < 0.001$). Patients with PsO with clinical nail disease had also significantly higher NVRI than those without nail disease ($p < 0.05$).
	Patients with PsO with nail disease	NVRI Mean (SD): 0.58 (0.10)	
	Patients with PsO without nail disease	NVRI Mean (SD): 0.52 (0.45)	
	Controls	NVRI Mean (SD): 0.42 (0.04)	

IQR interquartile range, *LRI* Resistance Index in longitudinal plane, *NGS* standard trilaminar appearance of the nail bed, *NVRI* Nailfold Vessel Resistive Index, *PD* power Doppler, *PsA* psoriatic arthritis, *PsO* psoriasis, *RI* Resistive Index, *SD* standard deviation, *TRI* Resistive Index in transverse plane
[a]Only studies with quantitative results regarding nail thickness, trilaminar appearance, presence of PD signal, and nail RI were included in this table

assess severity of nail matrix and bed PsO by area of involvement in the nail unit) than those with true (i.e., marked) abnormalities on US (median mNAPSI, 10 [1–56] vs 17 [1–50]; $p = 0.03$), with a moderate absolute agreement between US and clinical assessment (76.3% with $\kappa = 0.52$, $p < 0.0001$) [37].

The studies also investigated nail thickness using US, reporting an increased thickness of nail plate, bed, and matrix in patients with PsO and/or PsA compared with controls [26, 28, 30, 31, 37, 39] (Table 3). Marina et al. was not able to demonstrate a difference in nail bed thickness between patients with PsO and controls [31]. Comparing 2 groups with PsO, one with nail disease and other with scalp PsO and/or inverse PsO, Acquitter et al. (2016) reported that the former group presented with statistically higher nail matrix thickness than patients in the latter group [30]. It was not possible to identify in the studies a comparison between PsO and PsA patients in terms of nail bed thickness with statistical significant differences.

Presence of vascularity within the nail unit by ultrasonography Nail bed PD signals were variable in both patients with PsO and PsA across the studies, with a range varying from 20 to 96% [27, 29, 30, 35, 44]. A high frequency of vascularisation was also observed in healthy controls, ranging from 20 to 81.6% [27, 35]. Some studies demonstrated increased blood flow in patients with PsO [31, 39]. Comparing patients with PsO plus nails disease and patients with scalp PsO and/or inverse PsO, a higher frequency of PD signal in the nail bed was found in the first group compared with the second group [30] (Table 4). PD signals were usually scored semiquantitavely on a scale between 0 and 3. Interestingly, PsO was associated with all grades of PD signal severity [31]. On the contrary, Aydin et al. (2017) reported that a diagnosis of PsO was associated with a less frequent severe (grade 3) PD signal on the nail bed than in healthy controls (healthy controls vs PsO, 65.8% vs 34.9%; $p = 0.002$, 27].

Resistive index measurements Three studies assessed RI measurements in patients with PsO or PsA compared with controls (Table 5) [31, 34, 40]. According to two of these studies, patients with PsO presented with statistically higher Nailfold Vessel RI (NVRI) measurements than healthy controls [31, 40]. Mendonça et al. (2014) assessed RI measurements in patients with PsA and reported that patients with PsA had lower RI measurements in both the nail bed in transverse and longitudinal planes than controls (PsA, mean of longitudinal plane measurement, 0.50 ± 0.13; mean of transverse plane measurement, 0.48 ± 0.09; controls, mean of longitudinal plane measurement, 0.86 ± 0.41; mean of transverse plane measurement, 0.70 ± 0.16). In addition, RI measurements in the nail bed in the longitudinal plane were correlated with RI measurements in the nail bed in the transverse plane ($r = 0.333$; $p = 0.013$) and with duration of medication use ($r = 0.578$; $p = 0.002$) and was negatively correlated with the presence of PD in the nail bed ($r = -0.213$; $p = 0.038$). RI measurements in the nail bed in the transverse plane were not correlated with the presence of PD in the nail bed, while the measure of nail bed was correlated with the trilaminar appearance of nail ($r = 0.472$; $p = 0.023$, 34].

One study evaluated the sensitivity and specificity of RI measurements in patients with PsA [32]. In this study, patients with PsA presented statistically significant lower RI measurements than controls ($p < 0.001$), with high sensitivity and specificity for RI measurements in PSA patients (receiver operating characteristic curve = 0.858; $p < 0.01$). Patients with PsA and no symptoms of nail involvement also had lower RI measurements. Considering a 0.395 cutoff point for RI measurements, the results showed that RI measurements < 0.4 points were associated with 100 and 99% of sensitivity and specificity, respectively, for ungueal inflammatory activity [32].

Discussion

This systematic review was conducted to evaluate the current knowledge about the use of US for the diagnosis of nail disease in patients with PsO and PsA. However, the heterogeneous methodologic approaches did not allow us to perform a comparison of studies.

Although US is a method of diagnosis widely used in clinical practice for several diseases including PsA, real-world data shows that the use of this technique for the diagnosis of nail disease is still scarcely investigated in the literature, probably reflecting that the techniques is not routinely used in patients with PsO and PsA. Enthesitis/enthesopathies, joint synovitis and effusion, bone changes, tenosynovitis, and dactylitis are the main pathologies examined by US in patients with PsO and PsA [21]. The selected studies were mainly focused on the assessment of parameters that can differentiate healthy subjects with and without PsO and patients with PsO and PsA with and without nail disease [28, 29, 31–43].

A lower Doppler signal in the nail bed was found as marker of nail disease in patients with PsO and PsA compared with healthy controls. However the selected studies showed a wide variability for the presence of Doppler signal in the nail unit, mostly due to differences in the US equipment sensitivity or other variables such as Doppler settings, experience of the observer, or room temperature [29, 31, 34, 35, 39].

Some of the secondary outcomes of this review were related to resistance in the nail bed, such as to assess data regarding artifacts that could alter the RI measurement in the nail bed, the use of resistance in the nail bed to characterize inflammation, and differences in RI measurements in the nail bed among patients with PsO and PsA. Four of the included studies reported the RI measurements in the nail bed with conflicting results among patients with PsO and PsA, indicating the need for further evaluation in future studies to better determine how to apply the measure in clinical practice, including potential differences among specific subgroups.

Regarding artifacts that could alter the RI, two studies have shown significant differences when patients with PsO were compared with healthy controls and also when patients with PsO were stratified by the presence of nail disease [31, 40]. El-Ahmed and colleagues (2011) tested whether there were significant differences on NVRI measurements among groups of individuals based on sex, age, family history of PsO, and Psoriasis Area and Severity Index scores and no associations were found [40]. Also not all studies assessing these parameters reached statistical significance. Thus, this aspect of the disease still needs to be further investigated.

Morphologic changes, such as the thickness of nail beds, and nail plate, seem to be important parameters to analyze [28, 31, 34, 35, 37–39, 41–43]. In fact, patients with PsA and PsO presented significantly higher nail bed and nail plate thickness than controls [28, 39]; however, no study was able to predict more severe disease or the development of PsA based on this unique parameter [38].

Our review have limitations that need to be addressed, particularly the number of databases assessed and language limits, adopted due to logistic restrictions. Despite these limitations, we consider that the review was able to gather relevant and updated data about the current knowledge about the use of US to assess nail disease in PsO and PsA patients and also highlight areas for further investigation.

Conclusion

In conclusion, a significant variability across studies assessing nail disease using US in patients with PsO and PsA was observed. Samples were very diverse in terms of severity, disease duration and age. The measurement of thickness was the most frequently assessed parameter. Conflicting results exist on the presence of Doppler signals in the nail unit. Further studies are needed for the evaluation of the diagnostic value of this technique.

Abbreviations

IQR: Interquartile range; LRI: Resistance Index in longitudinal plane; mNAPSI: Modified NAPSI score; NGS: Standard trilaminar appearance of the nail bed; NPD: Presence of power Doppler in the nail bed; NVRI: Nailfold Vessel Resistive Index; OA: Osteoarthritis; PD: Power Doppler; PsA: Psoriatic arthritis; PsO: Psoriasis; RI: Resistive Index; SD: Standard deviation; TRI: Resistive Index in transverse plane; US: Ultrasonography

Acknowledgments

The authors thank ANOVA Consultoria em Saúde LTDA for providing scientific review support, which was funded by AbbVie in accordance with Good Publication Practice (GPP3) guidelines (http://www.ismpp.org/gpp3).

Authors' contributions

All authors made substantial contributions to conception and design, as well as acquisition, synthesis, and interpretation of data, and were also involved in writing the manuscript and given final approval of the version to be published.

Author details

[1]Department of Rheumatology and Postgraduate Program of the Pontifical Catholic, University of Campinas, Rua da Fazenda, 125, Condomínio Dálias, casa 10, Residencial Vila Flora, Sumaré, São Paulo 13175665, Brazil. [2]The Ottawa Hospital Research Institute, Division of Rheumatology, University of Ottawa, Ottawa, ON, Canada. [3]APHP, Hôpital Ambroise Paré, Rheumatology Department, 92100 Boulogne-Billancourt, France. [4]INSERM U1173, Laboratoire d'Excellence INFLAMEX, UFR Simone Veil, Versailles-Saint-Quentin University, 78180 Saint-Quentin-en-Yvelines, France.

References

1. Al-Mutairi N, Al-Farag S, Al-Mutairi A, et al. Comorbidities associated with psoriasis: an experience from the Middle East. J Dermatol. 2010;37:146–55. https://doi.org/10.1111/j.1346-8138.2009.00777.x.
2. Armstrong AW, Schupp C, Bebo B. Psoriasis comorbidities: results from the National Psoriasis Foundation surveys 2003 to 2011. Dermatology. 2012;225: 121–6. https://doi.org/10.1159/000342180.
3. Azfar RS, Gelfand JM. Psoriasis and metabolic disease: epidemiology and pathophysiology. Curr Opin Rheumatol. 2008;20:416–22. https://doi.org/10.1097/BOR.0b013e3283031c99.
4. Gottlieb AB, Chao C, Dann F. Psoriasis comorbidities. J Dermatol Treat. 2008; 19:5–21.
5. Gudjonsson JE, Elder JT. Psoriasis: epidemiology. Clin Dermatol. 2007;25: 535–46. https://doi.org/10.1016/j.clindermatol.2007.08.007.
6. Meier M, Sheth PB. Clinical spectrum and severity of psoriasis. Curr Probl Dermatol. 2009;38:1–20. https://doi.org/10.1159/000232301.
7. Parisi R, Symmons DPM, Griffiths CEM, Ashcroft DM. Global epidemiology of psoriasis: a systematic review of incidence and prevalence. J Invest Dermatol. 2013;133:377–85. https://doi.org/10.1038/jid.2012.339.
8. Sociedade Brasileira de Dermatologia. Consenso Brasileiro de Psoríase 2012, 2 ed. Rio de Janeiro; 2012.
9. Weigle N, McBane S. Psoriasis. Am Fam Physician. 2013;87:626–33.
10. Pasch MC. Nail psoriasis: a review of treatment options. Drugs. 2016;76:675–705. https://doi.org/10.1007/s40265-016-0564-5.
11. Kaur I, Handa S, Kumar B. Natural history of psoriasis: a study from the Indian subcontinent. J Dermatol. 1997;24:230–4. https://doi.org/10.1111/j.1346-8138.1997.tb02779.x.
12. de Jong EM, Seegers BA, Gulinck MK, et al. Psoriasis of the nails associated with disability in a large number of patients: results of a recent interview with 1,728 patients. Dermatology. 1996;193:300–3.
13. Salomon J, Szepietowski JC, Proniewicz A. Psoriatic nails: a prospective clinical study. J Cutan Med Surg. 2003;7:317–21. https://doi.org/10.1007/s10227-002-0143-0.
14. Baran R. The burden of nail psoriasis: an introduction. Dermatology. 2010; 221:1–5. https://doi.org/10.1159/000316169.
15. Dogra A, Arora A. Nail psoriasis: the journey so far. Indian J Dermatol. 2014; 59:319. https://doi.org/10.4103/0019-5154.135470.
16. Raposo I, Torres T. Nail psoriasis as a predictor of the development of psoriatic arthritis. Actas Dermosifiliogr. 2015;106:452–7. https://doi.org/10.1016/j.ad.2015.02.005.
17. Kaeley GS, Eder L, Aydin SZ, et al. Enthesitis: a hallmark of psoriatic arthritis. Semin Arthritis Rheum. 2018. https://doi.org/10.1016/j.semarthrit.2017.12.008.
18. Bakewell CJ, Olivieri I, Aydin SZ, et al. Ultrasound and magnetic resonance imaging in the evaluation of psoriatic dactylitis: status and perspectives. J Rheumatol. 2013;40:1951–7. https://doi.org/10.3899/jrheum.130643.
19. Aydin SZ, Ash ZR, Tinazzi I, et al. The link between enthesitis and arthritis in psoriatic arthritis: a switch to a vascular phenotype at insertions may play a role in arthritis development. Ann Rheum Dis. 2013;72:992–5. https://doi.org/10.1136/annrheumdis-2012-201617.
20. De Agustín J, Moragues C, De Miguel E, et al. A multicentre study on high-frequency ultrasound evaluation of the skin and joints in patients with psoriatic arthritis treated with infliximab. Clin Exp Rheumatol. 2012;30:879 85.

21. Coates LC, Hodgson R, Conaghan PG, Freeston JE. MRI and ultrasonography for diagnosis and monitoring of psoriatic arthritis. Best Pract Res Clin Rheumatol. 2012;26:805–22. https://doi.org/10.1016/j.berh.2012.09.004.
22. Cunha JS, Amorese-O'Connell L, Gutierrez M, et al. Ultrasound imaging of nails in psoriasis and psoriatic arthritis. Curr Treat Options Rheumatol. 2017; 3:129–40. https://doi.org/10.1007/s40674-017-0067-x.
23. Bisi MC, do Prado AD, Piovesan DM, et al. Ultrasound resistive index, power Doppler, and clinical parameters in established rheumatoid arthritis. Clin Rheumatol. 2017;36:947–51. https://doi.org/10.1007/s10067-016-3507-3.
24. Munn Z, Moola S, Lisy K, et al. Methodological guidance for systematic reviews of observational epidemiological studies reporting prevalence and cumulative incidence data. Int J Evid Based Healthc. 2015;13:147–53. https://doi.org/10.1097/XEB.0000000000000054.
25. Joanna Briggs Institute. Joanna Briggs Institute Reviewer's Manual. Adelaide: Joanna Briggs Institute; 2017.
26. Arbault A, Devilliers H, Laroche D, et al. Reliability, validity and feasibility of nail ultrasonography in psoriatic arthritis. Jt Bone Spine. 2016;83:539–44. https://doi.org/10.1016/j.jbspin.2015.11.004.
27. Aydin SZ, Castillo-Gallego C, Ash ZR, et al. Vascularity of nail bed by ultrasound to discriminate psoriasis, psoriatic arthritis and healthy controls. Clin Exp Rheumatol. 2017;35:872.
28. Fassio A, Idolazzi L, Zabotti A, et al. AB0742 Ultrasonography of the nail unit in psoriasis and psoriatic arthritis: a qualitative and quantitative analysis. Ann Rheum Dis. 2017;76:1314. https://ard.bmj.com/content/76/Suppl_2/1314.2.citation-tools.
29. Paramalingam S, Taylor A, Keen H. FRI0672 Assessment of the nail bed in psoriatic arthritis (PSA) by ultrasound (US) and MRI. Ann Rheum Dis. 2017; 76:744. https://ard.bmj.com/content/76/Suppl_2/744.2.citation-tools.
30. Acquitter M, Misery L, Saraux A, et al. Detection of subclinical ultrasound enthesopathy and nail disease in patients at risk of psoriatic arthritis. Joint Bone Spine. 2017;84:703–7. https://doi.org/10.1016/j.jbspin.2016.10.005.
31. Marina ME, Solomon C, Bolboaca SD, et al. High-frequency sonography in the evaluation of nail psoriasis. Med Ultrason. 2016;18:312–7. https://doi.org/10.11152/mu.2013.2066.183.hgh.
32. Mendonça JA. High specificity of spectral nail assessment in psoriatic arthritis patients. In: 2015 ACR/ARHP Annual Meeting; November 6-11, 2015. San Francisco; 2015.
33. El Miedany Y, El Gaafary M, Youssef S, et al. Tailored approach to early psoriatic arthritis patients: clinical and ultrasonographic predictors for structural joint damage. Clin Rheumatol. 2015;34:307–13. https://doi.org/10.1007/s10067-014-2630-2.
34. Mendonça JA, Nogueira JP, Laurido IMM, et al. SAT0191 can spectral Doppler identify nail enthesitis in psoriatic arthritis? Ann Rheum Dis. 2014; 73:659. https://doi.org/10.1136/annrheumdis-2014-eular.4789.
35. Sandobal C, Carbó E, Iribas J, et al. Ultrasound nail imaging on patients with psoriasis and psoriatic arthritis compared with rheumatoid arthritis and control subjects. J Clin Rheumatol. 2014;20:21–4. https://doi.org/10.1097/RHU.0000000000000054.
36. Aydin SZ, Castillo-Gallego C, Ash ZR, et al. Potential use of optical coherence tomography and high-frequency ultrasound for the assessment of nail disease in psoriasis and psoriatic arthritis. Dermatology. 2013;227:45–51. https://doi.org/10.1159/000351702.
37. Aydin SZ, Castillo-Gallego C, Ash ZR, et al. Ultrasonographic assessment of nail in psoriatic disease shows a link between onychopathy and distal interphalangeal joint extensor tendon enthesopathy. Dermatology. 2013; 225:231–5. https://doi.org/10.1159/000343607.
38. Gisondi P, Idolazzi L, Girolomoni G. Ultrasonography reveals nail thickening in patients with chronic plaque psoriasis. Arch Dermatol Res. 2012;304:727–32. https://doi.org/10.1007/s00403-012-1274-9.
39. Haddad A, Thavaneswaran A, Chandran V, Gladman DD. Clinical and ultrasonographic features of nail disease in psoriasis and psoriatic arthritis. In: 2012 ACR/ARHP Annual Meeting; November 9-14, 2012. Washington, DC; 2012.
40. Husein El-Ahmed H, Garrido-Pareja F, Ruiz-Carrascosa JC, Naranjo-Sintes R. Vessel resistance to blood flow in the nailfold in patients with psoriasis: a prospective case-control echo Doppler-based study. Br J Dermatol. 2012; 166:54–8. https://doi.org/10.1111/j.1365-2133.2011.10579.x.
41. Gutierrez M, Filippucci E, De Angelis R, et al (2010) A sonographic spectrum of psoriatic arthritis: "the five targets." Clin Rheumatol 29:133–142. doi: https://doi.org/10.1007/s10067-009-1292-y.
42. Gutiérrez M, Restrepo JP, Filippucci E, Grassi W. La ultrasonografía con sondas de alta frecuencia en el estudio de la piel y la uña psoriática. Rev Colomb Reumatol. 2009;16:332–5. https://doi.org/10.1016/S0121-8123(09)70096-9.
43. Gutierrez M, Wortsman X, Filippucci E, et al. High-frequency sonography in the evaluation of psoriasis: nail and skin involvement. J Ultrasound Med. 2009;28:1569–74.
44. Mendonça JA. As diferenças do Doppler espectral, na artrite psoriática e onicomicose. Rev Bras Reumatol. 2014;54:490–3. https://doi.org/10.1016/j.rbr.2014.03.029.

Active human herpesvirus infections in adults with systemic lupus erythematosus and correlation with the SLEDAI score

Alex Domingos Reis[1†], Cristiane Mudinutti[1†], Murilo de Freitas Peigo[1†], Lucas Lopes Leon[1], Lilian Tereza Lavras Costallat[2], Claudio Lucio Rossi[3], Sandra Cecília Botelho Costa[1] and Sandra Helena Alves Bonon[1*]

Abstract

Background: Human herpesviruses (HHVs) are responsible for a significant number of clinical manifestations in systemic lupus erythematous (SLE) patients. The aim of this study was to determine the frequency of active HHV infections in SLE patients and correlating them with disease activity.

Methods: Serum samples were collected from 71 SLE patients and their DNAs were extracted and analyzed to detect HHV-DNA viruses using the nucleic acid amplification technique.

Results: Fifteen out of the 71 (21.1%) patients tested positive for the HHV-DNA virus. Of them, 11/15 HHV-DNA-positive patients (73.3%) had SLE activity index (SLEDAI – Systemic Lupus Erythematosus Disease Activity Index) ≥8 ($p = 0.0001$). Active HCMV infection was the mostly frequently observed infection, occurring in 6/15 patients (40%). The frequencies of other active viral infections were 22% for HSV-1, 16.7% for HHV-7, and 5.5% for HSV-2. Viral coinfection (two or more viruses detected in the same sample) occurred in three patients (16.7%). Active HHV infections in SLE patients are more frequent in those with active SLE (≥8), who is at high risk of HHV reactivation and HCMV disease.

Conclusion: Viral surveillance is important to identify active HHV infections that can cause clinical symptoms and other complication in SLE patients.

Keywords: *Herpesviridae*, Systemic lupus erythematosus, Polymerase chain reaction

Introduction

Herpesvirus (HHV) infections in patients with systemic lupus erythematosus (SLE) are an important cause of morbidity and mortality [1–6]. Primary HHV infections and reactivation can cause a large spectrum of diseases, some of which can be fatal for immunocompromised patients. The human herpesvirus simplex 1 (HSV-1), and 2 (HSV-2) can cause orolabial and genital infections as well as keratitis, encephalitis and neonatal infections [7]; the varicella-zoster virus (VZV) is the causative agent of varicella and herpes zoster [8]; the Epstein-Barr virus (EBV) is associated with infectious mononucleosis, nasopharyngeal carcinoma, Burkitt's lymphoma, non-Hodgkin B-cell lymphomas and post-transplant lymphoproliferative diseases [9]; and the human cytomegalovirus (HCMV) is responsible for mononucleosis-like syndromes as well as systemic and organ-specific diseases (e.g., pneumonitis, gastrointestinal lesions, hepatitis, retinitis, pancreatitis, myocarditis, encephalitis and peripheral neuropathy) in immunocompromised patients

* Correspondence: sbonon@unicamp.br
†Alex Domingos Reis, Cristiane Mudinutti and Murilo de Freitas Peigo contributed equally to this work.
[1]Laboratory of Virology, School of Medical Sciences, State University of Campinas (UNICAMP), Rua Tessália Vieira de Camargo, 126, Campinas, SP 13.083-887, Brazil
Full list of author information is available at the end of the article

[10], having also been described as a trigger for the development of SLE [11]. Infections with human herpesvirus 6 (HHV-6 A/B), and more rarely human herpesvirus 7 (HHV-7), result in *exanthem subitum* in infants, whereas primary infections with HHV-6A are generally asymptomatic [12]. HHV-6B and HHV-7 are also associated with severe diseases (e.g., encephalitis and pneumonitis) in immunocompromised patients. Finally, human herpesvirus 8 (HHV-8) is mainly associated with Kaposi's sarcoma, one of the neoplasms that is most frequently encountered in HIV-infected patients [13]. Few studies have evaluated the impact of HHV infections on patients with SLE, therefore infection remains as the main cause of death, mostly due to their immunosuppressive therapy (i.e., steroids, such as prednisone) and abnormal immune response [14, 15]. This transversal study was undertaken to determine the frequency of HHV infections in patients with SLE using the Nested PCR (NPCR) technique, and to evaluate the laboratorial findings with disease activity.

Study sample and methods

Study sample

Seventy-one patients aged from 18 to 62 years old, with SLE, who were treated in the Rheumatology Service of the University of Campinas' Clinical Hospital between September 2007 and April 2009, in any stage of treatment, were included in this study. The median age of the patients was 40 years old (Table 1). Two different groups of patients were analyzed based on their Systemic Lupus Erythematosus Disease Activity Index (SLEDAI) (Table 1), group 1 patients corresponding to those with active SLE (SLEDAI ≥8), and group 2 patients to those without active SLE (SLEDAI< 8) [16–18]. Patients with SLEDAI ≥8 were arbitrarily considered as showing disease activity [19]. All procedures performed were in accordance with the ethical standards for research involving human beings of the institutional and/or national research committee and with the 1964 Helsinki declaration and its later amendments.

Inclusion criteria

1. Patients with SLE diagnosis, with active SLE or not, according to the SLEDAI criterion; 2. Consent of the patient or guardian authorizing the collection of the serum sample for the study; 3. Laboratory analysis of the serum samples collected from the SLE patients for detection of the presence of HHVs-DNA.

Table 1 Patient's characteristics

Characteristics	n
Gender – Female	71 (100%)
Median age	40 years old (18–78 years old range)
Active SLE (SLEDAI ≥8)	20/71 (28%)
Inactive SLE (SLEDAI < 8)	51/71 (72%)

Legend: *SLE* Systemic Lupus Erythematosus, *SLEDAI* Systemic Lupus Erythematosus Disease Activity Index

Exclusion criteria

1. Patients who did not meet the criteria described above.

Criteria used to characterize lupus activity

Active SLE was considered when the patient's SLEDAI was greater than or equal to 8, as recommended by the American College of Rheumatology and internal protocols [16–18]. The active and non-active SLE data described in the study were collected from the patients' medical records.

Methods

This was a descriptive transversal single-center study. All data were collected from clinical reports stored in the medical clinical reports service of the Clinical Hospital of the State University of Campinas to evaluate their correlation with positive HHV-DNA, e.g., SLEDAI, hospitalization and symptoms, allowing the inference of a diagnostic status.

Biological samples were collected and serum samples were obtained after centrifugation. The samples were stored at – 80 °C until the time of analysis.

All procedures performed in this study were in accordance with the ethical standards for research involving human beings of the institutional ethical committee of State University of Campinas and Brazilian national research committee, and with the 1964 Helsinki declaration and its later amendments. The Research Ethics Committee (Comitê de Ética em Pesquisa - CEP) of the Faculty of Medical Science (Faculdade de Ciências Médicas – FCM) of State University of Campinas (Unicamp) approved this study under the 789/2006 project number.

All patients that the samples were included in this study have signed the written informed consent form at the beginning of the study allowing the usage of this material.

Nested PCR for detection of HHV-DNA

The DNA was extracted from 200 μL of serum sample, according to the manufacturer's instructions (QIAamp DNA Blood Mini Kit, Cologne, Germany). The resulting DNA was eluted in 20 μL of TE-buffer. Two primer sets were used for each conserved region of HSV-1, HSV-2, VZV, EBV, HCMV, HHV-6 (types A and B), HHV-7, and HHV-8 DNA. HHV-DNA was detected in the serum samples using the NPCR technique. The primers used were chosen according to the respective authors [20–25]. The sizes of the NPCR amplification products were 138, 101, 266, 209, 167, 195 (HHV-6 type A), 423 (HHV-6 type B), 264, and 213 base pairs, respectively. The same protocol was used to amplify the human β2-microglobulin gene sequence to ensure quality.

Degree of immunosuppression

The degrees of immunosuppression were estimated according to the protocol of the University of Campinas' Rheumatology Service: 0 – *No immunosuppression* = prednisone concentrations lower than 5 mg kg/day; 1 – *Low Immunosuppression* = prednisone concentrations greater than or equal to 5 mg kg/day and less than 30 mg kg/day; 2 – *Moderate Immunosuppression* = prednisone concentrations greater than or equal to 30 mg kg/day and less than or equal to 59 mg kg/day; 3 – *High Immunosuppression* = prednisone dosage greater than or equal to 60 mg kg/day and/or dosage of the following drugs: azathioprine, cyclophosphamide, methotrexate and methylprednisolone (pulse therapy) [26].

Criteria for confirming HHV infection or likely HCMV disease

In the studied patients' samples, the criterion for defining the presence of active HHV infection was the presence of one positive HHV-DNA result in the DNA extracted from the serum samples. HHV coinfection was considered in case of two or more positive HHV-DNA results in the same serum sample. The following isolated and/or combined symptoms were used to characterize active HHV infection, and/or likely HCMV disease: fever, headache, abdominal pain, seizure, changes in behavior, low levels of consciousness, mental confusion, motor dysfunction, neuropathy, paresthesia, drowsiness, vomiting, weakness, weight loss, myoclonus, memory loss, visual and psychomotor impairment, genital and orofacial herpesvirus, ocular infection, dermatitis, varicella, mononucleosis syndrome, Burkitt's lymphoma, nasopharyngeal carcinoma, Hodgkin's disease, HCMV colitis, retinitis, hepatitis, pneumonitis, *roseola infantum* or *exanthem subitum*, Kaposi's sarcoma, primary effusion lymphoma and Cattleman's disease [27–32].

Statistical methods

The data were analyzed using descriptive statistics (median and range for continuous variables and percentages for categorical variables). The significance level adopted for this study was 5%. Statistics were calculated using the SPSS 16.0 software.

Results

Table 1 shows the characteristics of the 71 patients included in the study.

It was observed that in patients with active SLE (SLEDAI equal to or greater than 8), HHVs-DNA detection in the DNA extracted from the serum samples occurred more frequently, and this difference was statistically significant between the serum samples extracted from the DNA of patients without active SLE (SLEDAI < 8), $p < 0.0001$ (Table 2).

Of these positive HHV results, 26.6% had HSV-1-DNA; 1/15 (6.6%) had HSV-2-DNA; 6/15 (40%) had HCMV-DNA; and 20% had HHV-7-DNA. Coinfection with HCMV+HHV-7 occurred in 2/15 (13.3%) of the DNA extracted from the serum samples; 1/15 (6.6%) patient tested positive for both HSV-1 and HHV-7-DNA.

Of the four patients with SLEDAI ≥8, three had HHV-1-DNA and one had HHV-7 + HCMV coinfection. These patients did not show viral symptoms.

Of the four patients with SLEDAI ≥8, two with HHV-7-DNA, one with HSV-1-DNA and one with HSV-2-DNA, none showed any HHVs symptoms (SLEDAI 8, 10, 12 and 9, respectively).

Table 3 presents the patients' HHV test results and correspondent SLEDAI score and clinical symptoms in case of positive HHV-DNA. More details can be seen supplementary materials.

Discussion

One of the most common viral infections in immunocompromised patients is that caused by HHV, due to the immunosuppressive therapy used to treat the disease itself in the cases of autoimmune diseases, favoring the activity and reactivation of these opportunistic agents, leading to severe diseases if the virus replicates [15].

Our main objective was to determine the presence of the genome of herpesviruses in DNA extracted from serum samples of patients with SLE attested in institutional protocols and receiving immunosuppressive treatment. High SLEDAI score and increased risk of development of HHV diseases, especially those caused by HCMV, could be observed (*p < 0.0001*).

NAAT (nucleic acid amplification test) was chosen for detection of the herpesvirus in the DNA samples (active infection). Nested PCR (NPCR) techniques were used for this purpose, due to their capacity of detection of viral HHV copies, low cost and fast diagnosis. These NAAT applications allowed the detection of viral DNA, which is a relevant indicator for patients with increased risk of developing viral diseases. Also, the use of serum samples avoids the detection of latent herpesvirus. HHV-DNA can only be found with NAAT in the serum

Table 2 Patients with Active HHV infection and the SLEDAI score

	Positive HHV	Negative HHV	p*
Patients with SLEDAI ≥8	11	9	*0.0001
Patients with SLEDAI< 8	4	47	

Legend: *HHV* Human Herpesvirus, *HSV* Herpesvirus Simplex Virus, *SLEDAI* Systemic Lupus Erythematosus Disease Activity Index; p = *Fisher's Exact test

Table 3 Active HHV infection detected via Nested-PCR in the DNA extracted from the serum samples

Patient	Age (years)	HHV-DNA	SLEDAI	Clinical symptoms in case of positive HHV-DNA	DI	Drug
MJBS	20	HCMV+HHV-7	12	CNS vasculitis, leukocyturia, headache, weakness, urinary tract infection.	3	Pred+Mtx
SRGS	45	HCMV	12	**Hospitalization**. Edema, fever, vomiting and diarrhea, **HCMV disease in GIT**; ganciclovir treatment.	3	Pred+CP + Aza
MPM	34	HSV-1	12	Abdominal pains and heart cramps when in the ventral decubitus position and bilateral paresthesia.	2	Pred
NDRS	43	HCMV	11	**Hospitalization** for UTI (antibiotic) and disseminated SLE.	2	Pred+CFF
LRM[a]	31	HCMV	10	**Hospitalization died of pulmonary HCMV**. Leucopenia, acute respiratory failure, sepsis and multiple organs failure, generalized edema, tachypnea, fever, anemia, high HSV, low C3 and C4, proteinuria, hematuria	3	Metpred, Pred, CP, Pred.100 mg
MMS	27	HHV-7	10	**Hospitalization. Died of sepsis and refractory shock**. *Pseudomonas aeruginosa*, skin with SLE, weakness, drowsiness, joint pain, and little urination with generalized edema, arthralgia in hands, shoulder, hips, knees and ankles	3	Aza
MFO	48	HHV-7	10	Arthralgia, headache	1	Pred
AMSA	33	HSV-2	9	Convulsion for more than 8 days. Severe headache and persistent joint pain in the lower limbs.	3	Pred
MPP	24	HCMV	8	Proteinuria, hypertension, obesity	3	Pred+Aza
LSR	41	HHV1 + HHV-7	8	Proteinuria, *Candida albicans* onychomycosis, multipolar dermatofibroma, psoriasis versicolor	3	Metilpred
SM	33	HHV-7	8	Headache, photosensitivity	3	Aza
FDO	34	HCMV+ HHV-7	4	Articular pains in the hands, lumbar spine with edema; pain in the sacral region when moving	3	Mtx
MASP	47	HSV-1	1	Joint pain mainly in the hands, limb femoral arthralgia, asthma and idiopathic thrombocytopenic purpura	3	Pred
MAB	46	HSV-1	0	Arthritis, photosensitivity, autoimmune hepatitis, neutrophilic cutaneous vasculitis, esophageal varices, aseptic leukocyturia	3	Pred/Aza
CMT	23	HSV-1	0	Intermittent joint and lumbar pain, cough with mucoid expectoration	3	Pred/Aza

Legend: *DI* Degree of Immunosuppression, *HCMV* human cytomegalovirus, *HHV* human herpesvirus, *HSV* herpesvirus simplex, *SLEDAI* Systemic Lupus Erythematosus Disease Activity Index, *GIT* gastrointestinal tract, *UTI* urinary tract infection, *Pred* prednisone, *Mtx* pethotrexate, *CFF* ciprofloxacin, *Aza* pzathioprine, *Metpred* Pulse dosing of methylprednisolone, *CP* cyclophosphamide; [a]death by HCMV pneumonitis

of viremic patients, making it a useful tool for identifying patients with active infection [33–36].

Our main finding in this study was that patients with SLE are at increased risk of development of active infection and disease caused by these agents. Also, all patients who were hospitalized and those who died during the study had both HHV and SLEDAI ≥8.

Despite the fact some symptoms and classifications could have an association with a higher SLEDAI score, the replication of viral genetic material and the detection of this nucleic acids by NAAT can only be performed in patients in whom the virus is present and in circulation. However, distinguishing SLE manifestations from infection symptoms remains a challenge. Some authors mention the importance of new scores, which could include the use of biomarkers and other factors to make a more accurate determination of the worsening of patients with SLE, and allow a better differentiation of infections [15].

One of these patients was a 31-year-old woman with severe HCMV disease, who showed a series of symptoms (Table 3), such as fever, oral ulcers and edema, but also tachypnea, which leads to respiratory insufficiency. The pulmonary manifestation of HCMV disease, SLEDAI 10, was responsible for the death of this patient, showing the importance of medical monitoring to avoid the aggravation of SLEDAI score.

It is important to note that HHVs are ubiquitous viruses, HCMV being present in almost 100% of adults in developing countries (based on seroprevalence). In SLE reports, these HHV rates can achieve high levels, close to 90%. If a higher SLEDAI score actually leads to a higher probability of complications due to HCMV infection, and considering the prevalence of these viruses in some populations, this relation could mean an undesirable prognosis. The monitorization of SLE patients avoiding deleterious manifestations of the disease by seeking for a balance of SLE manifestations and the immunological status of the patient associated to the immunosuppressors intake, may propitiate a reduction of the SLE manifestations and allows the immunological response reduce the HHV infection risks and, consequently, lower the risk of death and morbidities [37].

The most studied interaction is that between EBV-SLE and VZV-SLE [38]. However, in this study, neither of these viruses were observed. The lack of EBV-DNA-positive patients was also demonstrated in the study by Kosminsky, 2006 [39]. Besides the absence of VZV, HHV-6 (A and B) and HHV-8, the detection could be performed in patients with the latent form of these viruses, and a follow-up study observing the viral kinetics in determined circumstances, especially more severe immunosuppression, could propitiate these detections.

The importance of HHV in SLE patients comes from a dysregulated immune response against these viruses. A likely molecular mimicry between EBV antigens and those targeted in SLE combined with increased seroconversion to EBV is also suggested, indicating higher viral reactivation in patients with SLE [38]. Several studies reposted a possible modulation of the immune system by EBV, which would cause an increase in the autoimmune activity [40–44].

Recent studies have suggested that the association between HHV-7 and HCMV may raise the level of immunosuppression and increase the incidence of graft rejection, possibly due to it potentiating the effect of HCMV or modulating the recipient immune system [44–46]. This immunomodulation may predispose other opportunistic infections such as fungal invasion and other viral infections [47].

Immunomodulation is an important factor for the development of opportunistic infections, and therefore it is impossible to affirm which was the role of HHV-7 in a patient with blood culture positive for *Pseudomonas aeruginosa* who died of septic shock. HHV-7-DNA was detected but, the role of this viral detection is unclear.

HHV-7 seems to be more associated with solid organ transplants. HHV-7 and HCMV coinfection and immune modulation are important factors for this virus' pathogenic potential [48].

HHV-7 DNA was detected in the plasma of 6 patients, and in 5 of them, SLE was active. The other patient, whose SLE was not active (SLEDAI 4), had active infection with HHV-7, but also had active HCMV infection (identified as the 12th patient in Table 3). Symptoms associated with these infections were not observed in this patient.

Regarding HCMV, in this study, active HCMV infection was observed in 6 of 15 (40%) patients with active HHV infection, and of these, 5/6 (83%) had active lupus.

It was found that 28.6% of the children with SLE (6/21) tested positive for HCMV, also showing that the infection can occur prior to immunosuppressive therapy, but becomes more common after it [3].

This study detected the presence of HSV-1 and HHV-2-DNA in 5/71 patients (7%) in total, of whom 2/5 (40%) had active SLE disease. Infection caused by HSV-1, although uncommon, should be considered in patients with SLE showing atypical symptoms. SLE can be a serious condition and often requires prolonged intense immunosuppressive therapy, which may predispose to infections, particularly those with unusual organisms, such as patients affected by HSV-1. A delay and/or inadequate therapy can lead to life-threatening situations. The only patient with active HSV-2 infection also had active SLE disease, proving that HSV-1 and 2 must not be neglected when considering infections in SLE patients.

DNA virus detection in serum can be very useful for the clinical assessment of patients with SLE and for monitoring the disease's progression, which is important for clinical practice so as to avoid unnecessary immunosuppressive treatments and allow a better prognosis.

The main limitation of this study is the lack of multivariate analysis, especially by the fact that in SLE any occurrence of infection determines an increase in disease activity, which in turn requires a step-forward in the immunosuppressive treatment.

Finally, this study provides the basis for developing further studies on SLE and HHV. Tests for detection of HHV-DNA should be performed, especially in SLE patients with SLEDAI greater than or equal to 8 (lupus activity), with the clinical surveillance and laboratory detection of active HHV infection and a longitudinal follow-up.

Conclusion

This study suggests that patients with active SLE are at increased risk for the development of active HHV infections or reactivation, especially HCMV. Laboratorial screening to detect HHV-DNA using NAAT can be a tool for obtaining a more accurate diagnosis and a better prognosis, which may lead to a more suitable use of antiviral therapy.

Supplementary information

Additional file 1. Information about the 15 patients with active viral infection and systemic lupus erythematosus (SLE).

Acknowledgments
We would like to thank the entire staff of the Laboratory of Virology (LABVIR) for their valuable support; the Rheumatology team that was involved in this study and all the patients who participated in the study. The authors thank Espaço da Escrita – Pró-Reitoria de Pesquisa - UNICAMP - for the language services provided.

Authors' contributions
ADR, CM, MFP and SHAB designed the experimental procedure and conducted the data analysis, having also drafted and proofread the manuscript; LTLC, CLR, SCBC and LLL reviewed the design of this study and proofread the manuscript; SHAB coordinated all phases of the research in the Laboratory of Virology/FCM/UNICAMP, conceptualized and designed the

study, reviewed its design and proofread the manuscript. All authors approved the final manuscript prior to submission.

Author details

[1]Laboratory of Virology, School of Medical Sciences, State University of Campinas (UNICAMP), Rua Tessália Vieira de Camargo, 126, Campinas, SP 13.083-887, Brazil. [2]Department of Internal Medicine, Discipline of Rheumatology, School of Medical Sciences, State University of Campinas (UNICAMP), Campinas, SP, Brazil. [3]Department of Clinical Pathology, School of Medical Sciences, State University of Campinas (UNICAMP), Campinas, SP, Brazil.

References

1. Costa SC, Miranda SRP, Alves G, Rossi CL, Figueiredo LT, Costa FF. Donated organs as a source of Cytomegalovirus (CMV) in renal transplant patients. Bras J Med Biol Res. 1994;27:2573–8.
2. Costa SCB, Miranda SRP, Alves G, Rossi CL, Figueiredo LTM, Costa FF. Detection of Cytomegalovirus infection by PCR in renal transplant patients. Bras J Med Biol Res. 1999;32:953–9.
3. Zhang C, Shen K, Jiang Z, He X. Early diagnosis and monitoring of active HCMV infection in children with Systemic lupus erythematosus. Chin Med J. 2001;114(12):1309–12.
4. Bonon SH, Menoni SM, Rossi CL, De Souza CA, Vigorito AC, Costa DB, Costa SC. Surveillance of cytomegalovirus infection in haematopoietic stem cell transplantation patients. J Inf Secur. 2005;50(2):130–7.
5. Katagiri A, Ando T, Kon T, Yamada M, Iida N, Takasaki Y. Cavitary lung lesion in a patient with lupus erythematous: an unusual manifestation of Cytomegalovirus pneumonitis. Mod Rheumatol. 2008;18(3):285–9.
6. Tanaka Y, Seo R, Nagai Y, Mori M, Togami K, Fujita H, Kurata M, Matsushita A, Maeda A, Nagai K, Kotani H, Takahashi T. Systemic lupus erythematosus complicated by cytomegalovirus-induced hemophagocytic syndrome and pneumonia. Nihon Rinsho Meneki Gakkai Kaishi. 2008;31(1):71–5.
7. Fatahzadeh M, Schwartz RA. Human herpes simplex virus infections: epidemiology, pathogenesis, symptomatology, diagnosis, and management. J Am Acad Dermatol. 2007;57(5):737–63 quiz 764-6. Review.
8. Gershon AA, Gershon MD. Pathogenesis and current approaches to control of varicella-zoster virus infections. Clin Microbiol Rev. 2013;26(4):728–43. https://doi.org/10.1128/CMR.00052-13.
9. Jha HC, Pei Y, Robertson ES. Epstein - Barr virus: diseases linked to infection and Transformation. Front Microbiol. 2016;7:1602 ECollection. Review.
10. Steininger C. Novel therapies for cytomegalovirus disease. Recent Pat Antiinfect Drug Discov. 2007;2(1):53–72 Review.
11. Amel R, Monia K, Anis M, Fatma BF, Chadia L. Systemic lupus erythematous revealed by cytomegalovirus infection. Pan Afr Med J. 2016;24:241 eCollection.
12. Agut H, Bonnafous P, Gautheret-Dejean A. Update on infections with human herpesviruses 6A, 6B, and 7.Med. Mal Infect. 2017;47(2):83–91. https://doi.org/10.1016/j.medmal.2016.09.004 Epub 2016 Oct 20. Review.
13. Dittmer DP, Damania B. (2016) Kaposi sarcoma-associated herpesvirus: immunobiology, oncogenesis, and therapy. J Clin Invest. 1; 126 (9):3165-75. doi: https://doi.org/10.1172/JCI84418. Epub Sep 1. Review.
14. Ramos-Casals M, Cuadrado MJ, Alba P, Sanna G, Brito-Zerón P, Bertolaccini L, Babini A, Moreno A, D'Cruz D, Khamashta MA. Acute viral infections in patients with systemic lupus erythematosus: description of 23 cases and review of the literature. Medicine (Baltimore). 2008;87(6):311–8. https://doi.org/10.1097/MD.0b013e31818ec711 Review.
15. Ospina FE, Echeverri A, Zambrano D, Suso JP, Martínez-Blanco J, Cañas CA, Tobón GJ. Distinguishing infections VS flares in patients with systemic lúpus erythematosus. Rheumatology. 2017;56-1:i46–54.
16. Lam GK, Petri M. Assessment of systemic lupus erythematosus. Clin Exp Rheumatol. 2005;23(5 Suppl 39):S120–32 Review.
17. Urowitz MB, Gladman DD. Measures of disease activity and damage in SLE. Clin Rheumatol. 1998;12(3):405–13 Baillieres. Review.
18. Petri M, Genovese M, Engle E, Hochberg M. Definition, incidence, and clinical description of flare in systemic lupus erythematosus. A prospective cohort study. Arthritis Rheum. 1991;34(8):937–44.
19. Pasoto SG, Mendonça BB, Bonfá E. Menstrual disturbances in patients with systemic lupus erythematosus without alkylating therapy: clinical, hormonal and therapeutic associations. Lupus. 2002;11:175–80.
20. Danise A, Cinque P, Vergani S, Candino M, Racca S, et al. Use of polymerase chain reaction assays of aqueous humor in the differential diagnosis of retinitis in patients infected with human immunodeficiency virus. Clin Infect Dis. 1997;24:1100–6.
21. Cinque P, Brytting M, Vago L, Castagna A, Parravicini C, et al. EpsteinBarr virus DNA in cerebrospinal fluid from patients with Aids related primary lymphoma of the central nervous system. Lancet. 1993;342:398–401.
22. Ehrnst A, Barkholt L, Lewensohhn-Fuchs I, Ljungman P, Teodosiu O, et al. CMV PCR monitoring in leukocytes of transplant patients. Clin Diagn Virol. 1995;3:139–53.
23. Fz W, Dahl H, Linde A, Brytting M, et al. Lymphotropic herpesviruses in allogeneic bone marrow transplantation. Blood. 1996;88:3615–20.
24. Yalcin S, Karpuzoglu T, Suleymanlar G, Mutlu G, Mukai T, et al. Human herpesvirus 6 and human herpesvirus 7 infections in renal transplant recipients and healthy adults in Turkey. Arch Virol. 1994;136:183–90.
25. Chan PK, Ho-Keung NG, Cheung JLK, Cheng AF. Survey for presence and distribution of human herpesvirus 8 in healthy brain. J Clin Microbiol. 2000;38(7):2772–3. https://doi.org/10.1128/jcm.38.7.2772-2773.2000.
26. Borba EF, Latorre LC, Brenol JCT, Kayser C, Silva NA, et al. Consensus of Systemic lupus erythematosus. Rev Bras Reumatol. 2008;48(4):169–207.
27. Evans CM, Kudesia G, McKendrick M. Management of herpesvirus infections. Int J Antimicrob Agents. 2013;42(2):119–28. https://doi.org/10.1016/j.ijantimicag.2013.04.023.
28. Ljungman P, Plotkin SA. Workshop on CMV disease; definition, clinical severity scores, and new syndromes. Scand J Infect Dis. 1995;99:87–9.
29. Ljungman P, Boeckh M, Hirsch HH, Josephson F, Lundgren J, Nichols G, Pikis A, Razonable RR, Miller V, Griffiths PD. Definitions of Cytomegalovirus infection and disease in transplant patients for use in clinical Trials.Disease definitions working Group of the Cytomegalovirus Drug Development Forum. Clin Infect Dis. 2017;64(1):87–91.
30. Costa FA, Soki MN, Andrade PD, Bonon SHA, Thomasini RL, et al. Simultaneous monitoring of CMV and human herpesvirus 6 infections and diseases in liver transplant patients: one-year follow-up. Clinics. 2011;66:949–53.
31. Thomasini RL, Martins JMM, Parola DC, Bonon SHA, Boin IFSF, et al. Detection of human herpesvirus-7 by qualitative nested-PCR: comparison between healthy individuals and liver transplant recipients. Rev Soc Bras Med Trop. 2008;41:556–9.
32. Peigo MF, Thomasini RL, Puglia ALP, Costa SHA, Bonon SHA, et al. Human herpesvirus-7 in Brazilian liver transplant recipients: a follow-up comparison between molecular and immunological assays. Transpl Infect Dis. 2009;11: 497–502.
33. Polstra AM, Van Den Burg R, Goudsmit J, Cornelissen M. Human herpesvirus 8 load in matched serum and plasma samples of patients with AIDS-associated Kaposi's sarcoma. J Clin Microbiol. 2003;41(12):5488–91.
34. Van Den Berg AP, Klompmaker IJ, et al. Antigenemia in the diagnosis and monitoring of active cytomegalovirus infection after liver transplantation. J Infect Dis. 1991;164(2):265–70.
35. Humar A, O'rourke K, et al. The clinical utility of CMV surveillance cultures and antigenemia following bone marrow transplantation. Bone Marrow Transplant. 1999;23(1):45–51.
36. Goossens VJ, Blok MJ, et al. Early detection of cytomegalovirus in renal transplant recipients: comparison of PCR, NASBA, pp65 antigenemia, and viral culture. Transplant Proc. 2000;32(1):155–8.
37. Antoni H, Dariusz K, Urszula M, Tadeusz W. Human cytomegalovirus in patients with systemic lupus erythematosus. Autoimmunity. 2005;38(7):487–91.
38. Doaty S, Agrawal H, Bauer E, Furst DE. Infection and lupus: which causes which? Curr Rheumatol Rep. 2016;18(3):13. https://doi.org/10.1007/s11926-016-0561-4.
39. Kosminsky S, de Menezes RC, Coêlho MR. Epstein-Barr virus infection in patients with systemic lupus erythematosus. Rev Assoc Med Bras. 2006;52(5):352–5.
40. James JA, Robertson JM. Lupus and Epstein-Barr. Curr Opin Rheumatol. 2012;24(4):383–8. https://doi.org/10.1097/BOR.0b013e3283535801 Review.
41. Gross AJ, Hochberg D, Rand WM, Thorley-Lawson DA. EBV and systemic lupus erythematosus: a new perspective. J Immunol. 2005;174(11):6599–607.
42. Harley JB, Harley IT, Guthridge JM, James JA. The curiously suspicious: a role for Epstein-Barr virus in lupus. Lupus. 2006;15(11):768–77.
43. Toussirot E, Roudier J. Epstein-Barr virus in autoimmune diseases. Best Pract Res Clin Rheumatol. 2008;22(5):883–96. https://doi.org/10.1016/j.berh.2008.09.007 Review.
44. Poole BD, Templeton AK, Guthridge JM, Brown EJ, Harley JB, James JA. Aberrant Epstein-Barr viral infection in systemic lupus erythematosus. Autoimmun Rev. 2009;8(4):3 37–42.

45. Tong CY, Bakran A, et al. Association of human herpesvirus 7 with cytomegalovirus disease in renal transplant recipients. Transplantation. 2000; 70(1):213–6.
46. Cunha BA, Gouzhva O, et al. Severe cytomegalovirus (CMV) community-acquired pneumonia (CAP) precipitating a systemic lupus erythematosus (SLE) flare. Heart Lung. 2009;38(3):249–52.
47. Razonable RR, Paya CV. The impact of human herpesvirus-6 and -7 infection on the outcome of liver transplantation. Liver Transpl. 2002;8(8):651–8.
48. White DW, Beard RS, Barton ES. Immune modulation during latent herpesvirus infection. Immunol Rev. 2012;245(1):189–208.

23

Altered Tregs and oxidative stress in pregnancy associated lupus

Naveet Pannu[1†], Rashmi Singh[1†], Sukriti Sharma[1], Seema Chopra[2] and Archana Bhatnagar[1*]

Abstract

Aim: SLE is a systemic autoimmune disease generally affecting woman in the reproductive age. It is associated with an altered level of Tregs and oxidative stress while an increase in Tregs, and different antioxidant mechanisms to combat oxidative stress are essential for successful pregnancy. Hence, this study aims to determine the level of $CD4^+$ and $CD8^+$ Tregs and oxidative stress in pregnant lupus patients.

Methods: Ten healthy and 10 pregnant lupus volunteers from the North Indian population, within the age group of 20–30 years were enrolled in the study. All the patients were non-smokers, non-alcoholics and were not associated or undergoing therapy for any other disease. They had a SLEDAI of 37.4 ± 7.32 with 5.2 ± 1.93 years of disease duration. Oxidative stress was determined by measuring the enzyme activity of anti-oxidant enzymes (catalase, superoxide dismutase and glutathione peroxidase) and the level of reduced glutathione and lipids peroxidised, spectrophotometrically. Flowcytometry was performed for immunophenotyping to determine $CD8^+$ and $CD4^+$ Tregs.

Results: Elevated $CD8^+$ Tregs and diminished $CD4^+$ Tregs were observed in pregnant lupus patients. Oxidative stress was significantly increased as the activities of anti-oxidant enzymes and level of reduced glutathione was considerably diminished. There was a substantial increase in the amount of lipids peroxidised.

Conclusion: Pregnant lupus patients undergo considerable level of oxidative stress in comparison to healthy pregnant woman. The decreased level of $CD4^+$ Tregs and an increase in $CD8^+$ Tregs might be another important factor responsible for pregnancy associated complications. Hence, lupus leads to alterations in the necessary conditions for a successful pregnancy, which might eventually cause higher mortality, morbidity and associated complications.

Keywords: Systemic lupus erythematosus, Oxidative stress, Pregnancy, $CD4^+$ Tregs, $CD8^+$ Tregs

Introduction

Systemic autoimmunity is primarily characterized by the loss of immunological tolerance and inability of the immune system to discriminate self antigens from non self antigens, hence rendering it a complex disease process. Systemic lupus erythematosus (SLE) is one such autoimmune disease characterized by the presence of high titer of auto-antibodies against nuclear antigens [1]. These auto-antibodies are produced against a broad range of antigens and as a consequence the manifestations of the disease are diverse. Wide arrays of factors are responsible for its etiology including genetic, hormonal and environmental triggers but the fundamental molecular mechanisms behind this systemic autoimmune response remain primarily indefinite. It involves multiple organ failure and is also harmful to the fetus during pregnancy. SLE mainly affects women in their reproductive years. Pregnancy in lupus patients often leads to higher maternal and fetal mortality, morbidity, pre-eclampsia and disease flares [2]. Higher risk of fetal loss, pre-term birth [3], intra-uterine growth restriction and neonatal lupus syndromes are major fetal complications during pregnancy in SLE patients [4].

A key issue in the pathogenesis of lupus is how intracellular antigens become exposed and targeted by the immune system. In this regard, excessive production of reactive oxygen species (ROS), altered redox state [5]

* Correspondence: bhatnagar.archana@gmail.com
†Naveet Pannu and Rashmi Singh contributed equally to this work.
[1]Department of Biochemistry, Panjab University, Chandigarh 160014, India
Full list of author information is available at the end of the article

and a defect in regulation of apoptosis [6] are considered as imperative factors. Despite the diverse clinical features, imbalance in oxidative state is considered to be a key feature in the development of SLE [7, 8]. Oxidative stress alters serum proteins, eventually leading to the establishment of autoimmunity and organ damage associated with lupus [9].

ROS target double bonds in polyunsaturated fatty acids of the cell membrane leading to lipid peroxidation (LPO) causing the associated complications of oxidative damage in SLE [5] Intracellular depletion of glutathione (GSH) levels are also one of the reason for the formation of ROS which causes oxidative damage and may be involved in deregulation of apoptosis in lupus. Delayed clearance of apoptotic cells may prolong interaction between ROS and apoptotic cells generating neoepitopes. Autoantibody are formed against these neoepitopes as well, eventually leading to the generation of a wide array of antibodies which causes tissue damage [9]. An increase in Malondialdehyde (MDA: a byproduct of lipid peroxidation), anti-superoxide dismutase (SOD) and anti-catalase (CAT) antibodies in the sera of SLE patients support a critical role for oxidative stress in disease development and progression. The positive relationships between oxidative stress markers and apoptosis marks the implications of oxidative stress in lupus [10].

Along with oxidative stress there has been growing evidence suggesting that infiltration of T-lymphocytes and other leukocytes into the sites of inflammation play a critical role in organ involvement during autoimmune diseases [11]. The altered functions of lymphocytes are a hallmark of SLE. T cells have been recognized to be crucial in the pathogenicity of SLE through their capabilities to communicate with and offer enormous help to B cells for driving autoantibody production [12]. Considerable attempts are focused on understanding the process by which self-reactive lymphocytes escape tolerance and induce autoimmune diseases. While it is well established that $CD4^+$ helper T cells play an important role in the process of B cell activation during antibody-mediated autoimmunity and in cell-mediated disease, the role of Tregs also holds enormous significance.

The aim of the study was to explore the state of oxidative stress, $CD4^+$ Tregs and $CD8^+$ Tregs in SLE, which may have further implications in better understanding of pathology of lupus and in the therapeutic management of the disease.

Materials and methods

Participants

Patients enrolled in the study were from Gynecology/Obstetrics Out-Patient Department of Post Graduate Institute of Medical Education and Research (PGIMER), Chandigarh. The parameters considered for this study have been approved by Institutional Ethical Clearance Committee, PGIMER, Chandigarh (PGI/IEC/2015/911). A total of twenty female volunteers were enrolled in the study, within the age group of 20–30 years and a mean age 28.1 ± 2.33 years. Of the total twenty, ten were healthy pregnant females and remaining were pregnant females with SLE. Disease activity of SLE patients was determined using SLE Disease Activity Index (SLEDAI) score [13] (maximum score of 105; severe score > 20; moderate score 10–20; mild score < 10). All the patients enrolled in the present study were non-smokers and non-alcoholics, not associated with any other autoimmune disease and were not undergoing therapy for any other disease. The patients were allowed to continue their drug regimens during the period of study. The Laboratory findings of pregnant SLE patients and pregnant healthy controls are listed in Table 1.

Blood samples

Venous blood samples were obtained from patients and controls. Samples were collected into heparinized vacutainers (Becton Dickinson, USA). Heparinized blood samples were used for separation of plasma for the estimation of reduced glutathione (GSH), LPO, and antioxidant enzymes SOD, CAT and glutathione peroxidase (GPx) and for the isolation of peripheral blood mononuclear cells (PBMCs) for T cell profiling.

Cell surface staining

PBMCs were isolated using red blood cell (RBC) lysis buffer. T-lymphocytes in the PBMCs were labelled with antibodies against specific cell surface markers for immunophenotyping. CD3 FITC, CD8 PE-Cy5, CD4 FITC and CD25 PE (BD Biosciences) antibodies were added to the cell suspension and incubated in dark at room temperature for 45 min. Cells were washed and acquired on flowcytometer (BD FACS LSR, BD Biosciences, USA) and analysed using FACSDiva 6.1.3 software (BD Biosciences, USA).

Table 1 Demographic characteristics of pregnant SLE patients and pregnant healthy controls

Parameters	SLE patients	Controls
Age	28.1 ± 2.33	25.5 ± 0.84
Month of pregnancy	5.4 ± 3.02	5.1 ± 2.18
Duration of disease (years)	5.2 ± 1.93	NA
ESR	29 ± 4.11***	16.4 ± 5.05
ANA (positive/negative)	9/1	NA
dsDNA (positive/negative)	9/1	NA
SLEDAI score	37.4 ± 7.32	NA

***Erythrocyte sedimentation rate (ESR) of SLE patients was significantly higher than control ($p < 0.001$). 90% of the SLE patients enrolled in the study were positive for anti-nuclear antibodies (ANA) and ds-DNA antibodies, with high Systemic Lupus Erythematosus Disease activity Index (SLEDAI)

Biochemical analysis

Protein estimation

Plasma protein was estimated by the method of Lowry [14] using bovine serum albumin as standard. The protein concentration was determined by comparing the optical density of the test sera with the standard plot and the result was expressed as mg/ml.

Lipid peroxidation

Lipid peroxidation was quantified in the plasma samples by measuring the levels of a secondary product of lipid peroxidation, malondialdehyde (MDA) [15]. MDA thiobarbituric acid adducts formed were measured spectrophotometrically at 532 nm. The results were expressed as nmol MDA/mg protein using molar extinction coefficient of MDA–thiobarbituric chromophore ($1.56 \times 10^5\ M^{-1}\ cm^{-1}$).

Determination of SOD activity

The method is based on the determination of the rate of reduction of nitroblue tetrazolium (NBT) to blue formazan dye in the plasma [16]. The decrease in absorbance was followed for 3 min at 560 nm. The enzyme activity was expressed as Units (U)/mg protein, where one unit of enzyme activity was defined as the amount of enzyme required to inhibit the rate of formazan formation by 50%.

Determination of CAT activity

Catalase activity was evaluated in the plasma samples and the reaction analysed the decrease in absorbance at 240 nm for 3 min [17]. Results were expressed as amount of hydrogen peroxide (H_2O_2) decomposed per min/mg protein using molar extinction coefficient of H_2O_2 ($71\ M^{-1}\ cm^{-1}$).

Determination of GSH levels

GSH was measured determining the yellow coloured complex formed by the conversion of 5,5′-dithio-bis 2-nitrobenzoic acid (DTNB) to 2-nitro-5-mercaptobenzoic acid in the plasma, which was measured spectrophotometrically at 412 nm [18]. The concentration was calculated against glutathione standard and was expressed as nmol GSH/mg protein.

Determination of GPx activity

GPx activity was assayed in the plasma samples. The assay determines the decrease in absorbance of the reaction mixture at 340 nm for 3 min [19]. Results were expressed as nmoles of NADPH oxidized per min per mg of protein, using molar extinction coefficient of NADPH ($6.22 \times 10^3\ M^{-1}\ cm^{-1}$).

Statistical analysis

Statistical analysis was performed using GraphPad Prism (Graphpad Software version 5.01, San Diego, USA). Values were expressed as Mean ± SD. Two tailed Student's t-test was used to determine statistical difference between the groups. The p value of 0.05 or less was considered significant.

Results

Demographic profile of subjects

The clinical and demographic characteristics of pregnant patients with SLE and healthy controls are stated in Table 1. 4 pregnant SLE patients were found to have severe SLEDAI score while 6 patients were in the moderate score category. The erythrocytes sedimentation rate (ESR) was significantly higher in pregnant SLE patients in comparison to healthy pregnant individuals (Fig. 1). The patients suffered from general manifestations like fatigue, headache; skin manifestations like alopecia, photosensitivity; nausea and vomiting, muscle weakness, lachrymal gland enlargement, severe manifestations like thrombocytopenia, etc. Previous history of child loss due to heart block was also reported in a patient. The SLE patients were being treated with low dose glucocorticosteroids (60%), non-steroidal anti-inflammatory drugs (NSAIDs) (25%), hydroxychloroquine (52%) and methotrexate and cyclophosphamide (15%).

T cell profiling

The percentage of $CD3^+CD8^+$ cells and $CD3^+CD8^+CD25^+$ cells were assessed in both the groups. The percentage of $CD3^+CD8^+$ cells and $CD3^+CD8^+CD25^+$ cells increased remarkably in SLE patients (43.85 ± 9.58% and 56.21 ± 2.96%) in comparison to the control group (23 ± 5.85% and 27.45 ± 1.06% respectively) (p value = 0.0023) Fig. 2.

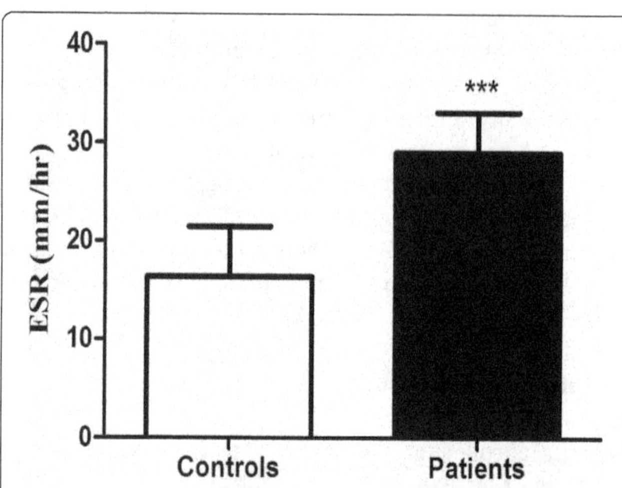

Fig. 1 Erythrocyte sedimentation rate of pregnant healthy controls and pregnant SLE patients. Values are expressed as Mean ± SD. ***$p < 0.001$

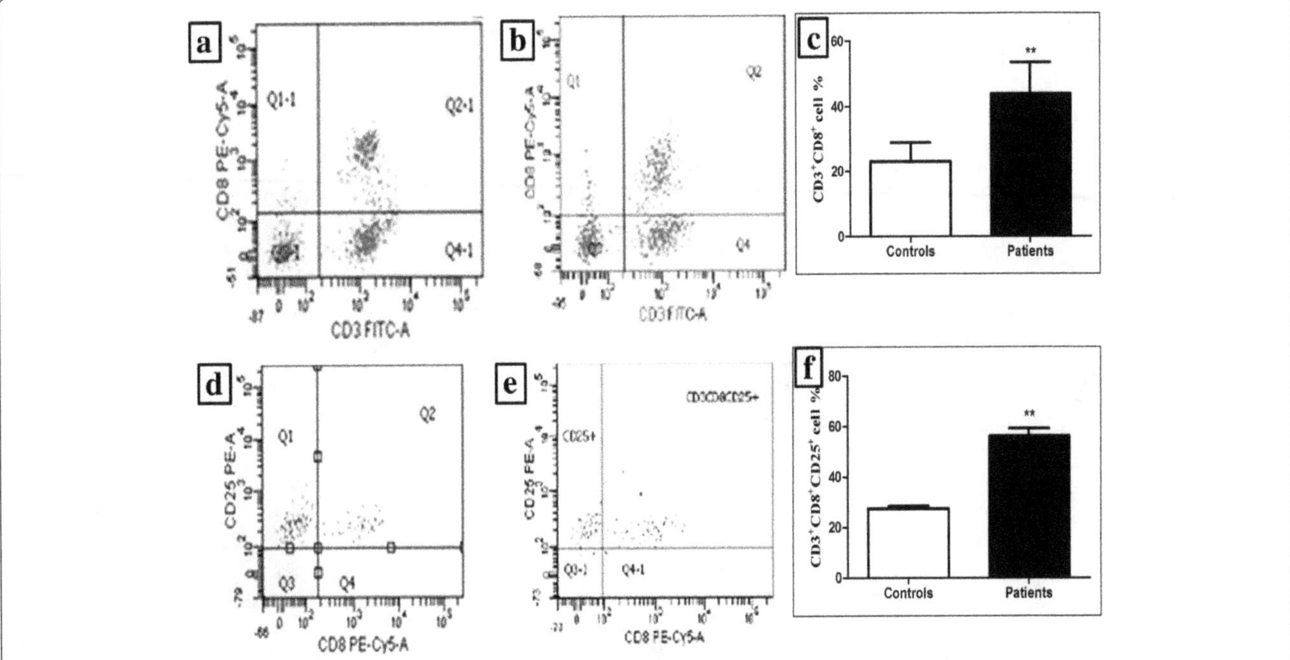

Fig. 2 a Dot plot of CD3$^+$CD8$^+$ T cells in controls (**b**) Dot plot of CD3$^+$CD8$^+$ T cells in patients (**c**) Statistical analysis of CD3$^+$CD8$^+$ T cells in controls and patients (**d**) Dot plot of CD3$^+$CD8$^+$CD25$^+$ T cells in controls (**e**) Dot plot of CD3$^+$CD8$^+$CD25$^+$ T cells in patients (**f**) Statistical analysis of CD3$^+$CD8$^+$CD25$^+$ T cells in controls and patients. All values are calculated as Mean ± SD. **$p < 0.01$

Unlike the CD3$^+$CD8$^+$ T-cells levels, the level of CD3$^+$CD4$^+$ T-cells were significantly lower in pregnant SLE patient (15.75 ± 1.89%) in comparison to healthy pregnant women (26.36 ± 2.62%). Diminished levels of CD3$^+$CD4$^+$CD25$^+$ T-cells were observed in pregnant lupus patients as compared to healthy controls. The CD3$^+$CD4$^+$CD25$^+$ T cell levels in pregnant lupus patients were 15.39 ± 1.94% which was remarkably lower than healthy controls 27.43 ± 1.74% (p value = 0.0002) Fig. 3.

Plasma protein estimation

Plasma protein levels were determined as the plasma of pregnant lupus patients and compared to healthy pregnant controls. A significant ($p = 0.0003$) elevation was seen in the level of proteins in case of SLE patients (5.247 ± 0.38 mg/ml) as compared to controls (3.694 ± 0.086 mg/ml) Fig. 4a.

Estimation of oxidative stress markers

It has been found that the activities of antioxidant enzymes such as SOD, CAT, GPx and the level of GSH are significantly reduced in patients with SLE as compared to controls. SOD is an antioxidant enzyme that plays role in neutralizing superoxide radicals (O_2^-). SOD activity was assessed in both controls and patients and as shown in Fig. 4b, it was found that SOD activity in patients was 23.29 ± 1.602 U/mg protein whereas, in control samples the SOD activity was found to be 43.16 ± 2.260 U/mg protein. This clearly demonstrated diminished SOD activity in patients as compared to control. When the data was analysed statistically, the p value was found to be 0.0001 which depicts a significant difference between both the values.

Catalase is another antioxidant enzyme that is responsible for scavenging H_2O_2 from cellular systems and thus protecting against cellular damage. In the study control samples showed a specific activity of 4.34 ± 0.73 U/mg protein. On the other hand, in SLE patients the specific activity was found to be 1.64 ± 0.08 U/mg protein. Figure 4c shows a significant decrease in the catalase activity in patients as compared to controls with a p value of 0.0001.

GPx activity was measured in both controls as well as patient samples and as shown in Fig. 4d SLE patients showed an enzyme activity of 2.73 ± 0.01 U/mg protein whereas in control samples the enzyme activity was measured to be 6.24 ± 0.23 U/mg protein. Statistical analysis of the data revealed significant decrease in enzyme activity in SLE patients with a p value of 0.0015.

GSH is an antioxidant molecule which protects the body from oxidative damage by neutralizing free radicals produced during biological processes. As shown in Fig. 5a it was found that the amount of GSH levels in SLE patients was significantly reduced (9.87 ± 0.38 nmoles/mg protein) as compared to GSH levels in control samples (18.28 ± 0.67 nmoles/mg protein), with a p value of 0.0001.

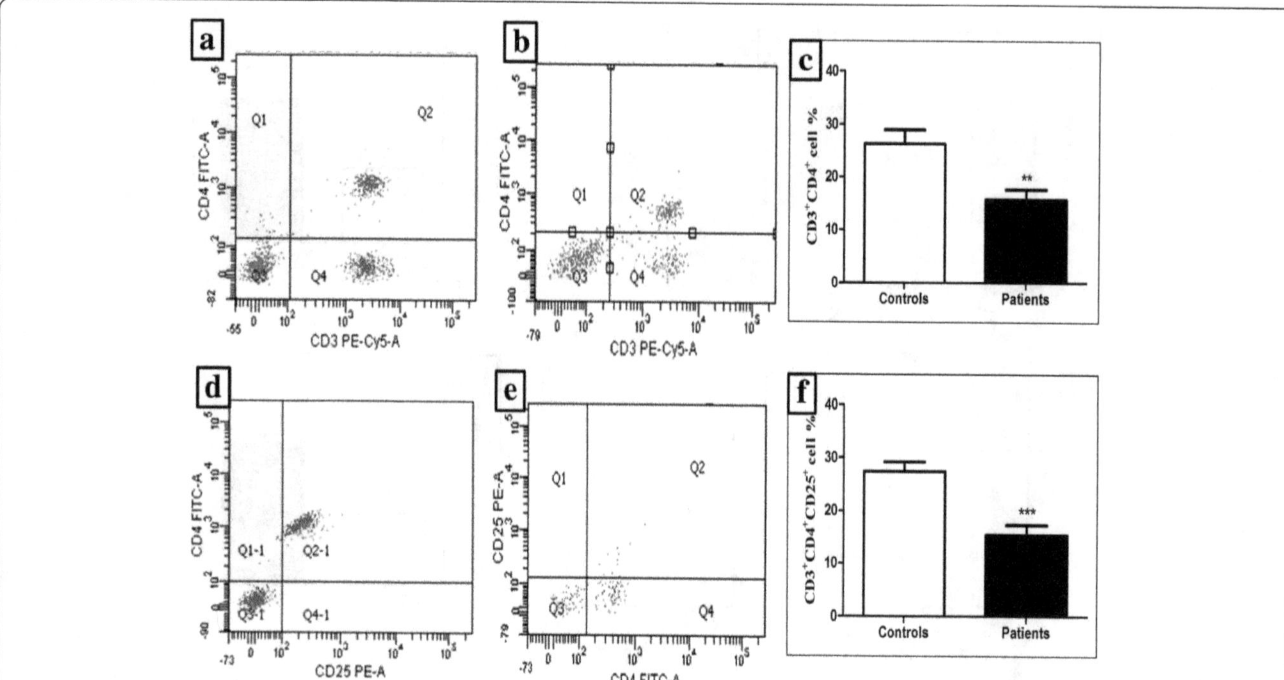

Fig. 3 **a** Dot plot of $CD3^+CD4^+$ T cells in controls (**b**) Dot plot of $CD3^+CD4^+$ T cells in patients (**c**) Statistical analysis of $CD3^+CD4^+$ T cells in controls and patients (**d**) Dot plot of $CD3^+CD4^+CD25^+$ T cells in controls (**e**) Dot plot of $CD3^+CD4^+CD25^+$ T cells in patients (**f**) Statistical analysis of $CD3^+CD4^+CD25^+$ T cells in controls and patients. All values are calculated as Mean ± SD. $^{**}p < 0.01$; $^{***}p < 0.001$

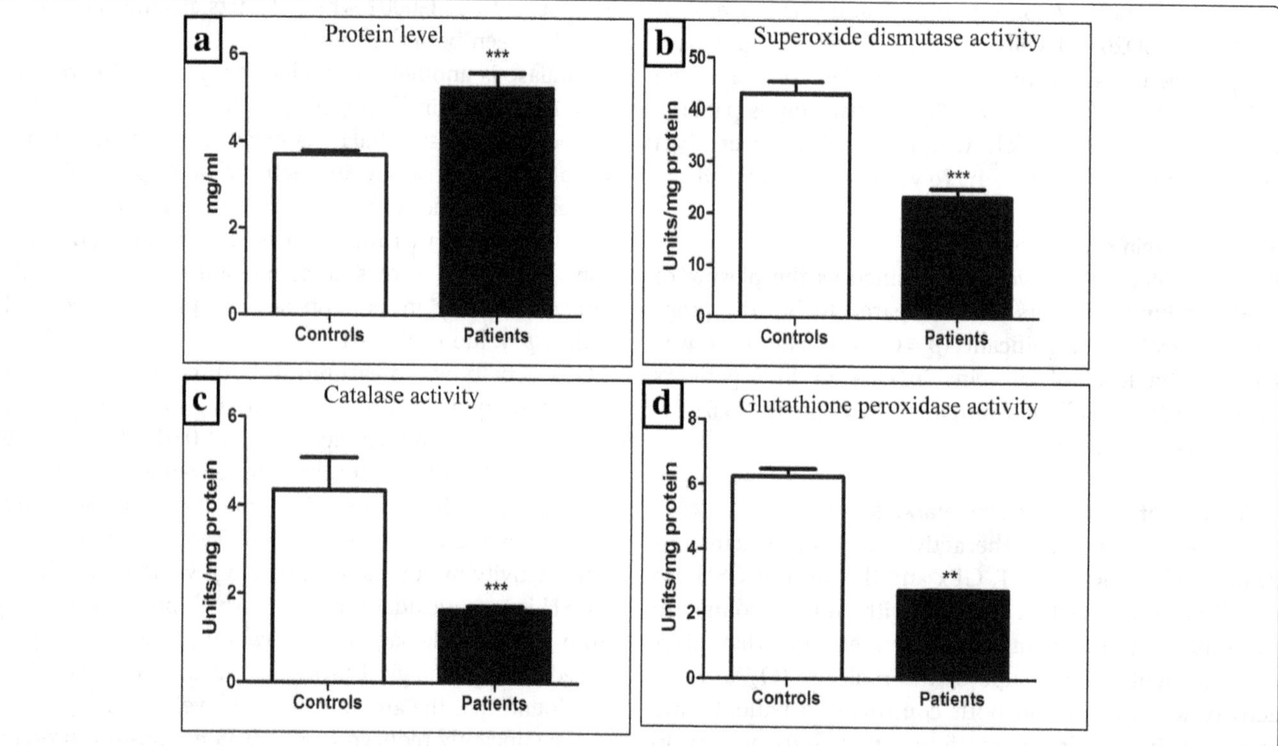

Fig. 4 Statistical analysis of (**a**) protein levels (**b**) activity of superoxide dismutase (**c**) activity of catalase (**d**) activity of glutathione peroxidase in plasma sample of controls and patients. All values are calculated as Mean ± SD. $^{**}p < 0.01$; $^{***}p < 0.001$

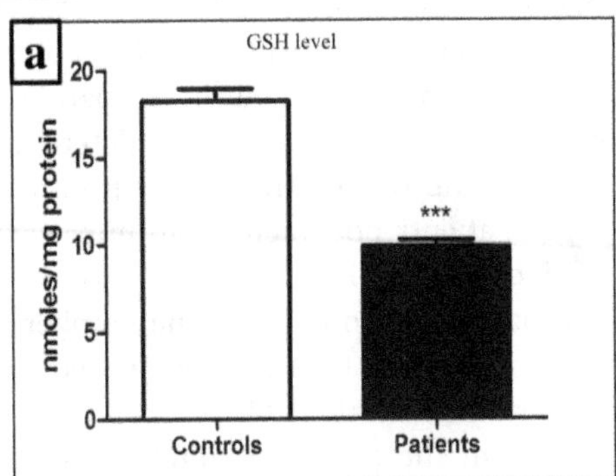

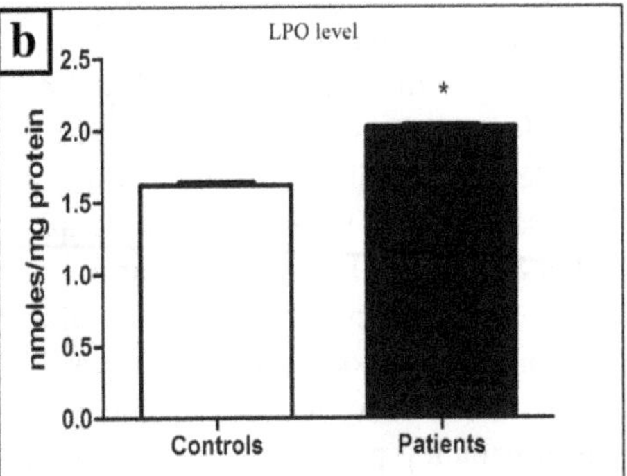

Fig. 5 Statistical analysis of the amount of (**a**) reduced glutathione (**b**) lipid peroxidation in plasma samples of controls and patients. All values are calculated as Mean ± SD. $*p < 0.05$; $***p < 0.001$

The extent of lipid peroxidation was assessed by measuring the amount of MDA-thiobarbituric acid adduct formation. SLE patients showed MDA level of 2.03 ± 0.01 nmoles/mg protein whereas the controls measured 1.62 ± 0.02 nmoles/mg protein. As shown in Fig. 5b, the amount of MDA production in SLE patients is significantly higher than the amount of MDA production in controls with a p value of 0.0112.

Discussion

This study led to some intriguing observations which enhanced the understanding of the role of oxidative stress, and Treg cells in the pathogenesis of pregnancy associated systemic lupus erythematosus. Flow cytometry of labelled PBMCs in pregnant lupus patients showed diminished levels of $CD3^+CD4^+CD25^+$ Treg cells and a significant elevation of $CD3^+CD8^+CD25^+$ Tregs cells in comparison to healthy pregnant women.

Treg cells are regulatory cells which play a pivotal role in the maintenance of immune tolerance regardless of their origin [20]. $CD4^+CD25^+$ Treg cells have been implicated in peripheral tolerance and regulation of autoimmune response [21]. Their reduced levels in SLE have been reported and it has been documented that these reduced levels may be responsible for the loss of self-tolerance and generation of autoimmune response [22]. On the other hand a successful pregnancy has to ensure fetal tolerance for which Tregs are hastily employed to the uterus-draining lymph nodes for successful implantation on the embryo [23]. A decrease in the levels of Tregs may be associated with loss of fetal tolerance and a pre-term cessation of pregnancy [24]. Results from our study state that pregnant women with lupus are at a high risk of loss of fetal tolerance due to depletion of $CD4^+CD25^+$ Tregs.

While Tregs have garnered much thought for their role in the preservation of immune homeostasis, studies have shown that subset of cells called $CD8^+$ Tregs also play immune regulatory functions [25]. These cells are known for their role in preventing autoantibody production and decreasing accumulation of autoimmune cells in organ that face prime manifestations in lupus [26]. On the other hand, during pregnancy human placental trophoblasts recruit $CD8^+$ Tregs to prevent fetal rejection [27] and pregnancy is associated with an expansion in these cells. Our study witnessed a significant increase in the level of $CD8^+CD25^+$ Tregs in pregnant lupus patients in comparison to healthy pregnant women. The altered interleukin-2 profile during pregnancy activates $CD8^+$ Tregs more than $CD4^+$ Tregs [28], hence $CD8^+$ Tregs might be experiencing higher level of stimulation than $CD4^+$ Tregs to maintain pregnancy. The increase in their number can also be associated with the fact that these cells have the role of complementing the function of $CD4^+$ Tregs [29], which are low in number hence, the number of T suppressor cells increases to compensate this decrease to allow a successful pregnancy.

Oxidative stress is increased in systemic lupus erythematosus (SLE), and it contributes to immune system dysregulation, abnormal activation and processing of cell-death signals, autoantibody production and fatal co morbidities. Oxidative modification of self antigens triggers autoimmunity, and the degree of such modification of plasma proteins shows striking correlation with disease activity and organ damage in SLE [9]. In this study the activities of antioxidant enzymes- catalase, superoxide dismutase, glutathione peroxidase, the amount of antioxidant molecule reduced glutathione and the extent of lipid peroxidation was measured. A significant decrease in the activity of CAT, SOD and GPx was observed in SLE patients as compared to controls. In addition to this, our results show significantly increased levels of lipid peroxidation in SLE patients. Lipid peroxidation in mitochondrial, lysosomal and cell membranes by ROI generates reactive aldehydes including malondialdehyde and 4- hydroxy-2-nonenal (HNE), which can spread oxidative damage through circulation. MDA and HNE, two major lipid peroxidation products, have extensively been used as the biomarkers of oxidative stress [30]. These products are highly reactive and can form adduct with proteins, making them highly immunogenic. Increased formation and subsequent accumulation of such aldehyde-modified protein adducts were found in various pathological states including autoimmune diseases like SLE [30]. Lipid peroxidation is associated with several pregnancy complications like preeclamsia [31]. Compiling these observations it can be stated that lupus is associated with increase in lipid peroxidation, hence, the pregnancy pathogenesis associated with lupus may also stem from the increase in lipid peroxidation.

Our observations also witnessed a decrease in enzyme activity of antioxidant enzymes like catalase, superoxide dismutase and glutathione peroxidase. Normal pregnancy is marked by an increase in oxidative state but this state is balanced by the increase in the enzyme activity of anti-oxidant enzymes for successful pregnancy [32]. As oxidative stress is associated with miscarriages and preeclampsia, it is very essential to combat oxidative stress [33]. On the other hand lupus is associated with a decrease in enzyme activities of catalase, superoxide dismutase, glutathione peroxidase and levels of reduced glutathione [34]. Pregnant lupus patients in our study manifested an increase in oxidative stress and the inability of the antioxidant defense mechanisms to combat this increased stress. These manifestations state that the various pregnancy complications like preeclampsia and miscarriages associated with lupus associated pregnancy may be due the inability of the anti-oxidative system to combat the increase in oxidative stress.

The role of oxidative stress and Tregs in lupus pathogenesis has been extensively researched. Findings suggest that lupus is associated with an increase in oxidative stress [35] and the associated mitochondrial hyperpolarisation [36]. The activation, proliferation and autophagy are T-cell is influenced by the state of ROS and ATP, which in turn is regulated by mitochondrial membrane potential [37]. Mitochondrial hyperpolarisation leads to a state of ATP depletion, which is sensed by FKBP12-rapamycin associated protein (FRAP, also known as mTOR or RAFT). mTOR is a member of phosphatidylinositol kinase-related kinase family and functions as a sensor to altered energy homeostasis and leads to the autophagy of T-cells during ATP depletion [38]. A similar state of increased ROS, mitochondrial hyperpolarisation, ATP depletion and T-cell apoptosis and necrosis has been reported in lupus patients [39].

Therapeutic interventions to regulate the altered state of oxidative stress and the associated T-cell autophagy in lupus have been given paramount interest by scientists. Studies have shown that the use of N-acetyl cysteine helps in reducing disease activity in lupus by inhibitor mTOR in T-cell [40]. NAC is a precursor of GSH and is hence a potent antioxidant whose potential has not only been proven in lupus but in idiopathic pulmonary fibrosis as well [41]. Another trial determining the effect of 6–15 ng/mL of sirolimus (Rapamycin) for 12 months on lupus patients documented an improvement in the state of T-cells [42]. Rapamycin is another mTOR inhibitor and has shown to improve the number of Tregs in lupus patients but this trial also manifested side effects such as nausea and infections [43].

Though the present finding has reported an increase in oxidative stress and a deregulating in the number of Tregs, but extending the above mentioned treatment regimens is another challenge. The beneficial effects of such treatments can only be extended to pregnant lupus patients after a thorough examination in pre clinical studies. Generating a suitable mouse model which replicates these manifestations is a challenge.

A remarkable elevation in the plasma protein concentrations were observed in pregnant SLE patients as compared to healthy controls. A high level of protein concentration, owing to the increase in interleukins, antibodies, Matrix metalloproteins, etc. has been reported earlier. Their association with organ damage has also been documented [44]. A similar finding in pregnant lupus patients hints to an increase in susceptibility to different organ complications, particularly to lupus nephritis.

Conclusion

Compiling the findings of this study it can be concluded that pregnancy associated with lupus is marked by an increase in plasma proteins, $CD8^{+}CD25^{+}$ Tregs, oxidative stress and a decrease in $CD4^{+}CD25^{+}$ Tregs. The two essential conditions for safe pregnancy i.e., low oxidative stress and an altered $CD4^{+}CD25^{+}$ Tregs are breached in pregnant lupus patients. Therefore, the patients are at a high risk of developing the associated complications i.e. preeclampsia and miscarriages. These findings state that there is potential for therapies targeting oxidative stress and Tregs in ameliorating the lupus associated complications in pregnancy.

Acknowledgements

The authors are grateful to University Grant Commission- Basic Scientific Research (UGC-BSR), New Delhi and Department of Science & Technology - Promotion of University Research and Scientific Excellence (DST-PURSE) and University Grants Commission- Special Assistance Programme (UGC-SAP) for financial support. The authors also like to thank all patients and healthy subjects participating in this investigation.

Authors' contributions

NP and AB have designed the work plan, RS and SS have executed the work, SC has provided the required samples and NP, RS and AB have drafted the manuscript. All authors read and approved the final manuscript.

Author details

[1]Department of Biochemistry, Panjab University, Chandigarh 160014, India.
[2]Department of Obstetrics and Gynaecology, PGIMER, Chandigarh 160012, India.

References

1. Pathak S, Mohan C. Cellular and molecular pathogenesis of systemic lupus erythematosus: lessons from animal models. Arthritis Res Ther. 2011;13(5):30.
2. Clowse ME, Jamison M, Myers E, James AH. A national study of the complications of lupus in pregnancy. Am J Obstet Gynecol. 2008;199(2):5.
3. Bramham K, Hunt BJ, Bewley S, Germain S, Calatayud I, Khamashta MA, et al. Pregnancy outcomes in systemic lupus erythematosus with and without previous nephritis. J Rheumatol. 2011;38(9):1906–13.
4. Lateef A, Petri M. Managing lupus patients during pregnancy. Best Pract Res Clin Rheumatol. 2013;27(3):435–47.
5. Kurien BT, Scofield RH. Free radical mediated peroxidative damage in systemic lupus erythematosus. Life Sci. 2003;73(13):1655–66.
6. Montalvão TM, Miranda-Vilela AL, Roll MM, Grisolia CK, Santos-Neto L. DNA damage levels in systemic lupus erythematosus patients with low disease activity: An evaluation by comet assay. Adv Biosci Biotechnol. 2012;3(07):6.
7. Cimen MY, Cimen OB, Kacmaz M, Ozturk HS, Yorgancioglu R, Durak I. Oxidant/antioxidant status of the erythrocytes from patients with rheumatoid arthritis. Clin Rheumatol. 2000;19(4):275–7.
8. Taysi S, Gul M, Sari RA, Akcay F, Bakan N. Serum oxidant/antioxidant status of patients with systemic lupus erythematosus. Clin Chem Lab Med. 2002; 40(7):684–8.
9. Perl A. Oxidative stress in the pathology and treatment of systemic lupus erythematosus. Nat Rev Rheumatol. 2013;9(11):674–86.
10. Mansour RB, Lassoued S, Gargouri B, El Gaid A, Attia H, Fakhfakh F. Increased levels of autoantibodies against catalase and superoxide dismutase associated with oxidative stress in patients with rheumatoid arthritis and systemic lupus erythematosus. Scand J Rheumatol. 2008;37(2):103–8.
11. Hoffman RW. T cells in the pathogenesis of systemic lupus erythematosus. Clin Immunol. 2004;113(1):4–13.
12. Mak A, Kow NY. The pathology of T cells in systemic lupus erythematosus. J Immunol Res. 2014;2014:8.
13. Bombardier C, Gladman DD, Urowitz MB, Caron D, Chang CH. Derivation of the SLEDAI. A disease activity index for lupus patients. The committee on prognosis studies in SLE. Arthritis Rheum. 1992;35(6):630–40.
14. Lowry OH, Rosebrough NJ, Farr AL, Randall RJ. Protein measurement with the Folin phenol reagent. J Biol Chem. 1951;193(1):265–75.
15. Buege JA, Aust SD. Microsomal lipid peroxidation. Methods Enzymol. 1978; 52:302–10.
16. Kono Y. Generation of superoxide radical during autoxidation of hydroxylamine and an assay for superoxide dismutase. Arch Biochem Biophys. 1978;186(1):189–95.
17. Luck H. Quantitative determination of catalase activity of biological material. Enzymologia. 1954;17(1):31–40.
18. Beutler E, Duron O, Kelly BM. Improved method for the determination of blood glutathione. J Lab Clin Med. 1963;61:882–8.
19. Paglia DE, Valentine WN. Studies on the quantitative and qualitative characterization of erythrocyte glutathione peroxidase. J Lab Clin Med. 1967; 70(1):158–69.
20. Chavele K-M, Ehrenstein MR. Regulatory T-cells in systemic lupus erythematosus and rheumatoid arthritis. FEBS Letters. 2011;585(23):3603–10.
21. Broere F, Apasov SG, Sitkovsky MV, van Eden W. A2 T cell subsets and T cell-mediated immunity. In: Nijkamp FP, Parnham MJ, editors. Principles of Immunopharmacology: 3rd revised and extended edition. Basel: Birkhäuser Basel; 2011. p. 15–27.
22. Bonelli M, Savitskaya A, von Dalwigk K, Steiner CW, Aletaha D, Smolen JS, et al. Quantitative and qualitative deficiencies of regulatory T cells in patients with systemic lupus erythematosus (SLE). Int Immunol. 2008;20(7):861–8.
23. Ruocco MG, Chaouat G, Florez L, Bensussan A, Klatzmann D. Regulatory T-cells in pregnancy: historical perspective, state of the art, and burning questions. Front Immunol. 2014;5:389.
24. Hsu P, Santner-Nanan B, Dahlstrom JE, Fadia M, Chandra A, Peek M, et al. Altered decidual DC-SIGN+ antigen-presenting cells and impaired regulatory T-cell induction in preeclampsia. Am J Pathol. 2012;181(6):2149–60.
25. Dinesh RK, Skaggs BJ, Cava AL, Hahn BH, Singh RP. CD8(+) Tregs in lupus, autoimmunity, and beyond. Autoimmun Rev. 2010;9(8):560–8.
26. Kang HK, Datta SK. Regulatory T cells in lupus. Int Rev Immunol. 2006;25 (1–2):5–25.
27. Shao L, Jacobs AR, Johnson V, Mayer L. Activation of CD8+ regulatory T cells by human placental trophoblasts. J Immunol. 2005;174(12):7539–47.
28. Churlaud G, Pitoiset F, Jebbawi F, Lorenzon R, Bellier B, Rosenzwajg M, et al. Human and Mouse CD8+CD25+FOXP3+ Regulatory T Cells at Steady State and during Interleukin-2 Therapy. Frontiers Immunol. 2015;6:171 [Original Research].
29. Smith TR, Kumar V. Revival of CD8+ Treg-mediated suppression. Trends Immunol. 2008;29(7):337–42.
30. Wang G, Pierangeli SS, Papalardo E, Ansari GA, Khan MF. Markers of oxidative and nitrosative stress in systemic lupus erythematosus: correlation with disease activity. Arthritis Rheum. 2010;62(7):2064–72.
31. Hubel CA, Roberts JM, Taylor RN, Musci TJ, Rogers GM, McLaughlin MK. Lipid peroxidation in pregnancy: new perspectives on preeclampsia. Am J Obstet Gynecol. 1989;161(4):1025–34.
32. Leal CA, Schetinger MR, Leal DB, Morsch VM, da Silva AS, Rezer JF, et al. Oxidative stress and antioxidant defenses in pregnant women. Redox Rep. 2011;16(6):230–6.
33. Burton GJ, Jauniaux E. Placental oxidative stress: from miscarriage to preeclampsia. J Soc Gynecol Investig. 2004;11(6):342–52.
34. Shah D, Mahajan N, Sah S, Nath SK, Paudyal B. Oxidative stress and its biomarkers in systemic lupus erythematosus. J Biomed Sci. 2014;21(1):23.
35. Lightfoot YL, Blanco LP, Kaplan MJ. Metabolic abnormalities and oxidative stress in lupus. Curr Opin Rheumatol. 2017;29(5):442–9.
36. Gergely P Jr, Grossman C, Niland B, Puskas F, Neupane H, Allam F, et al. Mitochondrial hyperpolarization and ATP depletion in patients with systemic lupus erythematosus. Arthritis Rheum. 2002;46(1):175–90.
37. Perl A, Gergely P Jr, Nagy G, Koncz A, Banki K. Mitochondrial hyperpolarization: a checkpoint of T-cell life, death and autoimmunity. Trends Immunol. 2004;25(7):360–7.
38. Desai BN, Myers BR, Schreiber SL. FKBP12-rapamycin-associated protein associates with mitochondria and senses osmotic stress via mitochondrial dysfunction. Proc Natl Acad Sci U S A. 2002;99(7):4319–24.
39. Perl A, Hanczko R, Doherty E. Assessment of mitochondrial dysfunction in lymphocytes of patients with systemic lupus erythematosus. Methods Mol Biol. 2012;900:61–89.
40. Lai Z-W, Hanczko R, Bonilla E, Caza TN, Clair B, Bartos A, et al. N-acetylcysteine reduces disease activity by blocking mammalian target of rapamycin in T cells from systemic lupus erythematosus patients: a randomized, double-blind, placebo-controlled trial. Arthritis Rheumatism. 2012;64(9):2937–46.
41. Demedts M, Behr J, Buhl R, Costabel U, Dekhuijzen R, Jansen HM, et al. High-dose acetylcysteine in idiopathic pulmonary fibrosis. N Engl J Med. 2005;353(21):2229–42.
42. Lai Z-W, Kelly R, Winans T, Marchena I, Shadakshari A, Yu J, et al. Sirolimus in patients with clinically active systemic lupus erythematosus resistant to, or intolerant of, conventional medications: a single-arm, open-label, phase 1/2 trial. Lancet. 2018;391(10126):1186–96.
43. Eriksson P, Wallin P, Sjöwall C. Clinical Experience of Sirolimus Regarding Efficacy and Safety in Systemic Lupus Erythematosus. Front Pharmacol. 2019;10:82 [Original Research].
44. Petrackova A, Smrzova A, Gajdos P, Schubertova M, Schneiderova P, Kromer P, et al. Serum protein pattern associated with organ damage and lupus nephritis in systemic lupus erythematosus revealed by PEA immunoassay. Clin Proteomics. 2017;14(32):017–9167.

24

Comparison of urinary parameters, biomarkers and outcome of childhood systemic lupus erythematosus early onset-lupus nephritis

Daniele Faria Miguel[1], Maria Teresa Terreri[2], Rosa Maria Rodrigues Pereira[3], Eloisa Bonfá[3], Clovis Artur Almeida Silva[4], José Eduardo Corrente[5], Claudia Saad Magalhaes[6*] and for the Brazilian Childhood-onset Systemic Lupus Erythematosus Group

Abstract

Background: Urinary parameters, anti-dsDNA antibodies and complement tests were explored in patients with childhood-Systemic Lupus Erythematosus (cSLE) early-onset lupus nephritis (ELN) from a large multicenter cohort study.

Methods: Clinical and laboratory features of cSLE cases with kidney involvement at presentation, were reviewed. Disease activity parameters including SLEDAI-2 K scores and major organ involvement at onset and follow up, with accrued damage scored by SLICC-DI, during last follow up, were compared with those without kidney involvement. Autoantibodies, renal function and complement tests were determined by standard methods. Subjects were grouped by presence or absence of ELN.

Results: Out of the 846 subjects enrolled, mean age 11.6 (SD 3.6) years; 427 (50.5%) had ELN. There was no significant difference in the ELN proportion, according to onset age, but ELN frequency was significantly higher in non-Caucasians ($p = 0.03$). Hematuria, pyuria, urine casts, 24-h proteinuria and arterial hypertension at baseline, all had significant association with ELN outcome ($p < 0.001$). With a similar follow up time, there were significantly higher SLICC-DI damage scores during last follow up visit ($p = 0.004$) and also higher death rates ($p < 0.0001$) in those with ELN. Low C3 (chi-square test, $p = 0.01$), but not C3 levels associated significantly with ELN. High anti-dsDNA antibody levels were associated with ELN ($p < 0.0001$), but anti-Sm, anti-RNP, anti-Ro, anti-La antibodies were not associated. Low C4, C4 levels, low CH50 and CH50 values had no significant association. High erythrocyte sedimentation rate (ESR) was associated with the absence of ELN ($p = 0.02$).

Conclusion: The frequency of ELN was 50%, resulting in higher morbidity and mortality compared to those without ELN. The urinary parameters, positive anti-dsDNA and low C3 are reliable for discriminating ELN.

Keywords: Anti-dsDNA antibodies, Childhood-onset systemic lupus erythematosus, Complement, C3, C4, Lupus nephritis

* Correspondence: claudia.saad@unesp.br
[6]Pediatric Rheumatology Division, Faculdade de Medicina de Botucatu, Universidade Estadual Paulista (UNESP), Botucatu, Brazil
Full list of author information is available at the end of the article

Background

Childhood systemic lupus erythematosus (cSLE) accounts for nearly 10–15% of all cases of SLE. It affects multiple organ systems including the kidneys, central nervous system, hematopoietic cells and skin [1] .

Lupus nephritis has been identified in 20–75% of childhood patients, indicating the worse prognosis when compared to adult patients [2–6]. However, most of the reported series evaluated lupus nephritis along the disease course. Only two series correlated silent lupus nephritis identified by renal biopsies at disease onset with serum biomarkers, including products of complement activation, as C3 and C4 levels [3, 7].. Ethnicity is one of the parameter associated to disease severity and systemic involvement [7] and there was no similar study in Latin America population. Therefore, we addressed the issue, exploring urinary parameters, renal function, anti dsDNA antibodies and complement tests in patients with childhood-Systemic Lupus Erythematosus (cSLE) and early-onset lupus nephritis (ELN), from a large multicenter national cohort study.

Methods

A large multicentric database including historical cohorts of cSLE cases, classified by the American College of Rheumatology (ACR) 1997 criteria, in 10 of the Brazilian cSLE Study Group centers, from 2013 to 2016, was analyzed for secondary data [8]. Parameters of cSLE activity were SLE Disease Activity Index 2000 (SLEDAI-2 K) scores at disease onset [9], major organ involvement such as glomerulonephritis, vasculitis, neuropsychiatric lupus, hematologic and cardio-vascular involvement and disease damage scores by Systemic Lupus International Collaborating Clinics/ACR-Damage Index (SLICC/DI) [10], at the last follow up visit.

Laboratory data, including antibody tests, urinary parameters and complement tests were obtained using standard methods in each laboratory of participating centres. Renal involvement status was defined according to pediatric definitions and guidelines [11, 12], as estimated by the physicians in the retrospective data collection. Glomerulonephritis was considered if either urine leukocytes, red blood cells, casts or renal function impairment above the normal range were present. Acute renal failure was defined as any sudden increase of serum creatinine above 2 mg/dl. Chronic renal failure was established with glomerular filtration rate lower than 60 ml/min/1.73 m2 of body surface, with or without any structural or functional damage, observed by abnormal biomarker or imaging, and occurring beyond 3 month of duration.

Initial c-SLE renal and extra-renal manifestations, including events recorded during the first six months after the diagnosis, the presence of arterial hypertension, abnormal urinalysis results, 24-h urinary protein excretion, renal function, acute and chronic renal failure status were used for comparison of the groups of cSLE with and without ELN. C3, C4, CH50, antinuclear antibodies (ANA), anti-double-stranded DNA (anti-dsDNA), anti-Sm, RNP, Ro/SSA and La/SSB tests results were also compared [8]. The clinical diagnosis of ELN required the presence of active urinary sediment based on SLEDAI-2 K criteria by Gladman et al. [9] during the first six month of the diagnosis. We selected the SLEDAI-2 K tool in order to standardize comparison of nephritis activity over time. Renal biopsy and histopathology evaluations by light microscopy and immunofluorescence, were performed independently, in each of the centres, and evaluated by local pathologists, classifying renal lesions by the World Health Organization (WHO) criteria or 2004 ISN/RPS criteria, scoring active and chronic lesions [11]. Subjects were classified according to the presence or absence of ELN, estimated by either clinical or biopsy findings.

Descriptive and parametric statistics, T-test and chi-square, were used for comparison of the groups of cSLE with and without ELN, at disease onset. The statistics tests were performed using SAS software v. 9.2 and values were considered significant if $p < 0.05$.

Results

Out of 852 subjects selected in the primary study from Gomes et al. [8], 846 with mean age of 11.6 (SD 3.6) years, with a comprehensive clinical assessment, were enrolled. Of those, 427 (50.5%) presented early-onset ELN and 419 (49,5%) did not present with ELN. Renal biopsy was performed in 228 of the cases, but only 181 were classified according to WHO criteria or 2004 ISN/RPS criteria, in addition to standard histopathology parameters [13]. Of those with renal biopsy, histopathology classification by WHO-2004 resulted in the proportion of 11 (6%) class I, 45 (25%) class II, 25 (14%) class III, 76 (42%) class IV, 21 (11%) class V and 3 (2%) class VI.

Table 1 illustrates demographic data, clinical features, laboratory, urinary parameters and outcome, in cSLE patients with and without ELN. No significant difference was found between male and female subjects, and no significant difference was found in each group of onset age, < 6 years, 6–12 and > 12 years. But, there was a significant difference related to the ethnic background. ELN frequency was significantly higher in non-Caucasian ($p = 0.03$). For ethnic classification, 20 subjects had missing data. Renal parameters, as 24 h-proteinuria, hematuria, pyuria, urine casts and arterial hypertension were compared, resulting in significant difference for those with ELN ($p < 0.001$), as well as presentation with acute renal failure (p < 0.001) and chronic renal failure ($p < 0.0002$). Low complement, defined by low C3, C4 or CH50 activity, was found in nearly 70% of those tested. Low C3 ($p = 0.01$) but not C3 levels, was associated significantly with ELN. Low C4, C4 levels or

Table 1 – Demographic and clinical features, laboratory parameters, disease activity, damage scores and death rates comparison in childhood-onset Systemic Lupus Erythematosus (c-SLE) patients with and without early onset lupus nephritis (ELN)

Variables	n of cases 427	cSLE with ELN	n of cases 419	cSLE without ELN	*p*-Value
Onset age (y)		11.6 ± 2.8		11.7 ± 3.2	0.65
0–6 y *n* (%)		17 (3.9)		21 (5)	0.74
6–12 y *n* (%)		206 (48.2)		196 (46.7)	0.74
> 12 y *n* (%)		198 (46.3)		194 (46.3)	0.74
Female *n* (%)		357 (83.6)		360 (86)	0.18
Caucasian *n* (%)	407	274 (67.3)	405	304 (72.5)	0.03*
Non-Caucasian *n* (%)	407	133 (32.7)	405	101 (24.9)	0.03*
SLEDAI-2 K (mean, SD) median		(20 ± 8) 20		(12 ± 7) 11	< 0.001*
Acute renal failure (ARF) *n* (%)		94 (22)		0	< 0.001*
Chronic renal failure (CRF) *n* (%)		17 (4)		0	0.0002*
Arterial hypertension n (%)		181 (42.3)		18 (4.2)	< 0.001*
Haematuria *n* (%)		309 (72.3)		56 (13.36)	< 0.001*
Pyuria *n* (%)		223 (52.2)		49 (11.7)	< 0.001*
Urine Casts *n* (%)		153 (35.8)		21 (5)	< 0.001*
Proteinuria *n* (%)		191 (44.7)		67 (16)	< 0.001*
24 h Proteinuria (g/day) (mean, SD)	191	(1.5 ± 2.9)	225	(0.12 ± 0.18)	< 0.001*
Low C3 *n* (%)	301	198 (65.7)	303	174 (57.4)	0.01*
Low C4 *n* (%)	265	183 (69)	280	183 (65.3)	0.07
Low CH50 *n* (%)	91	62 (68.1)	54	35 (65)	0.07
C3 (mg/dl) (mean, SD)	301	(60 ± 36)	303	(73 ± 38)	0.05
C4 (mg/dl) (mean, SD)	265	(12 ± 14)	280	(12 ± 10)	0.18
CH50 (U/ml) (mean, SD)	91	(87 ± 79)	54	(110 ± 84)	0.07
ESR mm/h (mean, SD)	343	(42 ± 35)	346	(49 ± 32)	0.02*
CRP mg% (mean, SD)	179	(5 ± 7)	217	(4 ± 6)	0.49
Anti-dsDNA antibodies *n* (%)	381	286 (75)	397	253 (63.7)	0.0001*
Anti-Sm antibodies *n* (%)	312	106 (34)	317	124 (39)	0.14
Anti-RNP antibodies *n* (%)	295	73 (24.7)	298	79 (26.5)	0.46
Anti-Ro/SSA antibodies *n* (%)	280	88 (31.4)	298	93 (31.2)	0.88
Anti-La/SSB antibodies *n* (%)	274	37 (13.5)	290	41 (14)	0.90
SLICC/DI (range) median		(0–9) 1		(0–3) 0	0.004*
Disease duration (y) (mean, SD)		(4.2 ± 3.6)		(4.2 ± 3.5)	0.80
Death n (%)	404	99 (24)	419	18 (4)	< 0.0001*

CH50–50% hemolytic activity of Complement, SLEDAI-2 K- SLE Disease Activity Index 2000, SLICC/DI - Systemic Lupus International Collaborating Clinics/ACR-Damage Index, anti-dsDNA - anti-double-stranded DNA
* significant values of p< 0.05

CH50 activity had no significant difference in the same comparison (Table 1).

Positive anti-dsDNA antibody test was associated with ELN ($p < 0.0001$), but all other autoantibodies, such as positive anti-Sm, anti-RNP, anti-Ro/SSA, anti-La/SSB, were not associated with early-onset ELN. Erythrocyte sedimentation rate (ESR) was significantly lower in cSLE with ELN compared to those without ELN ($p = 0.02$). We found no statistically significant difference in other major organ involvement in those with ELN compared to those without ELN. Only statistical trend was observed in the comparison of neuropsychiatric manifestations in those with ELN, tested by chi-square test ($p = 0.06$).

Further analysis of these patients, during the last follow-up, revealed that death rates were significantly higher in the group with ELN ($p < 0.0001$). Overall cSLE median follow up time was nearly four years; it was comparable between those with and without ELN (Table 1). SLICC-DI scored during the last follow up visit had significant difference, being higher in those with ELN ($p = 0.004$).

Discussion

This large multicenter study confirms and expands the findings of previous reports ponting to lupus nephritis as a relevant feature of cSLE. It further demonstrates that ELN is characterized by high frequency arterial hypertension, hematuria proteinuria, low C3, anti-dsDNA and a significant proportion of acute renal failure. It is in keeping with recent reports comparing renal involvement in cSLE versus adult onset SLE [14, 15]. The clinical picture mostly likely represents proliferative glomerular lesions. In fact, more than half of the patients had class III to V by WHO classification categories. This is in accordance with former case series reports, from different ethnic backgrounds populations. Comparable death rates and end-stage renal disease were also seen [2, 3, 14].

Our study contributes to the current knowledge of ELN in cSLE, reflecting in accrued damage, scored by SLICC damage index and mortality. In our series and previous reports, ELN is a predominant feature of cSLE, in particular when compared to adult series [14, 15]. ELN was confirmed by a comprehensive assessment of standardized clinical and laboratory measures, in a large multicentric study, from a population of mixed ethnic background, where non-Caucasians had higher frequency of ELN.

The role of complement as biomarker of ELN was explored. Complement and immunoglobulin deposition is a characteristic finding in ELN renal biopsies and low serum C3 and C4 have been considered as disease activity biomarkers. But, it was rarely reported in pediatric patients [7, 16, 17]. Activation of the classical complement system by immune complex contributes to inflammation and tissue injury. However, the measurement of C3 and C4 serum levels has several drawbacks. The range of C3 and C4 in the normal plasma is wide, consumption during activation can lead to increased synthesis due to acute phase reaction, resulting in no net change. Although complement serum levels do not differentiate between consumption and production, they are used worldwide for assessing lupus activity.

Our study has the limitations of a retrospective assessment, diagnosis delay or limitation of obtaining renal biopsy, as well as classifying those renal biopsies in different centers and also limited resources for laboratory tests as C3, C4 and CH50 determination. Other study limitations were those of retrospective assessments where new biomarkers were not studied. Also, the longitudinal comparison of final renal outcome as association with chronic renal failure, dyalisis and transplantation could not be addressed in this sample, but there is work is in progress in the expanded database, addressing this research question. In spite of these caveats, paired comparison between those presenting with ELN and without ELN was possible in a robust sample, in a series with a medium follow up time of four years.

Conclusion

The frequency of ELN was 50%, it was predominant in non Caucasians and resulted in higher morbidity and mortality. The urinary parameters, positive anti-dsDNA and low C3 are practical and reliable biomarkers, for discriminating ELN.

Acknowledgements
DF Miguel is undergraduate FAPESP scholar (2016/09092-3). We thank all contribution from all 27 Pediatric Rheumatology members of the Brazilian Childhood-onset Systemic Lupus Erythematosus Group and to the UNESP research office (EAP) at Botucatu Medical School.

Authors' contributions
All the authors provided substantial contribution to the study design, data acquisition, analysis, data interpretation and final approval of the manuscript.

Authors information
Not applicable.

Author details
[1]Universidade Estadual Paulista (UNESP) Faculdade de Medicina de Botucatu, Botucatu, Brazil. [2]Pediatric Rheumatology Division, Faculdade de Medicina de Botucatu, Universidade Estadual Paulista (UNESP), São Paulo, Brazil. [3]Rheumatology Division, Hospital das Clinicas HCFMUSP, Faculdade de Medicina, Universidade de São Paulo, São Paulo, Brazil. [4]Children's Institute, Hospital das Clinicas HCFMUSP, Faculdade de Medicina, Universidade de São Paulo, São Paulo, Brazil. [5]Biostatistic Department, Instituto de Biociencias, Universidade Estadual Paulista (UNESP), Botucatu, Brazil. [6]Pediatric Rheumatology Division, Faculdade de Medicina de Botucatu, Universidade Estadual Paulista (UNESP), Botucatu, Brazil.

References

1. Hiraki LT, Benseler SM, Tyrrell PN, Hebert D, Harvey E, Silverman ED. Clinical and laboratory characteristics and long-term outcome of pediatric systemic lupus Erythematosus: a longitudinal study. J Pediatr. 2008;152:550–6.
2. Hiraki LT, Lu B, Alexander SR, Shaykevich T, Alarcon GS, Solomon DH, Winkelmayer WC, Costenbader KH. End-stage renal disease due to lupus nephritis among children in the US, 1995-2006. Arthritis Rheum. 2011;63: 1988–97.
3. Frankovich JD, Hsu JJ, Sandborg CI. European ancestry decreases the risk of early onset, severe lupus nephritis in a single center, multiethnic pediatric lupus inception cohort. Lupus. 2012;21:421–9.
4. Lee PY, Yeh KW, Yao TC, Lee WI, Lin YJ, Huang JL. The outcome of patients with renal involvement in pediatric-onset systemic lupus erythematosus--a 20-year experience in Asia. Lupus. 2013;22:1534–40.
5. Wu JY, Yeh KW, Huang JL. Early predictors of outcomes in pediatric lupus nephritis: focus on proliferative lesions. Semin Arthritis Rheum. 2014;43:513–20.
6. Smith EMD, Lewandowski LB, Jorgensen AL, Phuti A, Nourse P, Scott C, Beresford MW. Growing international evidence for urinary biomarker panels identifying lupus nephritis in children - verification within the south African Paediatric lupus cohort. Lupus. 2018;27:2190–9.
7. Wakiguchi H, Takei S, Kubota T, Miyazono A, Kawano Y. Treatable renal disease in children with silent lupus nephritis detected by baseline biopsy: association with serum C3 levels. Clinical Rheumatol. 2017;36:433–7.
8. Gomes RC, Silva MF, Kozu K, Bonfa E, Pereira RM, Terreri MT, Magalhaes CS, Sacchetti SB, Marini R, Fraga M, et al. Features of 847 childhood-onset systemic lupus erythematousus patients in three age groups at diagnosis: a

Brazilian multicenter study. Arthritis Care Res. 2016;68:1736–41.
9. Gladman DD, Ibanez D, Urowitz MB. Systemic lupus erythematosus disease activity index 2000. J Rheumatol. 2002;29:288–91.
10. Sutton EJ, Davidson JE, Bruce IN. The systemic lupus international collaborating clinics (SLICC) damage index: a systematic literature review. Semin Arhritis Rheum. 2013;43:352–61.
11. Chan JC, William DM, Roth KS. Kidney failure in infants and children. Pediatric Rev. 2002;23:47–60.
12. National Kidney Foundation K/DOQI clinical practice guidelines for chronic kidney disease: evaluation, classification, and stratification. Am J Kidney Dis Suppl 2002, 39:S1–S266.
13. Marks SD, Sebire NJ, Pilkington C, Tullus K. Clinicopathological correlations of paediatric lupus nephritis. Pediatr Nephrol. 2007;22:77–83.
14. Ambrose N, Morgan TA, Galloway J, Ionnoau Y, Beresford MW, Isenberg DA. Differences in disease phenotype and severity in SLE across age groups. Lupus. 2016;25:1542–50.
15. Bundhun PK, Kumari A, Huang F. Differences in clinical features observed between childhood-onset versus adult-onset systemic lupus erythematosus: a systematic review and meta-analysis. Medicine. 2017;96:e8086.
16. Ting CK, Hsieh KH. A long-term immunological study of childhood onset systemic lupus erythematosus. Ann Rheum Dis. 1992;51:45–51.
17. Lewandowski LB, Schanberg LE, Thielman N, Phuti A, Kalla AA, Okpechi I, Nourse P, Gajjar P, Faller G, Ambaram P, et al. Severe disease presentation and poor outcomes among pediatric systemic lupus erythematosus patients in South Africa. Lupus. 2017;26:186–94.

Neutrophil/lymphocyte and platelet/lymphocyte ratios as potential markers of disease activity in patients with Ankylosing spondylitis

Mohammed Hadi Al-Osami[1], Nabaa Ihsan Awadh[2*], Khalid Burhan Khalid[3] and Ammar Ihsan Awadh[4]

Abstract

Background: The neutrophil/ lymphocyte ratio (NLR) and platelet/lymphocyte ratio (PLR) have the potential to be inflammatory markers that reflect the activity of many inflammatory diseases. The aim of this study was to evaluate the NLR and PLR as potential markers of disease activity in patients with ankylosing spondylitis.

Methods: The study involved 132 patients with ankylosing spondylitis and 81 healthy controls matched in terms of age and gender. Their sociodemographic data, disease activity scores using the Bath Ankylosing Spondylitis Disease Activity Index (BASDAI), erythrocyte sedimentation rate (ESR), and white blood cell, neutrophil, lymphocyte and platelet counts were recorded. The patients with ankylosing spondylitis were further divided according to their BASDAI scores into patients with inactive disease (BASDAI < 4) and patients with active disease (BASDAI ≥4). The correlations between the NLR, PLR and disease activity were analysed.

Results: There was a statistically significant difference in the NLR and PLR between the active and inactive ankylosing spondylitis patients (2.31 ± 1.23 vs. 1.77 ± 0.73, $p = 0.002$), (142.04 ± 70.98 vs. 119.24 ± 32.49, $p < 0.001$, respectively). However, there was no significant difference in both the NLR and PLR between the healthy control group and ankylosing spondylitis patients ($p > 0.05$). In addition, the PLR was significantly higher in both the active and inactive groups compared to those in the healthy control group (142.04 ± 70.98 vs. 99.32 ± 33.97, $p = 0.014$), (119.24 ± 32.49 vs. 99.32 ± 33.97, $p = 0.019$). The BASDAI scores were positively correlated with the PLR ($r = 0.219$, $p = 0.012$) and the NLR, but they were not statistically significant with the later ($r = 0.170$, $p = 0.051$). Based on the ROC curve, the best NLR cut-off value for predicting severe disease activity in ankylosing spondylitis patients was 1.66, with a sensitivity of 61.8% and a specificity of 50.6%, whereas the best PLR cut-off value was 95.9, with a sensitivity of 70.9% and a specificity of 55.5%.

Conclusion: The PLR may be used as a useful marker in the assessment and monitoring of disease activity in AS together with acute phase reactants such as the ESR.

Keywords: Ankylosing spondylitis, Neutrophil/lymphocyte ratio (NLR), Platelet/lymphocyte ratio (PLR), BASDAI

* Correspondence: dr.nabaaihsan@yahoo.com
[2]Rheumatology Unit, Department of Internal Medicine, Baghdad Teaching Hospital, Baghdad, Iraq
Full list of author information is available at the end of the article

Background

Ankylosing spondylitis (AS) is the main subtype of spondyloarthritides [1]. AS is a chronic, progressive, inflammatory rheumatic disease that primarily affects the sacroiliac joints and the axial skeleton. Oligoarthritis of the hips and shoulders, enthesopathy, and anterior uveitis are common conditions that can progress to significant functional disabilities that affect the quality of life with increased risk of comorbid conditions [2]. Disease activity is normally measured by using the Bath Ankylosing Spondylitis Activity Index (BASDAI), which is a patient-based questionnaire [3]. The neutrophil/lymphocyte ratio (NLR) and platelet/lymphocyte ratio (PLR) indicate the proportions of absolute neutrophil count and platelet count, respectively, to the lymphocyte count, and are derived from a routine complete blood count (CBC) test. Elevated values of the NLR and PLR denote increased inflammation [4–6]. The NLR has a diagnostic value in certain conditions with systemic or local inflammatory responses such as diabetes mellitus, coronary artery disease, ulcerative colitis, inflammatory arthritis, familial Mediterranean fever (FMF) and different malignancies [7–11]. The PLR plays a key role in atherosclerosis and atherothrombosis in peripheral arterial occlusive disease [12]. In addition, it was found that the value of the PLR is not affected by smoking, unlike the value of the NLR, which is correlated with the pack/year [13].

Elevated levels of c-reactive protein (CRP) (or erythrocyte sedimentation ratio (ESR) have been found in only about 60% of clinically-active AS patients [14]. The clinical assessment of disease activity and response to treatment in AS is complex and difficult. Although the two traditional markers of an acute phase response, ESR and CRP, have been used for assessment, they may not often correlate with the patient's symptoms or radiological progression. Thus, it is important to find a new monitoring marker that can reflect disease activity. The NLR and PLR are readily available, simple, and inexpensive tools that may indicate disease activity in AS patients. This study was aimed to evaluate the differences between the NLR, PLR and disease activity among AS patients and the control group, and to examine the correlation between the NLR, PLR and disease activity in AS patients. In addition, this study was also conducted to assess the validity of the NLR and PLR in differentiating between active and inactive AS.

Methods

Study design

This was a case-control study conducted among AS patients at the Rheumatology Unit of the Baghdad Teaching Hospital/Medical City from August 2017 to the end of April 2018. A signed informed consent form was obtained from each participant in the study. The study protocol was approved by the University of Baghdad, College of Medicine, Rheumatology and Medical Rehabilitation Unit in accordance with the Declaration of Helsinki with ethical approval reference no.: 2017070-EA-7189.

Participants

A total of 132 Iraqi patients diagnosed with ankylosing spondylitis after fulfilling the modified New York criteria for ankylosing spondylitis [15] were consecutively selected. Eighty-one (81) healthy control participants matched for age and gender were obtained from medical staff volunteers. Subjects with acute or chronic infections, hypertension, diabetes mellitus, a history of coronary heart disease or impairment in thyroid functions, renal/hepatic dysfunction, malignancy, history of surgery in the last 3 months, current smokers or with a history of smoking in the past year, hematologic disorders or receiving blood transfusion during the past 3 months, steroid therapy, chronic obstructive pulmonary disease (COPD), and overlapping with other autoimmune diseases such as rheumatoid arthritis, psoriatic arthritis and inflammatory enteritis were excluded from the study.

Age, gender, disease duration, and disease activity was evaluated by using the Bath Ankylosing Spondylitis Disease Activity Index score [3], while the laboratory results for white blood cell count (WBC count), neutrophil count, lymphocyte count, platelet count and ESR were recorded. The blood neutrophil/lymphocyte ratio (NLR) and platelet/lymphocyte ratio (PLR) for each participant were calculated manually by dividing the neutrophil count and platelet count, respectively by the lymphocyte count after obtaining the laboratory results. The patients were categorized into 2 groups according to their BASDAI scores. Patients with BASDAI scores of less than 4 were considered to be having inactive or mild disease activity, while patients with scores of 4 or above were considered to be displaying active disease.

The BASDAI is a composite index ranging from 0 (no symptoms) to 10 (maximal symptoms) on a numeric scale. It is a patient-based questionnaire that includes questions about fatigue, pain in the spine, pain at the peripheral joints and entheses, and the quality and quantity of morning stiffness. A cut-off value of 4 has been accepted in the BASDAI scale and scores, equal to or above the cut-off value, indicate that the disease is more active. The Nihon Kohden®Japan (Celltacα) and Vital Microsed-System®Germany ESR automated analysers were used to obtain the final results of the CBC and ESR, respectively.

Statistical analysis

The statistical analysis was performed using the Statistical Package for Social Sciences (SPSS) software for Windows version 20. The descriptive statistics were presented as the mean ± standard deviation (SD) for the continuous variables, and as frequencies and proportions (%) for the categorical variables. A student's t-test was used to compare the means of the continuous variables between the AS patients and the control group, and between the active and inactive AS patients. The parametric data of the three groups were compared using the one-way ANOVA test. For differences between the three groups, the post-hoc Tukey Test was utilized. The Pearson's correlation test was performed to determine the relationship between the NLR, PLR and BASDAI scores. A Receiver Operating Characteristic curve was used to assess the validity of the NLR and PLR to differentiate between the AS patients and the control group, and between the active and inactive AS. If the area under the curve (AUC) is 1.0, it is a perfect test; 0.9–0.99 indicates an excellent test; 0.8–0.89 is a good test; 0.7–0.79 is a fair test, 0.51–0.69 is a poor test, and 0.5 is of no value (Carter J V, 2016). $P < 0.05$ was considered as significant.

Results

Demographic, clinical and laboratory characteristics of the study population

The current study involved 213 participants comprised of 132 AS patients as well as 81 matched healthy controls. The ESR, and WBC, lymphocyte and platelet counts were significantly higher in the AS patients compared to the healthy controls ($p < 0.05$), whereas there was no significant difference with regard to their neutrophil count, NLR and PLR ($p > 0.05$). The other demographic and clinical characteristics are shown in Table 1.

Differences in mean values of NLR and PLR between active and inactive AS patients

The ankylosing spondylitis patients were categorised according to their disease activity into active disease ($n = 55$), and inactive or mild disease activity ($n = 77$). The mean BASDAI for the active group was 5.14 ± 0.92, range: 4–7.6, and for the inactive group it was 2.34 ± 0.91, range: 0.20–3.90.

The mean values of the NLR and PLR in the active AS group were significantly higher than the values in those with inactive or mild disease activity (2.31 ± 1.23 vs. 1.77 ± 0.73, $p = 0.002$), (142.04 ± 70.98 vs. 119.24 ± 32.49, $p < 0.001$), respectively, as shown in Figs. 1 and 2.

Disease activity and laboratory parameters

The laboratory parameters of the AS patients according to their BASDAI scores and the healthy controls are shown in Table 2. There were significantly different levels of WBC, neutrophil, lymphocyte and platelet counts, NLR, PLR and ESR among the three groups ($p < 0.05$).

By comparing the control group with the patients with BASDAI scores of < 4, there was a significant difference in the lymphocyte count, PLR and ESR ($p < 0.001$, $p = 0.019$, $p < 0.001$, respectively). Also, there was a significant difference in the WBC, neutrophil, lymphocyte and platelet counts, PLR and ESR on comparing the controls with those patients with BASDAI scores of ≥4 ($p < 0.001$, $p = 0.001$, $p = 0.019$, $p < 0.001$, $p = 0.014$, $p = 0.013$, respectively).

By comparing the two groups of AS patients (BASDAI ≥4 vs. BASDAI < 4), there was a significant difference in the WBC, neutrophil and platelet counts, NLR, PLR and ESR ($p = 0.040$, $p = 0.002$, $p < 0.001$, $p = 0.001$, $p < 0.001$, $p < 0.001$, respectively).

Correlation between BASDAI scores and laboratory parameters in ankylosing spondylitis patients

The BASDAI scores were moderately correlated with the platelet count and ESR in the AS patients (r = 0.304, $p < 0.001$; r = 0.394, p < 0.001, respectively). In addition, there was a weak correlation between the BASDAI scores and the WBC, neutrophil counts and PLR (r =

Table 1 Demographic, clinical and laboratory characteristics of AS patients and controls

	AS patients ($n = 132$)	Control ($n = 81$)	P value [a]
Age (years)	37.61 ± 10.0	35.98 ± 9.8	0.249
Male, n (%)	120 (90.9)	73(90.1)	0.849
Disease duration (years)	9.54 ± 7.3	–	–
BASDAI	3.51 ± 1.66	–	–
White blood cell count (10^9/L)	8.15 ± 1.75	7.31 ± 1.49	**< 0.001**
Neutrophil count (10^9/L)	4.85 ± 1.45	4.51 ± 0.98	0.066
Lymphocyte count (10^9/L)	2.71 ± 0.83	2.30 ± 0.51	**< 0.001**
Platelet count (10^9/L)	288.57 ± 89.47	263.08 ± 50.56	**0.020**
NLR	1.99 ± 1.00	2.02 ± 0.55	0.801
PLR	117.12 ± 56.51	119.24 ± 32.49	0.759
ESR (mm/hr.)	22.78 ± 21.03	8.24 ± 5.67	**< 0.001**

Values are means ± SD or numbers and percentages. [a], student t-test; AS, ankylosing spondylitis; BASDAI, Bath Ankylosing Spondylitis Activity Index; ESR, erythrocyte sedimentation rate; n, number; NLR, neutrophil/lymphocyte ratio; PLR, platelet/lymphocyte ratio; P value, probability value (< 0.05)

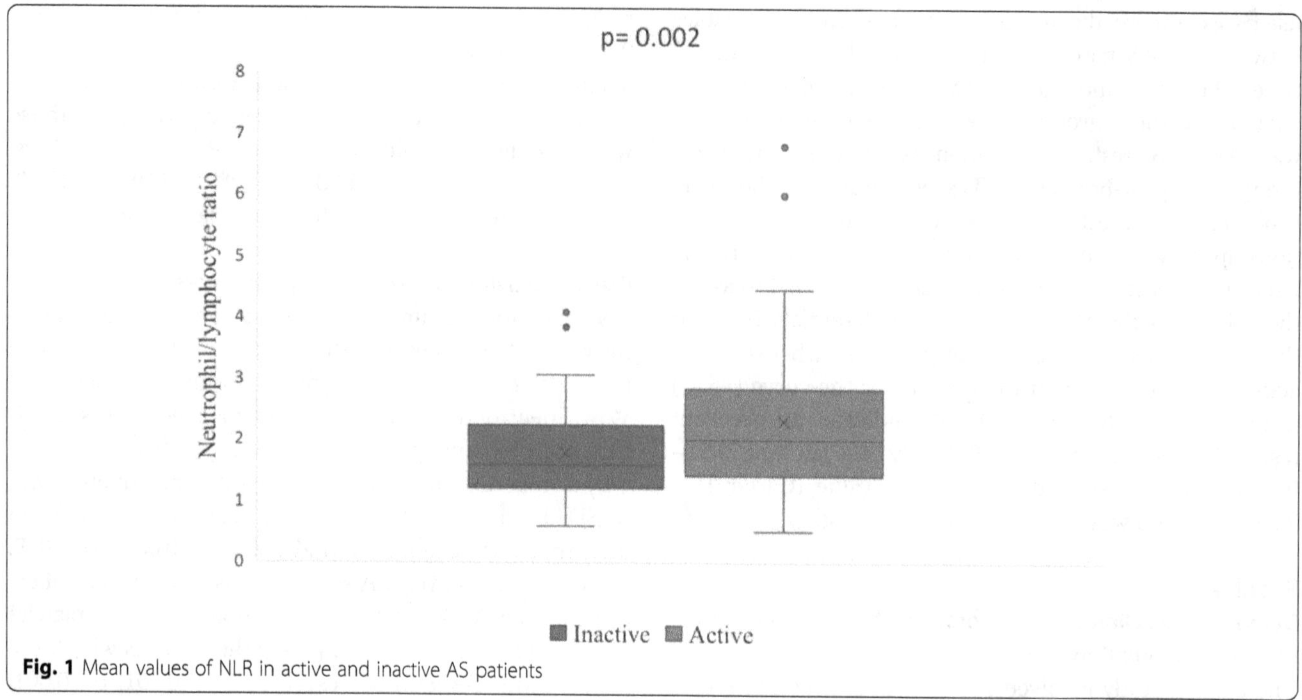

Fig. 1 Mean values of NLR in active and inactive AS patients

0.201, $p = 0.021$; r = 0.228, $p = 0.009$; r = 219, $p = 0.012$, respectively), while the NLR showed a very weak positive correlation with the BASDAI scores but it did not achieve statistical significance (Table 3, Figs. 3 and 4).

ROC analysis and validity of NLR, PLR and ESR between AS patients according to disease activity

Furthermore, the ESR and PLR were valid fair tests to differentiate the active AS from inactive AS, where the AUC for them were 0.726 and 0.702, respectively, with $p < 0.001$ (Fig. 5). The optimum cut-off value for the ESR was ≥15.5 mm/hr. (sensitivity of 70.9%, specificity 64.9%) and 95.9 for the PLR (sensitivity 70.9%, specificity 55.5%). However, the AUC for the NLR was 0.626 with a cut-off value of ≥1.66, sensitivity of 61.8%, and specificity of 50.6%. These validity parameters are shown in Table 4.

Discussion

The main findings of the current study were that the NLR, PLR and ESR were significantly higher in the active

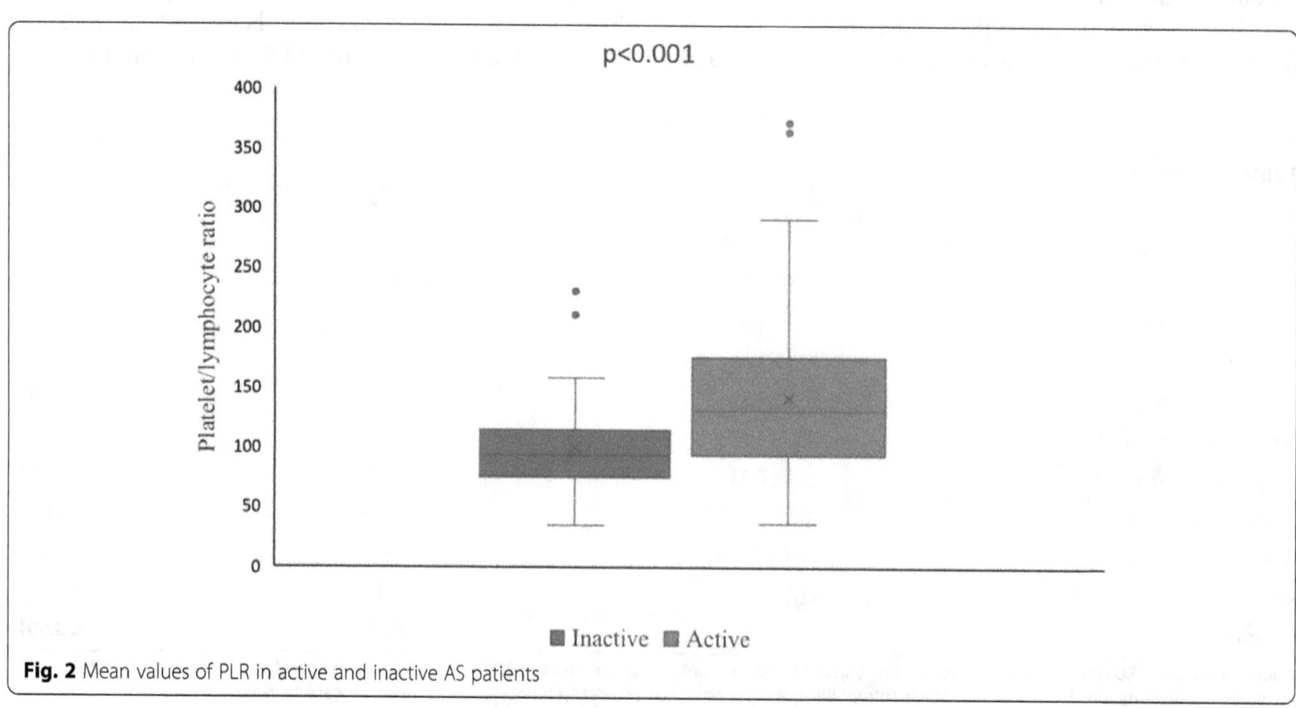

Fig. 2 Mean values of PLR in active and inactive AS patients

Table 2 Laboratory parameters of study groups based on disease activity

	Control ($n = 81$)	BASDAI< 4 ($n = 77$)	BASDAI≥4 ($n = 55$)	P value
White blood cell count (10^9/L)	7.31 ± 1.49	7.85 ± 1.65	8.56 ± 1.81	**< 0.001** P1 = 0.097 **P2 < 0.001** **P3 = 0.040**
Neutrophil count (10^9/L)	4.51 ± 0.98	4.53 ± 1.33	5.30 ± 1.51	**0.001** P1 = 0.994 **P2 = 0.001** **P3 = 0.002**
Lymphocyte count (10^9/L)	2.30 ± 0.51	2.76 ± 0.76	2.65 ± 0.92	**< 0.001** **P1 < 0.001** **P2 = 0.019** P3 = 0.661
Platelet count (10^9/L)	263.08 ± 50.56	257.58 ± 62.38	331.96 ± 103.22	**< 0.001** P1 = 0.879 **P2 < 0.001** **P3 < 0.001**
NLR	2.02 ± 0.55	1.77 ± 0.73	2.31 ± 1.23	**0.002** P1 = 0.138 P2 = 0.131 **P3 = 0.001**
PLR	99.32 ± 33.97	119.24 ± 32.49	142.04 ± 70.98	**< 0.001** **P1 = 0.019** **P2 = 0.014** **P3 < 0.001**
ESR (mm/hr.)	1.40 ± 3.48	15.31 ± 33.23	12.31 ± 25.86	**< 0.001** **P1 < 0.001** **P2 = 0.013** **P3 < 0.001**

AS, ankylosing spondylitis; BASDAI, Bath Ankylosing Spondylitis Disease Activity Index; ESR, erythrocyte sedimentation rate; *n*, number; NLR, neutrophil/lymphocyte ratio; PLR, platelet/lymphocyte ratio; *P* value, probability value (< 0.05); P1, Control vs. BASDAI < 4; P2, Control vs. BASDAI ≥4; P3, BASDAI ≥4 vs. BASDAI < 4
Comparisons of parametric data of three groups were performed with One-Way ANOVA test. Post-hoc Tukey Test was used for differences between the three groups

disease patients compared to the inactive disease patients. However, there was an insignificant difference between the healthy controls and AS patients in terms of the NLR and PLR, whereas the ESR was significantly higher in the group of AS patients. In addition, the ESR and PLR were significantly higher in the active and inactive disease patients compared to the healthy control group. Also, it was found that there was a significant but weak positive correlation between the BASDAI scores and the PLR, and a moderate correlation with the ESR values. Also, there was a very weak positive correlation between the BASDAI scores and the NLR, but it was not statistically significant. ESR and PLR were fair valid significant tests that can differentiate between active and inactive AS.

Table 3 Correlation between BASDAI scores and laboratory parameters in ankylosing spondylitis patients ($n = 132$)

Parameter	Pearson's correlation	P value
White blood cell count (10^9/L)	0.201	**0.021**
Neutrophil count (10^9/L)	0.228	**0.009**
Lymphocyte count (10^9/L)	−0.014	0.876
Platelet count (10^9/L)	0.304	**< 0.001**
NLR	0.170	0.051
PLR	0.219	**0.012**
ESR	0.394	**< 0.001**

ESR, erythrocyte sedimentation rate; *n*, number; NLR, neutrophil/lymphocyte ratio; PLR, platelet/lymphocyte ratio; *P* value, probability value (< 0.05)

The patients' demographic data in this study showed no significant difference when compared with the healthy control individuals. This indicated that the patients were correctly matched with the control group, and the effect of confounding variables that may influence the results was avoided.

This study showed that males were more predominant than females at a ratio of 10:1 with regard to AS. This was comparable with another Iraqi study conducted at a Baghdad teaching hospital by Abdul-Wahid K. M. et al. [16] in which a ratio of 11:1 was obtained. However, the findings of this study and the other Iraqi study [16] were inconsistent with those of other studies [17–19]. This inconsistency might be attributed to the following factors: the small sample size, and the fact that the number of women diagnosed with AS is less than the men, since,

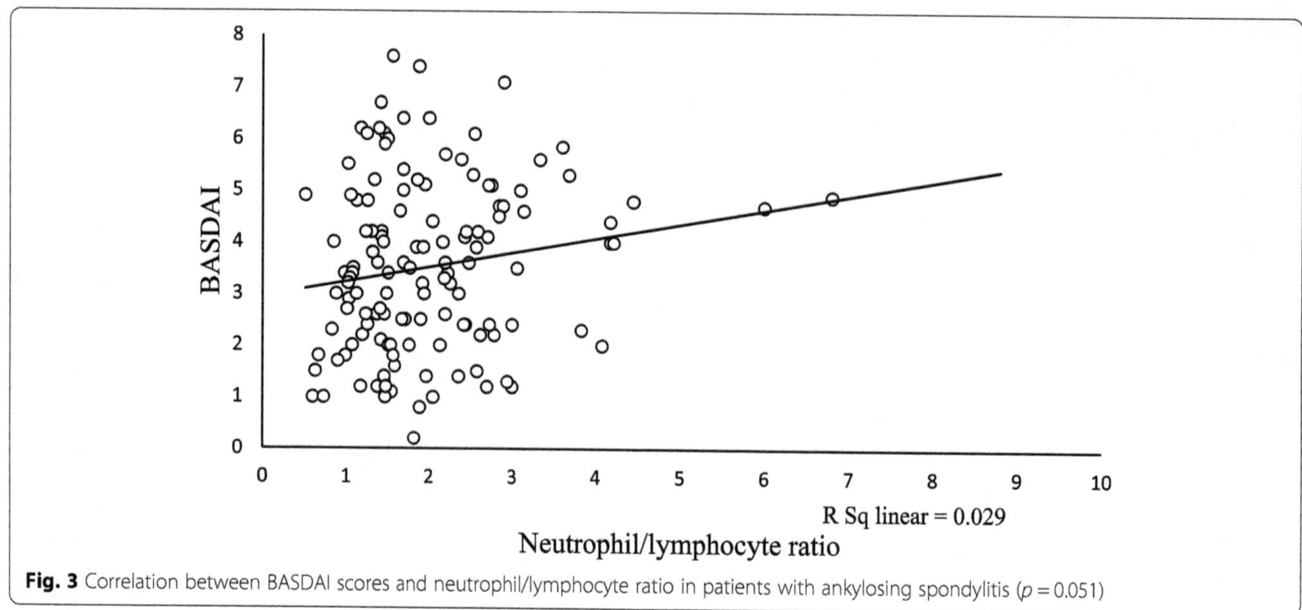

Fig. 3 Correlation between BASDAI scores and neutrophil/lymphocyte ratio in patients with ankylosing spondylitis ($p = 0.051$)

for reasons that are unclear, women seem to develop chronic changes later and less often [1]. In addition, some female patients were excluded from this study due to either their use of steroids or their being diabetic.

Although the pathogenesis of AS is unknown, some studies have suggested that neutrophils and lymphocytes may play a role in the pathogenesis of AS [1, 20]. In the literature, five studies [21–25] showed no significant difference in the NLR when comparing the AS patients with the healthy controls, and similar findings were also obtained with regard to the PLR [21, 25, 26], which were consistent with the results of this study. However, these results disagreed with the findings of four other studies with regard to the NLR [27–30] and one study concerning the PLR [24], which might have been related to the involvement of either newly-diagnosed patients with no previous treatment or only patients with active AS in their studies.

For individual AS patients, a disease activity assessment is a critical step in the management of the disease. Currently, the CRP and ESR are the most widely used laboratory indices for the estimation of AS disease activity. However, an increase in these indices may relate more to disease activity in the peripheral joints than to axial disease [31]. Therefore, a novel index is needed to improve the accuracy of currently available disease activity estimation tools. To further assess whether the higher NLR and PLR in AS were associated with clinical disease activity, the patients were divided into active and inactive subgroups based on the BASDAI scores. The patients with high BASDAI scores had significantly higher NLR and PLR levels. These results were in agreement

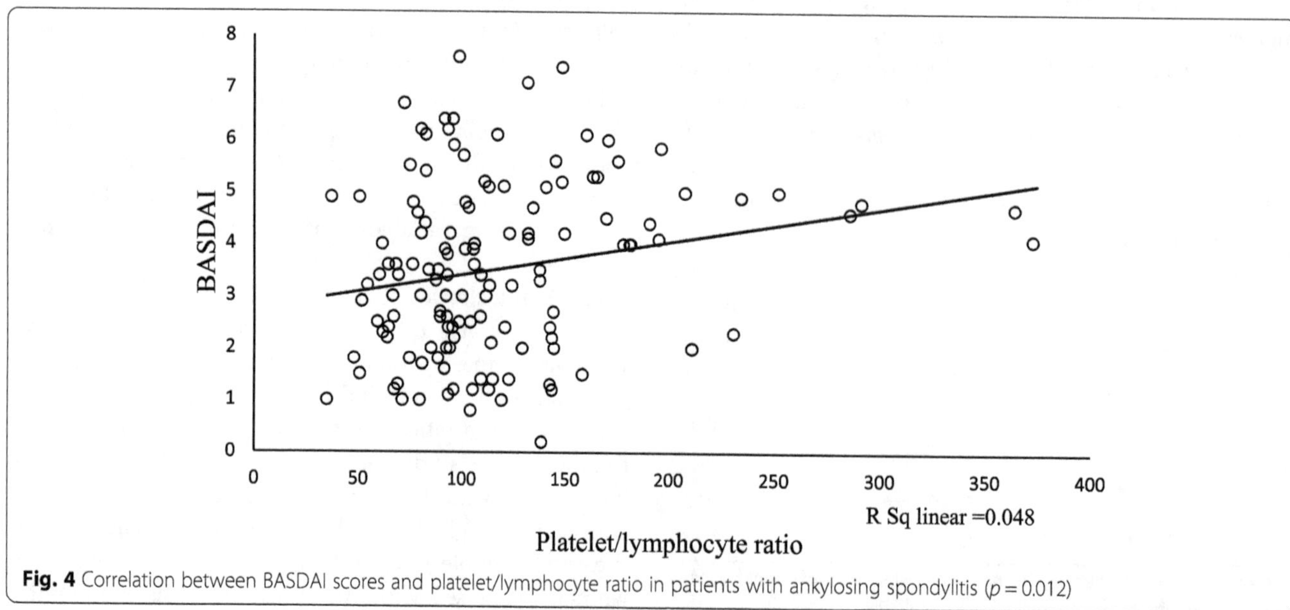

Fig. 4 Correlation between BASDAI scores and platelet/lymphocyte ratio in patients with ankylosing spondylitis ($p = 0.012$)

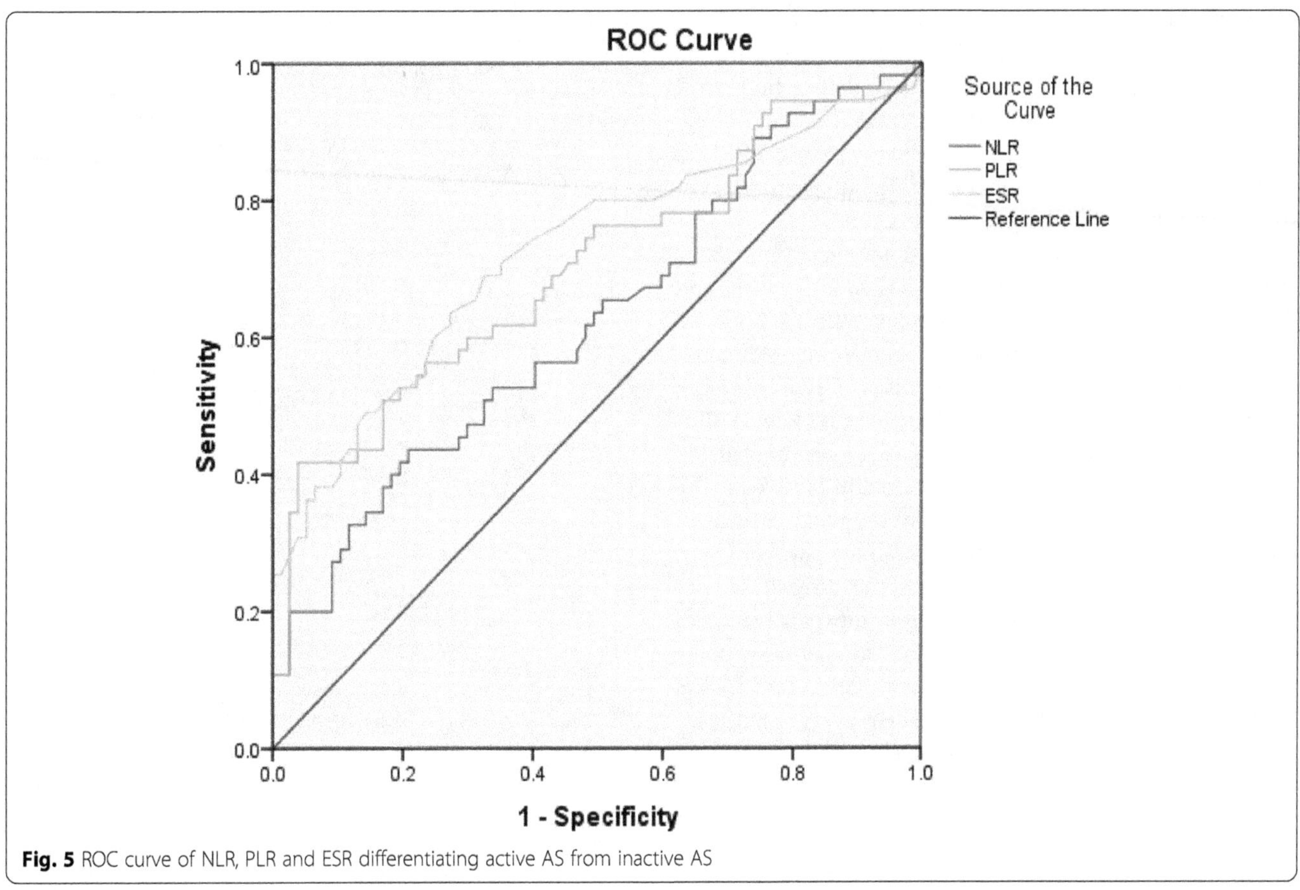

Fig. 5 ROC curve of NLR, PLR and ESR differentiating active AS from inactive AS

with the finding of Esraa et al. [21] and Kucuk et al. [30] that the NLR and PLR were significantly higher in patients with severe disease activity compared to mild disease activity.

There was a very weak positive correlation between the BASDAI scores and NLR but it was not statistically significant (r = 0.170, $p = 0.051$). This result was in agreement with the finding of Mercan et al. [22] and Gokmen et al. [29], but was in contrast to the findings of three other studies [21, 28, 30]. Meanwhile, there was a weak positive correlation between the PLR and the BASDAI scores, and this result was in agreement with the finding of Esraa et al. [21]. A further analysis showed a strong overall performance characteristic of the PLR in the diagnosis of severe AS patients. Based on the ROC curve, it was found that the PLR had an optimal sensitivity of 70.9%, specificity of 55.5%, and accuracy of 61.36%, and these were nearly similar to the sensitivity and accuracy of the ESR, which were 70.91 and 61.61%, respectively. Meanwhile, the NLR at a cut-off value of 1.66 showed poor validity as an inflammatory marker of severe disease activity in AS patients with an AUC of 0.626, sensitivity of 61.8%, specificity of 50.6%, and accuracy 56.82%. In addition, the ESR showed a moderate positive correlation with the BASDAI scores. This suggested that the PLR together with the ESR can be used as potential complementary assessment tools for the diagnosis of disease activity in AS patients. Similar findings regarding the NLR were reported by other two studies [30, 32]. Moreover, there is a lack of data in the literature about the performance of the PLR and the severity of disease activity in AS.

An estimation of patients with increased systemic inflammation would be useful to predict those patients with severe disease activity and who have developed comorbidities. Therefore, it is believed that it is important

Table 4 ROC curve analysis and validity of NLR, PLR and ESR to differentiate between active and inactive AS patients

Variable	AUC	95% CI	Cut-off value	Sensitivity	Specificity	Accuracy	*P* value
NLR	0.626	0.528–0.723	1.66	61.8%	50.6%	56.82%	**0.014**
PLR	0.702	0.608–0.795	95.9	70.9%	55.5%	61.36%	**< 0.001**
ESR	0.726	0.634–0.817	15.5	70.9%	64.9%	61.61%	**< 0.001**

AS, ankylosing spondylitis; AUC, area under curve; CI, confidence interval; ESR, erythrocyte sedimentation rate; NLR, neutrophil/lymphocyte ratio; PLR, platelet/lymphocyte ratio; *P* value, probability value (< 0.05)

to practically demonstrate the level of systemic inflammation in patients with AS. Thus, combined with the findings of this study, it is suggested that a high PLR level in AS may correlate with heightened disease activity in AS patients. The PLR together with the ESR are useful markers in the assessment of the inflammatory response and disease activity in AS patients.

There were some limitations to this study. This was a cross-sectional case-control study in a single centre, and the sample was smaller than samples used in previous studies, which did not permit the establishment of causality between the NLR, PLR and disease activity. Also, the possible effects of treatment on the NLR and PLR were not considered due to incomplete or unavailable treatment records, and the relationship between the NLR, PLR and cytokines was not investigated. However, this was the first study in Iraq to evaluate the NLR and PLR as potential tools for assessing the disease activity of AS. These are simple, rapid and inexpensive tools whose values can be easily calculated as common components of the complete blood count (CBC) test that is nowadays widely carried out in nearly every healthcare facility and by an automated machine.

Conclusions

There was a significant statistical difference in the neutrophil/lymphocyte ratio (NLR) and platelet/lymphocyte ratio (PLR) between active and inactive AS patients. However, there was no statistically significant difference in these ratios between the patients and the control group. There was a significant weak positive correlation between ankylosing spondylitis disease activity with the platelet/lymphocyte ratio (PLR), whereas there was no statistically significant correlation with the neutrophil/lymphocyte ratio (NLR). The PLR proved to be a fair and valid significant test that can differentiate between active and inactive AS. However, the NLR was shown to have poor validity. The PLR might be integrated into an assessment of AS disease activity. Further studies with a larger sample size and longer follow-up periods should be designed to validate the findings of this study and to further demonstrate their relation to the medications received and the disease outcome.

Acknowledgements

The authors would like to thank Prof. Dr. Nizar Abdulateef, Asst. Prof. Dr. Faiq Isho Gorial and Dr. Adil S. Dakhil for their valuable inputs and support in this study and also the participants in this study.

Authors' contributions

This paper is a part of NA board certification of rheumatology and medical rehabilitation in Iraq. The research was conducted by NA and supervised by MO. NA, and MO designed the project. Date collection was done by NA. AA contributed in the statistical analysis, and KK helped in drafting the manuscript. All authors read and approved the final manuscript.

Author details

[1]Rheumatology Unit, Department of Internal Medicine, College of Medicine, University of Baghdad, Baghdad, Iraq. [2]Rheumatology Unit, Department of Internal Medicine, Baghdad Teaching Hospital, Baghdad, Iraq. [3]Oral Surgery Unit, Department of Dentistry, Dijlah University College, Baghdad, Iraq. [4]Clinical Pharmacy Unit, Department of Pharmacy, Al-Esraa University College, Baghdad, Iraq.

References

1. Braun J, Sieper J. Ankylosing spondylitis. Lancet. 2007;369:1379–90.
2. Bascherini V, Caso F, Costa L, et al. TNFα-inhibitors for ankylosing spondylitis and non-radiographic axial spondyloarthritis. Pharm J. 2017; 9: No 1, online | DOI: https://doi.org/10.1211/CP.2017.20202077
3. Garrett S, Jenkinson T, Kennedy LG, et al. A new approach to defining disease status in ankylosing spondylitis: the Bath Ankylosing spondylitis disease activity index. J Rheumatol. 1994;21(12):2286–91.
4. Tsiara S, Elisaf M, Jagroop IA, Mikhailidis DP. Platelets as predictors of vascular risk: is there a practical index of platelet activity? Clin Appl Thromb Hemost. 2003;9(3):177–90.
5. Azab B, Daoud J, Naeem FB, et al. Neutrophil-to-lymphocyte ratio as a predictor of worsening renal function in diabetic patients (3-year follow-up study). Ren Fail. 2012;34(5):571–6.
6. Azab B, Shah N, Akerman M, McGinn JT. Value of platelet/lymphocyte ratio as a predictor of all-cause mortality after non-ST-elevation myocardial infarction. J Thromb Thrombolysis. 2012;34(3):326–34.
7. Celikbilek M, Dogan S, Ozbakır O, et al. Neutrophil– lymphocyte ratio as a predictor of disease severity in ulcerative colitis. J Clin Lab Anal. 2013;27(1): 72–6.
8. Tousoulis D, Antoniades C, Koumallos N, Stefanadis C. Pro- inflammatory cytokines in acute coronary syndromes: from bench to bedside. Cytokine Growth Factor Rev. 2006;17(4):225–33.
9. Ahsen A, Ulu MS, Yuksel S, et al. As a new inflammatory marker for familial Mediterranean fever: neutrophil-to- lymphocyte ratio. Inflammation. 2013; 36(6):1357–62.
10. Li MX, Liu XM, Zhang XF, et al. Prognostic role of neutrophil-to-lymphocyte ratio in colorectal cancer: a systematic review and meta-analysis. Int J Cancer. 2014;134(10):2403–13.
11. Templeton AJ, McNamara MG, Šeruga B, et al. Prognostic role of neutrophil-to-lymphocyte ratio in solid tumors: a systematic review and meta-analysis. J Natl Cancer Inst. 2014;106(6):dju124.
12. Macey M, Hagi-Pavli E, Stewart J, et al. Age, gender and disease-related platelet and neutrophil activation ex vivo in whole blood samples from patients with Behcet's disease. Rheumatology. 2011;50(10):1849–59.
13. Tulgar Y, Cakar S, Tulgar S, et al. The effect of smoking on neutrophil/ lymphocyte and platelet/lymphocyte ratio and platelet indices: a retrospective study. Eur Rev Med Pharmacol Sci. 2016;20(14):3112–8.
14. Poddubnyy D, Rudwaleit M, Haibel H, et al. Rates and predictors of radiographic sacroiliitis progression over 2 years in patients with axial spondyloarthritis. Ann Rheum Dis. 2011;70(8):1369–74.
15. Linden SVD, Valkenburg HA, Cats A. Evaluation of diagnostic criteria for ankylosing spondylitis. Arthritis Rheum. 1984;27(4):361–8.
16. Abdul-Wahid K, Karhoot J, Al-Osami M, et al. Assessment of serum Calprotectin (S-100 protein) in Iraqi patients with Ankylosing spondylitis and its relation with treatment and disease activity. IOSR J Pharm Biol Sci. 2018; 13(2):14–7.
17. Sieper J, Poddubnyy D. Axial spondyloarthritis. Lancet. 2017;390(10089):73–84.
18. Rudwaleit M, Haibel H, Baraliakos X, et al. The early disease stage in axial spondylarthritis: results from the German Spondyloarthritis inception cohort. Arthritis Rheum. 2009;60(3):717–27.
19. Van Tubergen A. The changing clinical picture and epidemiology of spondyloarthritis. Nat Rev Rheumatol. 2015;11(2):110.
20. Bleil J, Maier R, Hempfing A, et al. Histomorphologic and histomorphometric characteristics of zygapophyseal joint remodeling in ankylosing spondylitis. Arthritis Rheum. 2014;66(7):1745–54.
21. Inal EE, Sunar I, SARATAŞ Ş, et al. May neutrophil- lymphocyte and platelet-lymphocyte ratios indicate disease activity in ankylosing spondylitis? Arch Rheumatol. 2015;30(2):130–7.
22. Mercan R, Bitik B, Tufan A, et al. The association between neutrophil/ lymphocyte ratio and disease activity in rheumatoid arthritis and ankylosing spondylitis. J Clin Lab Anal. 2016;30(5):597–601.

23. ÖzŞahin M, Demirin H, Uçgun T, et al. Neutrophil-lymphocyte ratio in patients with ankylosing spondylitis. Abant Med J. 2014;3(1):16–20.
24. Boyraz İ, Koç B, Boyacı A, et al. Ratio of neutrophil/lymphocyte and platelet/ lymphocyte in patient with ankylosing spondylitis that are treating with anti-TNF. Int J Clin Exp Med. 2014;7(9):2912–5.
25. Boyraz I, Onur CS, Erdem F, et al. Assessment of relation between neutrophil lympocyte, platelet lympocyte ratios and epicardial fat thickness in patients with ankylosing spondylitis. Med Glas (Zenica). 2016;13(1):14–7.
26. Bozan N, Alpaycı M, Aslan M, et al. Mean platelet volume, red cell distribution width, platelet-to-lymphocyte and neutrophil-to-lymphocyte ratios in patients with ankylosing spondylitis and their relationships with high-frequency hearing thresholds. Eur Arch Otorhinolaryngol. 2016;273(11):3663–72.
27. Zhu S, Cai M, Kong X, et al. Changes of neutrophil-to- lymphocyte ratio and red blood cell distribution width in ankylosing spondylitis. Int J Clin Exp Pathol. 2016;9(8):8570–4.
28. CoŞkun BN, Öksüz MF, Ermurat S, et al. Neutrophil lymphocyte ratio can be a valuable marker in defining disease activity in patients who have started anti-tumor necrosis factor (TNF) drugs for ankylosing spondylitis. Eur J Rheumatol. 2014;1(3):101–5.
29. Gökmen F, Akbal A, ReŞorlu H, et al. Neutrophil– lymphocyte ratio connected to treatment options and inflammation markers of Ankylosing spondylitis. J Clin Lab Anal. 2015;29(4):294–8.
30. Kucuk A, Uslu A, Ugan Y, et al. Neutrophil-to-lymphocyte ratio is involved in the severity of ankylosing spondylitis. Bratisl Lek Listy. 2015;116(12):722–5.
31. McVeigh CM, Cairns AP. Diagnosis and management of ankylosing spondylitis. BMJ. 2006;333(7568):581–5.
32. El Maghraoui A. Extra-articular manifestations of ankylosing spondylitis: prevalence, characteristics and therapeutic implications. Eur J Intern Med. 2011;22(6):554–60.

26

The Brazilian Society of Rheumatology guidelines for axial spondyloarthritis – 2019

Gustavo Gomes Resende[1*], Eduardo de Souza Meirelles[2], Cláudia Diniz Lopes Marques[3], Adriano Chiereghin[4], Andre Marun Lyrio[5], Antônio Carlos Ximenes[6], Carla Gonçalves Saad[2], Célio Roberto Gonçalves[2], Charles Lubianca Kohem[7], Cláudia Goldenstein Schainberg[2], Cristiano Barbosa Campanholo[8], Júlio Silvio de Sousa Bueno Filho[9], Lenise Brandao Pieruccetti[10], Mauro Waldemar Keiserman[11], Michel Alexandre Yazbek[12], Penelope Esther Palominos[7], Rafaela Silva Guimarães Goncalves[3], Ricardo da Cruz Lage[1], Rodrigo Luppino Assad[13], Rubens Bonfiglioli[5], Sônia Maria Alvarenga Anti[14], Sueli Carneiro[15], Thauana Luíza Oliveira[16], Valderílio Feijó Azevedo[17], Washington Alves Bianchi[18], Wanderley Marques Bernardo[19], Marcelo de Medeiros Pinheiro[16] and Percival Degrava Sampaio-Barros[19]

Abstract

Spondyloarthritis is a group of chronic inflammatory systemic diseases characterized by axial and/or peripheral joints inflammation, as well as extra-articular manifestations. The classification axial spondyloarthritis is adopted when the spine and/or the sacroiliac joints are predominantly involved. This version of recommendations replaces the previous guidelines published in May 2013.

A systematic literature review was performed, and two hundred thirty-seven studies were selected and used to formulate 29 recommendations answering 15 clinical questions, which were divided into four sections: diagnosis, non-pharmacological therapy, conventional drug therapy and biological therapy. For each recommendation the level of evidence supporting (highest available), the strength grade according to Oxford, and the degree of expert agreement (inter-rater reliability) is informed.

These guidelines bring evidence-based information on clinical management of axial SpA patients, including, diagnosis, treatment, and prognosis.

Introduction

According to recent definition, spondyloarthritis (SpA) is a group of diseases characterized by spine and peripheral joints inflammation, as well as extra-articular manifestations, including anterior uveitis, psoriasis and inflammatory bowel disease, with a genetic predisposition linked to the human leukocyte antigen B27 (HLA-B27). The SpA spectrum includes ankylosing spondylitis (AS), psoriatic arthritis (PsA), reactive arthritis (ReA), enteropathic arthritis (EA) and undifferentiated spondyloarthritis (uSpA). Based on the Assessment of SpondyloArthritis international Society (ASAS) classification criteria, the spine and/or the sacroiliac joints involvement is named as axial spondyloarthritis (axial SpA) [1, 2]. The exclusive appendicular joints involvement is called as peripheral spondyloarthritis (p-SpA). On the other hand, if a patient has both clinical features, he should be classified according to the predominance (i.e., predominantly axial or predominantly peripheral involvement).

The purpose of these guidelines is to bring evidence-based information on clinical management of axial SpA patients, including, diagnosis, treatment and prognosis, for rheumatologists, general physicians, allied-specialists (dermatology, ophthalmology and gastroenterology), and other allied-professionals, such as physiotherapists. This version replaces the previous guidelines published on May 26, 2013 [3] and should be updated every 4 years.

Methods

A systematic literature review was performed, with external review of an specialized group of the Brazilian

* Correspondence: gustavogomesresende@yahoo.com.br
[1]Universidade Federal de Minas Gerais (UFMG), Alameda Álvaro Celso, 175 / 2° Andar. Santa Efigênia. CEP 30.150-260, Belo Horizonte, MG, Brazil
Full list of author information is available at the end of the article

Medical Association. It was used keywords defined according to the PICO (Patient | Intervention | Comparison | Outcome) strategy and searching for records in the following databases: MEDLINE, EMBASE, SciELO/ LILACS, and Cochrane Library, since March 1st, 2012 until December 31, 2018. The target population included patients with 3-month or more back pain and less than 45 years old, according to the ASAS classification criteria in 2009 [1, 2]. Two hundred thirty-seven studies were selected and used to formulate 29 recommendations answering 15 clinical questions, which were divided into four sections: diagnosis, non-pharmacological therapy, conventional drug therapy and biological therapy. For each recommendation the level of evidence supporting (highest available) and strength grade according to Oxford Centre for Evidence-based Medicine Levels of Evidence of 2001 [4] is informed. The methodological details of the bibliographic research and a table with the Oxford levels of evidence are available in the Additional file 1. The degree of expert agreement (inter-rater reliability) was determined by the Delphi method through an online anonymous survey. Table 1 summarizes these recommendations and Fig. 1 shows a guide algorithm for axial SpA management.

Whenever possible, the results are presented as absolute values, followed by an effect size measure to highlight its clinical significance or practical relevance. In comparisons among treated and untreated (placebo) ratios, the number needed to treat (NNT) or the number needed to harm (NNH), and the respective confidence intervals (95% CI) were calculated using a normal approximation, the most statistically robust method. The data retrieved from each study used to define these intervals are available in Additional file 2. In comparisons between paired means (before and after treatment), the effect sizes were calculated using the Cohen method (difference between the means divided by the pooled standard deviation of the groups). Effect sizes were considered small ranging from 0.2 to 0.4, medium ranging from 0.4 to 0.8 and large greater than 0.8.

Clinical questions

1. What are the clinical criteria for considering someone affected by a spondyloarthritis?

In 2009, the ASAS group conducted a study based on the Delphi methodology, with the participation of all members, and selected all possible variables that should be evaluated in a patient with axial SpA. These variables were evaluated in a prospective study that included 647 patients who experienced back pain for more than three months without definite cause or known diagnosis, with or without peripheral symptoms, and an onset of symptoms before 45 years of age who were followed in 25 university centers from 16 countries.

The classification criteria based on two main variables were proposed (Table 2). The sensitivity based on these criteria was 82.9% and the specificity was 84.4% [1, 2] (**1B**). Although some cases of axial SpA may start after 45 years of age, this age is set as a cut-off point to emphasize that many other causes of back pain after this age, particularly degenerative disorders, can mimic the imaging changes characteristic of axial SpA. Despite the specific criticisms directed to the method used to establish the classification criteria for SpA, proposed by ASAS, they represented a considerable advance in our understanding regarding the SpA spectrum and have been since widely adopted by the international community.

A study designed to assess the performance of the axial SpA classification criteria proposed by ASAS in Chinese individuals complaining of chronic back pain without radiological evidence of sacroiliitis found that the diagnostic concordance of the ASAS criteria was better than the criteria established by the European Spondyloarthropathy Study Group (ESSG) and by Bernard Amor. The sensitivity values of the ESSG, Amor and ASAS criteria were 81.5, 87.7 and 89.4%, respectively, and the specificity values were 78.6, 76.7 and 86.4%, respectively [5] (**2B**).

Another study, known as PROSpA (PRevalence Of axial SpA), assessed the performance of the ASAS criteria in another population: American individuals over the age of 18 years and chronic back pain with onset before age 45. In this study, the direct application of classification criteria proposed by the ASAS group enabled the diagnosis of 47% individuals with axial SpA. The specificity and sensitivity of the ASAS criteria were 79 and 81%, respectively, which are slightly lower than the values reported in other, more "selected" populations and may be related to the lower prevalence of HLA-B27-positive individuals [6] (**2B**). In 2016, the long-term follow-up (mean of 4.4 years) data regarding axial SpA cohort (N = 394 patients), based on ASAS classification criteria, showed that the positive predictive value was from 86 to 96% [7] (**2B**).

Despite the ASAS criteria has had a good performance, as shown above, their efficacy in diagnosing different populations varies, particularly in individuals with chronic back pain and whose pretest probability of axial SpA is low. Considering patients with back pain started after 45 years old, the ASAS axial criteria had also the best performance to classify as late-onset axial SpA in the clinical practice [8] (**2B**).

Recommendation

The 2009 ASAS criteria should be used to classify patients with axial spondyloarthritis. The diagnosis should be performed by an experienced physician or rheumatologist. **Level of evidence: 1B; strength of recommendation: A (strong); Degree of agreement: 9.2.**

Table 1 Recommendations of the Brazilian Society of Rheumatology for the diagnosis and management of axial SpA with their respective levels of evidence, strength of recommendation, and degrees of agreement among experts (interrater reliability)

Clinical question	Recommendation	Level of evidence	Strength of recommendation	Degree of agreement
1- What are the clinical criteria for considering someone affected by a spondyloarthritis?	The 2009 ASAS criteria should be used to classify patients with axial spondyloarthritis. The diagnosis should be performed by an experienced physician or a rheumatologist.	1B	A (strong)	9.2
2- What is the role of magnetic resonance imaging (MRI) in the initial evaluation of axial SpA?	In patients with clinically suspected axial SpA, in which sacroiliac radiography is not conclusive, sacroiliac joints (SIJ) MRI is recommended.	1A	A (strong)	9.0
	SIJ MRI scans should be acquired in T1W and STIR and/or T2 fat saturation (FATSAT) sequences. Intravenous MRI contrast (gadolinium) is not recommended routinely.	2B	B (moderate)	9.5
	Spine MRI scans are not recommended on a routine basis for the diagnosis of patients with suspected axial SpA and no sacroiliitis on images.	1B	A (strong)	8.5
3 - What is the role of the HLA-B27 in spondyloarthritis?	HLA-B27 test is recommended for patients with clinically suspected axial SpA for prognostic reasons (more severe axial involvement, higher risk of anterior uveitis and family history of axial SpA). Although it is frequently used as a diagnostic tool in our population, there is very limited evidence of its value.	2A	B (moderate)	9.2
4 - What is the evidence for the use of physical rehabilitation in patients with axial SpA?	Physical rehabilitation programs should be indicated and offered to all patients diagnosed with axial spondyloarthritis during all stages of the disease.	1A	A (strong)	9.8
	Programs specifically focused on improving mobility are primarily recommended, although programs focused on improving endurance and cardiorespiratory fitness are also beneficial.	2A	A (strong)	9.6
5 - What is the evidence for the use of glucocorticoids in patients with axial SpA?	Long-term use of systemic glucocorticoids to treat axial spondyloarthritis is not recommended.	5	D (very weak)	9.6
	Patients with symptomatic peripheral enthesitis can undergo peritendinous glucocorticoid injections. Caution advised because the procedure may increase the risk of rupture, particularly in the Achilles tendon.	2A	B (moderate)	9.2
	Patients with isolated buttock pain who are unresponsive to treatment with nonsteroidal anti-inflammatory drugs (NSAIDs) may experience short-term benefits from an intra-articular injection of triamcinolone acetate in the sacroiliac joints.	2C	B (moderate)	8.5
6 - In which situations is the continuous use of NSAIDs recommended for patients with axial SpA?	NSAIDs should be indicated as the first-line treatment for active and symptomatic axial SpA.	1A	A (strong)	9.8
	There is no evidence that a specific NSAID can be considered superior to the other NSAIDs.	1A	A (strong)	9.3

Table 1 Recommendations of the Brazilian Society of Rheumatology for the diagnosis and management of axial SpA with their respective levels of evidence, strength of recommendation, and degrees of agreement among experts (interrater reliability) *(Continued)*

Clinical question	Recommendation	Level of evidence	Strength of recommendation	Degree of agreement
	Evidence on the effect of NSAIDs on reducing radiographic progression in patients with axial SpA is conflicting.	1B	B (moderate)	9.3
7 - What is the evidence for the use of synthetic disease-modifying antirheumatic drugs (methotrexate, sulfasalazine and leflunomide) in patients with axial SpA?	The use of methotrexate and sulfasalazine is recommended for the treatment of patients with axial SpA when peripheral arthritis is present or in the absence of another pharmacological treatment option due to toxicity, intolerance or contraindications.	2A	B (moderate)	8.4
	The routine use of methotrexate or sulfasalazine as a co-medication in patients with axial SpA who are using biologics is not recommended.	2B	B (moderate)	9.6
8 - What evidence of efficacy supports indications for the use of biologics in patients with axial SpA?	Based on the opinion of the rheumatologist, the use of biologics (TNFα inhibitors or interleukin-17 inhibitors) to treat active (BASDAI≥4 or ASDAS≥2.1) and symptomatic axial SpA is recommended when the initial treatment with NSAIDs fails (disease persistence, toxicity or contraindications).	1A	A (strong)	8.9
	Biologics should be used to treat axial SpA when objective signs of inflammation are detected, such as elevated C-reactive protein (CRP) levels and/or the presence of sacroiliitis on MRI, as these parameters predict the response, particularly in the context of non-radiographic axial SpA.	1B	A (strong)	9.6
	Anti-TNF inhibitors (adalimumab, etanercept, golimumab and certolizumab pegol) are recommended for the treatment of non-radiographic axial SpA since they had an evidence-based approval.	1B	A (strong)	9.7
9 - Are there any differences regarding efficacy among the biologic agents to treat axial SpA patients?	The biologics TNFα inhibitors and the IL17A inhibitors exhibit similar effect sizes for controlling inflammatory activity in patients with axial SpA.	1A	A (strong)	8.9
10 - Does the safety of biologics differ in patients with axial SpA?	The biologics TNFα inhibitors and the IL17A inhibitors have similar effect sizes for the risk of adverse effects and short-term discontinuation.	1A	A (strong)	9.1
11 - Is the use of biological therapy able to reduce structural damage (radiographic progression) in patients with axial SpA?	The reduction in the progression rate of structural damage (observed on spinal radiographies) in patients with axial SpA can be observed in the long-term use of TNF inhibitors.	2B	B (moderate)	8.2
	A similar effect on radiographic progression seems to be observed with the continuous use of anti-IL17 (secukinumab) but need to be confirmed in long-term studies.	2C	B (moderate)	9.6
12 - What is the evidence regarding efficacy of biologic agents on extra-articular manifestations in patients with axial SpA?	In the case of recurrent anterior uveitis or active inflammatory bowel disease in the setting of axial SpA, anti-TNF monoclonal antibodies (infliximab, adalimumab, golimumab, and certolizumab pegol) have shown the best response rates among the biologics. Therefore, it is recommended to choose it, preferably to others.	2A	B (moderate)	9.4
	Monoclonal anti-TNF inhibitors (infliximab, adalimumab, golimumab, and certolizumab pegol) and ant-IL17 inhibitors have shown be the most effective, among the biologics, for the control of active psoriasis	2B	B (moderate)	9.4

Table 1 Recommendations of the Brazilian Society of Rheumatology for the diagnosis and management of axial SpA with their respective levels of evidence, strength of recommendation, and degrees of agreement among experts (interrater reliability) *(Continued)*

Clinical question	Recommendation	Level of evidence	Strength of recommendation	Degree of agreement
	in the setting of axial SpA. Therefore, it is recommended to choose it, preferably to others.			
13- What is the evidence that supports the switching among biologic agents in patients with axial SpA?	Patients with axial SpA who fail to show an initial response to a biological therapy (primary treatment failure), loss of efficacy (secondary treatment failure) or adverse effects may switch to another approved biologic, regardless mechanism of action.	2A	B (moderate)	9.4
	After the first biologic switch, the response rates decrease slightly but remain significant. The little available evidence on the second biologic switch suggest response rates even lower than the second-line treatment.	2A	B (moderate)	9.1
14 - For how long should a biologic be used during the follow-up of a patient with axial SpA?	In those who have reached the proposed treatment target, for at least 6 months, an attempt may be made to reduce the anti-TNFα dose or increase the interval between doses. Data on other mechanisms of action remains insufficient. However, the risk of long-term radiographic progression should be considered.	1B	B (moderate)	8.9
15 - Is there evidence for the use of biologics and/or target-specific small molecules with other mechanisms of action in patients with axial SpA?	The use of other biologics and/or target-specific small molecules (abatacept, tocilizumab, rituximab, sarilumab, ustekinumab and apremilast) is not recommended for the treatment of patients with axial SpA.	1B	A (strong)	9.5
	The Janus kinase (JAK) inhibitors tofacitinib and filgotinib showed promising clinical results in the treatment of ankylosing spondylitis, but more definitive evidence (phase III randomized clinical trials) is still needed prior to their recommendation.	2B	B (moderate)	9.1

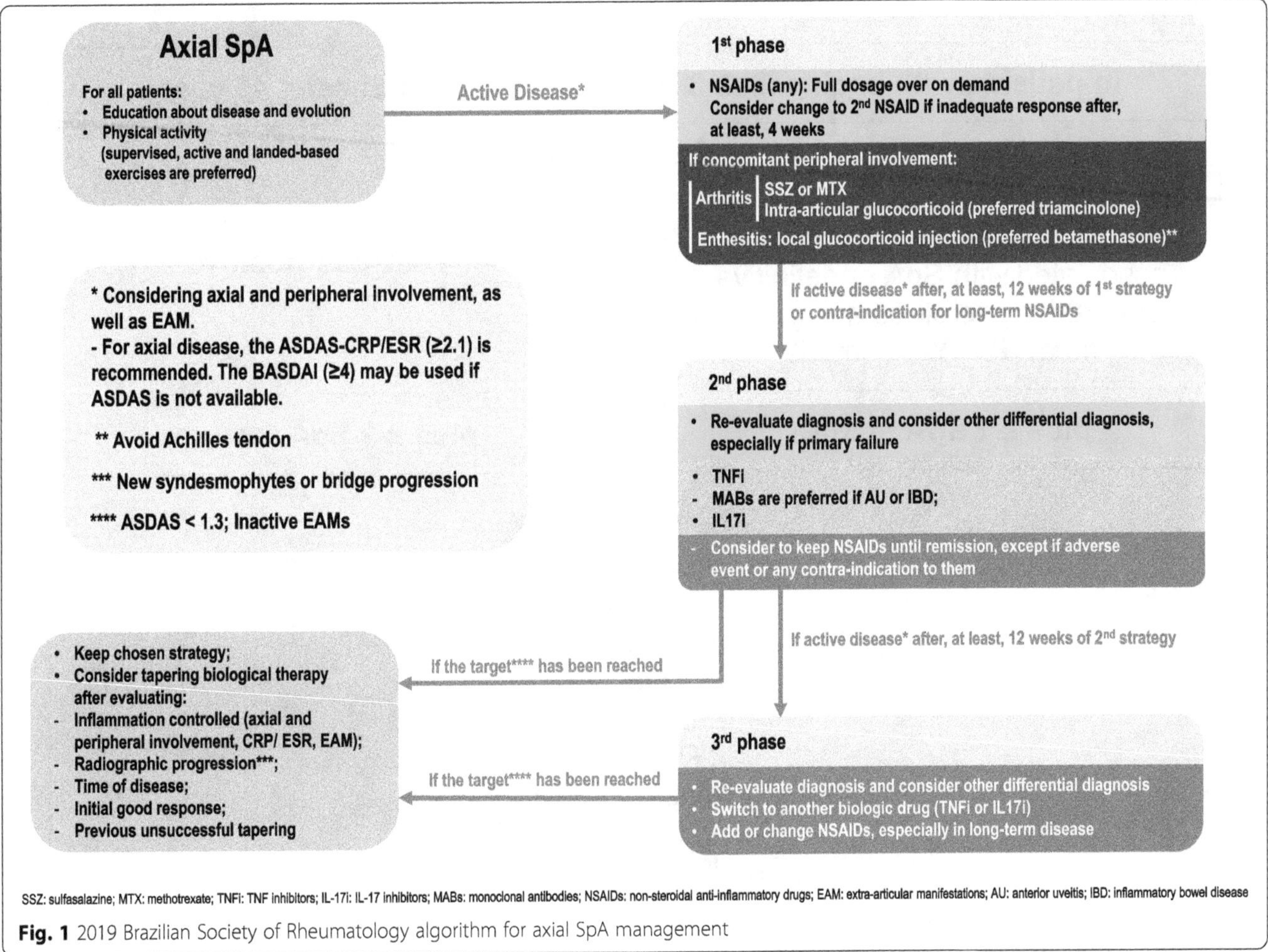

Fig. 1 2019 Brazilian Society of Rheumatology algorithm for axial SpA management

2. What is the role of magnetic resonance imaging (MRI) for the initial evaluation of axial SpA?

Sacroiliac joints (SIJ) and spine imaging plays a key role for the diagnosis, classification, monitoring and prognosis of axial SpA patients. Bone structural changes, usually with a late onset, are clearly identified using conventional radiography [9] (**2C**), whereas inflammatory changes, often with an early onset, are better evaluated using MRI [10, 11] (**2B**).

Diagnosis

In 2009, the ASAS/Outcome Measures in Rheumatology (OMERACT) MRI working group published that the unequivocal presence of bone marrow edema and osteitis (in at least two sites in one slice or in one site in two consecutive slices) is essential to define active sacroiliitis for diagnostic purposes. Active inflammatory lesions have been visualized with both short tau inversion-recovery (STIR) images and T1-weighted (T1W) sequences with fat suppression (FS) after administration of intravenous (IV) contrast (gadolinium) (T1 with FS post-Gd) [12] (**5**). In 2012, a study evaluated the baseline SIJ MRI scans of 29 patients with early inflammatory back pain (IBP) who were subsequently diagnosed with axial SpA according to the ASAS criteria, to validate the ASAS definition of active sacroiliitis. The study reported a 79% sensitivity, 89% specificity, a positive likelihood ratio (LR+) of 7.1 and a negative likelihood ratio (LR-) of 0.2 [13] (**2B**). In another study employing a retrospective design that analyzed 110 patients who were referred for SIJ MRI (of whom 28 were later diagnosed with axial SpA), the presence of bone marrow edema located in the sacral area and in both sacral and iliac areas was an independent predictor of diagnosis with odds ratios (ORs) of 7.07 (95% CI 1.05–47.6) and 36 (95% CI 5.61–23.1), respectively [14] (**2B**).

A multicenter study to evaluate the diagnostic utility of SIJ MRI scans from 187 people (75 patients with ankylosing spondylitis (AS), 27 patients with pre-radiographic IBP, 26 patients with non-specific back pain and 59 healthy controls) showed that bone marrow edema, erosion, fat metaplasia and ankylosis had 90% of sensitivity and 97% of specificity for diagnosis of axial SpA, with a LR+ = 30 and, therefore, 97% diagnostic certainty for positive axial SpA

Table 2 2009 ASAS classification criteria for axial spondyloarthritis

In patients with back pain ≥ 3 months and age at onset < 45 years		
Sacroiliitis on image Active (acute) inflammation on MRI highly suggestive of sacroiliitis associated with SpA or definitive radiographic sacroiliitis according to mod. New York criteria	**or**	**HLA-B27 positive**
plus ≥ 1 SpA feature		**plus ≥ 2 SpA features**
SpA features: Inflammatory back pain Arthritis Enthesitis (heel) Uveitis Dactylitis Psoriasis Crohn´s disease / ulcerative colitis Good response to NSAID Family history for SpA HLA-B27 Elevated CRP		

and 91% diagnostic certainty for negative axial SpA [11] (**1A**). The inclusion of erosions, but not fat metaplasia, for the definition of sacroiliitis (in addition to bone marrow edema) increased the sensitivity without a loss of specificity, according to three other studies [15–17] (**2B**). In the DESIR cohort that included patients with short-term axial SpA (IBP ≥ 3 months and ≤ 3 years), the structural lesions (≥5 erosions or fat metaplasia) on SIJ MRI were reliably used instead of positive radiography [18] (**2B**). Conversely, in the SPACE cohort, any combination of 5 chronic lesions (erosions or fat metaplasia) ensured a specificity >95% in discriminating patients with and without axial SpA [19] (**2B**). Regarding the SIJ MRI in the same cohort (SPACE), the use of an IV MRI contrast agent (gadolinium), which is essential for the detection of synovitis and/or capsulitis, failed to increase the sensitivity of the test compared with STIR alone, because these acute lesions were only observed in patients who also presented bone marrow edema (visible on STIR) [20] (**2B**). In addition, the acquisition of diffusion-weighted images (DWI) is an alternative to the use of contrast agents, reducing the risk of nephrotoxicity, albeit without showing better performance than STIR imaging analyses [21, 22] (**2B**).

Regarding spine MRI scans, the value and the best definition for a positive MRI related to axial SpA remains open to debate, with rather data heterogeneity in different studies. In 2012, the ASAS/OMERACT MRI working group defined a positive spine MRI (inflammation) when there were the presence of bone marrow edema (BME) in 3 or more sites (corner inflammatory lesions) [23] (**5**). Some findings corroborate its use as a diagnostic tool, suggesting some value of spine MRI when sacroiliitis is absent. The findings include the observation of more than five corner fatty lesions (CFL) identified by hypersignals in T1W images in association with the diagnosis of axial SpA in patients with back pain, with 86% diagnostic certainty (LR of 12.6) [24] (**2B**); identification of lesions (both inflammatory and structural) in the spine MRI scans of 50% of the 20 patients without sacroiliitis (on XR or MRI) of a total of 60 patients with a confirmed diagnosis of axial

SpA [25] (**2B**); and spinal inflammation in 53 of 109 (49%) patients with non-radiographic axial SpA, without sacroiliitis, who were included in a clinical trial [26] (**2B**). Conversely, some evidence also questions the value of spine MRI in patients with suspected axial SpA, without sacroiliitis. In the SPACE and DESIR cohorts, the inclusion of spinal MRI as an imaging criterion into the ASAS criteria resulted in the reclassification of a very small percentage of patients (1–2%) [27] (**2B**). In another study of 130 patients with chronic back pain who were younger than 50 years and 20 healthy controls, the combination of spine MRI (using the ASAS/OMERACT definition and several other alternatives) with SIJ MRI had little effect on the final accuracy, mainly due to the large number of false-positives (11–16% of the patients were diagnosed with non-specific back pain and 17.5% of the healthy controls had spine lesions) [28] (**2B**). In the ASAS cohort, in which the 2009 criteria were validated, only 5.4% of 235 patients with SIJ and spine MRI exclusively had spinal inflammation [2] (**2B**).

Prognosis

For the evaluation of patients with recent-onset IBP (<2 years), the combination of MRI-evident severe sacroiliitis, according to the Leeds scoring system (>75% of any SIJ quadrant affected by bone marrow edema), added to positive HLA-B27 predicts the future development of radiographically evident AS at eight years with 62% sensitivity, 92% specificity, 80% positive post-test probability and 83% negative post-test probability. Severe sacroiliitis alone predicted this diagnosis with 50% positive post-test probability and 84% negative post-test probability [10] (**2B**). Based on 2 to 7 years of follow-up of axial SpA patients, the evaluation of SIJ MRI changes (Danish score: erosion, edema and fat infiltration) revealed that chronic changes at baseline are related to the future development of AS. At baseline, the SIJ MRI scans with activity scores ≥2, total chronic scores ≥1, erosion scores ≥1 and fatty metaplasia scores ≥4 had predictive ability for the radiographic sacroiliitis of 74, 77, 79 and 68% accuracy, respectively [29] (**1B**). In another study, radiographic progression (measured using the modified Stoke Ankylosing Spondylitis Spinal Score [mSASSS]) was significantly greater during the follow-up period in patients with fat metaplasia and ankylosis at baseline SIJ MRI scans than in patients without these lesions [30] (**2B**). Also regarding spine MRI, the presence of corner inflammatory lesions (CILs) in AS patients after 2 years of follow-up predicted a 14.9% increase for developing new syndesmophytes (NNH = 7). After TNF inhibitors, this risk was 11.4% higher for vertebral corners with no inflammation than in those with inflammation (NNH = 9) [31] (**1B**). Higher Bath Ankylosing Spondylitis Metrology Index (BASMI; an index of the degree of functional limitation in patients with AS) scores have already been associated with higher Ankylosing Spondylitis spine Magnetic Resonance Imaging-activity (ASspiMRI-a; an index of spinal inflammatory activity on MRI) scores, particularly in patients who have suffered from the disease for ≤3 years and with higher mSASSS scores (an index of radiographic progression). In conclusion, spinal mobility is independently determined by both reversible spinal inflammation (on MRI) and irreversible structural damage (on XR) [32] (**2B**).

Recommendation

In patients with clinically suspected axial SpA, in which sacroiliac radiography is not conclusive, sacroiliac joints (SIJ) MRI is recommended. ***Level of evidence: 1A; Strength of recommendation: A (strong); Degree of agreement: 9.0.***

SIJ MRI scans should be acquired in T1W and STIR and/or T2 fat saturation (FATSAT) sequences. Intravenous MRI contrast (gadolinium) is not recommended routinely. ***Level of evidence: 2B; Strength of recommendation: B (moderate); Degree of agreement: 9.5.***

Spine MRI scans are not recommended on a routine basis for the diagnosis of patients with suspected axial SpA and no sacroiliitis on images. ***Level of evidence: 1B; Strength of recommendation: A (strong); Degree of agreement: 8.5.***

3. What is the role of HLA-B27 in axial spondyloarthritis?

Diagnosis

HLA-B27 represents an important arm (also known as clinical arm) of the ASAS classification criteria. When combined with other variables (such as imaging and other clinical criteria), HLA-B27 allows the classification of axial SpA [2] (**2B**). The presence of HLA-B27, when associated with sacroiliitis diagnosed on MRI, increases the diagnostic specificity for AS of the latter from 62 to 77% compared with MRI alone, without changing the sensitivity. A positive HLA-B27 test alone predicted the disease with 48% probability, and negative HLA-B27 test excluded the disease with 88% probability [10] (**2B**). The value of HLA-B27 as a diagnostic tool in the Brazilian population remains unknown due to lack of evidence.

Genetic factors have already been associated with susceptibility to AS, as shown in a meta-analysis of studies that measured the risk of occurrence of AS in relatives of patients with AS. A 63% risk was observed among monozygotic twins, an 8.2% risk was observed among first-degree relatives, and 1.0 and 0.7% risks were observed among second- and third-degree relatives, respectively [33] (**2A**). According to a study enrolled 348 blood donors of whom 20 were diagnosed with SpA, the relative risk (RR) of developing SpA was 20 (95% CI 4.6–94) among HLA-B27-positive individuals. In the same study, 50% of HLA-B27-positive individuals with IBP had sacroiliitis on SIJ MRI [34] (**2B**). The overall incidence and prevalence of AS and SpA strongly depend on and are directly correlated with the prevalence of HLA-B27 in a specific population. Indeed, in various countries, their prevalence rates vary widely: 0.14–1.4% for AS; 0.30–1.73% for SpA; and 5.4–16% for HLA-B27 [35, 36] (**2B**). Currently, more than 160 HLA-B27 subtypes have been identified (HLA-B*27:01 to HLA-B*27:161) and coded by 213 allelic variants, with wide variation related to ethnicity [37] (**5**).

Prognosis

In HLA-B27-positive AS patients, the data have shown longer disease duration (earlier onset of symptoms and diagnosis), higher frequency of NSAIDs intake, higher frequency of biologic agents therapy, higher disease severity (including extra-articular manifestations) and higher functional (Bath Ankylosing Spondylitis Functional Index – BASFI) and disease activity (BASDAI) scores [38, 39] (**2B**). In another study, HLA-B27-positive AS patients showed significantly more axial and hip involvement; higher positive family history frequency; and higher percentage of men among HLA-B27-positive AS patients than among HLA-B27-negative AS patients [40] (**2B**). There was significant association between HLA-B27 and BASMI (metrological index) in AS patients (worse prognosis) [41] (**2B**). In Chinese AS patients there was significant association between HLA-B27 positivity and severe SIJ involvement and earlier-onset disease [42] (**2B**). In fact, when AS patients were classified according to onset-disease age (<20 years, 21–30 years, 31–40 years and > 40 years), the positivity for HLA-B27 was found in 94.6, 90.2, 74.1, and 61.2%, respectively. The same pattern was also observed in non-radiographic axial SpA patients [43] (**2B**). A systematic literature review included almost 30,000 patients reported 4-times higher likely for uveitis in HLA-B27 positive AS patients [44] (**2A**).

Recommendation

> HLA-B27 test is recommended for patients with clinically suspected axial SpA for prognostic reasons (more severe axial involvement, higher risk of anterior uveitis and family history of axial SpA). Although it is frequently used as a diagnostic tool in our population, there is very limited evidence of its value. ***Level of evidence: 2A; Strength of recommendation: B (moderate); Degree of agreement: 9.2.***

4. What is the evidence for the use of physical rehabilitation in patients with axial SpA?

According to the Assessment of Spondyloarthritis International Society/ European League Against Rheumatism (ASAS/EULAR) group, the optimal management of patients with axial SpA requires a combination of non-pharmacological and pharmacological treatment modalities [45] (**1A**). Among non-pharmacological therapies, exercise is considered an important tool for maintaining or improving mobility and physical function and for preventing deformities [46–48] (**1A**).

Supervised exercise

A randomized controlled trial (RCT) compared the treatment of patients with AS (n = 40) using the Global Postural Reeducation (GPR) method or conventional exercise; both exercise interventions were conducted in weekly 1-h sessions in groups of 6–8 patients for 4 months. The outcomes were mobility, as assessed using the BASMI, activity assessed using the BASDAI and physical function scored with the BASFI. After 4 months (15 sessions), the BASFI (effect size of 0.32) and all BASMI parameters (effect sizes ranging from 0.36 to 1.1), but not the BASDAI, significantly improved in the GPR group. Only the tragus to wall distance and lumbar side flexion were significantly improved in the control group. The comparison between the two forms of treatment revealed better results in the group treated with postural rehabilitation using the GPR method than in the group treated with conventional training over a one-year follow-up period [49, 50] (**2B**). Similar results were obtained in another study in which patients with AS were subjected to a 16-week supervised GPR program (n = 22) or unsupervised training (n = 16). Morning stiffness, pain, spinal mobility, physical function (Health Assessment Questionnaire – Spondyloarthropathies – HAQ-S), quality of life (Medical Outcomes Study 36 - Item Short-Form Health Survey – SF-36) and disease activity (BASDAI) were evaluated, with significant improvements in all study parameters between the pre- and posttreatment periods in both groups. The GPR group reported significantly better results for morning stiffness, spinal mobility and the physical component of the SF-36 than the control group [51] (**2B**). Consistent with these findings, significant improvements in the BASDAI, BASMI and BASFI indices were observed in a group of patients with AS (n = 48) subjected to training combining the Pilates, McKenzie and Heckscher techniques compared to a group (n = 48) subjected to conventional physical therapy (classical kinesiotherapy) [52] (**2B**).

In-patient exercise

Patients with AS (n = 107) who were subjected to 4-week, in-patient rehabilitation programs were assessed for health status (patient global assessment, pain, morning stiffness, spinal mobility, BASFI, BASDAI and fatigue) according to the Assessments in Ankylosing Spondylitis working group's Improvement Criteria (ASAS-IC; the response criterion most commonly used in clinical trials, consisting of four domains: physical function, spinal pain, patient global assessment and inflammation). The programs offered a personalized assessment of physical therapy, group exercise, passive therapy, relaxation and patient education, with a difference in two components – endurance training (centers located in Norway) or mobility (centers located in the Mediterranean). After 16 weeks, all variables (except question 2 of the BASDAI (spinal pain), thoracic expandability and erythrocyte sedimentation rate (ESR)) were significantly improved by both modalities. The numbers of patients who achieved ASAS20 and ASAS40 were 27% (NNT = 4) and 19% (NNT = 5) higher after mobility-focused rehabilitation than after endurance training-focused rehabilitation at week 16. This difference, although not significant, persisted until the final assessment (week 28) [53] (**2B**). Another randomized clinical trial also reported evidence favoring a 3-week in-patient rehabilitation program (n = 46) over the "usual treatment", without systematic rehabilitation (n = 49). The results showed significant improvements of BASDAI (effect size = 1.38) and physical, emotional and vitality and pain components of the SF-36 after 4 months of follow-up. However, after 12 months, no significant differences were observed in any study outcome, thus indicating a transient effect of rehabilitation [54] (**2B**).

Education and home-based exercise

A non-randomized clinical trial (n = 66) compared patients with AS who underwent a home-based exercise program (after theoretical and practical counseling by a physical therapist) five times a week (at least 30 min per session) with patients who exercised less than five times a week (control group). After 3 months of follow-up, all assessed parameters, such as pain, morning stiffness, spinal mobility, BASFI, BASDAI, Ankylosing Spondylitis Quality of Life Questionnaire (ASQol) and the pulmonary function measures forced vital capacity (FVC) and forced expiratory volume in 1 s (FEV1) significantly improved in the treatment group compared to the baseline values, but not in the control group, which even showed worsening of some parameters (stiffness, mobility and ASQol). In the intergroup comparison, only the quality of life scores (ASQol) at 3 months differed significantly, in favor of the treatment group [55] (**2B**). Another RCT compared a short-term (5-day) education and exercise program, followed by unsupervised training, with conventional treatment (no exercise). This trial included 41 patients with AS and, after 3 months of follow-up, observed significant improvements (BASDAI, BASFI, ASQol and SF-36) compared to the baseline only in the education+exercise group. No improvements regarding BASMI or inflammatory markers were observed [56] (**2B**). The educational intervention effectiveness (a 2-h session, with guidance on the disease and an unsupervised physical activity program) was also investigated in another RCT (n = 756) in which 381 patients were allocated to the experimental group and 375 to the control group (without any specific intervention). After 6 months, the experimental group showed significantly better quality of life (ASQoL), physical function (BASFI), global pain and disease activity scores (BASDAI) than the control group, even after adjusting for baseline values, sex, age and education. The effect sizes ranged from 0.20 to 0.28 [57] (**2B**). A 2015 meta-analysis included data from six studies including 1098 patients and concluded that exercise, even unsupervised, significantly improves physical function (measured using the BASFI), disease activity (measured using the BASDAI) and depression and pain scores [58] (**2A**).

Aerobic exercise

A RCT compared the effect of aerobic exercise (a 50-min walk, 3 times per week for 3 months) followed by stretching exercises (intervention group) with stretching alone (control group) on 70 patients with AS (35 in each group). The BASMI, BASFI, HAQ-S, BASDAI and ASDAS scores improved in both groups, with no significant differences between groups. The 6-min walk test and aerobic capacity (as assessed using ergospirometry on a treadmill) were significantly improved in the intervention group compared with the control group [59] (**2B**). Another clinical trial included 106 patients with AS who were randomly allocated to the aerobic exercise group (3 times per week) or control group (both with a weekly session of stretching exercises). After 3 months, physical fitness (measured in watts) and the BASDAI peripheral pain component were significantly better in the aerobic exercise group than in the control group [60] (**2B**). In another nonrandomized trial, 46 patients with axial SpA were subjected to a 6-month physical exercise program, including aerobic training (60 min, twice a week), and compared with another 29 sex- and age-matched patients with axial SpA (controls, without any intervention). In the final evaluation, the ASDAS-CRP and BASMI values were significantly improved in both groups and were better in the exercise group than in the control group [61] (**2C**). Another study also reported benefits from aerobic exercise (40–60 min, 3 times per week) in 28 patients with axial SpA who were randomly allocated to the exercise group or to the control group. After 12 weeks, the exercise group showed significant differences in disease activity (BASDAI), physical function (BASFI), cardiorespiratory fitness (peak oxygen volume (VO_2)), body composition (% total and abdominal fat) and arterial stiffness markers (augmentation index and pulse wave velocity). Therefore, cardiovascular risk factors were reduced by this type of intervention [62] (**2B**).

Aquatic exercise

A clinical trial compared aquatic exercise (20 sessions: 5 sessions per week for 4 weeks) with home-based exercise after a practical demonstration in 69 patients with AS. All study parameters (pain, BASMI, BASFI, BASDAI and SF-36) were significantly improved after 4 and 12 weeks in both groups. The intergroup comparison showed significant differences in pain and in six of the eight components of the SF-36, favoring aquatic exercise [63] (**2B**). In another RCT, 30 patients with axial SpA were allocated to an aquatic exercise and stretching program (24 sessions: 3 sessions per week for 8 weeks) or to the control group (no training). Quality of life (SF-12), physical function (BASFI) and disease activity (BASDAI) only significantly differed between the pre- and post-intervention periods in the treatment group (effect sizes ranging from 0.44 to 0.66) [64] (**2B**).

However, it is important to emphasize that an exercise test could be requested before recommending some physical activity for AS patients, regardless disease activity, functional or mobility impairment, as well as concomitant diseases or other medications [65] (**2B**).

Recommendation

Physical rehabilitation programs should be indicated for and offered to all patients diagnosed with axial spondyloarthritis during all stages of the disease. ***Level of evidence: 1A; Strength of recommendation: A (strong); Degree of agreement: 9.8.***

Programs specifically focused on improving mobility are primarily recommended, although programs focused on improving endurance and cardiorespiratory fitness are also beneficial. ***Level of evidence: 2A; Strength of recommendation: B (moderate); Degree of agreement: 9.6.***

5. What is the evidence for the use of glucocorticoids in patients with axial SpA?

Systemic glucocorticoids

A double-blind study compared a single pulse therapy with two doses of methylprednisolone (375 mg *versus* 1000 mg in an IV injection for 3 days) in the treatment of 17 patients with AS who were unresponsive to NSAIDs with a 180-day follow-up. The study showed improvements in mobility, pain and morning stiffness following the administration of both doses, with less persistent effects on pain (the median time to requiring reintroduction of analgesics and/or NSAIDs was 8 days at the lowest dose and 25 days at the highest dose) than on morning stiffness (pretreatment levels were reached after 90 and 120 days of treatment with the lowest and highest dose, respectively) and mobility (improvement was observed throughout the follow-up period of 180 days). No significant difference in any outcome was observed between doses, but the very small sample size precluded this comparison. No serious adverse event was observed during the 180-day follow-up period [66] (**2B**). Another study with a retrospective design and a small sample size (n = 15) observed BASDAI improvement (7.4 ± 1.5 at baseline) after pulse therapy with methylprednisolone (250–500 mg per day for 3–5 days) from the first post-treatment evaluation (on the day after treatment, 3.9 ± 2.4, p < 0.001) to the 3-month (5.3 ± 1.8, p < 0.001) and 12-month (5.4, p < 0.001) evaluations [67] (**2C**). Conversely, the use of low-dose oral glucocorticoids (5.0 mg/day of modified-release prednisone) was evaluated in a 12-week uncontrolled study, which included 57 individuals with axial SpA who were refractory, intolerant to or contraindicated for NSAIDs. In the initial evaluation, 73.7% patients used a synthetic disease-modifying antirheumatic drug (DMARD; methotrexate (MTX), sulfasalazine (SSZ) or leflunomide (LFL)) and 7% used a TNFα inhibitor; the doses remained stable throughout the study. The results showed a significant decrease in disease activity (from 5.5 ± 2.6 to 3.0 ± 2.8 on the BASDAI; p = 0.001), but not concerning mobility (BASMI) or enthesitis index (Maastricht Ankylosing Spondylitis Enthesitis Score – MASES). No serious adverse event was observed during the 12-week follow-up period [68] (**2C**). Another short-term randomized, placebo-controlled trial, which included 34 patients with AS, found that daily treatment with two oral doses of prednisolone (20 or 50 mg) for two weeks improved activity indices compared with the placebo. Although the treatment group showed no significant improvement in the primary outcome (BASDAI50), the 50 mg/day dose led to significant decreases in BASDAI (2.39 [1.38–3.40], p = 0.03) and ASDAS-CRP scores (1.56 [0.93–2.20], p = 0.01), whereas the dose of 20 mg/day only produced a significant decrease in the ASDAS-CRP score (1.16 [0.45–1.88], p = 0.004) [69] (**2B**). A cohort study (n = 830) evaluated the safety of low daily oral doses (prednisone up to 10 mg or an equivalent dose) by comparing the incidence of adverse effects in AS patients users (n = 555) and nonusers (n = 275). The study found higher incidence of skin adverse effects, such as acne, hematomas and infections (22.2 *vs* 6.6/1000 patient-years (PY); p = 0.003) among users. However, when considering a mean follow-up period of 1.6 years (0.5–15) and a total of 1801 PY of exposure to glucocorticoids, the study did not detect differences related to low bone mass or lipids and glucose serum levels changes [70] (**2B**).

Infiltration with glucocorticoids

In an open-label and uncontrolled study, an ultrasound-guided retro-calcaneal bursa injection of 20 mg of methylprednisolone in 18 patients with SpA (27 cases of symptomatic Achilles enthesitis treated) improved pain (visual analog scale (VAS): 7 [4–10] *vs* 3 [0–7]; p < 0.0001) and ultrasound parameters (reduced tendon thickness and vascularity, peritendinous edema and bursitis and power Doppler signal intensity) after 6 weeks, without any complication documented until the last evaluation of each patient in the study (3 to 12 months) [71] (**2C**). A systematic literature review (which included only 5 studies, with only one RCT) questions the long-term effects of infiltration of glucocorticoids on the Achilles tendinopathy in general (not only in patients with SpA) and highlights the risk of tendon injuries and rupture [72] (**2A**).

An uncontrolled trial included 66 patients with axial SpA who experienced inflammatory back pain for at least two months without an improvement after 4 weeks of NSAID use and were treated with a computed tomography (CT)-guided intraarticular injection of 40 mg of triamcinolone acetate into the sacroiliac joints. The results showed a significant reduction in pain intensity (as assessed using the VAS) from 2 weeks (±1) to 10 months (±5) after the intervention. A reduction in the levels of serum inflammatory markers (ESR and CRP) and bone marrow edema on SIJ MRI were also observed [73] (**2C**).

Recommendation

Long-term use of systemic glucocorticoids to treat axial spondyloarthritis is not recommended. ***Level of evidence: 5; Strength of recommendation: D (very weak); Degree of agreement: 9.6.***
Patients with symptomatic peripheral enthesitis can undergo peritendinous glucocorticoid injections. Caution is advised because the procedure may increase the risk of rupture, particularly in the Achilles tendon. ***Level of evidence: 2A; Strength of recommendation: B (moderate); Degree of agreement: 9.2.***
Patients with isolated buttock pain who are unresponsive to treatment with nonsteroidal anti-inflammatory drugs (NSAIDs) may experience short-term benefits from an intraarticular injection of triamcinolone acetate in the sacroiliac joints. ***Level of evidence: 2C; Strength of recommendation: B (moderate); Degree of agreement: 8.5.***

6. In which situations is the continuous use of NSAIDs recommended for patients with axial SpA?

Based on evidence of high-to-moderate quality, an extensive systematic review and meta-analysis (Cochrane) published in 2015 (including 35 studies published until June 2014 and including 4356 patients with axial SpA) concluded that both traditional NSAIDs and cyclooxygenase-2 (COX-2) inhibitors (coxibs) are more effective than the placebo for improving pain, disease activity (BASDAI) and physical function (BASFI) in 6–12 weeks), with no significant differences in benefits or damages between the two classes of NSAIDs [74] (**1A**). Another systematic review and Bayesian network meta-analysis included 26 studies with 3410 patients (of whom approximately 60% overlapped with the Cochrane review mentioned above) by limiting the diagnosis to AS and compared 20 different NSAIDs. The authors also concluded that the evidence was insufficient to consider that any NSAID is more effective in treating AS than the other drugs [75] (**1A**). Other studies published after these reviews corroborate the similarity between coxibs and non-selective NSAIDs. A comparison between two doses of celecoxib (200 mg and 400 mg daily) and diclofenac (150 mg daily) did not detect differences in improving pain and adverse effects in 330 AS patients [76] (**1B**). The efficacy and tolerance/safety study of etoricoxib (daily doses of 60 and 90 mg) in AS patients had similar results to naproxen at dose of 1000 mg/day [77] (**1B**).

Inhibition of radiographic progression

Based on the current evidence, the continuous use of NSAIDs by AS patients might reduce the radiographic progression of spinal damage (new bone formation), although no clinical trial comparing the use of NSAIDs with placebo for this outcome has been published to date. A RCT compared continuous and on-demand use of NSAIDs (celecoxib). At the end of the study (after 24 months of follow-up), although significant differences in activity levels (BASDAI) and physical function (BASFI) were not observed between the two groups, radiographic progression, as assessed using the mSASSS, was three times higher in patients treated with the on-demand regimen than in patients treated with the continuous regimen (0.4 ± 1.7 *vs* 1.5 ± 2.5; $p = 0.002$). The frequency of adverse events, namely, hypertension, abdominal pain and dyspepsia, was higher in the continuous regimen group but was not significantly different from the on-demand regimen group [78]. Subgroup and *post hoc* analyses of this trial suggested that the benefit is greater in or even exclusive to patients at greater risk of radiographic progression (patients with elevated inflammatory tests, high rates of disease activity, and pre-existing syndesmophytes) [79] (**1B**). Another (retrospective) study reported similar results. In 88 patients with AS of the German Spondyloarthritis Inception Cohort (GESPIC), more intense use of NSAIDs (defined by the intake of doses ≥50% of the recommended maximum dose for each NSAID) compared with less intense use (NSAID index <50% of the maximum recommended dose) was associated with a lower likelihood of radiographic progression (defined as worsening ≥2 units on the mSASSS), with an OR of 0.15 (95% CI 0.02–0.96; $p = 0.045$), even after adjustment for baseline structural damage, CRP levels and smoking. Conversely, in 76 patients with non-radiographic axial SpA in the same cohort, the same difference in radiographic progression was not observed between intense or non-intense NSAID users, most likely due to the generally low frequency of new bone formation in this subgroup [80] (**2C**). However, opposite results were obtained in another prospective study known as ENRADAS (Effects of NSAIDs on Radiographic Damage in Ankylosing Spondylitis). In this randomized, multicenter trial, whose primary outcome was the difference in spinal radiographic progression measured using the mSASSS, patients with AS were randomly allocated to continuous treatment with diclofenac (150 mg/day) or to on-demand treatment. At the end of the two-year follow-up period, both groups showed significant radiographic progression, with no differences between individuals from the continuous regimen and on-demand regimen groups (OR = 1.3 with a 95% CI of 0.7–1.9 versus OR = 0.8 with a 95% CI of 0.2–1.4, respectively). No differences regarding adverse events were observed between the two groups [81] (**1B**). The evident contradiction between these results, including two clinical trials with very similar designs, indicates that the possible beneficial effect of NSAIDs on new bone formation is not clearly established.

Recommendation

NSAIDs should be indicated as the first-line treatment for active and symptomatic axial SpA. ***Level of evidence: 1A; Strength of recommendation: A (strong); Degree of agreement: 9.8.***
There is no evidence that a specific NSAID can be considered superior to the other NSAIDs. ***Level of evidence: 1A; Strength of recommendation: A (strong); Degree of agreement: 9.3.***
Evidence on the effect of NSAIDs on reducing radiographic progression in patients with axial SpA is conflicting. ***Level of evidence: 1B; Strength of recommendation: B (moderate); Degree of agreement: 9.3.***

7. What is the evidence for the use of synthetic disease-modifying antirheumatic drugs (methotrexate, sulfasalazine and leflunomide) in patients with axial SpA?

Methotrexate

A systematic review and meta-analysis showed the evidence regarding the effects of methotrexate in AS patients was insufficient. However, it is important to highlight that only 5 clinical trials were included (256 patients), with heterogeneity related to outcomes and treatments, hampering the its validity [82] (**2A**). Of the studies included in the review, only one randomized, placebo-controlled trial showed positive results in 35 patients with AS who were treated with methotrexate at a dose of 7.5 mg/week for 24 weeks. In this study, an improvement ≥20% in five of the eight following items was considered a response: a) morning stiffness intensity, b) physical well-being, c) BASDAI, d) BASFI, e) HAQ-S, f) physician global assessment (PGA), and g) patient-reported disease activity. The results showed a higher percentage of responsive patients in the treatment group than in the placebo group (53% *vs* 11%). In the intention-to-treat (ITT) analysis, an NNT = 3 was found, with BASDAI, BASFI and HAQ-S, and other PROs (patient-reported outcomes) improvements, with no differences in the reported frequency of adverse events [83] (**2B**). In a 1-year randomized clinical trial (RCT) with 51 AS patients, a weekly 7.5-mg dose of methotrexate had no additional benefit in improving activity, mobility or physical function parameters compared to the use of naproxen alone, with the exception of the PGA [84] (**2B**). Another 24-week RCT with 30 AS patients showed no significant difference between the groups [85] (**2B**). When comparing the use of methotrexate with placebo in patients with AS using infliximab, the results were also conflicting. An open-label, non-randomized, small-scale (n = 19) trial with a high risk of bias (the compared groups were heterogeneous with respect to previous exposure to treatments) observed a better BASDAI50 and ASAS50 response in the methotrexate group than in the placebo group [86] (**2C**). In another trial, 123 patients were allocated to an on-demand regimen of infliximab after conventional infusion. Of these individuals, 62 patients were treated with methotrexate (at a maximum dose of 12.5 mg per week) and 61 received anti-TNFα alone. After 52 weeks, no significant differences were found, according to the ASAS definition on improvement outcomes [87] (**2B**).

Thus, there is no agreement regarding the type of benefit or subpopulation in which the methotrexate could be used [88–90] (**2C**). Methotrexate also reduced the incidence of anterior uveitis (from 2.05/PY to 0.21/PY, p < 0.0001) in a small observational study that included 21 patients with recurrent acute anterior uveitis, 8 of whom (38%) had a positive HLA-B27 test [91] (**2C**).

Sulfasalazine

Eleven clinical trials were included in a systematic literature review (Cochrane) published in 2005 and updated in 2014, and the effects of sulfasalazine in patients with AS (n = 895) were assessed. The authors concluded that the evidence did not support any beneficial effect of the drug on reducing pain, disease activity or radiographic progression or on improving physical function or mobility. ESR and spinal stiffness were the only significantly improved outcomes, although with very small effect sizes and without clinical significance (−4.8 mm/h [95% CI −8.8 to −0.8] for ESR; and − 13.9 mm [95% CI −22.5 to −5.2] in a 100-mm visual scale for stiffness). In addition, the risk of treatment discontinuation due to adverse effects increased by 47%, with reports of severe adverse reactions (erythematous rash, nausea, anorexia and, insomnia) [92, 93] (**2A**).

Another study that was not included in the aforementioned review also assessed "non-radiographic patients". This RCT included 230 patients who showed no improvement after 24 weeks of treatment with 2 g of sulfasalazine per day compared to the placebo-treated group. Surprisingly, in the subgroup without peripheral arthritis, the BASDAI score improved significantly (due to the exclusive improvement in the spinal pain and spinal stiffness components) [94] (**2B**).

Two studies with the TNFα inhibitor etanercept used sulfasalazine (2–3 g per day) as an active comparator from which some evidence of efficacy was deduced. One trial allocated 187 patients with active AS to treatment with sulfasalazine. After 16 weeks, 52.9% of these patients achieved the ASAS20 response and 15.5% showed partial remission according to the ASAS definition [95] (**2C**). In the other trial (ESTHER), 36 patients with active, non-radiographic axial SpA received sulfasalazine for 48 weeks. At the end of the study, 42% of the treated patients achieved the ASAS20 response, 31% achieved the ASAS40 response, 19% achieved ASAS partial remission and 28% achieved the BASDAI50 response [96] (**2C**).

According to an observational study (NOR-DMARD), arthritis predicted the response (at 3 months) to sulfasalazine in 181 patients with axial SpA who received this drug as a first-line treatment (ΔBASDAI -1.4 [1.9] when arthritis was present *vs* − 0.3 [1.7] when absent; p = 0.008). In addition, the 3-year drug survival rate was higher in patients with peripheral arthritis than in patients without arthritis (0.22 vs. 0.10 respectively, p = 0.03) [97] (**2C**).

A RCT evaluated the efficacy of sulfasalazine (2.0 g/day target dose) combined with 90 mg/day etoricoxib compared with the NSAID alone in the treatment of 67 individuals with axial SpA. After 6 months of follow-up, a significant difference was observed between the percentage of responsive patients (clinical improvement: ΔASDAS>1.1) in the sulfasalazine (67.7%) and placebo (15.1%) groups, signifying a NNT = 1.90 (95%CI = 1.37–3.12). The mean improvements in the BASDAI (3.29 ± 0.97 vs 1.47 ± 0.99) and BASMI (3.10 ± 0.87 vs 1.32 ± 0.88) scores were also significantly higher in the sulfasalazine group than in the placebo group [98] (**2B**).

Another possible effect of sulfasalazine is to reduce the incidence of anterior uveitis flares in patients with axial SpA, according to data from two studies: an observational study (n = 10) in which the annual incidence dropped from 3.4 to 0.9 (p = 0.007) and a randomized clinical trial (n = 22) in which the relative risk of new episodes of acute anterior uveitis between the treatment (0.47/year) and placebo (1.06/year) groups was 0.44 (95% CI 0.30–0.64) [99, 100] (**2C**).

Leflunomide

Only one RCT has assessed the effects of leflunomide in patients with AS. After 24 weeks, the percentage of the 45 patients who responded to leflunomide was 27%, according to the ASAS20 criterion, a value that is similar to that of the placebo group (20%). Significant differences in the disease activity (BASDAI), functional (BASFI) and mobility (BASMI) indices, pain and joint edema were not observed. However, the risk of adverse events, such as gastrointestinal disorders, respiratory infections, dermatitis, fatigue, venous thrombosis and elevated liver enzyme levels increased by 20% (NNH = 5) [101] (**2B**). A 24-week open-label study with only 20 patients with AS was the only study to observe a significant (p = 0.039) improvement exclusively in the peripheral component (mean joint counts were 1.7 at baseline and 0.2 after 6 months), but no significant improvements regarding BASDAI, BASMI, BASFI and other PROs [102] (**2C**).

Effect of combined synthetic DMARDs on biological therapy survival

Two observational studies aimed to answer the still open question of whether synthetic DMARDs affect the retention rates (drug survival) of TNFα inhibitors in patients with axial SpA. The Swedish biologics registry ARTIS (Antirheumatic Therapies in Sweden) found that co-medication during the use of the first TNFα inhibitor (n = 2420) exerted a beneficial effect, as shown by a lower 5-year discontinuation rate in users than in nonusers (hazard ratio (HR) 0.71, 95% CI 0.59–0.85, p < 0.001 for AS; and HR 0.82, 95% CI 0.69–0.97, p = 0.020 for undifferentiated SpA) [103] (**2B**). Conversely, the Portuguese Rheumatic Diseases Register (n = 954) found no evidence of the same effect on retention after 13 years of follow-up (HR 1.07, 95% CI 0.68–1.68) [104] (**2B**).

Recommendation

The use of methotrexate and sulfasalazine is recommended for the treatment of patients with axial SpA when peripheral arthritis is present or in the absence of another pharmacological treatment option due to toxicity, intolerance or contraindications. ***Level of evidence: 2A; Strength of recommendation: B (moderate); Degree of agreement: 8.4.***

The routine use of methotrexate or sulfasalazine as a co-medication in patients with axial SpA who are using biologics is not recommended. ***Level of evidence: 2B; Strength of recommendation: B (moderate); Degree of agreement: 9.6.***

8. What evidence of efficacy supports indications for the use of biologics in patients with axial SpA?

Five TNFα inhibitors (anti-TNFα) are currently available as treatments for AS: the anti-TNFα monoclonal antibodies infliximab, adalimumab and golimumab; certolizumab pegol, which is only the fragment antigen-binding (Fab) portion of the antibody; and the TNFα receptor analog etanercept. The last four compounds are also approved for the treatment of non-radiographic axial SpA. The following interleukin-17 inhibitors (anti-IL17A) are also available: secukinumab, which is approved for AS, and ixekizumab (anti-IL17A/F), which has not yet been approved for axial SpA.

Anti-TNFα

A RCT including 69 patients with active AS (BASDAI≥4 and back pain ≥4 mm – VAS) who received IV infliximab therapy (5.0 mg/kg) or placebo at weeks 0, 2 and 6 performed a primary outcome evaluation (BASDAI50) at week 12. In this trial, 53% of patients in the treatment group showed this response, in contrast to 9% of patients in the placebo group (P < 0.0001, NNT = 2.3) [105] (**2B**). The open-label phase of this study, using the same dose administered every 6 weeks, confirmed a sustained response until the third year, based on the ITT analysis. In addition, 47% patients maintained the initial BASDAI50 response until week 54, 41% until week 102 and 47.1% until week 156 [106–108] (**2C**). Other publications from the same study (with data from 5 and 8 years of follow-up) confirmed the persistence of the long-term response, although without an ITT analysis, which tends to underestimate treatment effects within such long follow-up periods. Thirty-eight of the initial 69 patients (55%) completed the fifth year and 33 (47%) completed the eighth year. Of these patients, 25 (66%) and 21 (64%), respectively, maintained a BASDAI score < 50% of the initial BASDAI score [109, 110] (**2C**).

A much larger RCT (ASSERT study) evaluated 357 AS patients for 24 weeks using the same disease activity criteria, and patients were treated with infliximab (5.0 mg/kg) or placebo at weeks 0, 2, 6, 12 and 18. The drug effectively reduced the disease activity (ASAS20 responders: 61.2% vs. 19.2% in the placebo group, NNT =

2.4; ASAS40 responders: 47% vs. 12%, NNT = 2.8, ASAS partial remission: 22.4% vs 1.3%, NNT = 4.7, and BASDAI50: 51% vs. 10.7%, NNT = 2.5). Physical function also improved (reduction of ≥2 units of the BASFI score: 47.5% vs 13.3%, NNT = 2.9), as well as BASMI (−1.0 vs 0.0, p = 0.019), and the quality of life (physical component SF-36: −10.2 vs. 0.8, p < 0.001). No difference of the Mander enthesitis index (MEI) score was observed [111] (**1B**).

The first study assessing the efficacy of etanercept was an American study, in which 40 patients with active AS, defined as the presence of inflammatory back pain with morning stiffness for at least 45 min and PROs with moderate disease activity, were randomized to treatment with 25 mg of etanercept twice per week or placebo. At the end of the 4-month follow-up, there was a 50% increase (NNT = 2) in the response to treatment, as defined by a composite index that is very similar to ASAS20: improvement ≥20% in three of five measures of disease activity (duration of morning stiffness, intensity of night pain, BASFI, patient global assessment and joint edema score) [112] (**2B**). Another multinational 24-week RCT included 277 patients with active AS (score ≥ 30 mm for morning stiffness, as measured using a VAS, and greater than two of three parameters: patient global assessment, back pain and BASFI) who were treated with 25 mg of etanercept twice per week for 24 weeks or placebo. The results showed a 31% increase (NNT = 3.2) of ASAS20 after 12 weeks and a 35% increase (NNT = 2.9) of ASAS20 and a 13% increase (NNT = 7.7) of ASAS partial remission, as well as BASDAI, BASFI and BASMI [113] (**1B**). The open-label extension of this trial included 200 of the initially included patients (72%), who were followed until week 96. All patients who were initially treated with placebo started receiving etanercept. After 24 weeks, 70% of these patients also achieved ASAS20. At the end of two years, 74, 61, and 46% of patients who received the active drug (treatment group) for 96 weeks and 78, 54, and 38% of patients who received the drug for 72 weeks (placebo-treated group) achieved ASAS20, ASAS50 and ASAS70, respectively, suggesting a sustained response [114] (**2C**). Finally, the follow-up for up to week 192 consisted of 126 individuals of the 277 included in the original trial (45.5%). The percentages of patients who achieved ASAS20, ASAS40 and ASAS partial remission responses were 81, 69 and 44% in the treatment group (etanercept administered from the beginning of the trial) and 82, 68 and 28% in the placebo-treated group (etanercept administered after week 24) [115] (**2C**).

A small trial performed in four German centers included 30 patients, of whom 14 were randomly allocated to the treatment group (25 mg of etanercept twice per week) and 16 to the placebo group in a double-blind phase (6 weeks). After this phase, all patients received etanercept for 12 weeks and then discontinued this medication and were followed for another 12 weeks. The 6-week treatment resulted in a 51% improvement in BASDAI50 response (NNT = 2.0). The mean time (standard deviation) until reactivation (BASDAI≥4 and global assessment by the physician ≥4 in a 0–10-point VAS) was 6 (±3) weeks. Twenty-six of the 30 initial patients were included in the extension, of which all patients resumed the medication. In week 54, 58% patients had achieved a BASDAI50 response and 31% achieved ASAS partial remission. In addition, 21 of 26 (81%) patients completed 2 years of follow-up treatment, and 16 (62%) completed 7 years. Of these 16 patients, 31% achieved ASAS partial remission and 44% patients achieved the inactive disease criteria according to the ASDAS [116–118] (**2B**). Another RCT was conducted at 14 European centers and included 84 patients with active AS who received 25 mg of etanercept twice per week (n = 45) or placebo (n = 39) for 12 weeks. The results showed a 37% increase (NNT = 2.7) of ASAS20 response and a 50% increase (NNT = 2.0) of ASAS50 response, but no significant difference concerning ASAS70 response, despite the numerical difference favoring the drug group (24.4% vs 10.3%) [119] (**1B**). The effect of etanercept was also assessed on a subpopulation of patients with advanced and severe AS (namely, two intervertebral adjacent bridges and/or fusion at the lumbar spine, three intervertebral adjacent bridges and/or fusion at the thoracic spine, or two intervertebral adjacent bridges and/or fusion at the cervical spine). The patients were treated with 50 mg of etanercept per week (n = 39) or the placebo (n = 43) for 12 weeks. There was improved in the following parameters: 34% increase (NNT = 2.9) of ASAS20, 21% increase (NNT = 4.8) of ASAS40, 23% increase (NNT = 4.4) of BASDAI50 response, and 13% increase (NNT = 7.7) of ASAS partial remission. After 12 weeks, the results also showed significant BASDAI (−2.6), BASFI (−2.2), BASMI (−0.57) improvement. In addition, some lung function parameters were also improved: vital capacity (VC) of 2.88% (effect size = 0.17) and forced VC (FVC) of 3.75% (effect size = 0.24) [120] (**1B**). The ESTHER trial included patients with axial SpA (AS and non-radiographic axial SpA) who had experienced symptoms for less than five years and active inflammation in the axial skeleton on MRI. Patients were randomly allocated to treatment with 50 mg of etanercept/week (n = 40) or sulfasalazine (n = 36) for 12 months. At the end of this period, non-remitted patients continued in an open-label extension of the study, receiving long-term treatment with etanercept. Remitted patients discontinued the medication, resuming etanercept upon exacerbation. A significantly greater improvement in inflammation scores (SIJ and spinal MRI) was observed in the anti-TNFα-treated group than in the sulfasalazine-treated group. Significantly greater improvements were also observed regarding BASDAI, BASFI, MASES, EQ-5D and ASQoL. The efficacy and safety data from the two groups were similar. A similar long-term response level was also observed (3-year follow-up) [96, 121, 122] (**2C**). Another RCT (EMBARK) recruited 215 individuals with non-radiographic axial SpA who had experienced symptoms for up to five years. These individuals were randomly allocated to etanercept (50 mg/week) or placebo. After 12 weeks, the improvement of ASAS40 response was 16% better (NNT = 6.0) in the treatment group than placebo. The disease activity scores on SIJ and spinal MRI were also better in the treatment group than in the placebo group. A subgroup analysis observed correlations between CRP levels and sacroiliac inflammation on MRI (Spondyloarthritis Research Consortium of Canada (SPARCC) MRI scoring system) with an improved response. After 12 weeks, all patients received etanercept and were followed in an open-label extension study for another 36 weeks. The percentages of patients achieving the ASAS40 response who were initially allocated to etanercept and to placebo in week 48 were 52 and 53%, respectively [123, 124] (**1B**).

A systematic review with a meta-analysis involving 1570 participants compared the efficacy of etanercept in Caucasians with the Chinese population by calculating the relative risk (RR) of achieving ASAS20 (RR = 2.36, 95% CI 2.03–2.74) and ASAS40 (RR = 2.81, 95% CI 2.01–3.92) responses and ASAS partial remission (RR = 4.31, 95% CI 2.52–7.37) with treatment versus placebo [125] (**1A**).

The ATLAS study, a 24-week RCT with primary outcomes measured at week 12 and a 5-year open-label extension, included 315 patients with AS who were unresponsive to NSAIDs and treated with adalimumab at a dose of 40 mg every other week (n = 208) or placebo (n = 107). After 12 weeks, the results showed a 37.6% increase of the ASAS20 response (NNT = 2.7), a 26.8% increase of ASAS40 response (NNT = 3.7), and a 17% increase of ASAS partial remission (NNT = 5.9). In weeks 12 and 24, the treatment and control groups showed significant differences in improvement (BASDAI, BASFI, BASMI and MASES. The ASAS20 and ASAS40 responses and ASAS partial remission persisted for two years after treatment and were 64.5, 50.6 and 33.5%, respectively. A 3-year follow-up of these patients revealed a sustained response that was measured using the BASDAI, BASFI, SF-36 (summary of physical components) and ASQoL, and 125/208 (60%) patients of the group that was initially allocated to the adalimumab arm completed the 5th year of follow-up. Of these patients, 70 and 77% achieved ASDAS40 and BASDAI50 responses, whereas 51 and 56% met the ASAS partial remission and ASDAS inactive disease criteria [126–129], respectively (**1B**). A RCT published in 2008, even before the publication of the ASAS criteria (2009), which defined the concept of non-radiographic axial SpA, included patients (n = 46) with inflammatory back pain and a positive HLA-B27 test or inflammation on SIJ or spinal MRI and the absence of radiographic sacroiliitis. After 12 weeks, the use of adalimumab (40 mg every other week) led to a higher percentage of patients achieving the ASAS40 response compared to individuals treated with placebo (54.5% *vs* 12.5%, NNT = 2.4). The same level of response was observed in the placebo group after the switch to treatment and was maintained until week 52 of the open-label phase [130] (**1B**). Another large study (n = 185), which was already using the 2009 ASAS criteria, also evaluated the efficacy of 40 mg of adalimumab every two weeks for the treatment of active non-radiographic axial SpA (BASDAI≥4, axial pain VAS ≥ 4, and an inappropriate response, intolerance or contraindications to NSAIDs). Similar results were observed after 12 weeks. Compared with the placebo group, a significant 21% increase of ASAS40 response (NNT = 4.8), 11% increase of ASAS partial remission (NNT = 9), and 20% increase of remission according to ASDAS inactive disease (NNT = 5) were observed. Significant differences were also observed in the improvements in the BASDAI, ASDAS, HAQ-S, SF-36 and SPARCC activity scores on SIJ and spinal MRI. No differences in improvements regarding BASFI, BASMI and MASES were observed between the adalimumab and placebo groups. Elevated CRP levels at baseline and objective inflammation intensity on SIJ MRI were associated with an improved response [131] (**1B**). A meta-analysis included 8 clinical trials assessing the effects of adalimumab in AS. In the week 12, the risk ratio (or RR) of achieving ASAS20 and BASDAI50 was RR = 2.26 (95% CI 1.85–2.75) and RR = 2.82 (95% CI 2.14–3.71), respectively [132] (**1A**).

When subcutaneously treated with golimumab (50 mg/4 weeks), patients with active AS (BASDAI≥4, spinal pain VAS ≥ 4 and inadequate response to prior use of NSAIDs or synthetic DMARDs) achieved the following results compared with placebo: 37.6% increase of ASAS20 response (NNT = 2.7) and 30.5% increase in BASDAI50 (NNT = 3.3) as early as week 14; a 28.1% increase of ASAS40 response (NNT = 3.6) and 36.1% increase of BASDAI50 (NNT = 2.8) in week 24. Patients who received golimumab also showed significantly greater BASDAI, BASFI, SF-36 improvements, as well as sleep quality (Jenkins Sleep Evaluation Questionnaire (JSEQ). However, no improvement regarding the BASMI [133] (**1B**). The 5-year follow-up of those patients showed a sustained response [134, 135] (**2C**). Similar results were observed in a Chinese trial (n = 213) in which the treatment with golimumab increased the ASAS20 response by 24.3% (NNT = 4.1) after 14 weeks and by 27.1% (NNT = 3.7) after 24 weeks in a 1-year follow-up [136] (**2B**). The efficacy of golimumab in patients with non-radiographic axial SpA was also assessed in 198 patients (GO-AHEAD study RCT) with the disease for up to five years who were randomly allocated to treatment with golimumab (50 mg/4 weeks) or placebo. At week 16 of follow-up, more patients treated with golimumab achieved clinical responses than patients treated with placebo, with significant differences of 31.1% of ASAS20 (NNT = 3.2) and 33.7% of ASAS40 (NNT = 3) responses. Consistent with the results from other clinical trials analyzing this population of patients with non-radiographic axial SpA, no significant difference in ASAS20 or ASAS40 responses was observed between the golimumab and placebo treatments in the subgroup of patients without objective sings of inflammation (with normal CRP levels and without sacroiliitis on MRI) [137] (**1B**). Another route of administration of golimumab (IV injection) was tested in a 28-week RCT (40 centers from 8 countries) that included 208 patients with active AS (BASDAI≥4; axial pain VAS ≥ 4; ultrasensitive CRP ≥0.3 mg/dl) who were randomly allocated to treatment with 2 mg/kg golimumab at weeks 0, 4, 12 and every 8 weeks thereafter or with placebo. In this trial, 14.4% [30] of the individuals had already used another anti-TNFα antibody without primary treatment failure, and 5.8% (12) patients already showed complete spinal ankylosis at baseline. At week 16, the ASAS20, ASAS40 and BASDAI50 responses were achieved in the golimumab group, but not the placebo group: 73.3% *vs* 26.2% (NNT = 2.1), 47.6% *vs* 8.7% (NNT = 2.6), and 41% *vs* 14.6% (NNT = 3.8), respectively. Remission according to the ASDAS inactive disease criteria occurred in 17.1% patients (NNT = 5.8), as well as ASAS partial remission in 12.3% patients (NNT = 8.1). The BASFI score also improved to a significantly greater extent in the treatment group (−2.4 *vs* −0.5; $p < 0.001$) [138] (**1B**).

The efficacy of certolizumab pegol was assessed in the RAPID-axial SpA, which included 325 patients with active axial SpA, of whom \147 with non-radiographic axial SpA and they were randomly allocated to treatment with two certolizumab pegol dosing regimens (doses of 200 mg every two weeks and 400 mg every four weeks) or placebo. At baseline, 16% had already used another anti-TNFα antibody, without discontinuation due to primary treatment failures. At week 12, the ASAS20 response was achieved by 57.7 and 63.6% patients receiving doses of 400 and 200 mg of certolizumab pegol, respectively, compared with 38.3% patients treated with placebo (NNT = 5.2 and 3.95 for the two dosing regimens, respectively). Significant increases in ASAS40 responses of 25.4% (NNT = 3.9) and 31% (NNT = 3.2) were observed for patients receiving both dosing regimens, respectively. ASAS partial remission increased by 19.7% (NNT = 5.1) and 20.6% (NNT = 4.8) with the two certolizumab pegol dosing regimens compared to the placebo. In addition, the ASDAS inactive disease status was achieved by 25.2 and 20.6% patients receiving the two dosing regimens compared with 0% in the placebo group (NNT = 4 and 4.8). Altogether, the two arms of the treatment resulted in significant improvements of BASFI, BASDAI, BASMI and ASDAS compared with placebo, at both weeks 12 and 24 [139] (**1B**). A sustained response was assessed at the 96th week and up to the 4th year of follow-up, when 67% (218/325) participants continued receiving the drug in the study, of whom 31.4% met the ASDAS inactive disease criteria [140, 141] (**2C**).

Anti-IL17

In the MEASURE 1 and MEASURE 2 phase III trials, the anti-IL17A monoclonal antibody induced a significant reduction in signs and symptoms attributed to active AS (BASDAI≥4; axial pain VAS ≥ 4), at week 16 of follow-up. In the MEASURE 1 trial (n = 371), the patients in the treatment group received IV injections of 10 mg/kg secukinumab at weeks 0, 2 and 4, followed by maintenance therapy with 75 or 150 mg every 4 weeks. In the MEASURE 2 trial (n = 219), the antibody was subcutaneously (SC) injected (with 75 or 150 mg secukinumab) at weeks 0, 1, 2 and 3, followed by SC maintenance therapy every 4 weeks. In the MEASURE 1 trial, the ASAS20 response was reached at week 16 by 61, 60 and 29% patients treated with 150 mg, 75 mg and placebo, respectively ($p < 0.001$ for both comparisons with placebo [NNT = 3.1 for 150 mg and NNT = 3.2 for 75 mg]). Conversely, in the MEASURE 2 trial, these rates were 61, 41 and 28% ($p < 0.001$ for 150 mg *vs* placebo [NNT = 3] and $p = 0.10$ for 75 mg *vs* placebo). Therefore, SC injections (less intense and equally effective) and a 150-mg maintenance dose, but not a 75-mg dose (ineffective), were chosen as the best treatment. These response levels were maintained until week 52 in both studies (63% for both). In terms of the most clinically relevant secondary outcomes and considering only individuals who received the maintenance dose of 150 mg (which is the dose approved in Brazil for AS), 42 and 36% patients achieved ASAS40 at week 16 and 51 and 49% patients achieved this response at week 52 in the MEASURE 1 and MEASURE 2 trials, respectively. In terms of ASAS partial remission, 15% (MEASURE 1) and 14% (MEASURE 2) of patients achieved this condition at week 16 and 22% (in both studies) at week 52 [142] (**1B**). Comparing bio-naïve (n = 134) and anti-TNFα failure (n = 85) patients, it was shown good efficacy in both scenarios, although with smaller effect size (NNT = 2.7 for ASAS20 in the first group and NNT = 3.9 in the second group) [143] (**1B**). The levels of total spinal pain, night pain and fatigue (measured using the FACIT-fatigue scale) in individuals with or without elevated CRP levels at baseline and in patients who had or had not been treated with an anti-TNFα antibody were significantly decreased compared with patients treated with the placebo at week 16, with a sustained response until week 104 [144] (**1B**). The clinical responses observed at week 24 were sustained until the third year of follow-up [145–147] (**2C**).

Ixekizumab, another anti-IL17 antibody (specific for the IL17A homodimer and IL17A/F heterodimer), showed efficacy in treating AS in two published phase 3 trials, COAST-V and COAST-W. The former included 341 patients with an inadequate response or intolerance to NSAIDs who were randomly allocated (1:1:1:1) to receive 80 mg of ixekizumab SC every 2 or 4 weeks, 40 mg of adalimumab SC every 2 weeks or the placebo. The latter group included only patients with prior exposure (inadequate response or intolerance) to one or two anti-TNFα therapies (n = 316) and therefore the active comparator arm for this mechanism was not established. The NNTs for ASAS40 at week 16 were 3.2 (95% CI 2.3–4.9) in the bio-naïve subpopulation, with no significant difference for adalimumab, and 6.5 (95% CI 4.2–15.2) in the subpopulation that was previously exposed to anti-TNFα therapy [148, 149] (**1B**). This drug is not yet approved for the treatment of axial SpA.

Recommendation

Based on the opinion of the rheumatologist, the use of biologics (TNFα inhibitors or anti-IL17 antibodies) to treat active (BASDAI≥4 or ASDAS≥2.1) and symptomatic axial SpA is recommended when the initial treatment with NSAIDs fails (disease persistence, toxicity or contraindications). ***Level of evidence: 1A; Strength of recommendation: A (strong); Degree of agreement: 8.9.***

Biologics should be used to treat axial SpA when objective signs of inflammation are detected, such as elevated CRP levels and/or the presence of sacroiliitis on MRI, as these parameters predict the response, particularly in the context of non-radiographic axial SpA. ***Level of evidence: 1B; Strength of recommendation: A (strong); Degree of agreement: 9.6.***

Anti-TNF inhibitors (adalimumab, etanercept, golimumab and certolizumab pegol) are recommended for the treatment of non-radiographic axial SpA since had received an evidence-based approval. ***Level of evidence: 1B; Strength of recommendation: A (strong); Degree of agreement: 9.7.***

9. Do differences in efficacy exist among biologics used to treat axial SpA patients?

To date, only three trials have performed head-to-head comparisons between biological therapies in patients with axial SpA.

An open-label RCT analyzed 55 AS patients who were randomly allocated to treatment with infliximab or etanercept. At 12 weeks of follow-up, significant differences of BASDAI (3.5 *versus* 5.6, p < 0.005) and BASFI (3.5 *versus* 5.0, p < 0.005) in favor to infliximab. However, this difference was not sustained over time (104 weeks of follow-up). No difference of ASAS20 or ASAS40 responses was identified between groups at the 2nd, 12th or 104th weeks of follow-up [150] (**2B**).

A phase I (the primary endpoint was to show pharmacokinetic equivalence) randomized, double-blind, multicenter clinical trial (PLANETAS study) compared the efficacy of infliximab with one of its bio-similar (CT-P13) in patients with AS (n = 250, 125 in each treatment arm) for 30 weeks. The ASAS20 and ASAS40 responses observed at week 30 in the biosimilar and original groups, were: 70.5% *vs* 72.4% (OR = 0.91, 95% CI 0.51–1.62) and 51.8% *vs* 47.4% (OR = 1.19, 95% CI 0.70–2.00), respectively, with no significant differences between treatment groups [151] (**2B**).

Another open-label RCT compared the survival of patients receiving each drug and the disease activity, according to ASDAS-CRP, in patients with AS who were treated with etanercept (n = 163) or adalimumab (n = 82) in a real-life scenario (routine care). In a two-year follow-up period, no difference was observed between mean ASDAS-CRP (2.0 ± 0.9 for etanercept and 1.9 ± 1.1 for adalimumab, p = 0.624). However, the survival rate of patients treated with etanercept was significantly better than patients treated with adalimumab. The

Table 3 Increase in the relative frequency (%) of different outcomes and the number needed to treat (NNT) with respective 95% CIs calculated using a normal approximation compared to the placebo. - Data were not reported in the studies. Data from different studies were pooled when the same outcomes from the same treatments were available and when they referred to doses and/or regimens approved in Brazil

Outcome	ASAS20				ASAS40				ASAS PR			
	Follow-up time (weeks)											
	12 to 16		24		12 to 16		24		12 to 16		24	
Drug	%	NNT (95% CI)	%	NNT (95% CI)	%	NNT (95% CI)	%	NNT (95% CI)	%	NNT (95% CI)	%	NNT (95% CI)
Infliximab [111]	-	-	42	2.4 (1.9–3.2)	-	-	35	2.9 (2.2–4.0)	-	-	21	4.7 (3.7–6.7)
Etanercept [113, 119, 120, 123]	27	3.7 (2.9–5.1)	34	2.9 (2.2–4.3)	18	5.5 (3.6–11.7)	-	-	13	7.5 (3.7-∞)	13	7.6 (4.9–16.9)
Adalimumab [126, 130, 131]	27	3.7 (2.8–5.2)	-	-	26	3.8 (3.0–5.2)	26	3.8 (2.8–5.8)	16	6.4 (4.8–9.5)	17	6.1 (4.2–10.7)
Golimumab [133, 137, 138]	37	2.7 (2.3–3.4)	-	-	40	2.5 (2.1–3.2)	28	3.6 (2.5–6.0)	-	7.5 (4.8–16.3)	-	-
Certolizumab pegol [139]	22	4.5 (3.0–9.1)	-	-	28	3.6 (2.6–5.5)	-	-	20	5.0 (3.7–7.5)	-	-
Secukinumab [142]	36	2.8 (2.2–3.8)	-	-	30	3.3 (2.5–4.6)	-	-	12	8.1 (5.4–16.0)	-	-

HR of adalimumab discontinuation compared with etanercept discontinuation was 2.5 (95% CI 1.3–4.5, p = 0.006) [152] (**2B**).

The Table 3 outlines the relative frequencies (relative to the placebo group) of specific efficacy outcomes during treatment with different drugs. Although different studies with different populations are unable to be compared so simply, interestingly, all confidence intervals available for the same outcome overlap, at least in the short-term follow-up of the controlled period.

Another way to infer differences regarding efficacy among different agents is indirect comparisons meta-analysis, using the Bayesian network or Bayesian mixed treatment comparison (MTC). Recently, one of this methodology was used for analysis of data from 2574 AS patients from 16 RCTs wit adalimumab, etanercept, golimumab and infliximab, concluding that no evidence supported any difference in efficacy among these drugs concerning the following outcomes: ASAS20, ASAS40 and BASDAI50 responses [153] (**1A**). Another systematic review (28 eligible RCTs), including patients with non-radiographic axial SpA, also found no evidence of efficacy differences among different TNFα inhibitors [154] (**1A**). More recently, 18 RCTs (2971 AS patients), using secukinumab database and ASAS20 as main outcome, were indirectly compared (Bucher's method) and no differences were found [155] (**1A**).

Recommendation

The TNFα inhibitors and the IL17A inhibitors exhibit similar effect sizes for controlling inflammatory activity in patients with axial SpA. ***Level of evidence: 1A; Strength of recommendation: A (strong); Degree of agreement: 8.9.***

10. Does the safety of biologics differ in patients with axial SpA?

Similar to the efficacy comparison, safety differences among agents have been inferred using indirect comparisons and meta-analyses. Table 4 outlines the RRs of serious adverse events and treatment discontinuation (both in comparison with the placebo group) reported for different drugs. Interestingly, the confidence intervals of the RRs overlap in short-term, suggesting similar safety profiles.

Indirect comparisons and different meta-analyses (albeit with considerable data overlap) concluded that the data are similar among different biologics. Moreover, the rates of serious adverse events, including serious infections and malignancies associated with biological treatments, showed no significant differences from controls [153, 156, 157] (**1A**). The main limitation of the safety analysis, as shown in Table 4 and in the meta-analyses cited, is the low frequency of events due to the short follow-up (short exposure time) and to the selection of the exposed population according to the restrictive inclusion/exclusion criteria of RCTs. Long-term safety evidence and data that are closer to real-life scenarios are provided by registry studies and cohort studies. However, few of these studies have been performed specifically with patients with axial SpA, and in some studies presented below, other diagnoses, such as psoriatic arthritis (PsA) and rheumatoid arthritis (RA), were grouped in risk analyses.

A Canadian cohort study followed 440 patients with axial SpA for 1712 PY of observation. Two hundred sixty-four (60%) patients used some TNFα inhibitor in the study period, 124 (28.2%) used a DMARD (methotrexate-15%, sulfasalazine-10.9%, leflunomide-1.1%, and others-1.1%) and 42 (9.5%) used glucocorticoids, with a mean dose of 14 mg/day. The use of an anti-TNFα inhibitor did not exert significant effect on the incidence of infections in general compared with the lack of use of an anti-TNFα inhibitor. The incidence rates in the exposed and control groups were 19/100 PY *vs* 14/100 PY, respectively, with an OR adjusted for several cofactors (comorbidities, use of glucocorticoids and synthetic DMARDs) of 1.25 (95% CI

Table 4 Relative risks of different safety outcomes and respective 95% CIs calculated using a normal approximation. Data from different studies were pooled when the same outcomes from the same treatments were available and when they referred to doses and/or regimens approved in Brazil

Outcome	Serious adverse effects		Discontinuation for any cause	
	Follow-up time (weeks)			
	12 to 24			
Drug	Relative risk	95% CI	Relative risk	95% CI
Infliximab [111]	1.30	0.28–6.12	0.78	0.14–4.15
Etanercept [113, 119, 120, 123]	0.84	0.37–1.91	0.81	0.47–1.42
Adalimumab [126, 130, 131]	1.59	0.49–5.06	1.49	0.65–3.39
Golimumab [133, 137, 138]	0.94	0.35–2.56	1.19	0.52–2.75
Certolizumab pegol [139]	1.18	0.43–3.36	0.74	0.34–1.58
Secukinumab [142]	0.81	0.34–1.92	0.55	0.26–1.16

0.90–1.73). In the multivariate analysis, only the use of DMARDs increased the risk of infections with an OR of 1.73 (95% CI 1.21–2.48, p = 0.003) [158] (**2B**). A systematic review included 10 RCTs and 51 observational studies to compare the risk of adverse effects of 13 immunomodulators (biologics and target-specific molecules). The rates of adverse effects, discontinuation due to adverse effects, serious adverse effects, death, serious infections, tuberculosis, herpes zoster and malignancies were analyzed as outcomes of interest. However, 70% of the studies were conducted with patients diagnosed with RA, thus limiting the power of the analysis for axial SpA patients. Nevertheless, the outcome of discontinuation due to adverse effects was higher for infliximab than for adalimumab and etanercept in patients with AS, RA and PsA [159] (**2A**).

Two South Korean studies on the risk of tuberculosis (TB; South Korea is considered a country with an intermediate TB burden) have shown contradictory results regarding the effect of exposure to anti-TNFα therapy on the risk of TB. One of the studies calculated the TB incidence rates in patients with AS from a single center who were exposed (n = 354) or were not exposed (n = 919) to anti-TNFα therapy, with 308/100 thousand PY among nonusers and 168/100 thousand PY among users. A significant difference was not observed and the RR = 0.53 (95% CI 0.14–1.91), thus suggesting that exposure does not increase the risk [160] (**2B**). The other study also calculated the incidence of TB in 1322 patients with AS (336 users and 986 unexposed controls), finding an incidence of 600.2/100,000 PY among users and RR = 4.87 (95% CI 1.50–15.39) compared to nonusers [161] (**2B**). Two other observational studies, both of which were conducted in Turkey (a country with a high prevalence of TB), aimed to identify factors associated with an increased risk of developing TB among anti-TNFα drug users (in both studies, adalimumab, etanercept and infliximab alone were evaluated). The first study evaluated the medical records of 1887 patients receiving anti-TNFα therapy, 705 of whom (37.3%) had been diagnosed with AS. The overall incidence (all diagnoses) was 423/100,000 PY. The use of adalimumab (9.5-fold increase), male gender (15.6-fold increase) and a history of TB (11.5-fold increase) were indicated as risk factors for TB in the multivariate analysis [162] (**2B**). The other study is a case-control study in which 73 (52.1% patients with AS) cases of TB among anti-TNFα drug users were compared with 7695 (50.6% patients with AS) controls, namely, anti-TNFα drug users without TB. The prevalence of TB among patients with AS undergoing anti-TNFα therapy was 0.97%. The frequency of TB among infliximab users (considering all diagnoses) was 1.27%, which was significantly higher (OR = 3.4, 95% CI 1.88–6.10, p = 0.001) than adalimumab (0.57%) and etanercept (0.3%) [163] (**3B**).

Despite the limited data, the risk of tuberculosis in patients exposed to IL-17 inhibition seems to be low, as there are no cases described in clinical trials. In contrast, there is an increased risk of candida infections in patients treated with anti-IL-17 [142, 147–149] (**1B**). These small differences should be considered in the management of axial SpA patients.

Three publications with data from four registries did not detect increase in the risk of malignancies with the use of anti-TNFα therapy in patients with SpA. The BIOBADASER registry (761 Spanish patients with AS, among other diagnoses, who were undergoing anti-TNFα therapy and followed from 2001 to 2008) calculated a standardized incidence ratio of 0.92 (95% CI 0.44–1.70). The BIOSPAR registry (231 Belgian patients with SpA undergoing anti-TNFα therapy who were followed from 2000 to 2010) identified a nonsignificant increase in incidence among women, R = 1.99 (95% CI 0.54–3.82), but not in men, RR = 0.69 (95% CI 0.29–1.66), compared with the general population. The DANBIO registry (3255 Danish patients with SpA who were followed from 2001 to 2011) and ARTIS registry (5448 Swedish patients with SpA who were followed from 2001 to 2011) obtained a similar risk between patients undergoing anti-TNFα therapy and untreated patients, RR = 0.8 (95% CI 0.7–1.0) [164–166](**2B**).

Recommendation

The biologics TNFα inhibitors and the anti-IL17A inhibitors exhibit similar effect sizes for the short-term risks of serious adverse effects and discontinuation. ***Level of evidence: 1A; Strength of recommendation: A (strong); Degree of agreement: 9.1.***

11. Is the use of biological therapy able to reduce structural damage (radiographic progression) in patients with axial SpA?

Table 5 Mean mSASSS variations and respective 95% CIs calculated using a normal approximation (except for certolizumab pegol, whose 95% CI was reported by the authors of the original study). Data from different studies were pooled when the same outcomes from the same treatments were available and when they referred to doses and/or regimens approved in Brazil

Outcome	mSASSS variation (units)			
	Follow-up time (years)			
	0 to 2		0 to 4	
Drug	Δ mSASSS	95% CI	Δ mSASSS	95% CI
Infliximab [171, 172]	0.9	0.54–1.26	1.60	1.1–2.1
Etanercept [173]	0.91	0.62–1.21		
Adalimumab [174]	0.9	0.51–1.09		
Golimumab [175]	0.9	0.38–1.40	1.30	0.9–1.7
Certolizumab pegol [176]	0.67	0.21–1.13	0.98	0.34–1.63
Secukinumab [145, 177]	0.5	0.11–0.89	1.2	0.29–2.11

The reduction or even prevention of structural damage in patients with axial SpA is an important goal in the treatment of these diseases because, in addition to inflammation, the damage caused by bone new formation contributes to impaired mobility and function, particularly after the early phase (3 years of symptoms) [32] (**2B**). Observational studies have indicated a protective effect of anti-TNFα therapy on radiographic progression, particularly if it had been started early or extended for long periods (≥4 years) [167–170] (**2B**). However, a definitive demonstration that these agents are able to prevent or at least reduce progression is still expected, mainly because experimental studies (outlined in Table 5) have not yet provided definitive evidence of this property.

Infliximab

In the ASSERT study, the spinal radiographs of 201 patients with AS who received 5.0 mg/kg infliximab every 6 weeks after the induction dose for 96 weeks were analyzed (baseline and after week 96) for structural damage using the mSASSS. The radiographic progression (difference between mSASSS at weeks 0 and 96) of these patients was compared with patients with AS who had not been treated with biologics from a historical cohort (OASIS), with all the limitations of this type of comparison. No significant difference (p = 0.541) was observed between mean 2-year progression values in the ASSERT and OASIS cohorts, which were 0.9 ± 2.6 and 1.0 ± 3.2, respectively [171] (**2C**). Another cohort, in which 33 of the 69 patients with AS were initially included in the DIKAS (*Deutsche Infliximab Kohorte für AS*) study, also assessed radiographic progression using the mSASSS, but in two intervals: baseline-2 years; and 2–4 years. In this population, the mSASSS varied by 1.6 ± 2.6/4 years (lower than the variation in the OASIS cohort of 4.4/4 years). However, this study had notable limitations, including differences in baseline disease activity and methods for reading radiographs between the two groups. At the end of eight years of follow-up, 22 patients remained in the open-label extension using infliximab. The progression from baseline of these patients was then compared with 34 "controls" from another historic cohort (Herne) of patients with AS who had never undergone anti-TNFα therapy. Interestingly, although no difference in mean progression rates was observed between the two groups during the first 4 years (p = 0.18), a significant difference was detected in the last 4 years of follow-up (p = 0.01) favoring the infliximab group [172, 178] (**2C**).

Etanercept

Similarly, the effect of etanercept treatment on the progression of spinal structural damage was assessed by comparing 257 patients who were treated for up to two years (patients from the placebo-treated group were grouped with patients from the treatment group) with 175 patients from the OASIS cohort. Again, changes in radiological scores (mSASSS) of the cervical and lumbar spine after 96 weeks of treatment with etanercept were similar to the changes observed in patients from the historical cohort who were not treated with biological therapy (0.91 ± 2.45 *vs* 0.95 ± 3.18), thus suggesting a lack of a "disease-modifying" effect of etanercept [173] (**2C**).

Adalimumab

Using a similar study design, the ATLAS and M03–606 trials compared the radiographic progression of 307 patients with AS who were treated with adalimumab for two years with data from 169 patients of the historical OASIS cohort treated with non-biological drugs. Importantly, the patients enrolled in both RCTs who were initially allocated to the placebo group and started to receive adalimumab in the open-label phase were analyzed together with patients who were allocated to receiving biologics at the beginning of the trial. No difference in mSASSS variations was detected between groups, suggesting similar radiographic progression. The mean variation of the mSASSS from the start to the 2nd year of follow-up was 0.9 ± 3.3 and 0.8 ± 2.6 for patients from the historical OASIS cohort and for patients undergoing treatment with adalimumab, respectively (p = 0.771) [174] (**2C**).

Golimumab

The GO-RAISE study also led to the publication of an analysis of the 4-year radiographic progression of the 356 AS patients. Radiographs of 111 of the 138 (80%) patients initially allocated to the 50 mg golimumab group (the only subcutaneous dose approved in Brazil) were available for mSASSS analysis. The radiographic progression, as measured by calculating mSASSS variations, of the 50 mg golimumab group was, on average, 0.9 ± 2.7 in the first biennium and 1.3 ± 4.1 in the 4-year follow-up period. The 2-year analysis was performed using observed data, and the longer (4-year) analysis relied on 9% (26/299) of missing data that were completed by linear extrapolation. This difference in analyses considerably impairs the comparison between the two biennia. Nevertheless, the stability in mean rates of change in the two intervals (0–2 and 0–4 years) merely suggests that no acceleration in progression occurred [175] (**2C**).

Certolizumab pegol

A study of the effect of certolizumab pegol on the radiographic progression of axial SpA (one arm of the RAPID-axial SpA trial) included 174 patients with AS and 141 patients with non-radiographic axial SpA, whose radiographs of the cervical and lumbar spine were analyzed using the mSASSS at baseline and at weeks 96 and 204. In patients with non-radiographic axial SpA, damage progression was slow (0.06, 95% CI −0.17-0.28) during the 4 years of the study. In patients with AS, the mean change in mSASSS from week 0 to week 204 was 0.98 (95% CI 0.34–163). This change was greater in the first biennium (0.67, 95% CI 0.21–1.13) than in the second (0.31, 95% CI 0.02–0.60) biennium. This reduction in the progression rate between the two intervals suggests that long-term anti-TNFα therapy may inhibit the progression of structural damage [176] (**2C**).

Secukinumab

The MEASURE 1 trial also provided radiographic progression data for AS patients who were originally randomly allocated to secukinumab (75 and 150 mg) in 2 years. Eighty-six of the 97 patients included in the 150 mg group (88.7%) had radiographs available for mSASSS assessment. The mean change in this score from start to week 104 was 0.3 ± 2.53 units. Although this study reported the lowest mean radiographic progression among patients with AS treated with biologics and followed for 2 years differences in study design and populations preclude the comparison of these findings with results from other studies [145] (**2C**). In addition, 4-year data have already been published. seventy-one of the patients in the 150 mg group (73,2%) had at least baseline and week 208 radiographs. The rates of progression in the 0–2, 2–4, and 0–4 years intervals were, respectively, 0.5 ± 1.69; 0.7 ± 3.32; and 1.2 ± 3.91, respectively [177] (**2C**).

Recommendation

The reduction in the progression rate of structural damage (observed on spinal radiographies) in patients with axial SpA can be observed in the long-term use of TNF inhibitors. ***Level of evidence: 2B; Strength of recommendation: B (moderate); Degree of agreement: 8.2.***

A similar effect on radiographic progression seems to be observed with the continuous use of anti-IL17 (secukinumab) but need to be confirmed in long-term studies. ***Level of evidence: 2C; Strength of recommendation: B (moderate); Degree of agreement: 9.6.***

12. What is the evidence for the efficacy of biologics regarding the treatment of extra-articular manifestations in patients with axial SpA?

Uveitis

Despite the lack of RCTs addressed to assess the efficacy of biologics on uveitis associated with axial SpA, some observational, open-label and uncontrolled studies and subanalyses of RCTs reasonably bridges the gap of evidence regarding the efficacy of these treatments.

A subanalysis of data from seven studies including 397 patients with AS, whose cumulative exposure to placebo, infliximab and etanercept was 70, 147 and 430 PY, respectively, calculated the incidence of new episodes of uveitis in the three groups. The combined incidence of uveitis among patients treated with anti-TNFα drugs was 6.8/100 PY, in contrast to 15.6/100 PY in patients treated with placebo, which accounts for a 57% reduction in risk (RR = 0.43, 95% CI 0.23–0.81). The incidence of uveitis in patients treated with infliximab (3.4/100 PY) differed from patients treated with etanercept (7.9/100 PY), although the difference was not significant [179] (**2A**). An open-label, non-randomized clinical trial included 1250 patients with active AS who were treated with adalimumab for 20 weeks. The incidence of acute anterior uveitis in the year prior to treatment with adalimumab was 15/100 PY. Treatment with adalimumab decreased the short-term incidence (mean exposure of 106 days) to 7.4/100 PY, a 50% reduction in risk (RR = 0.50, 95% CI 0.34–0.73) [180] (**2C**). In a population with AS selected for an increased frequency of uveitis (77 patients with 52 attacks in the year before baseline), the reduction in risk was, as expected, even higher, from 68/100 to 14/100 PY after treatment with adalimumab for at least 12 weeks (RR = 0.20, 95% CI 0.13–0.32) [181] (**2C**). Another *post hoc* analysis of eight clinical trials of etanercept in patients with AS found a 55% lower incidence of uveitis in the etanercept group (8.6/100 PY) than in the placebo group (19.3/100 PY). In the long term, considering all patients treated with etanercept in the placebo-controlled period and in open-label extension studies, the incidence was 12/100 PY [182] (**2C**). Smaller (n ≤ 15) open-label and uncontrolled studies also reported the efficacy of the newer anti-TNFα drugs, golimumab and certolizumab pegol in the treatment of anterior uveitis associated with SpA, including in patients previously exposed to another anti-TNFα drugs [183–185] (**2C**). During the double-blind phase of the RAPID-axial SpA trial, the incidence of uveitis was lower in patients who received certolizumab pegol than in patients treated with the placebo (3/100 PY *versus* 10.3/100 PY). In the long-term follow-up period, the rate of uveitis remained low for up to week 96 (4.9/100 PY) and was similar between individuals with AS and non-radiographic axial SpA [186] (**2B**). An open-label, non-randomized trial included 93 patients with AS who were treated with golimumab for 12 months. The incidence of anterior uveitis was compared between the 12-month period prior to treatment and the treatment period. Treatment with golimumab reduced the risk of uveitis by 80% from 11.1 to 2.2/100 PY (RR = 0.20, 95% CI 0.04–0.91) [187] (**2C**). Finally, a meta-analysis published in 2015 used the inclusion criteria of RCTs of at least 12 weeks comparing anti-TNFα therapy with placebo and describing the rates of uveitis in both groups, and concluded that short-term anti-TNFα therapy was associated with fewer uveitis episodes in patients with AS (OR = 0.35, 95% CI 0.15–0.81). According to the results of a subgroup analysis, the effects of treatment with etanercept significantly differed from placebo, but not from monoclonal antibodies. Importantly, the statistical power (1-β) of this subanalysis in comparing etanercept with placebo, calculated *a posteriori*, was 99.8%. Conversely, in the comparison between monoclonal antibodies and placebo, the smaller sample size provided a statistical power of only 65.5% because only one trial of certolizumab pegol and two trials of infliximab met the inclusion criteria of the study [188] (**2A**). The incidence rates of

Table 6 Incidence (mean) of acute anterior uveitis (AAU) and inflammatory bowel disease (IBD) and respective 95% CIs calculated using a normal approximation. Data from different studies were pooled when the same outcomes from the same treatments were available and when they referred to doses and/or regimens approved in Brazil. * 95% CI reported by the authors of the original study. ** No new case or reactivation was reported in the study with golimumab IV. The incidence of this event was not described in studies with SC golimumab injections

Outcome	Incidence (events/100 PY)			
Drug	AAU Incidence	95% CI	IBD Incidence	95% CI
Infliximab [179, 189]	3.4	0.5–6.4	0.2	0–0.9*
Etanercept [179, 189]	7.9	5.4–10.5	1.3	0–4.2*
Adalimumab [180, 189]	7.4	4.7–10.1	0.8	0.6–2.5*
Golimumab [133, 138, 187]	2.2	0–5.2	0**	–
Certolizumab pegol [141, 186]	4.9	3.0–6.9	0.1	0–0.3
Secukinumab [142]	1.0	0.3–1.8	0.7	0.1–1.3

uveitis reported in the clinical trials analyzing the various biologics are outlined in Table 6.

The publication of a case series of paradoxical uveitis induced by anti-TNFα therapy highlighted possible differences in efficacy (or even safety) in the treatment of axial SpA-related uveitis between a fusion protein (etanercept) and monoclonal antibodies (including the antibody fraction certolizumab pegol) by suggesting that the incidence of new cases of uveitis increased following etanercept treatment [190] (**4**). Subsequently, evidence from several observational studies confirmed these findings. A study analyzed a large US health service claims database covering approximately 100 third-party payers and 170 million covered individuals. Of the more than 52,000 patients diagnosed with AS in the study period, 2115 initiated anti-TNFα therapy, with no prior history of uveitis. The incidence rates of (new) uveitis cases in patients receiving treatment with adalimumab, infliximab and etanercept were 2.4, 3.2 and 4.5%, respectively, with a significance difference only observed between adalimumab and etanercept, favoring the monoclonal antibody [191] (**2C**). A retrospective Chinese cohort study included 182 patients with AS and a previous history of uveitis. The treatments with the three anti-TNFα drugs available at that time (adalimumab, infliximab or etanercept) were equally effective, but the relapse rate with the soluble receptor (38%) was much higher than with the monoclonal antibodies (6 and 11% for adalimumab and infliximab, respectively). The combination of methotrexate with anti-TNFα therapy nullified the difference in efficacy observed between monotherapies [192] (**2B**). The Swedish registry also analyzed the incidence of anterior uveitis in more than 1600 patients with AS treated with adalimumab, infliximab and etanercept. The comparison of the incidence rates of uveitis before starting and in the first two years of treatment with each TNFα inhibitor showed a decrease in total rates for the treatments with adalimumab and infliximab. Conversely, the use of etanercept increased the incidence of anterior uveitis. The adjusted HR of uveitis in patients previously free of the disease (last two years before starting treatment with a TNFα inhibitor) were significantly higher for etanercept than adalimumab (HR = 3.86, 95% CI 1.85–8.06) and for etanercept than infliximab (HR = 1.99, 95% CI 1.23–3.22), with no differences between infliximab and adalimumab [193] (**2B**). A Korean cohort study of 1055 patients with AS analyzed the incidence of uveitis among users of an anti-TNFα antibody (adalimumab, infliximab or golimumab), soluble TNFα receptor (etanercept) and nonsteroidal anti-inflammatory drugs (NSAIDs). Compared with the group treated with NSAIDs alone, uveitis was less common in the group treated with anti-TNFα monoclonal antibodies (HR = 0.53, 95% CI 0.29–0.96), but more common in the group treated with etanercept (HR = 2.25, 95% CI 1.43–3.53) [194] (**2B**). Based on these data, among the anti-TNFα antibodies, monoclonal antibodies are more effective in preventing new episodes of uveitis than etanercept.

The data on secukinumab are insufficient to analyze its efficacy regarding this outcome. In the MEASURE 1 and 2 trials, no difference regarding uveitis incidence was observed between the treatment (regardless of dose or administration route) and placebo (RR = 1.20, 95% CI 0.25–5.73) groups [142] (**2B**).

Psoriasis and inflammatory bowel disease (IBD)

Among the biologics approved for the treatment of axial SpA in Brazil, the on-label use of adalimumab and infliximab is also approved for the treatment of psoriasis, Crohn's disease and ulcerative colitis; etanercept and secukinumab for plaque psoriasis; certolizumab pegol for Crohn's disease; and golimumab for ulcerative colitis. The incidence rates of cases of IBD reported in clinical trials of various biologics are outlined in Table 6.

No clinical trials have specifically assessed the efficacy of these drugs in treating psoriasis associated with axial

Table 7 Increase in the relative frequency (%), relative to placebo, in different outcomes, the corresponding number needed to treat (NNT) and 95% CIs calculated using a normal approximation. - Data were not available. Data from different studies were pooled when the same outcomes from the same treatments were available and when they referred to doses and/or regimens approved in Brazil

Outcome	PASI50		PASI75		PASI90	
	Follow-up time (weeks)					
	24		24		24	
Drug	%	NNT (95% CI)	%	NNT (95% CI)	%	NNT (95% CI)
Infliximab [195]	66.7	1.5 (1.3–1.8)	58.8	1.7 (1.4–2.1)	38.4	2.6 (2.0–3.6)
Etanercept [196, 197]	27.0	3.7 (2.6–6.3)	20.8	4.8 (3.5–7.8)	–	–
Adalimumab [198]	62.5	1.5 (1.2–1.8)	58.8	1.7 (1.4–2.2)	41.7	2.4 (1.9–3.3)
Golimumab [199]	66.7	1.5 (1.3–1.8)	55.5	1.8 (1.6–2.2)	32.2	3.1 (2.4–4.3)
Certolizumab pegol [200]	45.5	2.2 (1.7–2.9)	45.5	2.2 (1.8–2.8)	35.7	2.8 (2.2–3.7)
Secukinumab [201, 202]	–	–	37.0	2.1 (1.8–2.6)	35.7	2.7 (2.2–3.4)

SpA. However, the effects of these drugs are reasonably inferred, as surrogate markers, from the efficacy analysis of a clinical response known as the Psoriasis Area and Severity Index (PASI), which was 50, 75 and 90 in the respective studies of psoriatic arthritis. Table 7 outlines the relative frequencies (relative to the placebo group) of these responses in patients receiving treatment with different drugs. Again, despite differences between populations and even between profiles of prior exposure to treatment, the confidence intervals of the various studies available for the same outcome overlap, except for the etanercept results, suggesting that it is less effective in controlling psoriasis than monoclonal TNFα inhibitors and secukinumab (**2B**).

A meta-analysis of 9 RCTs and two open-label studies analyzed the incidence of IBD (Crohn's disease or ulcerative colitis) in patients with AS undergoing anti-TNFα therapy (infliximab, adalimumab or etanercept, n = 1130), of whom 6.7% (n = 76) had a history of one of these diseases. The treatment of these patients was associated with the incidence rates of reactivation and/or a new case of Crohn's disease or ulcerative colitis in 0.2/100 PY for infliximab, 2.3/100 PY for adalimumab and 2.2/100 PY for etanercept, whereas the incidence in the placebo group was 1.3/100 PY. Regarding flare-up prevention in patients with a history of IBD, infliximab was the most effective drug in this study. Regarding the onset of new cases, no differences were observed among the three drugs [189] (**2A**). In the MEASURE 1 and 2 trials, the pooled exposure-adjusted incidence rate of Crohn's disease alone in secukinumab-treated patients was 0.7/100 PY [142] (**1B**). In phase 2 clinical trials, etanercept and secukinumab showed no efficacy in treating Crohn's disease [203, 204] (**2B**).

Recommendation

In the case of recurrent anterior uveitis or active inflammatory bowel disease in the setting of axial SpA, anti-TNF monoclonal antibodies (infliximab, adalimumab, golimumab, and certolizumab pegol) have shown the best response rates among the biologics. Therefore, it is recommended to choose it, preferably to others. ***Level of evidence: 2A; Strength of recommendation: B (moderate); Degree of agreement: 9.4.***

Monoclonal anti-TNF inhibitors (infliximab, adalimumab, golimumab, and certolizumab pegol) and ant-IL17 inhibitors have shown be the most effective, among the biologics, for the control of active psoriasis in the setting of axial SpA. Therefore, it is recommended to choose it, preferably to others. ***Level of evidence: 2B; Strength of recommendation: B (moderate); Degree of agreement: 9.4.***

13. What evidence supports switching biologics in patients with axial SpA?

Switching biologics in patients with axial SpA either due to primary failure (those unresponsive since treatment initiation), secondary failure (those who stopped responding to treatment over time), or even toxicity, is frequently needed in the long-term use of biologic drugs in axial SpA. There are a limited number of studies with high-quality designs, particularly studies investigating more recently developed drugs, regarding this issue.

One uncontrolled trial included 23 patients with AS who were previously treated with infliximab (minimum 6 doses) and did not achieve the ASAS20 response. These patients were switched to treatment with etanercept 50 mg/ week for 54 weeks. By week 24, 78, 52 and 39% of patients had achieved ASAS20, ASAS50 and ASAS70, respectively. By week 54, 74% maintained at least the ASAS20 response, 61% maintained the ASAS50 response and 39% maintained the ASAS70 response [205] (**2C**). A retrospective analysis of a cohort of patients with AS who were treated with an anti-TNFα drug (infliximab, etanercept or adalimumab) reported a clinical response (BASDAI50) to a second anti-TNFα drug in 93% of 15 patients in whom the first anti-TNFα drug was switched due to primary or secondary treatment failure, adverse effects or patient preference [206] (**2C**). In another cohort, 16 patients with AS (15% of 108 users of anti-TNFα drugs) undergoing treatment with infliximab, etanercept or adalimumab switched to a different TNFα inhibitor due to inefficacy (67%) or to adverse events (28%). Of these patients, 67 and 86% achieved BASDAI50 response within six and 12 months, respectively. Patients who switched TNFα inhibitors due to adverse effects were more likely to show clinical responses than patients who switched due to a lack of efficacy [207] (**2C**). In a similar study, 11 (24%) of 46 patients with AS undergoing anti-TNFα therapy showed no clinical response or presented adverse effects. An adequate response was observed in 46% (n = 5) of patients treated with a second TNFα inhibitor and in 100% (n = 5) of patients treated with a third inhibitor [208] (**2C**). The Norwegian registry (NOR-DMARD) compared 437 patients with AS using a first anti-TNFα drug with another 77 patients with AS who switched to a second anti-TNFα drug. After 3 months, 50% and of 38% patients undergoing first-line treatment achieved BASDAI50 and ASAS40 responses, respectively, whereas the same response rates of patients undergoing second-line treatments (switchers) were 28% ($p = 0.007$ for intergroup difference) and 31% ($p = 0.41$), respectively. No significant efficacy difference of the second anti-TNFα drug was observed between switches due to inefficacy or to adverse effects [209] (**2B**). The Danish registry (DANBIO) also revealed worse responses to the second and third anti-TNFα drugs than the responses observed in naïve patients who were using an anti-TNFα drug for the first time, although half of the switches resulted in good responses. In addition, 432 patients with AS who switched once and 137 who switched twice were compared with 773 non-switchers. After 2 years of treatment, 79% patients who underwent first-line treatment and 54% of patients who underwent second- or third-line treatment maintained low disease activity with BASDAI<4 ($p < 0.0001$) and 71 and 37% has an ASDAS<2.1 ($p < 0.001$), respectively [210] (**2B**). Data on AS patients treated with an anti-TNFα drug (adalimumab, etanercept, infliximab or golimumab) were retrospectively analyzed, and 77 of the 175 patients included in the analysis received at least two anti-TNFα drugs (switchers). The main reason for switching the first medication was inefficacy. The BASDAI50 response 12 months after treatment initiation was achieved at a lower frequency among switchers than among non-switchers (47% *vs* 71%), corresponding to an OR of 0.37 (95% CI 0.26–0.52). Other evidence of a loss of response is the difference between the survival times of the first and second anti-TNFα therapy lines: 63 months (95% CI 57–69) and 39 months (95% CI 31–47), respectively, $p = 0.05$ [211] (**2B**).

More recently, two systematic literature reviews (SLRs) published results supporting the strategy of using a second anti-TNFα drug when treatment failure or adverse effects occur [212, 213] (**2A**). According to one of the reviews based on data from 21 studies, the NNT to achieve BASDAI50 response in patients undergoing first-line treatment with an anti-TNFα drug ranged from 1.6 to 2.0. Conversely, patients undergoing second-line treatment (with a second anti-TNFα drug) showed higher (worse) NNTs, although still significant, ranging from 2.5 to 4.0 [213] (**2A**).

In the phase 3 trials of the two most recently launched anti-TNFα drugs (golimumab and certolizumab pegol) in patients with axial SpA, a small portion of patients with prior exposure to anti-TNFα therapy, 16% in the RAPID-axial SpA trial of certolizumab pegol and 14.4% in the GO-ALIVE trial of IV administered golimumab, were analyzed. However, separate response data for this subpopulation were not reported in either case [138, 139] (**2C**).

In the MEASURE 2 trial of secukinumab for AS, 38.8% of the participants already used some anti-TNFα drug before starting the study. A subsequent publication compared the efficacy results between the two groups (anti-TNFα-naive and anti-TNFα-inadequate response/intolerance), and, not surprisingly, the clinical responses were also slightly worse in the group with prior exposure than in the group receiving the first-line biological therapy. The NNTs were calculated for first- and second-line treatments and were 2.7 (95% CI 1.8–5.6) and 3.9 (95% CI 2.0–60) for ASAS20; 3.9 (95% CI 2.3–14.3) and 4.0 (95% CI 2.4–11.2) for ASAS40; and 8.7 (95% CI 4.0–49) and 14 (95% CI 6.0–41) for ASAS partial remission, respectively [143] (**2B**). To date, no data on the efficacy of second- or third-line treatments after treatment failure or toxic response to secukinumab are available.

Recommendation

Patients with axial SpA who fail to show an initial response to a biological therapy (primary treatment failure), loss of efficacy (secondary treatment failure) or adverse effects should switch to another approved biologic, regardless of the mechanism of action. ***Level of evidence: 2A; Strength of recommendation: B (moderate); Degree of agreement: 9.4.***

After the first biologic switch, the response rates decrease slightly but remain significant. The little available evidence on the second biologic switch suggest response rates even lower than the second-line treatment. ***Level of evidence: 2A; Strength of recommendation: B (moderate); Degree of agreement: 9.1.***

14. For how long should a biologic be used during the follow-up of patients with axial SpA?

Considering the prevalence of axial SpA, the portion of patients who will require biologics and the costs involved (both financial and related to individual health), strategies for the reduction and/or discontinuation of these drugs in patients who are considered to have an inactive disease must be discussed. The lack of studies with adequate methodology and sufficient follow-up time further complicates the difficult task of defining remission in patients with axial SpA and the minimum time a patient should remain in this presumed inactive status before drug withdrawal begins.

Biological therapy discontinuation

A systematic review of biological therapy discontinuation in patients with axial SpA included 4 RCT extensions and an uncontrolled trial (n = 220) that were highly heterogeneous regarding the length of anti-TNFα therapy before discontinuation, use of co-medication in the post-discontinuation period and the definition of reactivation (flare-up). After 1-year follow-up, 76–100% (79% median) patients exhibited disease reactivation after a mean period ranging from 6 to 24 weeks after discontinuation. Importantly, in these studies, the probability of achieving a good clinical response similar to the response observed before discontinuation after resuming treatment with these drugs was high [214] (**2A**). A retrospective Polish study reported similar results. In that study, 74% of patients with axial SpA presenting low disease activity (LDA) and having completed anti-TNFα therapy withdrawal showed disease reactivation, which required a resumption of therapy, on average, after 14 weeks during an observation period ranging from 9 to 48 months [215] (**2C**). Conversely, the ABILITY-3 trial included 305 patients exclusively diagnosed with non-radiographic axial SpA axial who were using adalimumab and considered inactive (ASDAS<1.3) for at least 12 weeks in a randomized, double-blind controlled extension in which 152 of those patients continued to receive adalimumab and 153 received the placebo. After 40 weeks of follow-up, 70% of patients in the adalimumab group and 47% of patients in the placebo group remained without disease reactivation (defined as ASDAS≥2.1). The difference of 23% in the incidence of flare-ups at 40 weeks corresponds to a number needed to harm (NNH) of reactivation after withdrawal of 4.3 (95% CI 2.9–7.9) [216] (**1B**).

Dose reduction in biological therapy

The aforementioned systematic review also included data on gradual anti-TNFα dose reduction strategies from eight studies, mostly with low-grade evidence (six observational studies, one controlled but non-randomized trial and only one RCT) including 436 patients with AS who were followed for a median time of 12 months. The inclusion criteria, which were highly heterogeneous among the studies, ranged from three to six months in remission or LDA before starting anti-TNFα dose reduction. In most studies, remission was defined as BASDAI<2, normal CRP levels and LDA or as BASDAI<4 and normal CRP levels. The percentage of patients who maintained LDA or remission following the anti-TNFα dose reduction was reported in five studies and ranged from 53 to 100%. The remaining three studies reported mean changes in BASDAI and CRP levels after anti-TNFα dose reduction and found no relevant increase in these parameters. Patients with a longer remission time before dose reduction and patients without peripheral or extra-articular manifestations had higher success rates with anti-TNFα dose reduction [214] (**2A**). The Dutch cohort GLAS followed 58 patients with AS undergoing anti-TNFα therapy with LDA (BASDAI<4) for at least 6 months and for whom the treatment dose was reduced for 24 months. The etanercept dose was reduced from 50 mg/week to 25 mg/2 weeks in 4 reduction steps, infliximab was reduced from 5 mg/kg/8 weeks to 3 mg/kg/10 weeks in two steps and adalimumab was reduced from 40 mg/2 weeks to 40 mg/4 weeks in two steps. Dose reduction only continued if BASDAI remained <4 and the attending physician and patient agreed to the subsequent reduction. After 2 years, 53% patients remained on a reduced dose regimen (mean: 62 ± 11% of the standard dose) [217] (**2B**). Consistent with these findings, other studies reported success rates in anti-TNFα dose reduction (ranging from 50 to 75% of the standard dose) in patients with axial SpA who were in remission or LDA, ranging from 55 to 96% after one year of follow-up [218–221] and from 56 to 84% after 3 years [220, 222, 223].

Better results were observed among patients undergoing the same therapy and patients in remission for longer periods [219, 221] (**2C**). The drug survival remained unchanged during the four years (HR = 0.472, 95% CI 0.155–1.435) among 100 patients with AS for whom the dose of etanercept was reduced from 50 mg/week to 25 mg/week (or 50 mg/2 weeks) and among 34 controls who maintained the standard dose, thus supporting the efficacy of the reduced dose in patients in remission/LDA during the longest follow-up period [224] (**2B**). A South Korean study compared radiographic progression, using the mSASSS 2 and 4 years after the baseline between 116 patients with AS using a reduced anti-TNFα (etanercept or adalimumab) dose and 49 treated with a standard dose. The mean dose used by the reduction group was 68% of the standard dose, with no difference observed between groups. Only a small but significant difference was observed in patients at higher risk of progression (those with syndesmophytes since the baseline) in favor of the standard dose group (1.23 *vs* 1.72 units/year; p = 0.023) [225] (**2B**). No studies have examined a secukinumab dose reduction or withdrawal in patients with axial SpA.

Recommendation

In those who have reached the proposed treatment target, for at least 6 months, an attempt may be made to reduce the anti-TNFα dose or increase the interval between doses. Data on other mechanisms of action remains insufficient. However, the risk of long-term radiographic progression should be considered. ***Level of evidence: 1B; Strength of recommendation: B (moderate); Degree of agreement: 8.9.***

15. Is there evidence for the use of biologics and/or target-specific small molecules with other mechanisms of action (non-TNFαi and non-IL17i) in patients with axial SpA?

A non-negligible portion of patients with axial SpA will not achieve the desired activity control target, remission or at least LDA, despite the use of conventional drugs and biologicals approved for this indication. Here, we compile the currently available evidence for the efficacy of drugs with other action mechanisms, including target-specific small molecules.

Anti-CD20, anti-IL6R and CTLA4-Ig

A small (n = 20), open-label and uncontrolled trial reported a favorable response to rituximab (1000 mg IV combined with 100 mg methylprednisolone IV at weeks 0 and 2) in patients with AS and a history of anti-TNFα therapy failure (ASAS20, ASAS40, BASDAI50 and ASAS partial remission were only achieved by 30, 10, 0 and 0% patients, respectively). A modest response (ASAS20, ASAS40, BASDAI50 and ASAS partial remission were achieved by 50, 40, 50 and 30% patients, respectively) was observed only in bio-naïve individuals [226] (**2C**). The responsive patients (n = 9) were followed until week 48. Four maintained the response until the end of the study and five showed disease reactivation (defined by a worsening of the BASDAI corresponding to 1.5x the lowest value reached until week 24) and were retreated with the same dose, recovering their response within 48 weeks after retreatment [227] (**2C**). Negative results were also observed in two open-label and uncontrolled studies of abatacept in patients with active axial SpA, in which no difference was observed in any activity parameter assessed from baseline to week 24 [228, 229] (**2C**). Therapeutic blockade of the IL6 receptor (IL6R) was analyzed in the BUILDER-1 study, a phase II–III placebo-controlled randomized trial, which compared the efficacy of tocilizumab IV (n = 48) with placebo (n = 51) in the treatment of patients with AS in 24 weeks of follow-up. After 12 weeks, ASAS20 was achieved by 37.3 and 27.5% patients in the treatment and control groups (p = 0.28), respectively, and the study was discontinued [230] (**2B**). Another IL6R inhibitor, sarilumab, also failed to produce a clinical response in patients with AS in the ALIGN study, a randomized clinical trial with 301 patients. No differences in the ASAS20 response at week 12 were observed between the placebo group and the groups treated any dose of sarilumab tested in the trial [231] (**2B**).

Inhibitors of the IL23/IL17 axis

Despite the promising results of a phase II trial [232], ustekinumab, an antibody that specifically binds the p40 subunit of IL12 and IL23, three phase III studies (n = 1017) were interrupted early, after week 24, when the results showed no difference in the proportion of patients showing ASAS20, ASAS40 and BASDAI50 responses between the placebo and treatment groups or changes in ASDAS-CRP or BASFI scores [233] (**1B**).

Target-specific small molecules

The specific phosphodiesterase-4 (PDE-4) inhibitor apremilast did not induce significant differences in changes in BASDAI, BASFI and BASMI scores from baseline to week 12 compared with the placebo in a phase II study. Additionally, no difference in the frequency of the ASAS20 response was observed between the treatment and placebo groups [234] (**2B**). In turn, therapeutic blockade of Janus kinases (JAK), a family of non-receptor tyrosine kinases that transduce the intracellular signals of various cytokines, produced promising results in patients with AS. Tofacitinib, a JAK inhibitor selective for JAK-1 and JAK-3, was tested in a phase II trial with 207 patients randomly allocated to three treatment doses (2, 5 and 10 mg, 2 times per day) and placebo, whose primary outcome was the ASAS20 response at week 12. The groups of patients treated with 5 mg and 10 mg of tofacitinib differed significantly from the placebo group in the ASAS20, ASAS40 and BASDAI50 responses and non-significantly in the ASAS partial remission and ASDAS inactive disease responses. In addition, approximately one-third of the patients treated with tofacitinib showed reduced inflammation on sacroiliac joint and spinal MRI, which was the most common clinical response among those patients [235, 236] (**2B**). Another JAK inhibitor, filgotinib, which is selective for JAK-1, was also tested in the TORTUGA trial, a phase II clinical trial that included 116 patients with AS. At week 12, the change in the ASDAS from baseline was greater in the treatment group than in the placebo group: −1.47 (±1.04) and − 0.57 (0.82), respectively, with a mean difference of −0.85 (95% CI −1.17 to −0.53, p < 0.0001). At week 12, significantly greater proportions of patients in the treatment group achieved ASAS20 and ASAS40 responses, decreases in BASDAI, BASMI and BASFI scores and decreases in ultrasensitive CRP levels. Higher percentages of patients with ASDAS inactive disease and ASAS partial remission were observed in the treatment group than in the placebo group, but the differences were not significant [237] (**2B**).

Recommendation

The use of other biologics and/or target-specific small molecules (abatacept, tocilizumab, rituximab, sarilumab, ustekinumab and apremilast) is not recommended for the treatment of patients with axial SpA. ***Level of evidence: 1B; Strength of recommendation: A (strong); Degree of agreement: 9.5.***

The Janus kinase (JAK) inhibitors tofacitinib and filgotinib showed promising clinical results in the treatment of ankylosing spondylitis, but more definitive evidence (phase III randomized clinical trials) is still needed prior to their recommendation. ***Level of evidence: 2B; Strength of recommendation: B (moderate); Degree of agreement: 9.1.***

Conclusions

The recommendations presented herein seek to provide scientific evidence to rheumatologists and other agents involved in the care of patients with axial spondyloarthritis. In each situation chosen for response, were considered aspects as the therapeutic efficacy, safety, and costs, together with the critical assessment and experience of a panel of experts to standardize the management of these conditions in the national socioeconomic context but maintaining the autonomy of the physician in choosing different therapeutic options. These recommendations should be updated periodically because of the rapid development of this field of knowledge.

Supplementary information

Additional file 1. Bibliographic Research details.
Additional file 2. Data used in the Confidence Intervals.

Acknowledgements
Not applicable.

Authors' contributions
All authors made contributions to the acquisition of data, have been involved in drafting the manuscript or revising it critically for important intellectual content, participated in the voting rounds, gave final approval of the version to be published and have participated sufficiently in the work to take public responsibility for appropriate portions of the content.

Authors' information
Not applicable.

Competing interests
Gustavo Gomes Resende received lecture fees from Abbvie, Janssen, Novartis, Pfizer, and UCB; advisory board from Abbvie, Janssen, and Novartis; Research support from Brazilian Society of Rheumatology, FAPEMIG and UCB; clinical research payments from Abbvie and Pfizer; sponsorship for scientific events from Abbvie, Janssen, Lilly, Novartis, Pfizer, and UCB.
Eduardo de Souza Meirelles received payments as a speaker from Novartis, Abbvie, Abbott and Marjan; research grants from Novartis and Pfizer; support for conferences and courses from Aché, Pfizer, Novartis, Janssen, Abbvie, Roche, and Lilly; Advisory board fee from Novartis and Marjan.
Cláudia Diniz Lopes Marques received lecture fees from Abbvie, Janssen, Pfizer and Novartis; advisory board from Novartis and Abbvie; sponsorship for events from Abbvie, Janssen, Pfizer, Novartis, and Lilly.
Adriano Chiereghin received honoraria as a speaker from Janssen, Novartis, UCB, and Pfizer; support to courses and congresses from Abbvie, Janssen, Novartis, UCB, and Pfizer; advisory board from Novartis and Janssen.
Andre Marun Lyrio received payments from Speaker of Janssen and UCB; support to courses/congresses from Janssen, Abbvie, Pfizer, UBC, Novartis, and Lily.

Antônio Carlos Ximenes received payments for participation in clinical research from Abbvvie, Pfizer, Roche, BMS, and Amgen; on scientific board of Pfizer, and Abbivie; as a lecturer from AbbVie, Pfizer, and Abbott.
Carla Gonçalves Saad has no conflicts of interest.
Célio Roberto Gonçalves has no conflicts of interest.
Charles Lubianca Kohen received financial support for advisory board participation from Novartis; speaker fee from Janssen, Abbvie, Novartis, Pfizer, UCB; support to events from Janssen, Abbvie, Roche, Astra-Zeneca, Novartis.
Cláudia Goldenstein Schainberg has participated in the pharmaceutical advisory board of AbbVie, Janssen, Lilly, Novartis, and Pfizer; is a speaker invited by AbbVie, Janssen, Lilly, Novartis, Pfizer; has no stock of these pharmaceutical industries.

Cristiano Barbosa Campanholo received financial support for advisory board participation from Janssen, Abbvie, Bristol, Lilly, Novartis, Pfizer, UCB; speaker fee from Janssen, Abbvie, Lilly, Novartis, and Pfizer, UCB; support to events from Janssen, Abbvie, Bristol, Novartis, and Pfizer.
Júlio Silvio de Sousa Bueno Filho has no conflicts of interest.
Lenise Brandao Pieruccetti has no conflicts of interest.
Mauro Waldemar Keiserman received financial support for lectures, advisory bord and clinical research from Abbvie, Actelion, Biogen, Bristol, Celltrion, Lilly, Human Genome Sceiences, Janssen, Pfizer, Novartis, Roche, Sanofi, and UCB.
Michel Alexandre Yazbek received financial support from Abbvie, UCB, Novartis and Lilly.

Penelope Esther Palominos has no conflicts of interest.
Rafaela Silva Guimarães Goncalves received fees for lectures from Janssen, Novertis, Abbvie, Apsen, Bristol, and Pfizer; advisory board from Janssen.
Ricardo da Cruz Lage received speakers fee from Abbvie and Novartis; support to scientific events from Janssen, Novartis, Pfizer and Abbvie; clinical research payments from Abbvie.

Rodrigo Luppino Assad received fees for lectures and advisory board from Abbvie, Novartis, Janssen, UCB, Lilly, and Bristol; research support from Abbvie and UCB.

Rubens Bonfiglioli received financial support for clinical research from Roche, Pfizer, Amgen, and Novartis; for scientific advisory from Lilly, Abbvie, Roche, and UCB; for support to events from Roche, Pfizer, Abbvie and Novartis; for symposia and sponsored meetings from Roche, Pfizer, and Janssen.
Sônia Maria Alvarenga Anti received financial support from Abbvie, Jansen, Novartis, Lilly, and UCB.

Sueli Coelho da Silva Carneiro received honorary speaker from Abbvie, Janssen, Lilly, Novartis and Pfizer; support to research from CNPq and FAPERJ; support for congresses from Abbvie, Janssen, Novartis, Pfizer, CNPq and FAPERJ; advisory board from Janssen, Lilly, and Novartis.
Thauana Luíza Oliveira received lecturer fees from Abbvie, Novartis and Janssen; support to congresses from Abbvie and Janssen.
Valderílio Feijó Azevedo is GRAPPA member; Medical diretor of Edumed Biotech; received for clinical research from Pfizer, Roche, Janssen, Bristol, Abbvie, Medimmune, Boehringer, GSK, USB, Sanofi, Takeda, Bird Rock Bio, and NovoNordisk; financial support to events and lectures from Pfizer, Hospira, Roche, MSD, BMS, Merck Senoro, Janssen, Novertis, Celltrion, UCB, and AztraZeneca.

Washington Alves Bianchi has no conflicts of interest.
Wanderley Marques Bernardo has no conflicts of interest.

Marcelo de Medeiros Pinheiro received financial support for advisory board from Novartis and Janssen; by lectures from Novartis, Janssen, Abbvie.
Percival Degrava Sampaio-Barros received for participation in lectures, boards or scientific events from laboratories Abbvie, Janssen, Novartis, Pfizer and UCB.

Author details

[1]Universidade Federal de Minas Gerais (UFMG), Alameda Álvaro Celso, 175 / 2° Andar. Santa Efigênia. CEP 30.150-260, Belo Horizonte, MG, Brazil. [2]Universidade De São Paulo (USP), São Paulo, Brazil. [3]Universidade Federal de Pernambuco (UFPE), Recife, Brazil. [4]Pontifície Universidade Católica (PUC) de Sorocaba, Sorocaba, Brazil. [5]Pontifície Universidade Católica (PUC) de Campinas, Campinas, Brazil. [6]Hospital Estadual Geral de Goiania (HGG), Goiânia, Brazil. [7]Universidade Federal do Rio Grande do Sul (UFRS), Porto Alegre, Brazil. [8]Santa Casa de Misericórdia (SCM) de São Paulo, São Paulo, Brazil. [9]Departmento de Estatística, Universidade Federal de Lavras (UFLA), Lavras, Brazil. [10]Hospital Heliópolis, São Paulo, Brazil. [11]Pontifície Universidade Católica (PUC) de Porto Alegre, Porto Alegre, Brazil. [12]Universidade Estadual de Campinas (UNICAMP), Campinas, Brazil. [13]USP Ribeirão Preto, Ribeirão Preto, Brazil. [14]Hospital do Servidor Público do Estado de São Paulo, São Paulo, Brazil. [15]Universidade Federal do Rio De Janeiro (UFRJ), Rio de Janeiro, Brazil. [16]Universidade Federal de São Paulo (UNIFESP), São Paulo, Brazil. [17]Universidade Federal do Paraná (UFPR), Curitiba, Brazil. [18]Santa Casa de Misericórdia (SCM) do Rio De Janeiro, Rio de Janeiro, Brazil. [19]Universidade de São Paulo (USP), São Paulo, Brazil.

References

1. Rudwaleit M, Landewe R, van der Heijde D, Listing J, Brandt J, Braun J, et al. The development of Assessment of SpondyloArthritis international Society classification criteria for axial spondyloarthritis (part I): classification of paper patients by expert opinion including uncertainty appraisal. Ann Rheum Dis. 2009;68(6):770–6.
2. Rudwaleit M, van der Heijde D, Landewe R, Listing J, Akkoc N, Brandt J, et al. The development of Assessment of SpondyloArthritis international Society classification criteria for axial spondyloarthritis (part II): validation and final selection. Ann Rheum Dis. 2009;68(6):777–83.
3. Sampaio-Barros PD, Keiserman M, Meirelles Ede S, Pinheiro Mde M, Ximenes AC, Azevedo VF, et al. Recommendations for the management and treatment of ankylosing spondylitis. Rev Bras Reumatol. 2013;53(3):242–57.
4. Phillips B, Ball C, Sackett D, Badenoch D, Straus S, Haynes B, et al. Levels of Evidence. BJU Int. 2010; 106: 1424.
5. Lin Z, Liao Z, Huang J, Jin O, Li Q, Li T, et al. Evaluation of Assessment of Spondyloarthritis International Society classification criteria for axial spondyloarthritis in Chinese patients with chronic back pain: results of a 2-year follow-up study. Int J Rheum Dis. 2014;17(7):782–9.
6. Deodhar A, Mease PJ, Reveille JD, Curtis JR, Chen S, Malhotra K, et al. Frequency of Axial Spondyloarthritis Diagnosis Among Patients Seen by US Rheumatologists for Evaluation of Chronic Back Pain. Arthritis Rheumatol. 2016;68(7):1669–76.
7. Sepriano A, Landewe R, van der Heijde D, Sieper J, Akkoc N, Brandt J, et al. Predictive validity of the ASAS classification criteria for axial and peripheral spondyloarthritis after follow-up in the ASAS cohort: a final analysis. Ann Rheum Dis. 2016;75(6):1034–42.
8. Bendahan LT, Machado NP, Mendes JG, Oliveira TL, Pinheiro MM. Performance of the classification criteria in patients with late-onset axial spondyloarthritis. Mod Rheumatol. 2018;28(1):174–81.
9. Mau W, Zeidler H, Mau R, Majewski A, Freyschmidt J, Stangel W, et al. Clinical features and prognosis of patients with possible ankylosing spondylitis. Results of a 10-year followup. J Rheumatol. 1988;15(7):1109–14.
10. Bennett AN, McGonagle D, O'Connor P, Hensor EM, Sivera F, Coates LC, et al. Severity of baseline magnetic resonance imaging-evident sacroiliitis and HLA-B27 status in early inflammatory back pain predict radiographically evident ankylosing spondylitis at eight years. Arthritis Rheum. 2008;58(11): 3413–8.
11. Weber U, Lambert RG, Ostergaard M, Hodler J, Pedersen SJ, Maksymowych WP. The diagnostic utility of magnetic resonance imaging in spondylarthritis: an international multicenter evaluation of one hundred eighty-seven subjects. Arthritis Rheum. 2010;62(10):3048–58.
12. Rudwaleit M, Jurik AG, Hermann KG, Landewe R, van der Heijde D, Baraliakos X, et al. Defining active sacroiliitis on magnetic resonance imaging (MRI) for classification of axial spondyloarthritis: a consensual approach by the ASAS/OMERACT MRI group. Ann Rheum Dis. 2009;68(10): 1520–7.
13. Aydin SZ, Maksymowych WP, Bennett AN, McGonagle D, Emery P, Marzo-Ortega H. Validation of the ASAS criteria and definition of a positive MRI of the sacroiliac joint in an inception cohort of axial spondyloarthritis followed up for 8 years. Ann Rheum Dis. 2012;71(1):56–60.
14. Larbi A, Viala P, Molinari N, Lukas C, Baron MP, Taourel P, et al. Assessment of MRI abnormalities of the sacroiliac joints and their ability to predict axial spondyloarthritis: a retrospective pilot study on 110 patients. Skelet Radiol. 2014;43(3):351–8.
15. Weber U, Zubler V, Pedersen SJ, Rufibach K, Lambert RG, Chan SM, et al. Development and validation of a magnetic resonance imaging reference criterion for defining a positive sacroiliac joint magnetic resonance imaging finding in spondyloarthritis. Arthritis Care Res. 2013;65(6):977–85.
16. Weber U, Pedersen SJ, Zubler V, Rufibach K, Chan SM, Lambert RG, et al. Fat infiltration on magnetic resonance imaging of the sacroiliac joints has limited diagnostic utility in nonradiographic axial spondyloarthritis. J Rheumatol. 2014;41(1):75–83.
17. Weber U, Ostergaard M, Lambert RG, Pedersen SJ, Chan SM, Zubler V, et al. Candidate lesion-based criteria for defining a positive sacroiliac joint MRI in two cohorts of patients with axial spondyloarthritis. Ann Rheum Dis. 2015; 74(11):1976–82.
18. Bakker PA, van den Berg R, Lenczner G, Thevenin F, Reijnierse M, Claudepierre P, et al. Can we use structural lesions seen on MRI of the sacroiliac joints reliably for the classification of patients according to the ASAS axial spondyloarthritis criteria? Data from the DESIR cohort. Ann Rheum Dis. 2017;76(2):392–8.
19. de Hooge M, van den Berg R, Navarro-Compan V, Reijnierse M, van Gaalen F, Fagerli K, et al. Patients with chronic back pain of short duration from the SPACE cohort: which MRI structural lesions in the sacroiliac joints and inflammatory and structural lesions in the spine are most specific for axial spondyloarthritis? Ann Rheumatic Dis. 2016;75:1308–1314.
20. de Hooge M, van den Berg R, Navarro-Compan V, van Gaalen F, van der Heijde D, Huizinga T, et al. Magnetic resonance imaging of the sacroiliac joints in the early detection of spondyloarthritis: no added value of gadolinium compared with short tau inversion recovery sequence. Rheumatology. 2013;52(7):1220–4.
21. Zhao YH, Cao YY, Zhang Q, Mei YJ, Xiao JJ, Hu SY, et al. Role of Diffusion-weighted and Contrast-enhanced Magnetic Resonance Imaging in Differentiating Activity of Ankylosing Spondylitis. Chin Med J. 2017;130(11):1303–8.
22. Bradbury LA, Hollis KA, Gautier B, Shankaranarayana S, Robinson PC, Saad N, et al. Diffusion-weighted Imaging Is a Sensitive and Specific Magnetic Resonance Sequence in the Diagnosis of Ankylosing Spondylitis. J Rheumatol. 2018;45(6):771–8.
23. Hermann KG, Baraliakos X, van der Heijde DM, Jurik AG, Landewe R, Marzo-Ortega H, et al. Descriptions of spinal MRI lesions and definition of a positive MRI of the spine in axial spondyloarthritis: a consensual approach by the ASAS/OMERACT MRI study group. Ann Rheum Dis. 2012;71(8):1278–88.
24. Bennett AN, Rehman A, Hensor EM, Marzo-Ortega H, Emery P, McGonagle D. The fatty Romanus lesion: a non-inflammatory spinal MRI lesion specific for axial spondyloarthropathy. Ann Rheum Dis. 2010;69(5):891–4.
25. Lorenzin M, Ortolan A, Frallonardo P, Vio S, Lacognata C, Oliviero F, et al. Spine and sacroiliac joints on magnetic resonance imaging in patients with early axial spondyloarthritis: prevalence of lesions and association with clinical and disease activity indices from the Italian group of the SPACE study. Reumatismo. 2016;68(2):72–82.
26. van der Heijde D, Sieper J, Maksymowych WP, Brown MA, Lambert RG, Rathmann SS, et al. Spinal inflammation in the absence of sacroiliac joint inflammation on magnetic resonance imaging in patients with active nonradiographic axial spondyloarthritis. Arthritis Rheumatol. 2014;66(3):667–73.
27. Ez-Zaitouni Z, Bakker PA, van Lunteren M, de Hooge M, van den Berg R, Reijnierse M, et al. The yield of a positive MRI of the spine as imaging criterion in the ASAS classification criteria for axial spondyloarthritis: results from the SPACE and DESIR cohorts. Ann Rheum Dis. 2017;76(10):1731–6.
28. Weber U, Zubler V, Zhao Z, Lambert RG, Chan SM, Pedersen SJ, et al. Does spinal MRI add incremental diagnostic value to MRI of the sacroiliac joints

alone in patients with non-radiographic axial spondyloarthritis? Ann Rheum Dis. 2015;74(6):985–92.

29. Madsen KB, Schiottz-Christensen B, Jurik AG. Prognostic significance of magnetic resonance imaging changes of the sacroiliac joints in spondyloarthritis--a followup study. J Rheumatol. 2010;37(8):1718–27.
30. Maksymowych WP, Wichuk S, Chiowchanwisawakit P, Lambert RG, Pedersen SJ. Fat metaplasia on MRI of the sacroiliac joints increases the propensity for disease progression in the spine of patients with spondyloarthritis. RMD open. 2017;3(1):e000399.
31. Maksymowych WP, Chiowchanwisawakit P, Clare T, Pedersen SJ, Ostergaard M, Lambert RG. Inflammatory lesions of the spine on magnetic resonance imaging predict the development of new syndesmophytes in ankylosing spondylitis: evidence of a relationship between inflammation and new bone formation. Arthritis Rheum. 2009;60(1):93–102.
32. Machado P, Landewe R, Braun J, Hermann KG, Baker D, van der Heijde D. Both structural damage and inflammation of the spine contribute to impairment of spinal mobility in patients with ankylosing spondylitis. Ann Rheum Dis. 2010;69(8):1465–70.
33. Brown MA, Laval SH, Brophy S, Calin A. Recurrence risk modelling of the genetic susceptibility to ankylosing spondylitis. Ann Rheum Dis. 2000;59(11):883–6.
34. Braun J, Bollow M, Remlinger G, Eggens U, Rudwaleit M, Distler A, et al. Prevalence of spondylarthropathies in HLA-B27 positive and negative blood donors. Arthritis Rheum. 1998;41(1):58–67.
35. Schlosstein L, Terasaki PI, Bluestone R, Pearson CM. High association of an HL-A antigen, W27, with ankylosing spondylitis. N Engl J Med. 1973;288(14): 704–6.
36. Sieper J, Rudwaleit M, Khan MA, Braun J. Concepts and epidemiology of spondyloarthritis. Best Pract Res Clin Rheumatol. 2006;20(3):401–17.
37. Khan MA. An Update on the Genetic Polymorphism of HLA-B*27 With 213 Alleles Encompassing 160 Subtypes (and Still Counting). Curr Rheumatol Rep. 2017;19(2):9.
38. Freeston J, Barkham N, Hensor E, Emery P, Fraser A. Ankylosing spondylitis, HLA-B27 positivity and the need for biologic therapies. Joint Bone Spine. 2007;74(2):140–3.
39. Popescu C, Trandafir M, Badica A, Morar F, Predeteanu D. Ankylosing spondylitis functional and activity indices in clinical practice. J Med Life. 2014;7(1):78–83.
40. Yang M, Xu M, Pan X, Hu Z, Li Q, Wei Y, et al. Epidemiological comparison of clinical manifestations according to HLA-B*27 carrier status of Chinese ankylosing spondylitis patients. Tissue Antigens. 2013;82(5):338–43.
41. Fallahi S, Mahmoudi M, Nicknam MH, Gharibdoost F, Farhadi E, Saei A, et al. Effect of HLA-B*27 and its subtypes on clinical manifestations and severity of ankylosing spondylitis in Iranian patients. Iranian J Allergy Asthma Immunology. 2013;12(4):321–30.
42. Xiong J, Chen J, Tu J, Ye W, Zhang Z, Liu Q, et al. Association of HLA-B27 status and gender with sacroiliitis in patients with ankylosing spondylitis. Pakistan J Med Sciences. 2014;30(1):22–7.
43. Rudwaleit M, Haibel H, Baraliakos X, Listing J, Marker-Hermann E, Zeidler H, et al. The early disease stage in axial spondylarthritis: results from the German Spondyloarthritis Inception Cohort. Arthritis Rheum. 2009;60(3):717–27.
44. Zeboulon N, Dougados M, Gossec L. Prevalence and characteristics of uveitis in the spondyloarthropathies: a systematic literature review. Ann Rheum Dis. 2008;67(7):955–9.
45. van der Heijde D, Ramiro S, Landewé R, Baraliakos X, Van den Bosch F, Sepriano A, et al. 2016 update of the ASAS-EULAR management recommendations for axial spondyloarthritis. Ann Rheum Dis. 2017;76(6):978–91.
46. van den Berg R, Baraliakos X, Braun J, van der Heijde D. First update of the current evidence for the management of ankylosing spondylitis with non-pharmacological treatment and non-biologic drugs: a systematic literature review for the ASAS/EULAR management recommendations in ankylosing spondylitis. Rheumatology. 2012;51(8):1388–96.
47. Dagfinrud H, Kvien TK, Hagen KB. Physiotherapy interventions for ankylosing spondylitis. Cochrane Database Syst Rev. 2008;1:CD002822.
48. Regel A, Sepriano A, Baraliakos X, van der Heijde D, Braun J, Landewe R, et al. Efficacy and safety of non-pharmacological and non-biological pharmacological treatment: a systematic literature review informing the 2016 update of the ASAS/EULAR recommendations for the management of axial spondyloarthritis. RMD open. 2017;3(1):e000397.
49. Fernandez-de-Las-Penas C, Alonso-Blanco C, Morales-Cabezas M, Miangolarra-Page JC. Two exercise interventions for the management of patients with ankylosing spondylitis: a randomized controlled trial. Am J Physical Med Rehabilitation. 2005;84(6):407–19.
50. Fernandez-de-Las-Penas C, Alonso-Blanco C, Alguacil-Diego IM, Miangolarra-Page JC. One-year follow-up of two exercise interventions for the management of patients with ankylosing spondylitis: a randomized controlled trial. Am J Physical Med Rehabilitation. 2006;85(7):559–67.
51. Silva EM, Andrade SC, Vilar MJ. Evaluation of the effects of Global Postural Reeducation in patients with ankylosing spondylitis. Rheumatol Int. 2012; 32(7):2155–63.
52. Rosu MO, Topa I, Chirieac R, Ancuta C. Effects of Pilates, McKenzie and Heckscher training on disease activity, spinal motility and pulmonary function in patients with ankylosing spondylitis: a randomized controlled trial. Rheumatol Int. 2014;34(3):367–72.
53. Staalesen Strumse YA, Nordvag BY, Stanghelle JK, Roisland M, Winther A, Pajunen PA, et al. Efficacy of rehabilitation for patients with ankylosing spondylitis: comparison of a four-week rehabilitation programme in a Mediterranean and a Norwegian setting. J Rehabil Med. 2011;43(6):534–42.
54. Kjeken I, Bo I, Ronningen A, Spada C, Mowinckel P, Hagen KB, et al. A three-week multidisciplinary in-patient rehabilitation programme had positive long-term effects in patients with ankylosing spondylitis: randomized controlled trial. J Rehabil Med. 2013;45(3):260–7.
55. Aytekin E, Caglar NS, Ozgonenel L, Tutun S, Demiryontar DY, Demir SE. Home-based exercise therapy in patients with ankylosing spondylitis: effects on pain, mobility, disease activity, quality of life, and respiratory functions. Clin Rheumatol. 2012;31(1):91–7.
56. Kasapoglu Aksoy M, Birtane M, Tastekin N, Ekuklu G. The Effectiveness of Structured Group Education on Ankylosing Spondylitis Patients. J Clinical Rheumatol. 2017;23(3):138–43.
57. Rodriguez-Lozano C, Juanola X, Cruz-Martinez J, Pena-Arrebola A, Mulero J, Gratacos J, et al. Outcome of an education and home-based exercise programme for patients with ankylosing spondylitis: a nationwide randomized study. Clin Exp Rheumatol. 2013;31(5):739–48.
58. Liang H, Zhang H, Ji H, Wang C. Effects of home-based exercise intervention on health-related quality of life for patients with ankylosing spondylitis: a meta-analysis. Clin Rheumatol. 2015;34(10):1737–44.
59. Jennings F, Oliveira HA, de Souza MC, Cruz Vda G, Natour J. Effects of Aerobic Training in Patients with Ankylosing Spondylitis. J Rheumatol. 2015;42(12):2347–53.
60. Niedermann K, Sidelnikov E, Muggli C, Dagfinrud H, Hermann M, Tamborrini G, et al. Effect of cardiovascular training on fitness and perceived disease activity in people with ankylosing spondylitis. Arthritis Care Research. 2013; 65(11):1844–52.
61. Levitova A, Hulejova H, Spiritovic M, Pavelka K, Senolt L, Husakova M. Clinical improvement and reduction in serum calprotectin levels after an intensive exercise programme for patients with ankylosing spondylitis and non-radiographic axial spondyloarthritis. Arthritis Res Therapy. 2016;18(1):275.
62. Sveaas SH, Berg IJ, Provan SA, Semb AG, Hagen KB, Vollestad N, et al. Efficacy of high intensity exercise on disease activity and cardiovascular risk in active axial spondyloarthritis: a randomized controlled pilot study. PLoS One. 2014;9(9):e108688.
63. Dundar U, Solak O, Toktas H, Demirdal US, Subasi V, Kavuncu V, et al. Effect of aquatic exercise on ankylosing spondylitis: a randomized controlled trial. Rheumatol Int. 2014;34(11):1505–11.
64. Fernandez Garcia R, Sanchez Sanchez Lde C, Lopez Rodriguez Mdel M, Sanchez Granados G. [Effects of an exercise and relaxation aquatic program in patients with spondyloarthritis: A randomized trial]. Medicina Clinica 2015;145(9):380–384.
65. Klemz BN, Reis-Neto ET, Jennings F, Siqueira US, Klemz FK, Pinheiro HH, et al. The relevance of performing exercise test before starting supervised physical exercise in asymptomatic cardiovascular patients with rheumatic diseases. Rheumatology (Oxford). 2016;55(11):1978–86.
66. Peters ND, Ejstrup L. Intravenous methylprednisolone pulse therapy in ankylosing spondylitis. Scand J Rheumatol. 1992;21(3):134–8.
67. Rihl MBN, Wiese B, Schmidt RE, Zeidler H. Intravenous Glucocorticoid Pulse Therapy in Active, NSAID Refractory Axial Ankylosing Spondylitis: A Retrospective Analysis Spanning 12 Months. J Arthritis. 2018;7(1):266–9.
68. Bandinelli F, Scazzariello F, Pimenta da Fonseca E, Barreto Santiago M, Marcassa C, Nacci F, et al. Low-dose modified-release prednisone in axial spondyloarthritis: 3-month efficacy and tolerability. Drug Design Development Therapy. 2016;10:3717–24.
69. Haibel H, Fendler C, Listing J, Callhoff J, Braun J, Sieper J. Efficacy of oral prednisolone in active ankylosing spondylitis: results of a double-blind, randomised, placebo-controlled short-term trial. Ann Rheum Dis. 2014;73(1):243–6.

70. Zhang YP, Gong Y, Zeng QY, Hou ZD, Xiao ZY. A long-term, observational cohort study on the safety of low-dose glucocorticoids in ankylosing spondylitis: adverse events and effects on bone mineral density, blood lipid and glucose levels and body mass index. BMJ Open. 2015;5(6):e006957.
71. Srivastava P, Aggarwal A. Ultrasound-guided retro-calcaneal bursa corticosteroid injection for refractory Achilles tendinitis in patients with seronegative spondyloarthropathy: efficacy and follow-up study. Rheumatol Int. 2016;36(6):875–80.
72. Metcalfe D, Achten J, Costa ML. Glucocorticoid injections in lesions of the achilles tendon. Foot Ankle International. 2009;30(7):661–5.
73. Bollow M, Braun J, Taupitz M, Haberle J, Reibhauer BH, Paris S, et al. CT-guided intraarticular corticosteroid injection into the sacroiliac joints in patients with spondyloarthropathy: indication and follow-up with contrast-enhanced MRI. J Comput Assist Tomogr. 1996;20(4):512–21.
74. Kroon FPB, van der Burg LRA, Ramiro S, Landewé RBM, Buchbinder R, Falzon L, et al. Non-steroidal anti-inflammatory drugs (NSAIDs) for axial spondyloarthritis (ankylosing spondylitis and non-radiographic axial spondyloarthritis) (Review). Cochrane Libr. 2015;7.
75. Wang R, Dasgupta A, Ward MM. Comparative efficacy of non-steroidal anti-inflammatory drugs in ankylosing spondylitis: a Bayesian network meta-analysis of clinical trials. Ann Rheum Dis. 2015.
76. Walker C, Essex MN, Li C, Park PW. Celecoxib versus diclofenac for the treatment of ankylosing spondylitis: 12-week randomized study in Norwegian patients. J Int Med Res. 2016;44(3):483–95.
77. Balazcs E, Sieper J, Bickham K, Mehta A, Frontera N, Stryszak P, et al. A randomized, clinical trial to assess the relative efficacy and tolerability of two doses of etoricoxib versus naproxen in patients with ankylosing spondylitis. BMC Musculoskelet Disord. 2016;17(1):426.
78. Wanders A, Heijde D, Landewe R, Behier JM, Calin A, Olivieri I, et al. Nonsteroidal antiinflammatory drugs reduce radiographic progression in patients with ankylosing spondylitis: a randomized clinical trial. Arthritis Rheum. 2005;52(6):1756–65.
79. Kroon F, Landewe R, Dougados M, van der Heijde D. Continuous NSAID use reverts the effects of inflammation on radiographic progression in patients with ankylosing spondylitis. Ann Rheum Dis. 2012;71(10):1623–9.
80. Poddubnyy D, Rudwaleit M, Haibel H, Listing J, Marker-Hermann E, Zeidler H, et al. Effect of non-steroidal anti-inflammatory drugs on radiographic spinal progression in patients with axial spondyloarthritis: results from the German Spondyloarthritis Inception Cohort. Ann Rheum Dis. 2012;71(10):1616–22.
81. Sieper J, Listing J, Poddubnyy D, Song IH, Hermann KG, Callhoff J, et al. Effect of continuous versus on-demand treatment of ankylosing spondylitis with diclofenac over 2 years on radiographic progression of the spine: results from a randomised multicentre trial (ENRADAS). Ann Rheum Dis. 2015.
82. Yang Z, Zhao W, Liu W, Lv Q, Dong X. Efficacy evaluation of methotrexate in the treatment of ankylosing spondylitis using meta-analysis. Int J Clin Pharmacol Ther. 2014;52(5):346–51.
83. Gonzalez-Lopez L, Garcia-Gonzalez A, Vazquez-Del-Mercado M, Munoz-Valle JF, Gamez-Nava JI. Efficacy of methotrexate in ankylosing spondylitis: a randomized, double blind, placebo controlled trial. J Rheumatol. 2004;31(8):1568–74.
84. Altan L, Bingol U, Karakoc Y, Aydiner S, Yurtkuran M, Yurtkuran M. Clinical investigation of methotrexate in the treatment of ankylosing spondylitis. Scand J Rheumatol. 2001;30(5):255–9.
85. Roychowdhury B, Bintley-Bagot S, Bulgen DY, Thompson RN, Tunn EJ, Moots RJ. Is methotrexate effective in ankylosing spondylitis? Rheumatology. 2002;41(11):1330–2.
86. Perez-Guijo VC, Cravo AR, Castro Mdel C, Font P, Munoz-Gomariz E, Collantes-Estevez E. Increased efficacy of infliximab associated with methotrexate in ankylosing spondylitis. Joint Bone Spine. 2007;74(3):254–8.
87. Breban M, Ravaud P, Claudepierre P, Baron G, Henry YD, Hudry C, et al. Maintenance of infliximab treatment in ankylosing spondylitis: results of a one-year randomized controlled trial comparing systematic versus on-demand treatment. Arthritis Rheum. 2008;58(1):88–97.
88. Creemers MC, Franssen MJ, van de Putte LB, Gribnau FW, van Riel PL. Methotrexate in severe ankylosing spondylitis: an open study. J Rheumatol. 1995;22(6):1104–7.
89. Biasi D, Carletto A, Caramaschi P, Pacor ML, Maleknia T, Bambara LM. Efficacy of methotrexate in the treatment of ankylosing spondylitis: a three-year open study. Clin Rheumatol. 2000;19(2):114–7.
90. Sampaio-Barros PD, Costallat LT, Bertolo MB, Neto JF, Samara AM. Methotrexate in the treatment of ankylosing spondylitis. Scand J Rheumatol. 2000;29(3):160–2.
91. Bachta A, Kisiel B, Tłustochowicz M, Raczkiewicz A, Rękas M, Tłustochowicz W. High Efficacy of Methotrexate in Patients with Recurrent Idiopathic Acute Anterior Uveitis: a Prospective Study. Arch Immunol Ther Exp. 2017;65(1):93–7.
92. Chen J, Liu C. Sulfasalazine for ankylosing spondylitis. Cochrane Database Syst Rev. 2005;2:CD004800.
93. Chen J, Lin S, Liu C. Sulfasalazine for ankylosing spondylitis. Cochrane Database Syst Rev. 2014;11:CD004800.
94. Braun J, Zochling J, Baraliakos X, Alten R, Burmester G, Grasedyck K, et al. Efficacy of sulfasalazine in patients with inflammatory back pain due to undifferentiated spondyloarthritis and early ankylosing spondylitis: a multicentre randomised controlled trial. Ann Rheum Dis. 2006;65(9):1147–53.
95. Braun J, van der Horst-Bruinsma IE, Huang F, Burgos-Vargas R, Vlahos B, Koenig AS, et al. Clinical efficacy and safety of etanercept versus sulfasalazine in patients with ankylosing spondylitis: a randomized, double-blind trial. Arthritis Rheum. 2011;63(6):1543–51.
96. Song IH, Hermann K, Haibel H, Althoff CE, Listing J, Burmester G, et al. Effects of etanercept versus sulfasalazine in early axial spondyloarthritis on active inflammatory lesions as detected by whole-body MRI (ESTHER): a 48-week randomised controlled trial. Ann Rheum Dis. 2011;70(4):590–6.
97. Fagerli KM, van der Heijde D, Heiberg MS, Wierod A, Kalstad S, Rodevand E, et al. Is there a role for sulphasalazine in axial spondyloarthritis in the era of TNF inhibition? Data from the NOR-DMARD longitudinal observational study. Rheumatology. 2014;53(6):1087–94.
98. Khanna Sharma S, Kadiyala V, Naidu G, Dhir V. A randomized controlled trial to study the efficacy of sulfasalazine for axial disease in ankylosing spondylitis. Int J Rheum Dis. 2018;21(1):308–14.
99. Muñoz-Fernández S, Hidalgo V, Fernández-Melón J, Schlincker A, Bonilla G, Ruiz-Sancho D, et al. Sulfasalazine reduces the number of flares of acute anterior uveitis over a one-year period. J Rheumatol. 2003;30(6):1277–9.
100. Benitez-Del-Castillo JM, Garcia-Sanchez J, Iradier T, Bañares A. Sulfasalazine in the prevention of anterior uveitis associated with ankylosing spondylitis. Eye (Lond). 2000;14(Pt 3A):340–3.
101. van Denderen JC, van der Paardt M, Nurmohamed MT, de Ryck YM, Dijkmans BA, van der Horst-Bruinsma IE. Double blind, randomised, placebo controlled study of leflunomide in the treatment of active ankylosing spondylitis. Ann Rheum Dis. 2005;64(12):1761–4.
102. Haibel H, Rudwaleit M, Braun J, Sieper J. Six months open label trial of leflunomide in active ankylosing spondylitis. Ann Rheum Dis. 2005;64(1):124–6.
103. Lie E, Kristensen LE, Forsblad-d'Elia H, Zverkova-Sandstrom T, Askling J, Jacobsson LT, et al. The effect of comedication with conventional synthetic disease modifying antirheumatic drugs on TNF inhibitor drug survival in patients with ankylosing spondylitis and undifferentiated spondyloarthritis: results from a nationwide prospective study. Ann Rheum Dis. 2015;74(6):970–8.
104. Sepriano A, Ramiro S, van der Heijde D, Avila-Ribeiro P, Fonseca R, Borges J, et al. Effect of Comedication With Conventional Synthetic Disease-Modifying Antirheumatic Drugs on Retention of Tumor Necrosis Factor Inhibitors in Patients With Spondyloarthritis: A Prospective Cohort Study. Arthritis Rheumatol. 2016;68(11):2671–9.
105. Braun J, Brandt J, Listing J, Zink A, Alten R, Golder W, et al. Treatment of active ankylosing spondylitis with infliximab: a randomised controlled multicentre trial. Lancet. 2002;359(9313):1187–93.
106. Braun J, Brandt J, Listing J, Zink A, Alten R, Burmester G, et al. Long-term efficacy and safety of infliximab in the treatment of ankylosing spondylitis: an open, observational, extension study of a three-month, randomized, placebo-controlled trial. Arthritis Rheum. 2003;48(8):2224–33.
107. Braun J, Brandt J, Listing J, Zink A, Alten R, Burmester G, et al. Two year maintenance of efficacy and safety of infliximab in the treatment of ankylosing spondylitis. Ann Rheum Dis. 2005;64(2):229–34.
108. Braun J, Baraliakos X, Brandt J, Listing J, Zink A, Alten R, et al. Persistent clinical response to the anti-TNF-alpha antibody infliximab in patients with ankylosing spondylitis over 3 years. Rheumatology. 2005;44(5):670–6.
109. Braun J, Baraliakos X, Listing J, Fritz C, Alten R, Burmester G, et al. Persistent clinical efficacy and safety of anti-tumour necrosis factor alpha therapy with infliximab in patients with ankylosing spondylitis over 5 years: evidence for different types of response. Ann Rheum Dis. 2008;67(3):340–5.
110. Baraliakos X, Listing J, Fritz C, Haibel H, Alten R, Burmester GR, et al. Persistent clinical efficacy and safety of infliximab in ankylosing spondylitis

after 8 years--early clinical response predicts long-term outcome. Rheumatology. 2011;50(9):1690–9.

111. van der Heijde D, Dijkmans B, Geusens P, Sieper J, DeWoody K, Williamson P, et al. Efficacy and safety of infliximab in patients with ankylosing spondylitis: results of a randomized, placebo-controlled trial (ASSERT). Arthritis Rheum. 2005;52(2):582–91.
112. Gorman JD, Sack KE, Davis JC Jr. Treatment of ankylosing spondylitis by inhibition of tumor necrosis factor alpha. N Engl J Med. 2002;346(18):1349–56.
113. Davis JC Jr, Van Der Heijde D, Braun J, Dougados M, Cush J, Clegg DO, et al. Recombinant human tumor necrosis factor receptor (etanercept) for treating ankylosing spondylitis: a randomized, controlled trial. Arthritis Rheum. 2003;48(11):3230–6.
114. Davis JC, van der Heijde DM, Braun J, Dougados M, Cush J, Clegg D, et al. Sustained durability and tolerability of etanercept in ankylosing spondylitis for 96 weeks. Ann Rheum Dis. 2005;64(11):1557–62.
115. Davis JC Jr, van der Heijde DM, Braun J, Dougados M, Clegg DO, Kivitz AJ, et al. Efficacy and safety of up to 192 weeks of etanercept therapy in patients with ankylosing spondylitis. Ann Rheum Dis. 2008;67(3):346–52.
116. Brandt J, Khariouzov A, Listing J, Haibel H, Sorensen H, Grassnickel L, et al. Six-month results of a double-blind, placebo-controlled trial of etanercept treatment in patients with active ankylosing spondylitis. Arthritis Rheum. 2003;48(6):1667–75.
117. Brandt J, Listing J, Haibel H, Sorensen H, Schwebig A, Rudwaleit M, et al. Long-term efficacy and safety of etanercept after readministration in patients with active ankylosing spondylitis. Rheumatology. 2005;44(3):342–8.
118. Baraliakos X, Haibel H, Fritz C, Listing J, Heldmann F, Braun J, et al. Long-term outcome of patients with active ankylosing spondylitis with etanercept-sustained efficacy and safety after seven years. Arthritis Research Therapy. 2013;15(3):R67.
119. Calin A, Dijkmans BA, Emery P, Hakala M, Kalden J, Leirisalo-Repo M, et al. Outcomes of a multicentre randomised clinical trial of etanercept to treat ankylosing spondylitis. Ann Rheum Dis. 2004;63(12):1594–600.
120. Dougados M, Braun J, Szanto S, Combe B, Elbaz M, Geher P, et al. Efficacy of etanercept on rheumatic signs and pulmonary function tests in advanced ankylosing spondylitis: results of a randomised double-blind placebo-controlled study (SPINE). Ann Rheum Dis. 2011;70(5): 799–804.
121. Song IH, Weiss A, Hermann KG, Haibel H, Althoff CE, Poddubnyy D, et al. Similar response rates in patients with ankylosing spondylitis and non-radiographic axial spondyloarthritis after 1 year of treatment with etanercept: results from the ESTHER trial. Ann Rheum Dis. 2013;72(6): 823–5.
122. Song IH, Hermann KG, Haibel H, Althoff CE, Poddubnyy D, Listing J, et al. Consistently Good clinical response in patients with early axial spondyloarthritis after 3 years of continuous treatment with etanercept: longterm data of the ESTHER trial. J Rheumatol. 2014;41(10):2034–40.
123. Dougados M, van der Heijde D, Sieper J, Braun J, Maksymowych WP, Citera G, et al. Symptomatic efficacy of etanercept and its effects on objective signs of inflammation in early nonradiographic axial spondyloarthritis: a multicenter, randomized, double-blind, placebo-controlled trial. Arthritis Rheumatol. 2014;66(8):2091–102.
124. Maksymowych WP, Dougados M, van der Heijde D, Sieper J, Braun J, Citera G, et al. Clinical and MRI responses to etanercept in early non-radiographic axial spondyloarthritis: 48-week results from the EMBARK study. Ann Rheum Dis. 2016;75(7):1328–35.
125. Li ZH, Zhang Y, Wang J, Shi ZJ. Etanercept in the treatment of ankylosing spondylitis: a meta-analysis of randomized, double-blind, placebo-controlled clinical trials, and the comparison of the Caucasian and Chinese population. Eur J Orthopaedic Surg Traumatol. 2013;23(5):497–506.
126. van der Heijde D, Kivitz A, Schiff MH, Sieper J, Dijkmans BA, Braun J, et al. Efficacy and safety of adalimumab in patients with ankylosing spondylitis: results of a multicenter, randomized, double-blind, placebo-controlled trial. Arthritis Rheum. 2006;54(7):2136–46.
127. van der Heijde D, Schiff MH, Sieper J, Kivitz AJ, Wong RL, Kupper H, et al. Adalimumab effectiveness for the treatment of ankylosing spondylitis is maintained for up to 2 years: long-term results from the ATLAS trial. Ann Rheum Dis. 2009;68(6):922–9.
128. van der Heijde DM, Revicki DA, Gooch KL, Wong RL, Kupper H, Harnam N, et al. Physical function, disease activity, and health-related quality-of-life outcomes after 3 years of adalimumab treatment in patients with ankylosing spondylitis. Arthritis Res Therapy. 2009;11(4):R124.
129. Sieper J, van der Heijde D, Dougados M, Brown LS, Lavie F, Pangan AL. Early response to adalimumab predicts long-term remission through 5 years of treatment in patients with ankylosing spondylitis. Ann Rheum Dis. 2012; 71(5):700–6.
130. Haibel H, Rudwaleit M, Listing J, Heldmann F, Wong RL, Kupper H, et al. Efficacy of adalimumab in the treatment of axial spondylarthritis without radiographically defined sacroiliitis: results of a twelve-week randomized, double-blind, placebo-controlled trial followed by an open-label extension up to week fifty-two. Arthritis Rheum. 2008;58(7):1981–91.
131. Sieper J, van der Heijde D, Dougados M, Mease PJ, Maksymowych WP, Brown MA, et al. Efficacy and safety of adalimumab in patients with non-radiographic axial spondyloarthritis: results of a randomised placebo-controlled trial (ABILITY-1). Ann Rheum Dis. 2013;72(6):815–22.
132. Wang H, Zuo D, Sun M, Hua Y, Cai Z. Randomized, placebo controlled and double-blind trials of efficacy and safety of adalimumab for treating ankylosing spondylitis: a meta-analysis. Int J Rheum Dis. 2014;17(2):142–8.
133. Inman RD, Davis JC Jr, Heijde D, Diekman L, Sieper J, Kim SI, et al. Efficacy and safety of golimumab in patients with ankylosing spondylitis: results of a randomized, double-blind, placebo-controlled, phase III trial. Arthritis Rheum. 2008;58(11):3402–12.
134. Braun J, Deodhar A, Inman RD, van der Heijde D, Mack M, Xu S, et al. Golimumab administered subcutaneously every 4 weeks in ankylosing spondylitis: 104-week results of the GO-RAISE study. Ann Rheum Dis. 2012;71(5):661–7.
135. Deodhar A, Braun J, Inman RD, van der Heijde D, Zhou Y, Xu S, et al. Golimumab administered subcutaneously every 4 weeks in ankylosing spondylitis: 5-year results of the GO-RAISE study. Ann Rheum Dis. 2015;74(4):757–61.
136. Bao C, Huang F, Khan MA, Fei K, Wu Z, Han C, et al. Safety and efficacy of golimumab in Chinese patients with active ankylosing spondylitis: 1-year results of a multicentre, randomized, double-blind, placebo-controlled phase III trial. Rheumatology. 2014;53(9):1654–63.
137. Sieper J, van der Heijde D, Dougados M, Maksymowych WP, Scott BB, Boice JA, et al. A randomized, double-blind, placebo-controlled, sixteen-week study of subcutaneous golimumab in patients with active nonradiographic axial spondyloarthritis. Arthritis Rheumatol. 2015;67(10):2702–12.
138. Deodhar A, Reveille JD, Harrison DD, Kim L, Lo KH, Leu JH, et al. Safety and Efficacy of Golimumab Administered Intravenously in Adults with Ankylosing Spondylitis: Results through Week 28 of the GO-ALIVE Study. J Rheumatol. 2018;45(3):341–8.
139. Landewé R, Braun J, Deodhar A, Dougados M, Maksymowych WP, Mease PJ, et al. Efficacy of certolizumab pegol on signs and symptoms of axial spondyloarthritis including ankylosing spondylitis: 24-week results of a double-blind randomised placebo-controlled Phase 3 study. Ann Rheum Dis. 2013;73:39–47.
140. Sieper J, Landewe R, Rudwaleit M, van der Heijde D, Dougados M, Mease PJ, et al. Effect of certolizumab pegol over ninety-six weeks in patients with axial spondyloarthritis: results from a phase III randomized trial. Arthritis Rheumatol. 2015;67(3):668–77.
141. van der Heijde D, Dougados M, Landewe R, Sieper J, Maksymowych WP, Rudwaleit M, et al. Sustained efficacy, safety and patient-reported outcomes of certolizumab pegol in axial spondyloarthritis: 4-year outcomes from RAPID-axSpA. Rheumatology (Oxford). 2017;56(9):1498–509.
142. Baeten D, Sieper J, Braun J, Baraliakos X, Dougados M, Emery P, et al. Secukinumab, an Interleukin-17A Inhibitor, in Ankylosing Spondylitis. N Engl J Med. 2015;373(26):2534–48.
143. Sieper J, Deodhar A, Marzo-Ortega H, Aelion JA, Blanco R, Jui-Cheng T, et al. Secukinumab efficacy in anti-TNF-naive and anti-TNF-experienced subjects with active ankylosing spondylitis: results from the MEASURE 2 Study. Ann Rheum Dis. 2017;76(3):571–92.
144. Deodhar A, Conaghan PG, Kvien TK, Strand V, Sherif B, Porter B, et al. Secukinumab provides rapid and persistent relief in pain and fatigue symptoms in patients with ankylosing spondylitis irrespective of baseline C-reactive protein levels or prior tumour necrosis factor inhibitor therapy: 2-year data from the MEASURE 2 study. Clin Exp Rheumatol. 2018.
145. Braun J, Baraliakos X, Deodhar A, Baeten D, Sieper J, Emery P, et al. Effect of secukinumab on clinical and radiographic outcomes in ankylosing spondylitis: 2-year results from the randomised phase III MEASURE 1 study. Ann Rheum Dis. 2017;76(6):1070–7.
146. Marzo-Ortega H, Sieper J, Kivitz A, Blanco R, Cohen M, Martin R, et al. Secukinumab and Sustained Improvement in Signs and Symptoms of Patients With Active Ankylosing Spondylitis Through Two Years: Results From a Phase III Study. Arthritis Care Res. 2017;69(7):1020–9.

147. Baraliakos X, Kivitz AJ, Deodhar AA, Braun J, Wei JC, Delicha EM, et al. Long-term effects of interleukin-17A inhibition with secukinumab in active ankylosing spondylitis: 3-year efficacy and safety results from an extension of the Phase 3 MEASURE 1 trial. Clin Exp Rheumatol. 2018; 36(1):50–5.
148. van der Heijde D, Cheng-Chung Wei J, Dougados M, Mease P, Deodhar A, Maksymowych WP, et al. Ixekizumab, an interleukin-17A antagonist in the treatment of ankylosing spondylitis or radiographic axial spondyloarthritis in patients previously untreated with biological disease-modifying anti-rheumatic drugs (COAST-V): 16 week results of a phase 3 randomised, double-blind, active-controlled and placebo-controlled trial. Lancet. 2018; 392(10163):2441–51.
149. Deodhar A, Poddubnyy D, Pacheco-Tena C, Salvarani C, Lespessailles E, Rahman P, et al. Efficacy and Safety of Ixekizumab in the Treatment of Radiographic Axial Spondyloarthritis: 16 Week Results of a Phase 3 Randomized, Double-Blind, Placebo Controlled Trial in Patients with Prior Inadequate Response or Intolerance to Tumor Necrosis Factor Inhibitors. Arthritis Rheumatol. 2019;71(4):599-611.
150. Giardina AR, Ferrante A, Ciccia F, Impastato R, Miceli MC, Principato A, et al. A 2-year comparative open label randomized study of efficacy and safety of etanercept and infliximab in patients with ankylosing spondylitis. Rheumatol Int. 2010;30(11):1437–40.
151. Park W, Hrycaj P, Jeka S, Kovalenko V, Lysenko G, Miranda P, et al. A randomised, double-blind, multicentre, parallel-group, prospective study comparing the pharmacokinetics, safety, and efficacy of CT-P13 and innovator infliximab in patients with ankylosing spondylitis: the PLANETAS study. Ann Rheum Dis. 2013;72(10):1605–12.
152. Ruwaard J, l'Ami MJ, Marsman AF, Kneepkens EL, van Denderen JC, van der Horst-Bruinsma IE, et al. Comparison of drug survival and clinical outcome in patients with ankylosing spondylitis treated with etanercept or adalimumab. Scand J Rheumatol. 2018;47(2):122–6.
153. Liu W, Wu YH, Zhang L, Liu XY, Bin X, Bin L, et al. Efficacy and safety of TNF-alpha inhibitors for active ankylosing spondylitis patients: Multiple treatment comparisons in a network meta-analysis. Sci Rep. 2016;6:32768.
154. Corbett M, Soares M, Jhuti G, Rice S, Spackman E, Sideris E, et al. Tumour necrosis factor-alpha inhibitors for ankylosing spondylitis and non-radiographic axial spondyloarthritis: a systematic review and economic evaluation. Health Technol Assess. 2016;20(9):1–334 v-vi.
155. Ungprasert P, Erwin PJ, Koster MJ. Indirect comparisons of the efficacy of biological agents in patients with active ankylosing spondylitis: a systematic review and meta-analysis. Clin Rheumatol. 2017;36(7):1569–77.
156. Wang S, He Q, Shuai Z. Risk of serious infections in biological treatment of patients with ankylosing spondylitis and non-radiographic axial spondyloarthritis: a meta-analysis. Clin Rheumatol. 2018;37(2):439–50.
157. Hou LQ, Jiang GX, Chen YF, Yang XM, Meng L, Xue M, et al. The Comparative Safety of TNF Inhibitors in Ankylosing Spondylitis-a Meta-Analysis Update of 14 Randomized Controlled Trials. Clin Rev Allergy Immunol. 2018;54(2):234–43.
158. Wallis D, Thavaneswaran A, Haroon N, Ayearst R, Inman RD. Tumour necrosis factor inhibitor therapy and infection risk in axial spondyloarthritis: results from a longitudinal observational cohort. Rheumatology. 2015;54(1): 152–6.
159. Desai RJ, Thaler KJ, Mahlknecht P, Gartlehner G, McDonagh MS, Mesgarpour B, et al. Comparative Risk of Harm Associated With the Use of Targeted Immunomodulators: A Systematic Review. Arthritis Care Research. 2016; 68(8):1078–88.
160. Kim EM, Uhm WS, Bae SC, Yoo DH, Kim TH. Incidence of tuberculosis among korean patients with ankylosing spondylitis who are taking tumor necrosis factor blockers. J Rheumatol. 2011;38(10):2218–23.
161. Kim HW, Park JK, Yang JA, Yoon YI, Lee EY, Song YW, et al. Comparison of tuberculosis incidence in ankylosing spondylitis and rheumatoid arthritis during tumor necrosis factor inhibitor treatment in an intermediate burden area. Clin Rheumatol. 2014;33(9):1307–12.
162. Cagatay T, Bingol Z, Kiyan E, Yegin Z, Okumus G, Arseven O, et al. Follow-up of 1887 patients receiving tumor necrosis-alpha antagonists: Tuberculin skin test conversion and tuberculosis risk. Clin Respir J. 2018;12(4):1668–75.
163. Kisacik B, Pamuk ON, Onat AM, Erer SB, Hatemi G, Ozguler Y, et al. Characteristics Predicting Tuberculosis Risk under Tumor Necrosis Factor-alpha Inhibitors: Report from a Large Multicenter Cohort with High Background Prevalence. J Rheumatol. 2016;43(3):524–9.
164. Carmona L, Abasolo L, Descalzo MA, Perez-Zafrilla B, Sellas A, de Abajo F, et al. Cancer in patients with rheumatic diseases exposed to TNF antagonists. Semin Arthritis Rheum. 2011;41(1):71–80.
165. Westhovens I, Lories RJ, Westhovens R, Verschueren P, de Vlam K. Anti-TNF therapy and malignancy in spondyloarthritis in the Leuven spondyloarthritis biologics cohort (BIOSPAR). Clin Exp Rheumatol. 2014;32(1):71–6.
166. Hellgren K, Dreyer L, Arkema EV, Glintborg B, Jacobsson LT, Kristensen LE, et al. Cancer risk in patients with spondyloarthritis treated with TNF inhibitors: a collaborative study from the ARTIS and DANBIO registers. Ann Rheum Dis. 2017;76(1):105–11.
167. Haroon N, Inman R, Learch T, Weisman M, Lee M, Rahbar MH, et al. The Impact of Tumor Necrosis Factor Alfa Inhibitors on Radiographic Progression in Ankylosing Spondylitis. Arthritis Rheum. 2013;65(10):2645–54.
168. Molnar C, Scherer A, Baraliakos X, de Hooge M, Micheroli R, Exer P, et al. TNF blockers inhibit spinal radiographic progression in ankylosing spondylitis by reducing disease activity: results from the Swiss Clinical Quality Management cohort. Ann Rheum Dis. 2018;77(1):63–9.
169. Maas F, Spoorenberg A, Brouwer E, Bos R, Efde M, Chaudhry RN, et al. Spinal radiographic progression in patients with ankylosing spondylitis treated with TNF-alpha blocking therapy: a prospective longitudinal observational cohort study. PLoS One. 2015;10(4):e0122693.
170. Kim TJ, Shin JH, Kim S, Sung IH, Lee S, Song Y, et al. Radiographic progression in patients with ankylosing spondylitis according to tumor necrosis factor blocker exposure: Observation Study of Korean Spondyloarthropathy Registry (OSKAR) data. Joint Bone Spine. 2016;83(5): 569–72.
171. van der Heijde D, Landewe R, Baraliakos X, Houben H, van Tubergen A, Williamson P, et al. Radiographic findings following two years of infliximab therapy in patients with ankylosing spondylitis. Arthritis Rheum. 2008;58(10):3063–70.
172. Baraliakos X, Listing J, Brandt J, Haibel H, Rudwaleit M, Sieper J, et al. Radiographic progression in patients with ankylosing spondylitis after 4 yrs of treatment with the anti-TNF-alpha antibody infliximab. Rheumatology (Oxford). 2007;46(9):1450–3.
173. van der Heijde D, Landewe R, Einstein S, Ory P, Vosse D, Ni L, et al. Radiographic progression of ankylosing spondylitis after up to two years of treatment with etanercept. Arthritis Rheum. 2008;58(5):1324–31.
174. van der Heijde D, Salonen D, Weissman BN, Landewe R, Maksymowych WP, Kupper H, et al. Assessment of radiographic progression in the spines of patients with ankylosing spondylitis treated with adalimumab for up to 2 years. Arthritis Res Therapy. 2009;11(4):R127.
175. Braun J, Baraliakos X, Hermann KG, Deodhar A, van der Heijde D, Inman R, et al. The effect of two golimumab doses on radiographic progression in ankylosing spondylitis: results through 4 years of the GO-RAISE trial. Ann Rheum Dis. 2014;73(6):1107–13.
176. van der Heijde D, Baraliakos X, Hermann KA, Landewe RBM, Machado PM, Maksymowych WP, et al. Limited radiographic progression and sustained reductions in MRI inflammation in patients with axial spondyloarthritis: 4-year imaging outcomes from the RAPID-axSpA phase III randomised trial. Ann Rheum Dis. 2018;77(5):699–705.
177. Braun J, Baraliakos X, Deodhar A, Poddubnyy D, Emery P, Delicha EM, et al. Secukinumab shows sustained efficacy and low structural progression in ankylosing spondylitis: 4-year results from the MEASURE 1 study. Rheumatology (Oxford). 2019;58(5):859–868.
178. Baraliakos X, Haibel H, Listing J, Sieper J, Braun J. Continuous long-term anti-TNF therapy does not lead to an increase in the rate of new bone formation over 8 years in patients with ankylosing spondylitis. Ann Rheum Dis. 2014;73(4):710–5.
179. Braun J, Baraliakos X, Listing J, Sieper J. Decreased incidence of anterior uveitis in patients with ankylosing spondylitis treated with the anti-tumor necrosis factor agents infliximab and etanercept. Arthritis Rheum. 2005;52(8):2447–51.
180. Rudwaleit M, Rodevand E, Holck P, Vanhoof J, Kron M, Kary S, et al. Adalimumab effectively reduces the rate of anterior uveitis flares in patients with active ankylosing spondylitis: results of a prospective open-label study. Ann Rheum Dis. 2009;68(5):696–701.
181. van Denderen JC, Visman IM, Nurmohamed MT, Suttorp-Schulten MS, van der Horst-Bruinsma IE. Adalimumab significantly reduces the recurrence rate of anterior uveitis in patients with ankylosing spondylitis. J Rheumatol. 2014; 41(9):1843–8.
182. Sieper J, Koenig A, Baumgartner S, Wishneski C, Foehl J, Vlahos B, et al. Analysis of uveitis rates across all etanercept ankylosing spondylitis clinical trials. Ann Rheum Dis. 2010;69(1):226–9.

183. Yazgan S, Celik U, Isik M, Yesil NK, Baki AE, Sahin H, et al. Efficacy of golimumab on recurrent uveitis in HLA-B27-positive ankylosing spondylitis. Int Ophthalmol. 2017;37(1):139–45.
184. Calvo-Rio V, Blanco R, Santos-Gomez M, Rubio-Romero E, Cordero-Coma M, Gallego-Flores A, et al. Golimumab in refractory uveitis related to spondyloarthritis. Multicenter study of 15 patients. Semin Arthritis Rheum. 2016;46(1):95–101.
185. Hernández M, Mesquida M, Llorens V, Maza MSdl, Blanco R, Calvo V, et al. THU0381 Certolizumab pegol is effective in uveitis associated to spondyloarthritis refractory to other tumour necrosis factor inhibitors. Ann Rheumatic Dis. 2017;76(Suppl 2):350-.
186. Rudwaleit M, Rosenbaum JT, Landewe R, Marzo-Ortega H, Sieper J, van der Heijde D, et al. Observed Incidence of Uveitis Following Certolizumab Pegol Treatment in Patients With Axial Spondyloarthritis. Arthritis Care Research. 2016;68(6):838–44.
187. van Bentum RE, Heslinga SC, Nurmohamed MT, Gerards AH, Griep EN, Koehorst C, et al. Reduced Occurrence Rate of Acute Anterior Uveitis in Ankylosing Spondylitis Treated with Golimumab - The GO-EASY Study. J Rheumatol. 2019;46(2):153–159.
188. Wu D, Guo YY, Xu NN, Zhao S, Hou LX, Jiao T, et al. Efficacy of anti-tumor necrosis factor therapy for extra-articular manifestations in patients with ankylosing spondylitis: a meta-analysis. BMC Musculoskelet Disord. 2015;16:19.
189. Braun J, Baraliakos X, Listing J, Davis J, van der Heijde D, Haibel H, et al. Differences in the incidence of flares or new onset of inflammatory bowel diseases in patients with ankylosing spondylitis exposed to therapy with anti-tumor necrosis factor alpha agents. Arthritis Rheum. 2007;57(4):639–47.
190. Wendling D, Paccou J, Berthelot JM, Flipo RM, Guillaume-Czitrom S, Prati C, et al. New onset of uveitis during anti-tumor necrosis factor treatment for rheumatic diseases. Semin Arthritis Rheum. 2011;41(3):503–10.
191. Wendling D, Joshi A, Reilly P, Jalundhwala YJ, Mittal M, Bao Y. Comparing the risk of developing uveitis in patients initiating anti-tumor necrosis factor therapy for ankylosing spondylitis: an analysis of a large US claims database. Curr Med Res Opin. 2014;30(12):2515–21.
192. Lian F, Zhou J, Wei C, Wang Y, Xu H, Liang L, et al. Anti-TNFalpha agents and methotrexate in spondyloarthritis related uveitis in a Chinese population. Clin Rheumatol. 2015;34(11):1913–20.
193. Lie E, Lindstrom U, Zverkova-Sandstrom T, Olsen IC, Forsblad-d'Elia H, Askling J, et al. Tumour necrosis factor inhibitor treatment and occurrence of anterior uveitis in ankylosing spondylitis: results from the Swedish biologics register. Ann Rheum Dis. 2017;76(9):1515–21.
194. Kim MJ, Lee EE, Lee EY, Song YW, Yu HG, Choi Y, et al. Preventive effect of tumor necrosis factor inhibitors versus nonsteroidal anti-inflammatory drugs on uveitis in patients with ankylosing spondylitis. Clin Rheumatol. 2018; 37(10):2763–70.
195. Kavanaugh A, Krueger GG, Beutler A, Guzzo C, Zhou B, Dooley LT, et al. Infliximab maintains a high degree of clinical response in patients with active psoriatic arthritis through 1 year of treatment: results from the IMPACT 2 trial. Ann Rheum Dis. 2007;66(4):498–505.
196. Mease PJ, Kivitz AJ, Burch FX, Siegel EL, Cohen SB, Ory P, et al. Etanercept treatment of psoriatic arthritis: safety, efficacy, and effect on disease progression. Arthritis Rheum. 2004;50(7):2264–72.
197. Mease PJ, Goffe BS, Metz J, VanderStoep A, Finck B, Burge DJ. Etanercept in the treatment of psoriatic arthritis and psoriasis: a randomised trial. Lancet. 2000;356(9227):385–90.
198. Mease PJ, Gladman DD, Ritchlin CT, Ruderman EM, Steinfeld SD, Choy EH, et al. Adalimumab for the treatment of patients with moderately to severely active psoriatic arthritis: results of a double-blind, randomized, placebo-controlled trial. Arthritis Rheum. 2005;52(10):3279–89.
199. Kavanaugh A, McInnes I, Mease P, Krueger GG, Gladman D, Gomez-Reino J, et al. Golimumab, a new human tumor necrosis factor alpha antibody, administered every four weeks as a subcutaneous injection in psoriatic arthritis: Twenty-four-week efficacy and safety results of a randomized, placebo-controlled study. Arthritis Rheum. 2009;60(4):976–86.
200. Mease PJ, Fleischmann R, Deodhar AA, Wollenhaupt J, Khraishi M, Kielar D, et al. Effect of certolizumab pegol on signs and symptoms in patients with psoriatic arthritis: 24-week results of a Phase 3 double-blind randomised placebo-controlled study (RAPID-PsA). Ann Rheum Dis. 2014;73(1):48–55.
201. Mease PJ, McInnes IB, Kirkham B, Kavanaugh A, Rahman P, van der Heijde D, et al. Secukinumab Inhibition of Interleukin-17A in Patients with Psoriatic Arthritis. N Engl J Med. 2015;373(14):1329–39.
202. McInnes IB, Mease PJ, Kirkham B, Kavanaugh A, Ritchlin CT, Rahman P, et al. Secukinumab, a human anti-interleukin-17A monoclonal antibody, in patients with psoriatic arthritis (FUTURE 2): a randomised, double-blind, placebo-controlled, phase 3 trial. Lancet. 2015;386(9999):1137–46.
203. Sandborn WJ, Hanauer SB, Katz S, Safdi M, Wolf DG, Baerg RD, et al. Etanercept for active Crohn's disease: a randomized, double-blind, placebo-controlled trial. Gastroenterology. 2001;121(5):1088–94.
204. Hueber W, Sands BE, Lewitzky S, Vandemeulebroecke M, Reinisch W, Higgins PD, et al. Secukinumab, a human anti-IL-17A monoclonal antibody, for moderate to severe Crohn's disease: unexpected results of a randomised, double-blind placebo-controlled trial. Gut. 2012;61(12):1693–700.
205. Cantini F, Niccoli L, Benucci M, Chindamo D, Nannini C, Olivieri I, et al. Switching from infliximab to once-weekly administration of 50 mg etanercept in resistant or intolerant patients with ankylosing spondylitis: results of a fifty-four-week study. Arthritis Rheum. 2006;55(5):812–6.
206. Coates LC, Cawkwell LS, Ng NW, Bennett AN, Bryer DJ, Fraser AD, et al. Real life experience confirms sustained response to long-term biologics and switching in ankylosing spondylitis. Rheumatology. 2008; 47(6):897–900.
207. Pradeep DJ, Keat AC, Gaffney K, Brooksby A, Leeder J, Harris C. Switching anti-TNF therapy in ankylosing spondylitis. Rheumatology. 2008;47(11):1726–7.
208. Haberhauer G, Strehblow C, Fasching P. Observational study of switching anti-TNF agents in ankylosing spondylitis and psoriatic arthritis versus rheumatoid arthritis. Wien Med Wochenschr. 2010;160(9–10):220–4.
209. Lie E, van der Heijde D, Uhlig T, Mikkelsen K, Rodevand E, Koldingsnes W, et al. Effectiveness of switching between TNF inhibitors in ankylosing spondylitis: data from the NOR-DMARD register. Ann Rheum Dis. 2011;70(1): 157–63.
210. Glintborg B, Ostergaard M, Krogh NS, Tarp U, Manilo N, Loft AG, et al. Clinical response, drug survival and predictors thereof in 432 ankylosing spondylitis patients after switching tumour necrosis factor alpha inhibitor therapy: results from the Danish nationwide DANBIO registry. Ann Rheum Dis. 2013;72(7):1149–55.
211. Gulyas K, Bodnar N, Nagy Z, Szamosi S, Horvath A, Vancsa A, et al. Real-life experience with switching TNF-alpha inhibitors in ankylosing spondylitis. Eur Health Econ. 2014;15(Suppl 1):S93–100.
212. Cantini F, Niccoli L, Nannini C, Cassara E, Kaloudi O, Giulio Favalli E, et al. Second-line biologic therapy optimization in rheumatoid arthritis, psoriatic arthritis, and ankylosing spondylitis. Semin Arthritis Rheum. 2017;47(2):183–92.
213. Deodhar A, Yu D. Switching tumor necrosis factor inhibitors in the treatment of axial spondyloarthritis. Semin Arthritis Rheum. 2017;47(3):343–50.
214. Navarro-Compan V, Plasencia-Rodriguez C, de Miguel E, Balsa A, Martin-Mola E, Seoane-Mato D, et al. Anti-TNF discontinuation and tapering strategies in patients with axial spondyloarthritis: a systematic literature review. Rheumatology. 2016;55(7):1188–94.
215. Sebastian A, Wojtala P, Lubinski L, Mimier M, Chlebicki A, Wiland P. Disease activity in axial spondyloarthritis after discontinuation of TNF inhibitors therapy. Reumatologia. 2017;55(4):157–62.
216. Landewe R, Sieper J, Mease P, Inman RD, Lambert RG, Deodhar A, et al. Efficacy and safety of continuing versus withdrawing adalimumab therapy in maintaining remission in patients with non-radiographic axial spondyloarthritis (ABILITY-3): a multicentre, randomised, double-blind study. Lancet. 2018;392(10142):134–44.
217. Arends S, van der Veer E, Kamps FB, Houtman PM, Bos R, Bootsma H, et al. Patient-tailored dose reduction of TNF-alpha blocking agents in ankylosing spondylitis patients with stable low disease activity in daily clinical practice. Clin Exp Rheumatol. 2015;33(2):174–80.
218. Fong W, Holroyd C, Davidson B, Armstrong R, Harvey N, Dennison E, et al. The effectiveness of a real life dose reduction strategy for tumour necrosis factor inhibitors in ankylosing spondylitis and psoriatic arthritis. Rheumatology. 2016;55(10):1837–42.
219. Almirall M, Salman-Monte TC, Lisbona MP, Maymo J. Dose reduction of biological treatment in patients with axial spondyloarthritis in clinical remission: Are there any differences between patients who relapsed and to those who remained in low disease activity? Rheumatol Int. 2015;35(9): 1565–8.
220. Lian F, Zhou J, Wang Y, Chen D, Xu H, Liang L. Efficiency of dose reduction strategy of etanercept in patients with axial spondyloarthritis. Clin Exp Rheumatol. 2018;36(5):884–90.

221. Chen MH, Lee MH, Liao HT, Chen WS, Lai CC, Tsai CY. Health-related quality of life outcomes in patients with rheumatoid arthritis and ankylosing spondylitis after tapering biologic treatment. Clin Rheumatol. 2018;37(2): 429–38.
222. Redondo C, Martinez-Feito A, Plasencia-Rodriguez C, Navarro-Compan V, Nuno-Nuno L, Peiteado D, et al. Golimumab Tapering Strategy Based on Serum Drug Levels in Patients With Spondyloarthritis. Arthritis Rheumatol. 2018;70(8):1356–8.
223. Plasencia C, Kneepkens EL, Wolbink G, Krieckaert CL, Turk S, Navarro-Compan V, et al. Comparing Tapering Strategy to Standard Dosing Regimen of Tumor Necrosis Factor Inhibitors in Patients with Spondyloarthritis in Low Disease Activity. J Rheumatol. 2015;42(9):1638–46.
224. Park JW, Yoon YI, Lee JH, Park JK, Lee EB, Song YW, et al. Low dose etanercept treatment for maintenance of clinical remission in ankylosing spondylitis. Clin Exp Rheumatol. 2016;34(4):592–9.
225. Park JW, Kwon HM, Park JK, Choi JY, Lee EB, Song YW, et al. Impact of Dose Tapering of Tumor Necrosis Factor Inhibitor on Radiographic Progression in Ankylosing Spondylitis. PLoS One. 2016;11(12):e0168958.
226. Song IH, Heldmann F, Rudwaleit M, Listing J, Appel H, Braun J, et al. Different response to rituximab in tumor necrosis factor blocker-naive patients with active ankylosing spondylitis and in patients in whom tumor necrosis factor blockers have failed: a twenty-four-week clinical trial. Arthritis Rheum. 2010;62(5):1290–7.
227. Song IH, Heldmann F, Rudwaleit M, Listing J, Appel H, Haug-Rost I, et al. One-year follow-up of ankylosing spondylitis patients responding to rituximab treatment and re-treated in case of a flare. Ann Rheum Dis. 2013; 72(2):305–6.
228. Song IH, Heldmann F, Rudwaleit M, Haibel H, Weiss A, Braun J, et al. Treatment of active ankylosing spondylitis with abatacept: an open-label, 24-week pilot study. Ann Rheum Dis. 2011;70(6):1108–10.
229. Lekpa FK, Farrenq V, Canoui-Poitrine F, Paul M, Chevalier X, Bruckert R, et al. Lack of efficacy of abatacept in axial spondylarthropathies refractory to tumor-necrosis-factor inhibition. Joint Bone Spine : Revue Du Rhumatisme. 2012;79(1):47–50.
230. Sieper J, Porter-Brown B, Thompson L, Harari O, Dougados M. Assessment of short-term symptomatic efficacy of tocilizumab in ankylosing spondylitis: results of randomised, placebo-controlled trials. Ann Rheum Dis. 2014;73(1): 95–100.
231. Sieper J, Braun J, Kay J, Badalamenti S, Radin AR, Jiao L, et al. Sarilumab for the treatment of ankylosing spondylitis: results of a Phase II, randomised, double-blind, placebo-controlled study (ALIGN). Ann Rheum Dis. 2015;74(6): 1051–7.
232. Poddubnyy D, Hermann KG, Callhoff J, Listing J, Sieper J. Ustekinumab for the treatment of patients with active ankylosing spondylitis: results of a 28-week, prospective, open-label, proof-of-concept study (TOPAS). Ann Rheum Dis. 2014;73(5):817–23.
233. Deodhar A, Gensler LS, Sieper J, Clark M, Calderon C, Wang Y, et al. Three Multicenter, Randomized, Double-Blind, Placebo-Controlled Studies Evaluating the Efficacy and Safety of Ustekinumab in Axial Spondyloarthritis. Arthritis Rheumatol. 2018;71:258–270.
234. Pathan E, Abraham S, Van Rossen E, Withrington R, Keat A, Charles PJ, et al. Efficacy and safety of apremilast, an oral phosphodiesterase 4 inhibitor, in ankylosing spondylitis. Ann Rheum Dis. 2013;72(9):1475–80.
235. van der Heijde D, Deodhar A, Wei JC, Drescher E, Fleishaker D, Hendrikx T, et al. Tofacitinib in patients with ankylosing spondylitis: a phase II, 16-week, randomised, placebo-controlled, dose-ranging study. Ann Rheum Dis. 2017; 76(8):1340–7.
236. Maksymowych WP, Heijde DV, Baraliakos X, Deodhar A, Sherlock SP, Li D, et al. Tofacitinib is associated with attainment of the minimally important reduction in axial magnetic resonance imaging inflammation in ankylosing spondylitis patients. Rheumatology. 2018;57(8):1390–9.
237. van der Heijde D, Baraliakos X, Gensler LS, Maksymowych WP, Tseluyko V, Nadashkevich O, et al. Efficacy and safety of filgotinib, a selective Janus kinase 1 inhibitor, in patients with active ankylosing spondylitis (TORTUGA): results from a randomised, placebo-controlled, phase 2 trial. Lancet. 2018; 392(10162):2378–87.

Permissions

All chapters in this book were first published by BioMed Central; hereby published with permission under the Creative Commons Attribution License or equivalent. Every chapter published in this book has been scrutinized by our experts. Their significance has been extensively debated. The topics covered herein carry significant findings which will fuel the growth of the discipline. They may even be implemented as practical applications or may be referred to as a beginning point for another development.

The contributors of this book come from diverse backgrounds, making this book a truly international effort. This book will bring forth new frontiers with its revolutionizing research information and detailed analysis of the nascent developments around the world.

We would like to thank all the contributing authors for lending their expertise to make the book truly unique. They have played a crucial role in the development of this book. Without their invaluable contributions this book wouldn't have been possible. They have made vital efforts to compile up to date information on the varied aspects of this subject to make this book a valuable addition to the collection of many professionals and students.

This book was conceptualized with the vision of imparting up-to-date information and advanced data in this field. To ensure the same, a matchless editorial board was set up. Every individual on the board went through rigorous rounds of assessment to prove their worth. After which they invested a large part of their time researching and compiling the most relevant data for our readers.

The editorial board has been involved in producing this book since its inception. They have spent rigorous hours researching and exploring the diverse topics which have resulted in the successful publishing of this book. They have passed on their knowledge of decades through this book. To expedite this challenging task, the publisher supported the team at every step. A small team of assistant editors was also appointed to further simplify the editing procedure and attain best results for the readers.

Apart from the editorial board, the designing team has also invested a significant amount of their time in understanding the subject and creating the most relevant covers. They scrutinized every image to scout for the most suitable representation of the subject and create an appropriate cover for the book.

The publishing team has been an ardent support to the editorial, designing and production team. Their endless efforts to recruit the best for this project, has resulted in the accomplishment of this book. They are a veteran in the field of academics and their pool of knowledge is as vast as their experience in printing. Their expertise and guidance has proved useful at every step. Their uncompromising quality standards have made this book an exceptional effort. Their encouragement from time to time has been an inspiration for everyone.

The publisher and the editorial board hope that this book will prove to be a valuable piece of knowledge for researchers, students, practitioners and scholars across the globe.

List of Contributors

Andrea Y. Shimabuco, Celio R. Gonçalves, Julio C. B. Moraes, Mariana G. Waisberg, Ana Cristina de M. Ribeiro, Percival D. Sampaio-Barros, Eloisa Bonfa and Carla G. S. Saad
Faculdade de Medicina da Universidade de São Paulo, Av. Dr. Arnaldo, 455 3° andar - sala 3131 - Cerqueira César, São Paulo, SP Cep: 01246-903, Brazil

Céu Tristão Martins Conceição, Ivone Minhoto Meinão and Emília Inoue Sato
Rheumatology Division, Escola Paulista de Medicina, Universidade Federal de São Paulo, Rua Botucatu 740 – Disciplina de Reumatologia CEP 04023900, São Paulo, SP, Brazil

José Atilio Bombana
Department of Psychiatry, Escola Paulista de Medicina, Universidade Federal de São Paulo, São Paulo, Brazil

Imman Mokhtar Metwally and Nahla Naeem Eesa
Rheumatology and Rehabilitation Department, Faculty of Medicine, Cairo University, Cairo, Egypt

Mariam Halim Yacoub
Clinical and Chemical Pathology Department, Faculty of Medicine, Cairo University, Cairo, Egypt

Rabab Mahmoud Elsman
Rheumatology Department, Helwan University Hospital, Helwan, Egypt

Tatiana Vasconcelos Peixoto, Solange Carrasco, Domingos Alexandre Ciccone Botte, Natasha Ugriumov and Suzana Beatriz Veríssimo de Mello
Laboratório de Imunologia Celular (LIM-17) - Faculdade de Medicina FMUSP, Universidade de Sao Paulo, Sao Paulo, SP, Brazil

Sergio Catanozi
Laboratório de Lípides (LIM-10) - Faculdade de Medicina FMUSP, Universidade de Sao Paulo, Sao Paulo, SP, Brazil

Edwin Roger Parra
Departamento de Patologia Clínica - Faculdade de Medicina FMUSP, Universidade de Sao Paulo, Sao Paulo, SP, Brazil

Thaís Martins Lima and Francisco Garcia Soriano
Laboratório de Emergências Clínicas (LIM-51) - Faculdade de Medicina FMUSP, Universidade de Sao Paulo, Sao Paulo, SP, Brazil

Caio Manzano Rodrigues
Faculdade de Medicina de Botucatu (FMB), Universidade Estadual Paulista Júlio de Mesquita Filho (Unesp), Botucatu, SP, Brazil

Cláudia Goldenstein-Schainberg
Laboratório de Imunologia Celular (LIM-17) – Hospital das Clínicas HCFMUSP, Faculdade de Medicina, Universidade de Sao Paulo, Sao Paulo, SP, Brazil
Faculdade de Medicina da Universidade de São Paulo, Av. Dr. Arnaldo, 455 3° andar - sala 3131 - Cerqueira César, São Paulo, SP Cep: 01246-903, Brazil

Adriana Rodrigues Fonseca, Marta Cristine Felix Rodrigues, Flavio Roberto Sztajnbok and Sheila Knupp Feitosa de Oliveira
Pediatric Rheumatology Unit, Instituto de Puericultura e Pediatria Martagão Gesteira, Universidade Federal do Rio de Janeiro (UFRJ), Rua Bruno Lobo, 50– Cidade Universitária, Rio de Janeiro, Brazil

Marcelo Gerardin Poirot Land
Internal Medicine Post- graduation Program, Faculty of Medicine, Universidade Federal do Rio de Janeiro (UFRJ), Rio de Janeiro, Brazil

Wen Qi Cher
Yong Loo Lin School of Medicine, National University of Singapore, Singapore

Yu Heng Kwan
Program in Health Services and Systems Research, Duke-NUS Medical School, Singapore, Singapore

Warren Weng Seng Fong
Department of Rheumatology and Immunology, Singapore General Hospital, Singapore, Singapore

Hui Min Charlotte Choo
Yong Loo Lin School of Medicine, National University of Singapore, Singapore
Department of Internal Medicine, Singapore General Hospital, Academia Building, Level 4, 20 College Road, Singapore 169856, Singapore

Zhen-rui Shi, Yan-fang Han, Lin Zheng, Guo-zhen Tan and Liangchun Wang
Department of Dermatology, Sun Yat-sen Memorial Hospital, Sun Yat-sen University, 107 Yanjiang Rd W, Guangzhou 510120, China

Jing Yin
Affiliated Hospital of Shandong Academy of Medical Sciences, Jinan, China

Yu-ping Zhang
Department of Dermatology, Sun Yat-sen Memorial Hospital, Sun Yat-sen University, 107 Yanjiang Rd W, Guangzhou 510120, China
Department of Dermatology, Zhongshan People's Hospital, No.2 Sunwen East Road, Zhongshan 528403, Guangdong, China

Ze-xin Jiang
Department of Dermatology, Sun Yat-sen Memorial Hospital, Sun Yat-sen University, 107 Yanjiang Rd W, Guangzhou 510120, China
Department of Dermatology, The First People's Hospital of Foshan, Foshan 528000, China

Matheus Calil Faleiros
São Carlos School of Engineering, University of São Paulo, São Carlos, SP, Brazil

Marcello Henrique Nogueira-Barbosa
Ribeirão Preto Medical School, University of São Paulo, Ribeirão Preto, SP, Brazil
MAInLab Medical Artificial Intelligence Laboratory, Ribeirão Preto Medical School, Ribeirão Preto, Brazil
Ribeirão Preto Medical School Musculoskeletal Imaging Research Laboratory, Ribeirão Preto, Brazil
Radiology Division / CCIFM, Ribeirão Preto Medical School, Av. Bandeirantes, 3900, Ribeirão Preto, SP CEP 14048-900, Brazil

Vitor Faeda Dalto
Ribeirão Preto Medical School Musculoskeletal Imaging Research Laboratory, Ribeirão Preto, Brazil

José Raniery Ferreira Júnior and Paulo Mazzoncini de Azevedo-Marques
Ribeirão Preto Medical School, University of São Paulo, Ribeirão Preto, SP, Brazil
MAInLab Medical Artificial Intelligence Laboratory, Ribeirão Preto Medical School, Ribeirão Preto, Brazil

Ariane Priscilla Magalhães Tenório, Rodrigo Luppino-Assad and Paulo Louzada-Junior
Ribeirão Preto Medical School, University of São Paulo, Ribeirão Preto, SP, Brazil

Rangaraj Mandayam Rangayyan
Electrical and Computer Engineering Schulich School of Engineering University of Calgary, Calgary, Alberta, Canada

Juliana Delfino, Thiago Alberto F. G. dos Santos and Thelma L. Skare
Mackenzie Evangelical University Hospital, Curitiba, PR, Brazil

Kaline Medeiros Costa Pereira, Sandro Perazzio, Atila Granado A. Faria, Viviane C. Santos, Marcelle Grecco, Neusa Pereira da Silva and Luis Eduardo Coelho Andrade
Disciplina de Reumatologia, Universidade Federal de São Paulo, Rua Botucatu 740, 3o andar, São Paulo, SP, Brazil

Eloisa Sa Moreira
Departamento de Genética e Biologia Evolutiva, Centro de Estudos do Genoma Humano, Instituto de Biociências, Universidade de São Paulo, São Paulo, SP, Brazil

Penélope Esther Palominos, Andrese Aline Gasparin and Carla Saldanha
Serviço de Reumatologia, Hospital de Clínicas de Porto Alegre, Ramiro Barcelos 2350, sexto andar, Porto Alegre, Rio Grande do Sul CEP 90035-903, Brazil

Ana Paula Beckhauser de Campos
Serviço de Reumatologia, Hospital Universitário Evangélico, Alameda Augusto Stellfeld, 1908, Bigorrilho, Curitiba, Paraná CEP 80730-150, Brazil

Sandra Lúcia Euzébio Ribeiro
Serviço de Reumatologia, Hospital Universitário Getúlio Vargas, Universidade Federal do Amazonas, Avenida Apurinã 4, Manaus, Amazonas CEP 69020-170, Brazil

Charles Lubianca Kohem
Serviço de Reumatologia, Hospital de Clínicas de Porto Alegre, Ramiro Barcelos 2350, sexto andar, Porto Alegre, Rio Grande do Sul CEP 90035-903, Brazil
Faculdade de Medicina, Universidade Federal do Rio Grande do Sul, Ramiro Barcelos 2400, Porto Alegre, Rio Grande do Sul CEP 90035-903, Brazil

Jady Wroblewski Xavier, Felipe Borges de Oliveira and Bruno Guerra
Faculdade de Medicina, Universidade Federal do Rio Grande do Sul, Ramiro Barcelos 2400, Porto Alegre, Rio Grande do Sul CEP 90035-903, Brazil

Aline Castello Branco Mancuso
Departamento de Bioestatística, Hospital de Clínicas de Porto Alegre, Ramiro Barcelos 2350, Porto Alegre, Rio Grande do Sul CEP 90035-903, Brazil

Percival Degrava Sampaio-Barros
Serviço de Reumatologia, Faculdade de Medicina, Hospital das Clínicas HCFMUSP, Universidade de São Paulo, São Paulo, Brazil

Vanessa Hax, Ana Laura Didonet Moro, Ricardo Machado Xavier and Odirlei Andre Monticielo
Division of Rheumatology, Hospital de Clínicas de Porto Alegre, Universidade Federal do Rio Grande do Sul, 2350 Ramiro Barcelos St, Room 645, Porto Alegre, RS 90035-903, Brazil

Rafaella Romeiro Piovesan
Medical School Student, Universidade Federal do Rio Grande do Sul, Porto Alegre, Brazil

Luciano Zubaran Goldani
Division of Infectious Diseases, Hospital de Clínicas de Porto Alegre, Universidade Federal do Rio Grande do Sul, Porto Alegre, Brazil

Verena A. Balbi, Bárbara Montenegro, Ana C. Pitta, Ana R. Schmidt, Sylvia C. Farhat, Laila P. Coelho, Juliana C. O. Ferreira, Kátia Kozu, Lucia M. Campos and Adriana M. Sallum
Pediatric Rheumatology Unit, Children's Institute, Hospital das Clinicas HCFMUSP, Faculdade de Medicina, Universidade de Sao Paulo, Sao Paulo, SP, Brazil

Clovis A. Silva
Pediatric Rheumatology Unit, Children's Institute, Hospital das Clinicas HCFMUSP, Faculdade de Medicina, Universidade de Sao Paulo, Sao Paulo, SP, Brazil
Division of Rheumatology, Hospital das Clinicas HCFMUSP, Faculdade de Medicina, Universidade de Sao Paulo, Sao Paulo, SP, Brazil

Rosa M. R. Pereira
Division of Rheumatology, Hospital das Clinicas HCFMUSP, Faculdade de Medicina, Universidade de Sao Paulo, Sao Paulo, SP, Brazil

Daniela P. Piotto
Pediatric Rheumatology Unit, Universidade Federal de São Paulo, São Paulo, Brazil

Claudia Saad-Magalhães
Pediatric Rheumatology Unit, São Paulo State University (UNESP) - Faculdade de Medicina de Botucatu, São Paulo, Brazil

Virginia P. Ferriani
Pediatric Rheumatology Unit, Ribeirão Preto Medical School, University of São Paulo, São Paulo, Brazil

Gabriela Blay
Pediatric Rheumatology Unit, Children's Institute, Faculdade de Medicina da Universidade de São Paulo (FMUSP), Av. Dr. Eneas Carvalho Aguiar, 647 - Cerqueira César, São Paulo, SP 05403-000, Brazil
Pediatric Pulmonology Unit, Children's Institute, FMUSP, Av. Dr. Eneas Carvalho Aguiar, 647 - Cerqueira César, São Paulo, SP 05403-000, Brazil

Joaquim C. Rodrigues
Pediatric Pulmonology Unit, Children's Institute, FMUSP, Av. Dr. Eneas Carvalho Aguiar, 647 - Cerqueira César, São Paulo, SP 05403-000, Brazil

Gabriela N. Leal, Glaucia V. Novak, Beatriz C. Molinari, Lucia M. A. Campos and Eloisa Bonfá
Pediatric Rheumatology Unit, Children's Institute, Faculdade de Medicina da Universidade de São Paulo (FMUSP), Av. Dr. Eneas Carvalho Aguiar, 647 - Cerqueira César, São Paulo, SP 05403-000, Brazil

Natali W. Gormezano
Division of Rheumatology, FMUSP, Sao Paulo, Brazil

Nadia E. Aikawa
Pediatric Rheumatology Unit, Children's Institute, Faculdade de Medicina da Universidade de São Paulo (FMUSP), Av. Dr. Eneas Carvalho Aguiar, 647 - Cerqueira César, São Paulo, SP 05403-000, Brazil
Division of Rheumatology, FMUSP, Sao Paulo, Brazil

Maria T. Terreri, Ana P. Sakamoto, Gleice Clemente, Octavio A. B. Peracchi and Vanessa Bugni
Pediatric Rheumatology Unit, Universidade Federal de São Paulo, Sao Paulo, Brazil

Claudia S. Magalhães and Taciana A. P. Fernandes
São Paulo State University (UNESP), Faculdade de Medicina de Botucatu, Sao Paulo, Brazil

Roberto Marini
São Paulo State University of Campinas (UNICAMP), Sao Paulo, Brazil

Silvana B. Sacchetti
Irmandade da Santa Casa de Misericórdia de São Paulo, Sao Paulo, Brazil

Luciana M. Carvalho
Ribeirão Preto Medical School - University of São Paulo, Sao Paulo, Brazil

Melissa M. Fraga
Hospital Darcy Vargas, Sao Paulo, Brazil

Tânia C. M. Castro
Hospital Menino Jesus, Sao Paulo, Brazil

Valéria C. Ramos
Pontifical Catholic University of Sorocaba, Sao Paulo, Brazil

Mônica Verdier, Pedro Anuardo, Lucia Maria Arruda Campos, Juliana C. O. A. Ferreira, Marco Felipe Castro Silva and Mariana Ferriani
Pediatric Rheumatology Unit, Children's Institute, Hospital das Clinicas HCFMUSP, Faculdade de Medicina, Universidade de Sao Paulo, Sao Paulo, SP, BR, Brazil

Nadia Emi Aikawa and Rosa Maria Rodrigues Pereira
Division of Rheumatology, Hospital das Clinicas HCFMUSP, Faculdade de Medicina, Universidade de Sao Paulo, Av. Dr. Eneas Carvalho Aguiar, 647 - Cerqueira César, São Paulo, SP 05403-000, Brazil

Natali Weniger Spelling Gormezano and Clovis Artur Silva
Pediatric Rheumatology Unit, Children's Institute, Hospital das Clinicas HCFMUSP, Faculdade de Medicina, Universidade de Sao Paulo, Sao Paulo, SP, BR, Brazil
Division of Rheumatology, Hospital das Clinicas HCFMUSP, Faculdade de Medicina, Universidade de Sao Paulo, Av. Dr. Eneas Carvalho Aguiar, 647 - Cerqueira César, São Paulo, SP 05403-000, Brazil

Ricardo Romiti
Division of Dermatology, Hospital das Clinicas HCFMUSP, Faculdade de Medicina, Universidade de Sao Paulo, Sao Paulo, SP, BR, Brazil

Ana Paula Sakamoto
Pediatric Rheumatology Unit, Universidade Federal de São Paulo, São Paulo, Brazil

Maria Teresa Terreri
Pediatric Rheumatology Division, Faculdade de Medicina de Botucatu, Universidade Estadual Paulista (UNESP), São Paulo, Brazil

Claudia Saad Magalhães and Juliana Sato
São Paulo State University (UNESP) - Faculdade de Medicina de Botucatu, Botucatu, Brazil

Virginia Paes Leme Ferriani
Pediatric Rheumatology Unit, Ribeirão Preto Medical School - University of São Paulo, Ribeirão Preto, Brazil

Maraísa Centeville
São Paulo State University of Campinas (UNICAMP), Campinas, Brazil

Maria Carolina Santos
Irmandade da Santa Casa de Misericórdia de São Paulo, São Paulo, Brazil

Juliana Fernandes Sarmento Donnarumma
Rheumatology Division, Medicine Department, Escola Paulista de Medicina, Universidade Federal de São Paulo (UNIFESP), São Paulo, SP, Brazil

Eloara Vieira Machado Ferreira and Jaquelina Ota-Arakaki
Division of Pneumology, Medicine Department, Escola Paulista de Medicina, Universidade Federal de São Paulo (UNIFESP), São Paulo, SP, Brazil

Cristiane Kayser
Rheumatology Division, Medicine Department, Escola Paulista de Medicina, Universidade Federal de São Paulo (UNIFESP), São Paulo, SP, Brazil
Disciplina de Reumatologia da Universidade Federal de São Paulo, Rua Botucatu 740, 3 ° andar, São Paulo, SP 04023-062, Brazil

Narjes Soleimanifar and Behrouz Nikbin
Molecular immunology research center, Tehran University of Medical Sciences, Tehran, Iran
Department of Molecular Medicine, School of Advanced Technologies in Medicine, Tehran University of Medical Sciences, Tehran, Iran
Department of Immunology, Tehran University of Medical Sciences, Tehran, Iran.

Zahra Hosseini-khah
Department of Molecular Medicine, School of Advanced Technologies in Medicine, Tehran University of Medical Sciences, Tehran, Iran

Mohammad Hossein Nicknam
Molecular immunology research center, Tehran University of Medical Sciences, Tehran, Iran
Department of Immunology, Tehran University of Medical Sciences, Tehran, Iran.

Katayoon Bidad
Immunology, Asthma and Allergy Research Institute, Tehran University of Medical Sciences, Tehran, Iran

Ahmad Reza Jamshidi and Mahdi Mahmoudi
Rheumatology Research Center, Tehran University of Medical Sciences, Tehran, Iran

Shayan Mostafaei
Department of Community Medicine, Faculty of Medicine, Kermanshah University of Medical Sciences, Kermanshah, Iran

William Dario Mcewen Tamayo and Libia Maria Rodriguez Padilla
Universidad Pontificia Bolivariana, Calle 78B # 72a-109, Medellín, Antioquia, Colombia

Daniel Montoya Roldan
Hospital la Maria, Calle 92 EE #67-61, Medellín, Antioquia, Colombia

Carlos Jaime Velasquez Franco and Miguel Antonio Mesa Navas
Universidad Pontificia Bolivariana, Calle 78B # 72a-109, Medellín, Antioquia, Colombia
Cínica Universitaria Bolivariana, Cra 72A #78b -50, Medellín, Antioquia, Colombia

Maria Fernanda Alvarez Barreneche
Clínica Cardiovid, Calle 78 # 75-21, Medellín, Antioquia, Colombia Medellin, Colombia

Thauana Luiza de Oliveira and Marcelo M. Pinheiro
Rheumatology Division, Spondyloarthritis Section, Universidade Federal de São Paulo, Rua Leandro Dupré, 204, Conjunto 74, Vila Clementino, São Paulo, SP CEP 04025-010, Brazil

Hilton Telles Libanori
Hospital Israelita Albert Einstein, São Paulo, Brazil

Tassia Catiuscia da Hora
Faculdade Metropolitana de Camaçari- Jorge Amado, Ponto Certo, Camaçari, BA 42.801-120, Brazil

Kelly Lima
Centro Universitário Estácio da Bahia, Xingu Street, 179 - Stiep, Salvador, BA, Brazil

Roberto Rodrigues Bandeira Tosta Maciel
Universidade do Estado da Bahia- Silveira Martins, 2555 - Cabula, Salvador, BA 41150-000, Brazil

José Alexandre Mendonça
Department of Rheumatology and Postgraduate Program of the Pontifical Catholic, University of Campinas, Rua da Fazenda, 125, Condomínio Dálias, casa 10, Residencial Vila Flora, Sumaré, São Paulo 13175665, Brazil

Sibel Zehra Aydin
The Ottawa Hospital Research Institute, Division of Rheumatology, University of Ottawa, Ottawa, ON, Canada

Maria-Antonietta D'Agostino
APHP, Hôpital Ambroise Paré, Rheumatology Department, 92100 Boulogne-Billancourt, France
INSERM U1173, Laboratoire d'Excellence INFLAMEX, UFR Simone Veil, Versailles-Saint-Quentin University, 78180 Saint-Quentin-en-Yvelines, France

Alex Domingos Reis, Cristiane Mudinutti, Murilo de Freitas Peigo, Lucas Lopes Leon, Sandra Cecília Botelho Costa and Sandra Helena Alves Bonon
Laboratory of Virology, School of Medical Sciences, State University of Campinas (UNICAMP), Rua Tessália Vieira de Camargo, 126, Campinas, SP 13.083-887, Brazil

Lilian Tereza Lavras Costallat
Department of Internal Medicine, Discipline of Rheumatology, School of Medical Sciences, State University of Campinas (UNICAMP), Campinas, SP, Brazil

Claudio Lucio Rossi
Department of Clinical Pathology, School of Medical Sciences, State University of Campinas (UNICAMP), Campinas, SP, Brazil

Naveet Pannu, Rashmi Singh, Sukriti Sharma and Archana Bhatnagar
Department of Biochemistry, Panjab University, Chandigarh 160014, India

Seema Chopra
Department of Obstetrics and Gynaecology, PGIMER, Chandigarh 160012, India

Daniele Faria Miguel
Universidade Estadual Paulista (UNESP) Faculdade de Medicina de Botucatu, Botucatu, Brazil

Clovis Artur Almeida Silva
Children's Institute, Hospital das Clinicas HCFMUSP, Faculdade de Medicina, Universidade de São Paulo, São Paulo, Brazil

José Eduardo Corrente
Biostatistic Department, Instituto de Biociencias, Universidade Estadual Paulista (UNESP), Botucatu, Brazil

Claudia Saad Magalhaes
Pediatric Rheumatology Division, Faculdade de Medicina de Botucatu, Universidade Estadual Paulista (UNESP), Botucatu, Brazil

Mohammed Hadi Al-Osami
Rheumatology Unit, Department of Internal Medicine, College of Medicine, University of Baghdad, Baghdad, Iraq

Nabaa Ihsan Awadh
Rheumatology Unit, Department of Internal Medicine, Baghdad Teaching Hospital, Baghdad, Iraq

Khalid Burhan Khalid
Oral Surgery Unit, Department of Dentistry, Dijlah University College, Baghdad, Iraq

Ammar Ihsan Awadh
Clinical Pharmacy Unit, Department of Pharmacy, Al-Esraa University College, Baghdad, Iraq

Gustavo Gomes Resende and Ricardo da Cruz Lage
Universidade Federal de Minas Gerais (UFMG), Alameda Álvaro Celso, 175 / 2° Andar. Santa Efigênia. CEP 30.150-260, Belo Horizonte, MG, Brazil

Eduardo de Souza Meirelles, Carla Gonçalves Saad, Célio Roberto Gonçalves and Cláudia Goldenstein Schainberg
Universidade De São Paulo (USP), São Paulo, Brazil

Cláudia Diniz Lopes Marques and Rafaela Silva Guimarães Goncalves
Universidade Federal de Pernambuco (UFPE), Recife, Brazil

Adriano Chiereghin
Pontifície Universidade Católica (PUC) de Sorocaba, Sorocaba, Brazil

Andre Marun Lyrio and Rubens Bonfiglioli
Pontifície Universidade Católica (PUC) de Campinas, Campinas, Brazil

Antônio Carlos Ximenes
Hospital Estadual Geral de Goiania (HGG), Goiânia, Brazil

Penelope Esther Palominos
Universidade Federal do Rio Grande do Sul (UFRS), Porto Alegre, Brazil

Cristiano Barbosa Campanholo
Santa Casa de Misericórdia (SCM) de São Paulo, São Paulo, Brazil

Júlio Silvio de Sousa Bueno Filho
Departmento de Estatística, Universidade Federal de Lavras (UFLA), Lavras, Brazil

Lenise Brandao Pieruccetti
Hospital Heliópolis, São Paulo, Brazil

Mauro Waldemar Keiserman
Pontifície Universidade Católica (PUC) de Porto Alegre, Porto Alegre, Brazil

Michel Alexandre Yazbek
Universidade Estadual de Campinas (UNICAMP), Campinas, Brazil

Rodrigo Luppino Assad
USP Ribeirão Preto, Ribeirão Preto, Brazil

Sônia Maria Alvarenga Anti
Hospital do Servidor Público do Estado de São Paulo, São Paulo, Brazil

Sueli Carneiro
Universidade Federal do Rio De Janeiro (UFRJ), Rio de Janeiro, Brazil

Thauana Luíza Oliveira and Marcelo de Medeiros Pinheiro
Universidade Federal de São Paulo (UNIFESP), São Paulo, Brazil

Valderílio Feijó Azevedo
Universidade Federal do Paraná (UFPR), Curitiba, Brazil

Washington Alves Bianchi
Santa Casa de Misericórdia (SCM) do Rio De Janeiro, Rio de Janeiro, Brazil

Wanderley Marques Bernardo
Universidade de São Paulo (USP), São Paulo, Brazil

Index

A

Albumin, 19-25, 172

Ankylosing Spondylitis, 1-5, 7-8, 71, 86-88, 92, 126-128, 130-131, 139-141, 143, 183-185, 187-192, 196, 199-203, 219-226

Anti-nucleosome Antibody, 19, 21-22, 24

Anti-rheumatic Drugs, 1, 127-128

Anxiety, 9-17, 147-149

Artificial Intelligence, 63-64, 70-71

Autoantibodies, 20, 25-26, 28, 30, 38, 41-42, 46, 56-59, 61-62, 73, 94, 96-98, 100, 103, 121, 177-178, 180

Autoimmune Disease, 9, 39, 49-50, 52-53, 98, 106, 116, 129, 170

Autoimmune Hepatitis, 99-104, 166

Autotolerance Failure, 27-28

B

Bariatric Surgery, 139-140, 142

Behavioral Therapy, 144-148, 150

C

Classification Criteria, 40-41, 44-48, 60, 76, 78, 85-88, 92, 94, 98, 100, 112, 117, 133, 151, 192-193, 198-199, 220

Coping Strategies, 9, 11, 14, 16-17

Correlation Coefficient, 66, 69, 80, 89, 127, 130

Cytomegalovirus, 49-50, 52, 55, 96, 166, 168-169

D

Damage Index, 9, 11, 13, 17, 73, 75-80, 83, 93, 95, 102, 138, 179, 181-182

Depression, 9-15, 17, 147-149

Dermatitis, 142, 165, 205

Diffuse Alveolar Hemorrhage, 105-110

Disease Activity, 1-9, 11-12, 14, 17, 19-20, 24-26, 28, 35, 37, 39, 41, 47, 52, 117, 119, 122-124, 126-128, 130-131, 133-138, 140-141, 149-150, 163-166, 168, 171, 176-191, 200-203, 205-207, 209, 212, 216-217, 220-221, 223-226

Disease Course, 40, 46-47, 72, 111, 138, 179

Disease Duration, 1-4, 6, 9, 12-13, 16, 21, 45, 49, 52-53, 79, 88, 99, 101-102, 105-108, 111-114, 116, 127-128, 141, 161, 170, 180, 184-185, 200

E

Enthesitis, 1, 85-92, 140-141, 161-162, 194, 202-203, 206

Etiology, 10, 116-117, 170

F

Fat Intake, 126-128

Fatigue, 10, 14, 149-150, 172, 184, 200, 205, 208, 223

Flow Cytometry, 27, 29, 32

Food Intake, 126-127

G

Gene Copy Number, 77, 79-83

H

Health Problem, 139

Hepatomegaly, 99-103

Human Immunodeficiency Virus, 54, 93, 95-96, 98, 168

Hypertension, 99-101, 116-117, 119-125, 132-133, 166, 178-180, 203

I

Immunosuppressants, 49, 51-53, 73, 121, 140

Intensive Care Unit, 108-109, 132, 138

Interleukin Profile, 27, 31, 35

Intravenous Immunoglobulin, 100, 112-113

L

Leukopenia, 42, 44, 52-53, 74, 93-95, 101, 111, 113-114

Lupus Nephritis, 19-26, 37, 39, 41-42, 61, 72-73, 75-76, 109-110, 115, 176-182

Lupus Patients, 17, 37, 58, 61, 72-75, 82, 93, 98, 124, 170, 173, 175-177

Lymphadenopathy, 93, 100

Lymphocyte, 28, 31, 35, 51-52, 54, 97, 130, 183-185, 187-191

Lymphopenia, 44, 51, 53-54, 56, 93-97, 134

M

Machine Learning, 63-64, 66, 69-71

Magnetic Resonance Imaging, 63-64, 71, 141-142, 157, 194, 197, 199, 220-221, 226

Meta-analysis, 24, 26, 45, 47-48, 50, 61, 130, 144-146, 148-150, 182, 190, 199, 201, 203-204, 207, 213, 215, 221-225

Monocytes, 29, 31-33, 35, 98, 131

Mortality, 23, 49, 54-55, 72, 74, 76, 93, 97, 105, 109-110, 117, 123, 126, 130, 132-133, 136-138, 163, 170, 178, 181, 190

Multicenter Study, 15, 61, 83, 99, 102-105, 107, 110-111, 115, 181-182, 197, 225

Multivariate Analysis, 1, 3, 5-6, 24-25, 116, 118, 120-121, 211

Mycophenolate, 21, 52-53, 55, 75, 94, 96, 98, 100, 106, 109, 112, 120-121, 134

N

Nail Disease, 151-154, 156, 158-162
Nailfold Capillaroscopy, 116-118, 120, 122, 124
Nephritis, 19-26, 37, 39, 41-42, 61, 72-76, 93-97, 101, 107-110, 114-115, 134, 138, 144, 176-182
Neuropsychiatric Lupus, 93, 97, 104, 106, 110, 112, 115
Neutrophil, 52, 183-185, 187-191

O

Opportunistic Infections, 93, 167
Oxidative Stress, 170-171, 173, 175-177

P

Pathogenesis, 20, 28, 54-55, 75, 121, 123, 126, 130-131, 168, 170, 175-177, 188
Pharmacological Treatment, 144-146, 148-149, 195, 200, 205, 221
Phenotype, 39, 77-79, 81, 103, 124, 151, 161, 182
Phytotherapy, 144-145, 148, 150
Pneumonia, 51-53, 55, 135-136, 168-169
Power Doppler, 151-152, 157-159, 161-162
Pregnancy, 119, 121-123, 170-171, 175-177
Prognosis, 55, 61, 72, 74, 76, 82, 93, 98, 117, 123-124, 133, 137, 166-167, 177, 179, 192, 197, 199-200, 220
Psoriasis, 91, 140, 151-155, 157-159, 161-162, 166, 192, 195, 214-215, 225
Psoriatic Arthritis, 2, 7-8, 86, 91-92, 151-152, 157-159, 161-162, 184, 215, 225
Psychoanalytic Psychotherapy, 9-10, 15, 17-18
Psychotherapy, 9-18

Q

Quality Assessment, 49-50, 55
Quality Of Life, 2, 4-5, 7-12, 14-15, 17, 64, 85-86, 92, 130, 138-139, 144-147, 150-152, 154, 184, 200-201, 206, 221, 226

R

Renal Biopsies, 179, 181
Renal Histopathology, 21-23
Resistive Index, 152, 157-162
Risk Factors, 49-55, 83, 98, 116-118, 120, 124, 126-127, 201, 211
Rituximab, 100, 112-113, 134, 136, 196, 218-219, 226

S

Spectral Doppler, 151-152, 157, 159, 162
Spondyloarthritis, 1-2, 7-8, 63-65, 71, 85-86, 88, 92, 126, 139-143, 190, 192-194, 198-200, 202-203, 207, 219-226
Systematic Review, 17, 26, 47-50, 54, 61, 121, 124-125, 130, 144-145, 148, 150, 160-161, 182, 190, 203-204, 207, 217, 224
Systemic Lupus Erythematosus, 9-11, 14-15, 17, 19, 25-27, 38-41, 47-49, 52, 55-56, 61, 72-81, 83-84, 93, 95-96, 98-111, 113-116, 119-125, 132, 137-138, 140, 144-145, 150, 163-171, 175, 177-182

T

Thrombocytopenia, 42, 44, 74, 93-97, 101, 105, 107, 109, 134-135, 137, 172
Thrombosis, 73, 96, 101-102, 106, 108, 112, 119, 121-123, 205

U

Ultrasonography, 151-157, 160-162

V

Viral Hepatitis, 61, 101-102
Viral Loads, 49, 51-52, 54

W

Weight Loss, 139, 140, 165